PROGRESS IN BRAIN RESEARCH

VOLUME 60

THE NEUROHYPOPHYSIS:
STRUCTURE, FUNCTION AND CONTROL

Recent volumes in PROGRESS IN BRAIN RESEARCH

PROGRESS IN BRAIN RESEARCH

VOLUME 60

THE NEUROHYPOPHYSIS: STRUCTURE, FUNCTION AND CONTROL

Proceedings of the 3rd International Conference on the Neurohypophysis,
held at Babraham, Cambridge (U.K.), on September 14–16th, 1982

edited by

B.A. CROSS

and

G. LENG

A.R.C. Institute of Animal Physiology, Babraham, Cambridge CB2 4AT (U.K.)

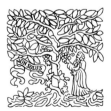

ELSEVIER
Amsterdam — New York
1983

PUBLISHED BY:
ELSEVIER SCIENCE PUBLISHERS B.V.
P.O. BOX 211
AMSTERDAM, THE NETHERLANDS

SOLE DISTRIBUTOR FOR THE U.S.A. AND CANADA:
ELSEVIER SCIENCE PUBLISHING CO., INC.
52 VANDERBILT AVENUE
NEW YORK, NY 10017, U.S.A.

Library of Congress Cataloging in Publication Data

International Conference on the Neurohypophysis (3rd: 1982: Babraham, Cambridgeshire)
The neurohypophysis, structure, function, and control.

(Progress in brain research; v. 60)
Bibliography: p.
Includes index.
1. Neurohypophysis—Congresses.   I. Cross, B.A. (Barry A.)   II. Leng, G.
(Gareth)   III. Title.   IV. Series.   [DNLM: 1. Pituitary gland,
Posterior—Congresses.   W1 PR667J v. 60/WK 520 I58 1982n]   QP376.P7 vol. 60   612'.82s
[599'.01'88]   83-5679 [QP188.P58]
ISBN 0-444-80479-X (U.S.)

ISBN FOR THE SERIES 0-444-80104-9
ISBN FOR THE VOLUME 0-444-80479-X

WITH 172 ILLUSTRATIONS AND 38 TABLES

© ELSEVIER SCIENCE PUBLISHERS B.V. 1983

PRINTED IN THE NETHERLANDS

List of Contributors

R. Acher, Laboratory of Biological Chemistry, University of Paris VI, 96 Bd Raspail, 75006 Paris, France

V.T.Y. Ang, Department of Medicine, St. George's Hospital Medical School, London SW17 ORE, U.K.

A.J. Baertschi, Department of Animal Biology, University of Geneva, 1211 Geneva 4, Switzerland

B.J. Barber, Department of Physiology, Medical College of Wisconsin, 8701 Watertown Plank Road, Milwaukee, WI 53226, U.S.A.

L. Ben, Department of Physiology, University of California, San Francisco, San Francisco, CAQ 94143, U.S.A.

J.-L. Bény, Department of Animal Biology, University of Geneva, 1211 Geneva 4, Switzerland

R.J. Bicknell, A.R.C. Institute of Animal Physiology, Babraham, Cambridge CB2 4AT, U.K.

S.D. Birkett, Department of Anatomy, The Medical School, University of Bristol, University Walk, Bristol B58 1TD, U.K.

G.J. Boer, Netherlands Institute for Brain Research, IJdijk 28, 1095 KJ Amsterdam, The Netherlands

B. Bohus, Department of Animal Physiology, University of Groningen, P.O. Box 14, 9750 AA Haren (Gn), The Netherlands

W. Bryan, Smith Kline & French Labs., Department of Pharmacology, Philadelphia, PA 19101, U.S.A.

R.M. Buijs, Netherlands Institute for Brain Research, IJdijk 28, 1095 KJ Amsterdam, The Netherlands

J.T. Chapman, Department of Physiology, Charing Cross Hospital Medical School, London W6 8RF, U.K.

J. Chauvet, Laboratory of Biological Chemistry, University of Paris VI, 96 Bd Raspail, 75006 Paris, France

M.T. Chauvet, Laboratory of Biological Chemistry, University of Paris VI, 96 Bd Raspail, 75006 Paris, France

S. Cheng, Department of Physiology, Dartmouth Medical School, Hanover, NH 03756, U.S.A.

G. Clarke, University of Bristol, Department of Anatomy, The Medical School, Bristol BS8 1TD, U.K.

A.W. Cowley, Jr., Department of Physiology, Medical College of Wisconsin, 8701 Watertown Plank Road, Milwaukee, WI 53226, U.S.A.

K. Cransberg, Rudolf Magnus Institute for Pharmacology, University of Utrecht, Vondellaan 6, 3521 GD Utrecht, The Netherlands

J.A. Creba, Department of Biochemistry, University of Birmingham, P.O. Box 363, Birmingham 815 2TT, U.K.

W. de Jong, Rudolf Magnus Institute for Pharmacology, University of Utrecht, Vondellaan 6, 3521 GD Utrecht, The Netherlands

G.J. de Vries, Netherlands Institute for Brain Research, IJdijk 28, 1095 KJ Amsterdam, The Netherlands

D. de Wied, Rudolf Magnus Institute for Pharmacology, Medical Faculty, University of Utrecht, Vondellaan 6, 3521 GD Utrecht, The Netherlands

J.J. Dreifuss, Département de Physiologie, Centre Médical Universitaire, Rue Michel Servet, 1211 Geneva 4, Switzerland

J.O. Drife, University Department of Obstetrics and Gynaecology, Bristol Maternity Hospital, Bristol, U.K.

R.E.J. Dyball, Department of Anatomy, Downing Street, Cambridge CB2 3DY, U.K.

R.G. Dyer, A.R.C. Institute of Animal Physiology, Babraham, Cambridge CB2 4AT, U.K.

A P F. Flint, A.R.C. Institute of Animal Physiology, Babraham, Cambridge CB2 4AT, U.K.

M.J. Freund-Mercier, Laboratoire de Physiologie Générale, LA 309 C.N.R.S., 21, rue René Descartes, F 67084 Strasbourg Cédex, France

B.H. Gähwiler, Preclinical Research, Sandoz Ltd., 4002 Basle, Switzerland

H. Gainer, Section on Functional Neurochemistry, Laboratory of Developmental Neurobiology, Nat. Inst. of Child Health and Human Development, N.I.H., Bldg. 36, Rm 2A21, Bethesda, MD 20205, U.S.A.

I.B. Gartside, Department of Physiology, Charing Cross Hospital Medical School, London W6 8RF, U.K.

D.M. Gash, Department of Anatomy, Box 603, School of Medicine and Dentistry, University of Rochester, Rochester, NY 14642, U.S.A.

C.B. González, Department of Anatomy, The Medical School, University of Bristol, University Walk, Bristol B58 1TD, U.K.

M. Gross, Smith, Kline & French Labs., Department of Pharmacology, Philadelphia, PA 19101, U.S.A.

Y. Guerne, Laboratoire de Physiologie Générale, LA 309 C.N.R.S., 21, rue René Descartes, F 67084 Strasbourg Cédex, France

G.R. Hardy, Department of Physiology, Dartmouth Medical School, Hanover, NH 03756, U.S.A.

P.T. Hawkins, Department of Biochemistry, University of Birmingham, P.O. Box 363, Birmingham B15 3TT, U.K.

J. Hawthorn, Department of Medicine, St. George's Hospital Medical School, London SW17 ORE, U.K.

M. Holzbauer, A.R.C. Institute of Animal Physiology, Babraham, Cambridge CB2 4AT, U.K.

M.G.R. Hull, University Department of Obstetrics and Gynaecology, Bristol Maternity Hospital, Bristol, U.K.

S.P. Hunt, MRC Neurochemical Pharmacology Unit, Medical Research Council Centre, Hills Road, Cambridge, CB2 2QH, U.K.

D. Hurpet, Laboratory of Biological Chemistry, University of Paris VI, 96 Bd Raspail, 75006 Paris, France

K. Inenaga, Department of Physiology, University of Occupational and Environmental Health, School of Medicine, Kitakyushu, Japan

S. Ishikawa, Jichi Medical School, 3311-1 Yakushiji, Minamikawachi-Machi, Tochigi 329-04, Japan

S. Jard, Centre CNRS-INSERM de Pharmacologie-Endocrinologie, rue de la Cardonille, B.P. 5055, 34033 Montpellier Cédex, France

J.S. Jenkins, Department of Medicine, St. George's Hospital Medical School, London SW17 ORE, U.K.

J. Jolles, University Psychiatric Clinic, Nicolaas Beetsstraat 24, 3511 HG Utrecht, The Netherlands

H. Kannan, Department of Physiology, University of Occupational and Environmental Health, School of Medicine, Kitakyushu, Japan.

B. Kavanagh, Smith Kline & French Labs., Department of Pharmacology, Philadelphia, PA 19101, U.S.A.

L.C. Keil, Ames Research Center, Moffett Field, CA 94035, U.S.A.

L.B. Kinter, Smith Kline & French Labs., Department of Pharmacology, Philadelphia, PA 19101, U.S.A.

C.J. Kirk, Department of Biochemistry, University of Birmingham, P.O. Box 363, Birmingham B15 2TT, U.K.

K. Koizumi, Department of Physiology — Box 31, Downstate Medical Center, S.U.N.Y., 450 Clarkson Avenue, Brooklyn, NY 11203, U.S.A.

E. Kolodziejczyk, Department of Animal Biology, University of Geneva, 1211 Geneva 4, Switzerland

J.G. Kooy, Rudolf Magnus Institute for Pharmacology, University of Utrecht, Vondellaan 6, 3521 GD Utrecht, The Netherlands

D. Lawrence, Department of Pharmacology and Therapeutics, Faculty of Medicine, University of Calgary, 3330 Hospital Dr. M.W., Calgary, Alberta, Canada T2N 4N1

J.F. Laycock, Department of Physiology, Charing Cross Hospital Medical School, London W6 8RF, U.K.

K. Lederis, Department of Pharmacology and Therapeutics, Faculty of Medicine, University of Calgary, 3330 Hospital Dr. N.W., Calgary, Alberta, Canada T2N 4N1

G. Leng, A.R.C. Institute of Animal Physiology, Babraham, Cambridge CB2 4AT, U.K.

S.L. Lightman, Medical Unit, Westminster Medical School, Page Street, London SW1P 2AP, U.K.

M. Manning, Department of Biochemistry, Medical College of Ohio, Toledo, OH 43699, U.S.A.

J. Maselli, Department of Physiology, University of California, San Francisco, San Francisco, CA 94143, U.S.A.

W.T. Mason, A.R.C. Institute of Animal Physiology, Babraham, Cambridge CB2 4AT, U.K.

R.H. Michell, Department of Biochemistry, University of Birmingham, P.O. Box 363, Birmingham B15 2TT, U.K.

G. J. Moore, Department of Medical Biochemistry, University of Calgary, Alberta, Canada T2N 1N4

F. Moos, Laboratoire de Physiologie Générale, LA 309 C.N.R.S., 21, rue René Descartes, F 67084 Strasbourg Cédex, France

J.F. Morris, Department of Human Anatomy, South Parks Road, Oxford OX1 3QX, U.K.

M. Mühlethaler, Département de Physiologie, Centre Médical Universitaire, Rue Michel Servet, 1211 Geneva 4, Switzerland

E. Muscholl, Pharmakologisches Institut der Universität, 65 Mainz, Obere Zahlbacher Str. 67, D-6500 Mainz, F.R.G.

M. Ninkovic, MRC Neurochemical Pharmacology Unit, Medical Research Council Centre, Hills Road, Cambridge, CB2 2QH, U.K.

R. Noble, University of Bristol, Department of Anatomy, The Medical School, Bristol BS8 1TD, U.K.

J.J. Nordmann, I.N.S.E.R.M., U. 176, Rue Camille Saint-Saëns, 33077 Bordeaux Cédex, France

W.G. North, Department of Physiology, Dartmouth Medical School, Hanover, NH 03756, U.S.A.

M.F.D. Notter, Department of Anatomy, Box 603, School of Medicine and Dentistry, University of Rochester, Rochester, NY 14642, U.S.A.

B.T. Pickering, Department of Anatomy, The Medical School, University of Bristol, University Walk, Bristol, BS8 1TD, U.K.

Q.J. Pittman, Department of Pharmacology and Therapeutics, Faculty of Medicine, University of Calgary, 3330 Hospital Dr. N.W., Calgary, Alberta, Canada T2N 4N1

D.G. Porter, Department of Anatomy, The Medical School, Bristol BS8 1TD, U.K.

D.A. Poulain, Unité de Recherches de Neurobiologie des Comportements, I.N.S.E.R.M., U. 176, Rue Camille Saint-Saëns, 33077 Bordeaux Cédex, France

K. Racké, Pharmakologisches Institut der Universität, 65 Mainz, Obere Zahlbacher Str. 67, D-6500 Mains, F.R.G.

D.J. Ramsay, Department of Physiology, University of California, San Francisco, San Francisco, CA 94143, U.S.A.

I.A. Reid, Department of Physiology, University of California, San Francisco, San Francisco, CA 94143, U.S.A.

Ph. Richard, Laboratoire de Physiologie Générale, LA 309 C.N.R.S., 21, rue René Descartes, F 67084 Strasbourg Cédex, France

D. Richter, Institut für Physiologische Chemie der Universität Hamburg, Martinistrasse 52, 2000 Hamburg 20, F.R.G.

A.G. Robinson, University of Pittsburgh, Medical School, 930 Scaife Hall, Pittsburgh, PA 15261, U.S.A.

I.C.A.F. Robinson, Laboratory of Endocrine Physiology and Pharmacology, National Institute for Medical Research, Mill Hill, London NW7 1AA, U.K.

J.C. Rosenior, Department of Medical Biochemistry, University of Calgary, Alberta, Canada T2N 1N4

M.N. Rossor, National Hospital for Nervous Diseases, Queen Square, London WC1, U.K.

J.A. Russell, Department of Physiology, University Medical School, Edinburgh EH8 9AG, Scotland, U.K.

P.E. Sawchenko, The Salk Institute, P.O. Box 85800, San Diego, CA 92138, U.S.A.

W.H. Sawyer, Department of Pharmacology, College of Physicians and Surgeons, Columbia University, New York, NY 10032, U.S.A.

H. Schmale, Institut für Physiologische Chemie der Universität Hamburg, Martinistrasse 52, 2000 Hamburg 20, F.R.G.

R.W. Schrier, Department of Medicine, University of Colorado Health Science Center, 4200 East Ninth Avenue, Denver, CO 80262, U.S.A.

J. Schwartz, Department of Physiology, University of California, San Francisco, San Francisco, CA 94143, U.S.A.

L. Share, Department of Physiology and Biophysics, University of Tennessee Center for the Health Sciences, Memphis, TN 38163, U.S.A.

D.F. Sharman, A.R.C. Institute of Animal Physiology, Babraham, Cambridge CB2 4AT, U.K.

F.D. Shaw, Department of Anatomy, King's College London, Strand, London WC2R 2LS, U.K.

E.L. Sheldrick, A.R.C. Institute of Animal Physiology, Babraham, Cambridge CB2 4AT, U.K.

D. Shue, Smith Kline & French Labs., Department of Pharmacology, Philadelphia, PA 19101, U.S.A.

A.-J. Silverman, Department of Anatomy and Cell Biology, College of Physicians and Surgeons, Columbia University, 630 W.168 St., New York, NY 10032, U.S.A.

C.D. Sladek, Department of Anatomy, University of Rochester School of Medicine and Dentistry, P.O. Box 603 Rochester, NY 14642, U.S.A.

J.R. Sladek, Jr., Department of Anatomy, Box 603, School of Medicine and Dentistry, University of Rochester, Rochester, NY 14642, U.S.A.

M.V. Sofroniew, Department of Human Anatomy, South Parks Road, Oxford OX1 3QX, U.K.

F.L. Stassen, Smith Kline & French Labs., Department of Pharmacology, P.O. Box 7929, Philadelphia, PA 19101, U.S.A.

L. Sulat, Smith Kline & French Labs., Department of Pharmacology, Philadelphia, PA 19101, U.S.A.

D.F. Swaab, Netherlands Institute for Brain Research, IJdijk 28, 1095 KJ Amsterdam, The Netherlands

R.W. Swann, Department of Anatomy, The Medical School, University of Bristol, University Walk, Bristol BS8 1TD, U.K.

L.W. Swanson, The Clayton Foundation for Research — California Division, La Jolla, CA 92037, U.S.A.

D.T. Theodosis, I.N.S.E.R.M., U. 176, Unité de Recherches de Neurobiologie des Comportements, Domaine de Carreire, Rue Camille Saint-Saëns, 33077 Bordeaux Cédex, France

T.N. Thrasher, Department of Physiology, University of California, San Francisco, San Francisco, CA 94143, U.S.A.

C.D. Tweedle, Department of Anatomy, Michigan State University, East Lansing, MI 48824, U.S.A.

H. Valtin, Department of Physiology, Dartmouth Medical School, Hanover, NH 03756, U.S.A.

F.W. van Leeuwen, Netherlands Institute for Brain Research, IJdijk 28, 1095 KJ Amsterdam, The Netherlands

J.G. Verbalis, University of Pittsburgh, Medical School, 930 Scaife Hall, Pittsburgh, PA 15261, U.S.A.

C.A.M. Versteeg, Rudolf Magnus Institute for Pharmacology, University of Utrecht, Vondellaan 6, 3521 GD Utrecht, The Netherlands

J.B. Wakerley, University of Bristol, Department of Anatomy, The Medical School, Bristol BS8 1 TD, U.K.

D.C. Wathes, Department of Anatomy, The Medical School, Bristol BS8 1TD, U.K.

V.D. Wiebelhaus, Smith Kline & French Labs., Department of Pharmacology, Philadelphia, PA 19101, U.S.A.

H. Yamashita, Department of Physiology, University of Occupational and Environmental Health, School of Medicine, Kitakyushu, Japan

N. Yim, Smith Kline & French Labs., Department of Medicinal Chemistry, Philadelphia, PA 19101, U.S.A.

E.A. Zimmerman, Department of Neurology, College of Physicians and Surgeons, Columbia University, 630 W. 168 St., New York, NY 10032, U.S.A.

Preface

The Third International Conference on the Neurohypophysis was held in the new Conference Centre at the Institute of Animal Physiology, Babraham, Cambridge, on 14–16th September 1982. This volume contains the papers of all the main contributors to the proceedings and also one from Dr. D. Richter who, although an invited participant, was prevented at the last minute from attending.

The Conference was sponsored by the International Society for Neuroendocrinology whose representatives, B. Donovan (U.K.) and J.D. Vincent (France), served on the Programme Committee. Other members of the Committee were B.A. Cross (U.K. Chairman), J.J. Dreifuss (Switzerland), W.H. Sawyer (U.S.A.), L. Share (U.S.A.) and D. de Wied (The Netherlands).

The local executive committee comprised B.A. Cross (Chairman), R.E.J. Dyball, A.P.F. Flint and G. Leng (Secretary), and they were supported by numerous colleagues at Babraham who assisted with the scientific, social and secretarial work of the Conference.

November 1982   Barry Cross and Gareth Leng

Chairman's Introductory Remarks

"The scientific world has not been overburdened by international meetings devoted to this important endocrine organ, for twenty years separated the first two, and six years the second and third. We have all been very modest and avoided the frequent and frenetic exchanges that characterize some of the more sensational branches of endocrinology.

That is not to deny that dramatic advances have occurred in the physiology and biochemistry of the neurohypophysis or their importance to human (and animal) welfare. I hope this meeting will assess these advances and reach a critical judgement of the present state of knowledge.

The programme committee have tried to put together a balanced agenda for discussion. But we recognize that such selectivity is bound to be highly subjective, and there must be those who feel we have signally failed in the task by omission of this or that speaker or topic. May I apologize on behalf of myself and my colleagues for these shortcomings and trust that sufficient unscheduled discussion time has been allowed in the programme to cover the more serious gaps.

There are quite a few present who will recollect with pleasure the last conference in Key Biscayne, which charted among other things the major developments in the biosynthesis, neurophysiology and mode of action of neurohypophysial hormones. It was a splendid meeting in an idyllic Caribbean setting. As you see Cambridge is trying its best to rival that sunshine and blue sky this week, but the price we pay is a few hours of total obscurity in the morning before the mist clears

I think only Bill Sawyer, Gordon Bisset and myself here today are survivors from the First Conference in 1956 in Bristol, but I should like to hang my text for this Introduction on remembrance of those times.

Hans Heller, Professor of Pharmacology at Bristol, organized that first meeting. You will recall his pioneering work on the secretion and metabolic inactivation of vasopressin and on the evolution of neurohypophysial hormones.

The most illustrious participant was undoubtedly Sir Henry Dale; discoverer of oxytocin, enunciator of Dale's Law, one time President of the Royal Society, and scientist extraordinary. He was 81 years old at the Bristol meeting but still in top form as I found to my cost when I incautiously crossed swords with him in discussion on the control of uterine contraction.

Another luminary was Harry van Dyke, who might be thought of as the father, or perhaps the grandfather, of the family of neurophysins, for the isolation and characterization of the Van Dyke protein gave the first hint that oxytocin and vasopressin might be release products rather than the stored form of the hormones.

My own teachers John Folley and Geoffrey Harris were also there. Harris was, of course, most famous for his great work on the pituitary portal system, but had used his celebrated remote control stimulation method to study in vivo effects of endogenous neurohypophysial hormones. Folley was best known for his work on galactopoiesis but he too had worked on the posterior pituitary and he reported experiments at the Bristol meeting which launched the so-called Benson and Folley hypothesis.

This postulated that oxytocin released by suckling in the milk-ejection reflex flowed through vascular connexions to the anterior pituitary to stimulate prolactin discharge. It was a nice unifying concept with much appeal since it provided an economical explanation of the potent effect of the suckling stimulus on both milk secretion and milk removal. But it was wrong, and I cite this case from the fifties lest we find ourselves in danger of similar error 25 years later.

Benson and Folley's principal evidence was that oxytocin injections had a similar effect in retarding weaning involution of rat mammary glands to that produced by treatment with prolactin. Much additional supporting evidence was accumulated, but it was all circumstantial. No amount of circumstantial evidence is worth as much as a single crucial experiment. Meites and colleagues showed that retardation of weaning involution could equally well be produced by oxytocin in hypophysectomized rats on standard replacement therapy, showing clearly that oxytocin could not be working at the pituitary level, but that the effect was a peripheral one in the mammary gland itself. It is always dangerous to argue from a distance with indirect evidence. Do we not sometimes make this mistake when we extrapolate from in vitro results to the whole animal?

I learnt my scientific scepticism from such masters as E. B. Verney and Geoffrey Harris, who both displayed to perfection those twin virtues of the good scientist, an active imagination coupled to a disbelieving nature. Verney discovered osmoreceptors but could not bring himself to believe in volume receptors. Harris was sceptical of the Scharrers' theory of neurosecretion, and both he and Verney felt vasopressin was a misnomer (for antidiuretic hormone) since the hormone had no demonstrable physiological role in cardiovascular homeostasis. Of course, it is much easier to be critical of other peoples' theories than one's own. The point is that all theories are suspect unless tested and retested, until destruction if necessary. Harris needed his Zuckerman. What endures from such controversy approaches more nearly the truth.

At this Conference we shall be treated to expositions of some concepts that have already won wide acceptance, and some novel ones that have yet to be assimilated. Old questions, like that of the location of osmoreceptors in the brain, will be given another airing with new data, and some new questions, such as the nature and function of opioid terminals in the neural lobe, will be brought up for examination.

Let us review and evaluate all this material in a mood of courteous scepticism, along with fraternal admiration for the ingenuity and fortitude of all the protagonists.''

B.A. Cross

List of Abbreviations

Abbreviations are explained on their first appearance in each chapter. The most commonly used abbreviations are:

AII	angiotensin II	5-HT	5-hydroxytryptamine
ACTH	adrenocorticotrophic hormone	i.c.v.	intracerebroventricular
AV3V	antero-ventral wall of the third ventricle	i.n.	intranasal
		i.v.	intravenous
AVP	arginine-vasopressin	LE rat	Long–Evans rat
AVT	arginine-vasotocin	LVP	lysine-vasopressin
BP	blood pressure	NA	noradrenaline
CNS	central nervous system	NIL	neurointermediate lobe
CRF	corticotropin releasing factor	Np	neurophysin
CSF	cerebrospinal fluid	NSG	neurosecretory granule
DA	dopamine	NTS	nucleus tractus solitarius
DGLVP	desglycin-amide^9-lysine-vasopressin	OVLT	organum vasculosum laminae terminalis
DI rat	Brattleboro rat homozygous for diabetes insipidus	OXT	oxytocin
		PVN	paraventricular nucleus
ECF	extracellular fluid	RIA	radioimmunoassay
EM	electron microscope	SCN	suprachiasmatic nucleus
GABA	γ-aminobutyric acid	SFO	subfornical organ
HNS	hypothalamo-neurohypophysial system	SHR	spontaneously hypertensive rats
HPLC	high performance liquid chromatography	SIADH	syndrome of inappropriate antidiuretic hormone secretion
HRP	horseradish peroxidase	SON	supraoptic nucleus

Contents

Section I — Afferent Pathways to Neurosecretory Neurones

Section V — Mechanisms of Release from the Neurohypophysis

Afferent Pathways to Neurosecretory Neurones

The Neurohypophysis: Structure, Function and Control, Progress in Brain Research, Vol. 60, edited by B.A. Cross and G. Leng
© *1983 Elsevier Science Publishers B.V.*

Organization of Neural Inputs to the Supraoptic and Paraventricular Nuclei: Anatomical Aspects

J.F. MORRIS

Department of Human Anatomy, South Parks Road, Oxford OX1 3QX (U.K.)

INTRODUCTION

The anatomists' first goal in the analysis of the organization of the neural inputs to the supraoptic (SON) and paraventricular (PVN) hypothalamic nuclei must be to determine the origin, course, and precise mode of termination of the pathways that project to the magnocellular oxytocin and vasopressin neurones of these nuclei. Methods of fibre tracing at the light and electron microscope level now put this goal within reach and cytochemical techniques make structural studies important also in the analysis of neurotransmitters within the afferent systems. Ideally an analysis of the neural inputs should provide a circuitry which not only explains the coupling between effective stimuli and the release of hormone but also such phenomena as the coordination of oxytocin cells during the milk ejection reflex.

In many animals the SON consists of a relatively homogeneous group of magnocellular neurones which project entirely to the neural lobe. Furthermore, the SON contains many more magnocellular neurones than does the PVN and is thus quantitatively, at least, more important in determining the output of oxytocin and vasopressin to peripheral blood.

By contrast the PVN contains a large number of different cell groups only some of which are magnocellular. Many of its oxytocin and vasopressin cells projects to sites other than the neural lobe. Particularly from the posterior part of the PVN, cells project to autonomic centres of the medulla and spinal cord (Armstrong and Hatton, 1980; Armstrong et al., 1980; Koh and Ricardo, 1980; Swanson and Kuypers, 1980; Swanson et al., 1980; Sawchenko and Swanson, this volume). Occasional cells project to both neural lobe and brainstem (Swanson and Kuypers, 1980). For this reason Swanson's group stress integration of autonomic (parvocellular) and neuroendocrine (magnocellular) controls by the PVN (e.g. Swanson and Sawchenko, 1980). The parvocellular part of the PVN contains other neurosecretory neurones such as those containing somatostatin (Dubois and Kolodziejczyk, 1975) and a corticotrophin releasing hormone (Bugnon et al., 1982) in addition to vasopressin cells that project to the median eminence rather than the neural lobe (see Silverman et al., 1981), and other neurones whose content and projections are unknown. The many accessory groups of magnocellular neurones also project primarily to the neurohypophysis, but their afferents have not been studied.

This review concentrates on recent contributions of anatomical studies to our understanding of the afferent control of oxytocin and vasopressin secretion, and highlights problems of interpretation and areas of expanding interest. Control of the other neurohormones of the PVN will not be considered except to note that, in many cases, definition of the termination of the afferents to the PVN is too imprecise to specify the cell type on which the fibres end. Many reviews which cover either broader or more specialized fields have already appeared (Cross and Dyball, 1974; Hayward, 1977; Harris, 1978; Palkovits and Zaborsky, 1980; Swanson and Sawchenko, 1980; Leng et al., 1982; Palkovits, 1981; Swanson and Mogenson, 1981; Poulain and Wakerley, 1982).

TOPOGRAPHY OF THE MAGNOCELLULAR NEURONES

Analysis of the termination of the afferent systems that contact magnocellular neurones requires that the topography of these neurones is understood, in particular the ramifications of their dendritic tree.

Only recently have visualizations of entire magnocellular neurones become available as a result of detailed Golgi-(Luqui and Fox, 1976; Dyball et al., 1979; Felten and Cashner, 1979; Armstrong et al., 1982; van den Pol, 1982), Golgi-like immunoperoxidase-(Sofroniew and Glassmann, 1981) and horseradish peroxidase-fillings of the neurones (e.g. Armstrong et al., 1980). Magnocellular oxytocin and vasopressin cells seem to have similar morphology (Sofroniew and Glassmann, 1981) but there is no agreed interpretation of the morphologic distinction of different types of process. The electron microscope is needed for unequivocal identification of synapses but, at the ultrastructural level, only the neurosecretory somata can be unequivocally identified. The identification of postsynaptic elements is complicated by the finding of both 170 nm neurosecretory granules and immunostaining for vasopressin, oxytocin and neurophysin in processes which appear to be dendrites, and synapses on the length of what appear to be neurosecretory axons, even in the neural lobe (see van den Pol, 1982). The difficulty is compounded by the projection into the SON of dendrites of lateral hypothalamic neurones (Millhouse, 1980) and the virtual impossibility of identifying dendrites of magnocellular PVN neurones unless they contain appropriately sized neurosecretory granules, or can be followed from a perikaryon, since some parvocellular neurones also contain vasopressin. Synapses on dendrites and on axons would be expected to have very different effects so that failure to identify them with certainty hampers any interpretation of function.

Light microscopic studies on the SON indicate that axons leave either the soma or a proximal dendrite to join the supraoptico-neurohypophysial tract and that a relatively simple tree of 2–4 dendrites extends down into the ventral glial lamina (Luqui and Fox, 1976; Dyball et al., 1979; Felten and Cashner, 1979; Armstrong et al., 1982). About 600 boutons contact the average SON neurone, the majority ending on dendritic shafts (Léránth et al., 1975).

In the PVN, axons from those groups that project to the neurohypophysis mostly pass laterally towards the fornix then ventrally towards SON. The dendritic trees of lateral and posterolateral groups of magnocellular neurones differ in the orientation of their 2–4 dendrites. Those of the more rostral lateral group stay within the PVN and traverse its medial parvocellular part, some running around its lateral perimeter, while those of the more caudal posterolateral PVN project laterally towards the fornix as well as medially (Armstrong et al., 1980; van den Pol, 1982). These observations, combined with the differential localization of oxytocin and vasopressin in the nuclei, make it clear that it is insufficient to describe an afferent pathway as ending "in the SON" and still less "in the PVN". A careful analysis of the site of termination in relation to the dendritic trees and neuronal subgroups is necessary if functional correlations are to be inferred.

NON-SYNAPTIC INPUTS TO THE MAGNOCELLULAR NEURONES

Before considering afferent neural inputs, it must be acknowledged that the output of magnocellular neurones is probably influenced by a variety of non-synaptic inputs. Some features, such as phasic firing of vasopressin neurones, may be intrinsic to the cells (see Poulain and Wakerley, 1982, for review).

The ventricles and CSF

Many substances will reach, and may affect, magnocellular neurones by diffusion from the CSF via the extracellular space. In addition, specialized, often dilated processes of PVN neurones pass close to, or possibly into, the 3rd ventricle (Sofroniew and Glassmann, 1981) but the function of such processes is unknown.

Hormonal inputs via the blood supply

Some magnocellular neurones in the PVN (and SON in the mouse but not the rat) accumulate oestrogen (Sar and Stumpf, 1980; Rhodes et al., 1981). At first sight this would appear to be linked to the oestrogen-stimulated release of oxytocin and vasopressin. However, the cells which accumulate oestrogen are found in the parts of PVN which project to the medulla and spinal cord rather than the pituitary (see above). Occasional PVN neurones may also accumulate testosterone but again this was not found in the SON in the rat (Sar and Stumpf, 1973). Cortisol raises the osmotic threshold for vasopressin release (Streeten et al., 1981), but whether this is a direct or indirect effect on the magnocellular neurones is unknown.

Osmosensitivity of magnocellular neurones

This contentious topic has recently been reviewed (Leng et al., 1982; Poulain and Wakerley, 1982; and see Sladek, and Mason, both this volume). The evidence for believing magnocellular neurones to be osmosensitive will not be reviewed here but it must be noted that, so far as the afferent inputs and their organization are concerned, the difficult question of the hierarchy of effect among the intrinsic and the various non-magnocellular receptors mediating osmoregulation remains unanswered.

Non-synaptic amine release and vascular control

Studies by Swanson's group (Swanson et al., 1977, 1978; Hartman et al., 1980) have shown that a number of aminergic terminals in the PVN end on blood vessels, and that amines control cerebral blood flow and permeability. The magnocellular nuclei have a profuse capillary bed and aminergic neurones could therefore exert large influences through vascular control. Swanson's group also suggest that, as in the cortex, some monoaminergic terminals in the PVN do not form synapses but rather release amine more generally into the extracellular fluid. This conclusion is based on the absence of a visible synaptic specialization in 81 % of sectioned aminergic terminals. The interpretation needs confirmation by serial section analysis, and the effect of amines released in this way is not known, though they could act on both glia (see below) and neurones.

The magnocellular neurones may therefore be influenced by a number of non-synaptic mechanisms. The extent to which such mechanisms interact with, or even take precedence over, synaptic neural inputs remains to be discovered, but the possibility adds a large unknown to the equation of afferent control of the magnocellular neurones.

LOCAL CIRCUITS IN THE CONTROL OF MAGNOCELLULAR NEURONES

In 1976 F.O. Schmitt et al. drew attention to the important role of local circuits in brain function. In the magnocellular neurosecretory system Sofroniew and Glassmann (1981) suggest that bulbous neurophysin-positive processes might be presynaptic dendrites. Large areas of soma to soma contact between magnocellular neurones have been recognized in both nuclei (Lafarga et al., 1975; Gregory et al., 1980; Theodosis et al., 1981; Hatton and Tweedle, 1982). Although their precise physiological significance is unclear at present, secretion-related changes in the degree of apposition suggest that insertion and withdrawal of glial processes between the cells can be functionally important in the nuclei as well as in the pituitary (see below).

Gap junctions have been reported in PVN slabs in vitro (Andrew et al., 1981) but the cells that they connect, their extent and number, their transience or permanence, and their relation to, for example, the coordination of oxytocin cells during the milk ejection reflex, are still unclear.

The existence of recurrent collaterals from magnocellular axons has been discussed in relation to both synchronous firing and recurrent inhibition and excitation of the cells. While there is some evidence for axonal branches which terminate within the nuclei (Sofroniew and Glassmann, 1981), no unequivocal evidence for locally terminating collaterals has been found (van den Pol, 1982). The PVN may receive afferents from SON and contralateral PVN (Silverman et al., 1981) so that an input from magnocellular neurones need not be restricted to the same nucleus. However, there have been no reports of presynaptic elements containing classical 170 nm neurosecretory granules despite numerous reports on the ultrastructure of the nuclei over two decades. Granulated vesicles in the synapses of the SON and PVN are usually 90–120 nm in diameter. Small granules of this size can be found in magnocellular neurones (Morris et al., 1977) but their content is unknown and it seems unlikely that collateral branches could select granules on the basis of their size. Vasopressin is found in granules of this size in the parvocellular PVN projection to the median eminence (see Silverman et al., 1981).

INTERNEURONES IN THE CONTROL OF MAGNOCELLULAR NEURONES

A spinal alpha motor neurone — the classical "final common pathway" — is contacted by very few fibres of the long afferent motor tracts, but receives the vast majority of its direct input from a pool of interneurones on which the long and local afferent pathways end. The magnocellular neurones are the final common pathway for vasopressin and oxytocin release. They are likewise subject to a wide range of inputs and produce a variety of responses depending on the totality of the combined input. For example, oxytocin is released as a pulse from virtually all the oxytocin neurones during the milk ejection reflex but its release during osmotic stimulation is probably more sustained (see Poulain and Wakerley, 1982). Interneurones could therefore play a large part in coordinating the responses to long afferent pathway stimuli. Discussions of recurrent inhibition and excitation have either assumed or predicted the presence of interneurones, but such cells have received little attention from morphologists. In the SON of the rat there are few cells that could be considered as interneurones but such cells are present in the SON of the rabbit and cat (Felten and Cashner, 1979; Sofroniew et al., 1982). In the PVN, by contrast, there are many cells that could fulfil this role. Interneurones might also be located around the nuclei, particularly in the case of the SON. Freund-Mercier et al. (1981) have identified two populations of parvocellular neurones in the periphery of PVN which show transsynaptic activation, and other neurones which show no response after neural stalk stimulation. Those PVN neurones which did not respond contained ca. 100 nm dense-cored granules, but whether these were interneurones, parvocellular neurosecretory neurones, or have no connection to the magnocellular system, cannot be determined. The cells influenced transsynaptically are said to contain no dense-cored granules. However, the alcian blue technique used would make such vesicles more difficult to see and, in my experience, virtually all PVN neurones which are not magnocellular or parvocellular neurosecretory in type contain just a few 90–110 nm granules, as do similar cells in the region around PVN. Also, it is not clear whether the cells are activated transsynaptically from antidromic impulses generated in magnocellular or in other axons projecting to the neurohypophysis. Sofroniew et al. (1982) have recently demonstrated choline acetyltransferase immunoreactivity in a population of neurones just dorsal to the SON and cells in a similar position have been implicated as interneurones by the electrophysiological studies of Leng (Leng and Wiersma, 1981; Leng, 1981a, b). Such cells could therefore be interneurones which provide the elusive excitatory cholinergic input to the magnocellular neurones. Consistent with this is the finding of Léránth et al. (1975) that deafferentation of the SON induced the least degeneration among synapses contacting SON dendrites, the site in which an excitatory input should be located.

The deafferentation study of Léránth et al. (1975) which reports that only ca. 25 % of synapses in SON degenerated after isolation of an island containing the SON is often quoted as evidence that supraoptic magnocellular neurones themselves form extensive interconnections. However, the islands investigated by Léránth et al. contained much more than just the SON and would have included the area of hypothalamus dorsal and dorsolateral to the SON that has been discussed above. The authors acknowledge this area as a possible source of afferents but comment that it is not rich in neurones. This appearance will be due, at least in part, to the small size of the cells by contrast with those of the SON. Lateral hypothalamic neurones seem to send dendrites and perhaps axons into the SON region (Millhouse, 1980), but much more precise information is needed.

The interpretation of many investigations of long afferent paths to the magnocellular system is crucially affected by the interneurone problem. If long afferent tracts do end to a significant extent on interneurones then our present ignorance of the location of these cells means that retrograde tracings from injections of label confined to the nuclei may reveal only a small part of the total picture.

TRANSMITTERS IN THE AFFERENT PATHWAYS

There is good evidence that magnocellular neurones are directly sensitive to acetylcholine, noradrenaline (NA), dopamine, angiotensin II and opioid peptides; and substance P, thyrotrophin releasing hormone and somatostatin terminals are also found in the nuclei (see Hayward, 1977; Palkovits and Brownstein, 1978; Poulain and Wakerley, 1982). We have already seen that interneurones might form the cholinergic input. Both nicotinic and muscarinic receptors are found in higher concentrations in PVN than in SON (Block and Billiar, 1981; Hoover et al., 1981) but the significance of this is difficult to determine in view of the heterogeneity of the PVN.

The foundations of our understanding of the aminergic input were laid by fluorescence studies (see Palkovits, 1981). More recently, the anatomy of the catecholamine input has been studied extensively by Sladek and McNeill and their colleagues (Sladek and McNeill, 1980; McNeill and Sladek, 1981a, b; see Sladek and Sladek, this volume) and by Swanson's group (Sawchenko and Swanson, 1981) in an elegant series of experiments which use combinations of techniques to provide the precision of information that is now required. These studies have yet to be extended to the ultrastructural level but the general pattern is clear.

In the SON the NA input, which is largely inhibitory, is most pronounced in the ventral part of the nucleus where vasopressin cells predominate, and is particularly rich in the ventral lamina where the magnocellular dendrites are found. In Brattleboro rats, which lack vasopressin, the NA input lies more dorsally (Scholer and Sladek, 1981) but the significance of this interesting finding has yet to be determined. Hypothalamic NA metabolism and magnocellular electrical activity are increased in animals limited in their access to water, but the increase is already abolished by 10 min access to water by which time the plasma osmolarity is unlikely to have been corrected (Luttinger and Seiden, 1981). The NA input ending within the SON originates almost entirely from the A1 cell group (Loewy et al., 1981; McKellar and Loewy, 1981; Sawchenko and Swanson, 1981; Sladek and Sladek, this volume). Jones and Moore (1977) and Iijima and Ogawa (1980a, b) suggest that the locus coeruleus also contributes an NA input to SON, but McKellar and Loewy (1981) claim that this represents a spread of label to the region dorsal to SON. Sawchenko and Swanson (1981) come to a similar conclusion since True Blue injections "centred on but not restricted to, the SON" labelled locus coeruleus and A2 cells, but proline/leucine injections into neither A2 nor locus coeruleus labelled terminals within SON. However, it is in this area dorsal to SON that interneurones projecting to SON may exist (see above) so such an input may be of significance.

In the PVN the NA input, which is derived from about three times the number of cells that provide afferents to SON, passes to both parvocellular and magnocellular zones. As in the SON, the ventral medullary A1 group contributes most (68 %) to the NA input and again they project primarily to the area containing magnocellular vasopressin neurones. Of aminergic cells labelled retrogradely from PVN, 26 % were found in the A2 group. These cells innervated periventricular, medial and dorsal periventricular parts of PVN but not the magnocellular region. Of labelled cells 6 % were found in locus coeruleus and their terminals were restricted to the periventricular parvocellular parts of PVN (Sawchenko and Swanson, 1981; McNeill and Sladek, 1980a).

The dorsal vagal complex (A2), A1 and locus coeruleus are extensively interconnected (Sawchenko and Swanson, 1981) and these cell groups also receive reciprocal peptidergic projections from the parvocellular PVN (see Sawchenko and Swanson; and Sladek and Sladek, this volume).

Little is known of the pathways using adrenaline or dopamine, but recent studies by Mason (personal communication) showing heterogeneity among oxytocin neurones in their response to dopamine should warn against assuming that all cells of one hormonal type will have the same synaptic input or receptors. Serotonin (5-HT) may be present in afferents from the raphe of the ventral medulla (Loewy et al., 1981) but has received little attention.

Opioid peptides appear to affect magnocellular neurones at the hypothalamic level (see, e.g., Baertschi et al., 1981). The origin of this projection is unknown, though enkephalins are known to occur in arcuate neurones. Recently, however, Charnay et al. (1982) have co-localized enkephalin and tyrosine hydroxylase immunoreactivities in locus coeruleus neurones so that enkephalins might reach the PVN (and SON?) with catecholamine fibres, although the locus coeruleus does not appear to project to the magnocellular neurones directly.

Substance P also appears to affect the system at hypothalamic level (Baertschi et al., 1981), though again the pathway is unknown.

THE SOURCE OF THE AFFERENTS TO THE PVN AND SON

Before considering the afferent paths in terms of their functions in the various neuroendocrine reflexes the origin of fibres projecting to the PVN and SON as determined by various fibre tracing techniques will be reviewed.

Any tracing technique is only as good as the precision with which the label injected can be localized. Careful analyses of the injection sites such as that reported by Tribollet and Dreifuss (1981) are crucial to interpretation. By contrast, comments that an injection site was "essentially confined to the nucleus" only create uncertainty. However, even the most careful analysis could not localize uptake to one cell group within a nucleus as heterogenous as the PVN and combinations of anterograde and retrograde techniques are needed. Unfortunately, the afferent input to the more homogenous SON has been less studied, presumably for technical reasons.

It is difficult to assess the extent to which the prominence of a particular afferent pathway will be reflected in prominence of its functional effect. The glial sheaths of dendrites, and long dendritic and short perikaryal spinous appendages could influence the effect of various synapses. Also, the relative geometry of the afferent arborizations with respect to the dendritic trees may allow repeated contacts between a single incoming axon and a magnocellular dendrite giving functional prominence to what is quantitatively a small input (van den Pol, 1982). Also, the finding that the incidence of single boutons contacting two cells increases in lactation reminds us that the afferent input may be more plastic than is usually considered (Hatton and Tweedle, 1982; Theodosis et al., 1981).

Spinal cord afferents

Although afferents from the nipples and cervix pass up the spinal cord (Cross and Dyball, 1974), spinal cord projection neurones have not been retrogradely labelled from either PVN or SON thus far (Tribollet and Dreifuss, 1981). It would appear likely that most spinal afferents relay in the brainstem (probably in the nucleus tractus solitarius (NTS)), but more studies with different degrees of labelling are needed before a direct spinal projection can be excluded.

Brainstem afferents to the magnocellular nuclei

The synapse degeneration study of Záborsky et al. (1975) showed that about 33 % of SON synapses probably arise from the brainstem. Table I summarizes the results of a number of tracing studies virtually all of which refer to the rat. Noradrenergic fibres pass via a dorsal and a ventral pathway to the diencephalon and most of the afferents probably pass into the hypothalamus via either the medial forebrain bundle or the dorsal longitudinal fasciculus and seem to be predominantly ipsilateral. These aspects of the pathways have received rather less attention than the sites of origin of the afferents.

The origin of the brainstem NA afferents has already been discussed above. Lack of structural evidence for direct afferents from the NTS to SON is interesting in view of the electrophysiological evidence that about half the SON neurones are influenced by NTS stimulation (Kannan and Koizumi, 1981). The NTS does, however, project heavily via

TABLE I

STRUCTURAL STUDIES TRACING BRAINSTEM AFFERENTS TO THE PARAVENTRICULAR AND
SUPRAOPTIC HYPOTHALAMIC NUCLEI

Brainstem site	SON	PVN
	Reference[a]	
Ventral medulla	4, 5, 9	4, 5, 9
A1 catecholamine group	4, 5, 9	4, 5, 9
Tractus solitarius		1, 4, 5, 7, 12
A2 catecholamine group	(8)	10
Locus coeruleus	3, (8)	5, 9, 11, 12
Other catecholamine groups		10
Nucl. raphe magnus		4
Lateral dorsal tegmental nucleus		4
Central grey and parabrachial nucleus	(8)	4, 5, 12

[a] Key to references

1. Ciriello and Calarescu, 1980a — Anterograde radioautography (AR)
2. Iijima and Ogawa, 1980a, b — Retrograde HRP (RHRP)
3. Jones and Moore, 1977 — AR
4. Loewy et al., 1981 — AR, RHRP
5. McKellar and Loewy, 1981 — AR
6. McNeill and Sladek, 1980a, b — Catecholamine fluorescence with peptide immunocytochemistry
7. Ricardo and Koh, 1978 — AR, RHRP
8. Rogers et al., 1979 — RHRP; abstract only
9. Sawchenko and Swanson, 1981 — AR and retrograde True Blue with dopamine-β-hydroxylase immunocytochemistry.
10. Sladek and Sladek (this volume)
11. Swanson and Hartman, 1980 — RHRP
12. Tribollet and Dreifuss, 1981 — RHRP

(mainly) non-noradrenergic fibres (1) to the A1 and other cell groups of the ventral medulla which in turn project to parvo- and magnocellular PVN, and (2) to the locus coeruleus which projects to parvocellular PVN and possibly to magnocellular PVN and SON via interneurones (Sawchenko and Swanson, 1981). Connections between the NTS neurones and A1 cells in the dorsal vagal complex would be difficult to define by tracing techniques, but both the dorsal vagal complex and the locus coeruleus receive a heavy reciprocal projection from A1. A direct connection from NTS to PVN neurones exists, though its mode of termination is unknown (Ciriello and Calarescu, 1980b, and see Table I). The non-A1 ventral medulla projection to PVN and SON may contain 5-HT since it is abolished by pretreatment with 5,7-dihydroxy-tryptamine (McKellar and Loewy, 1981). In addition to those tabulated, Rogers et al. (1979) also claim projections to SON from the nuclei centralis superior, reticularis tegmenti pontis, reticularis parvocellularis, reticularis lateralis and raphe pontis. Orthograde studies (McKellar and Loewy, 1981; Sawchenko and Swanson, 1981) indicate that the magnocellular PVN neurones receive directly only from A1 and ventral medulla, an input which therefore parallels that to SON since a locus coeruleus projection direct to SON is disputed (see above).

Forebrain afferents to PVN and SON

Table II summarizes the results of studies tracing the forebrain afferents to the PVN and SON.

TABLE II

STRUCTURAL STUDIES TRACING FOREBRAIN AFFERENTS TO THE SUPRAOPTIC AND PARAVEN-
TRICULAR NUCLEI

Forebrain site	SON	PVN
	Reference[a]	
Limbic:		
Lateral septum	(8), 17	7, 12, 16
Bed nucleus of stria terminalis	(8)	2, 3(?), 7
Ventral subiculum	17	12, 14, 16
Medial amygdala	(8), 17	12, 16
Preoptic area:		
Medial preoptic area	(8)	3, 12, 13
Lateral preoptic area	(8)	12
Periventricular preoptic area	(8), 13	3, 13
Hypothalamus:		
Anterior hypothalamic area	(8)	4, 9
Ventromedial hypothalamus	5	5, 10, 12
Periventricular hypothalamus		12
Arcuate nucleus		12
Lateral hypothalamus	(8)	11
Contralateral PVN		12
Ispilateral SON		3, 6, 12
Suprachiasmatic nucleus		15
Zona incerta		12
Circumventricular organs:		
OVLT	6	12
Subfornical organ	6, (8)	1, 12

[a] Key to references:
1. Carithers et al., 1980a, b — EM degeneration
2. Conrad and Pfaff, 1976a — Anterograde radioautography (AR)
3. Conrad and Pfaff, 1976b — AR
4. Conrad and Pfaff, 1976c — AR
5. Kaelber and Leeson, 1967 — Nauta and EM degeneration
6. Miselis et al., 1979 — AR retrograde HRP (RHRP)
7. Powell and Rorie, 1967 — EM degeneration
8. Rogers et al., 1979 — RHRP; abstract only
9. Saper et al., 1978 — AR
10. Saper et al., 1976 — AR
11. Saper et al., 1979 — AR
12. Silverman et al., 1981 — RHRP
13. Swanson, 1976 — AR
14. Swanson and Cowan, 1975a — AR
15. Swanson and Cowan, 1975b — AR
16. Tribollet and Dreifuss, 1981 — RHRP
17. Záborsky et al., 1975 — EM degeneration

Záborsky et al. (1975) have proposed from degeneration studies that 12 % of all SON synapses (or 50 % of long afferents) arise from limbic structures. Of the limbic inputs, that from the lateral septum appears to be the strongest (5 % of total; but N.B. the lesions were mainly of medial septum) and has supportive electrophysiological data (see Poulain, this volume). The medial amygdala contributes ca. 3 % of the SON synapses and these fibres may follow the ventral amygdalofugal pathway (Záborsky et al., 1975). Rogers et al. (1979) also suggest an input from CA1–3 of the hippocampus but other retrograde studies suggest that this is unlikely (Swanson and Cowan, 1975a; Meibach and Siegel, 1977a, b; Silverman et al., 1981). The retrograde studies show inputs from subiculum and septal nuclei, but the antero-grade radioautographic studies of Meibach and Siegel (1977a, b) do not mention the PVN or SON by name among the projections from the septum. If the problem is not merely one of nomenclature precision ("midline hypothalamic terminals" are noted) this may reflect a difference due to technique (Silverman et al., 1981). The medial preoptic area gives more projections than the lateral preoptic area, but both inputs pass primarily to the periventricular regions of PVN. The periventricular preoptic area also projects to the lateral hypothalamus dorsal to SON where interneurones related to the SON might be located.

Connections within the hypothalamus are perhaps the most difficult to analyse with tracing techniques. Záborsky et al. (1975) calculate that 4–5 % of SON synapses arise within the hypothalamus. Saper et al. (1978) found no input to SON from ventromedial hypothalamus, but three other reports (see Table II) show a projection to PVN, though again more detail of the projections is necessary before inputs to the nuclei can be said to differ in this respect.

Of the periventricular organs, the subfornical organ (SFO) seems to contain many more cells projecting to both PVN and SON than does the organum vasculosum laminae terminalis (OVLT). Also, in distinction to virtually all other afferents, the projection of the SFO to the SON is much more marked than that to the PVN (Silverman et al., 1981).

The projection to the PVN (but not the SON) from the suprachiasmatic nucleus (Swanson and Cowan, 1975b) may contain vasoactive intestinal peptide (Sims et al., 1980) and is interesting in the light of Kaufman's (1981) report of a diurnal rhythm in osmotic drinking threshold in addition to likely diurnal rhythms in corticotrophin control (see Silverman et al., 1981).

It is tempting to conclude from Tables I and II that the magnocellular neurones of the SON receive fewer afferents than those of the PVN. However, since many afferents to PVN end in parvocellular regions, this conclusion is invalid until we have a far better understanding of which pathways end on which type of PVN neurone, and more studies on the afferents to the SON are available.

CONTROL IN THE NEURAL LOBE

It is perhaps fitting that this analysis of the afferents to the PVN and SON should end by acknowledging that the neurohypophysis itself almost certainly has "the last word" in determining the output of oxytocin and vasopressin. A detailed analysis of controls in the neural lobe is outside the remit of this review (but see Pittman et al., and Tweedle, this volume). It must be noted, however, that a large number of possible presynaptic neuromodu-lators are reported to exist in the neural lobe. These include acetylcholine and dopamine, GABA, the enkephalins and dynorphin, substance P, angiotensin II, CCK/gastrin, neurotensin and calcitonin. Evidence has been presented that enkephalins, dynorphin, CCK, angiotensin II and renin might be co-packaged in magnocellular neurones, though, by contrast, quite separate fibres containing opioids and apparently ending on glia have also been reported (see van Leeuwen and de Vries, this volume). As in the hypothalamus the glia appear to exert a more dynamic role than had been expected, and so the neuromodulators might act directly on the magnocellular terminals, or influence their output via either the glia or the vasculature.

FUNCTIONAL ASPECTS OF AFFERENT PATHWAYS

Now that the afferents to the nuclei have been reviewed, the extent to which these can be related to the functional neuroendocrine reflexes involving vasopressin and oxytocin can be considered.

Milk ejection reflex

Relatively little has been added to our understanding of the anatomy of the afferent pathways since Cross and Dyball's (1974) review. It appears likely that ascending spinal afferents synapse in the brainstem since no direct spinal afferents to the SON or PVN have been found. The lateral tegmentum of the midbrain is clearly a crucial part of the pathway for without it the milk ejection reflex does not occur. A pathway via the ventral tegmentum of the midbrain is implicated by Juss and Wakerley (1981) but its effect seems to be modulatory, altering the timing of the reflex. The septal input to PVN also appears to be modulatory, since lesions do not abolish the reflex but stimulation of the septum lengthens the intervals between milk ejections (see Poulain, this volume). The connections between SON and PVN and between the PVN of the two sides, the contacts between adjacent magnocellular neurones, and the synapses which affect more than one neurone may, in part, explain the coordination of the oxytocin cells in milk ejection. However, the mechanism whereby the reflex is "gated" to provide different temporal patterns of milk ejection in different animals is quite unknown and provides a challenge to experimenters of all disciplines.

Oxytocin release during labour

On general principles termination of the ascending spinal afferents from the cervix in the tractus solitarius complex would be expected. This complex projects to PVN and SON via interconnected catecholamine and non-catecholamine pathways, but which projections are important, and how this afferent path differs from that connecting the nipples to the PVN and SON thereby producing different patterns of oxytocin release, are not known.

Release of oxytocin and vasopressin in cardiovascular reflexes

The cardiovascular afferent pathway undoubtedly involves the IX and X cranial nerves, the NTS and its efferent pathways discussed above. As for the other ascending projections, it would be possible for neurohormone release to be controlled via changes in an inhibitory pathway alone. However, the absence of any structural evidence for an excitatory pathway from NTS to the SON is a big gap in our understanding, since it seems unlikely that the reflex release of vasopressin is mediated solely via the PVN, which does receive a direct projection from the NTS.

Osmotic release of vasopressin and oxytocin

The projections to SON and PVN from the SFO and OVLT must be related to osmotic control since lesions in the anterior part of the third ventricle (e.g. Eng and Miselis, 1981; Carithers et al., 1980) or anterior disconnections of the hypothalamus (Dyball and Prilusky, 1981) prevent not only drinking behaviour and osmotically stimulated release of vasopressin, but also the activation of synthesis in the SON neurones (see Carithers et al., 1981). That the

SFO provides a quantitatively greater input to SON than PVN must also be significant. However, the mechanism whereby these inputs are integrated with other osmotically sensitive inputs from a variety of sources is still unknown.

Role of PVN in feeding behaviour

Large lesions of the PVN region cause overeating and obesity in the rat (Leibowitz et al., 1981) in the same way as do ventromedial hypothalamic lesions. The input from the ventromedial hypothalamus to parvocellular PVN presumably plays a role in this.

Role of oxytocin and vasopressin in memory and behaviour

The limbic afferents to the PVN (and SON?) are prime candidates for afferent pathways involved in the role of the magnocellular neuropeptides on behaviour and memory processing (see de Wied, this volume). Again, however, much more precise information is needed on the localization of neuroendocrine effects on these processes before analysis of the limbic connections of the nuclei provides more than an interesting correlation.

CONCLUSION

The widespread use of tracing techniques since the 1976 Neurohypophysis Conference has considerably enhanced our understanding of sites which project afferents to the PVN and SON. Such techniques have given particularly precise information when used in combination with one another and with identification of the peptides, transmitters, or enzymes characterizing the cells. However, there are still many gaps in our knowledge. The definition of the terminals often lacks precision in terms of the type of cell contacted — a particular problem in the PVN. The whole question of interneurones controlling the magnocellular neurones has yet to be investigated experimentally. Moreover, the classical afferent inputs to the nuclei clearly form only one of a number of factors controlling the output of the cells. This is beautifully exemplified by the ability of grafted vasopressin neurones to restore normal urine output in Brattleboro rats (Gash et al., 1980, and this volume). Intrinsic sensitivity of the cells to hormones and osmotic pressure, relations with the glia in both the hypothalamus and pituitary, and control within the neural lobe all offer exciting challenges for the investigator who wishes to unravel the way in which neuroendocrine and autonomic functions are controlled by these fascinating nuclei.

SUMMARY

The anatomists' first goal in the analysis of the organization of neural inputs to the paraventricular (PVN) and supraoptic nuclei (SON) must be to determine the origin, course and mode of termination of the pathways and individual fibres that project to oxytocin and vasopressin neurones. Cytochemical techniques make structural studies important also in the analysis of neurotransmitters in those systems. Ideally such analyses should provide a circuitry which explains the coupling between effective stimuli and the release of hormone, including such phenomena as the coordinated multicellular release of oxytocin in milk ejection.

Despite three decades of study of the nuclei this goal has not been achieved in that we know with certainty the origin of few of the fibres that synapse directly onto vasopressin- or oxytocinergic neurones of either PVN or SON. The extent of progress in delineating the various afferent systems is discussed. The analysis is complicated by the finding that, while most SON neurones project to the neurohypophysis, many neurones of the PVN (especially its parvocellular portion) project to other parts of the central nervous system, in some cases to sites from which afferent inputs are derived. Furthermore, many PVN neurones are neither oxytocinergic nor vasopressinergic, making the demonstration that an afferent system ends within the nucleus insufficient to permit a precise functional interpretation. Immediate afferents to the magnocellular neurones arise from both long projection systems and local interneurones. They form synapses on dendrites, somata and axons, and may also influence the neurones by non-synaptic release of transmitter in the hypothalamus or actions on the neurohypophysial neurosecretory terminals.

ACKNOWLEDGEMENTS

Neuroendocrine studies in the author's laboratory are generously supported by Grants ARC AG43/94 and MRC G608/263.

REFERENCES

Andrew, R.D., MacVicar, B.A., Dudek, F.E. and Hatton, G.I. (1981) Dye transfer through gap junctions between neuroendocrine cells of rat hypothalamus. *Science*, 211: 1187–1189.

Armstrong, W.E. and Hatton, G.I. (1980) The localization of projection neurons in the rat hypothalamic paraventricular nucleus following vascular and neurohypohyseal injections of HRP. *Brain Res. Bull.*, 5: 473–477.

Armstrong, W.E., Warach, S., Hatton, G.I. and McNeill, T.H. (1980) Subnuclei in the rat hypothalamic paraventricular nucleus: a cytoarchitectural, horseradish peroxidase and immunocytochemical analysis. *Neuroscience*, 5: 1931–1958.

Armstrong, W.E., Scholer, J. and McNeill, T.H. (1982) Immunocytochemical, Golgi, and electron microscopic characterisation of putative dendrites in the ventral glial lamina of the rat supraoptic nucleus. *Neuroscience*, 7: 679–694.

Baertschi, A.J., Zingg, H.H. and Dreifuss, J.J. (1981) Enkephalins, substance P, bradykinin and angiotensin II: different sites of action on the hypothalamo-neurohypophyseal system. *Brain Res.*, 220: 107–119.

Block, G.A. and Billiar, R.B. (1981) Properties and regional distribution of nicotinic cholinergic receptors in the rat hypothalamus. *Brain Res.*, 212: 152–158.

Bugnon, C., Fellmann, D., Gouget, A. and Carot, J. (1982) Ontogeny of the corticoliberin neuroglandular system in rat brain. *Nature (Lond.)*, 298: 159–161.

Carithers, J., Bealer, S.L., Brody, M.J. and Johnson, A.K. (1980) Fine structural evidence of degeneration in supraoptic nucleus and subfornical organ of rats with lesions in the anteroventral third ventricle. *Brain Res.*, 201: 1–12.

Carithers, J., Dellmann, H.D., Bealer, S.L., Brody, M.J. and Johnson, A.K. (1981) Ultrastructural effects of anteroventral third ventricle lesions on supraoptic nuclei and neural lobes of rats. *Brain Res.*, 220: 13–29.

Charnay, Y., Leger, L., Dray, F., Berod, A. Jouvet, M., Pujol, J.F. and Dubois, P.M. (1982) Evidence for the presence of enkephalin in catecholaminergic neurones of cat locus coeruleus. *Neurosci. Lett.*, 30: 147–151.

Ciriello, J. and Calaresu, F.R. (1980a) Autoradiographic study of ascending projections from cardiovascular sites in the nucleus tractus solitarius in the cat. *Brain Res.*, 186: 448–453.

Ciriello, J. and Calaresu, F.R. (1980b) Monosynaptic pathway from cardiovascular neurons in the nucleus tractus solitarii to the paraventricular nucleus in the cat. *Brain Res.*, 193: 529–533.

Conrad, L.C. and Pfaff, D.W. (1976a) Autoradiographic tracing of nucleus accumbens efferents in the rat. *Brain Res.*, 113: 589–596.

Conrad, L.C. and Pfaff, D.W. (1976b) Efferents from medial basal forebrain and hypothalamus in the rat. I. An autoradiographic study of the medial preoptic area. *J. comp. Neurol.*, 169: 185–220.

Conrad, L.C. and Pfaff, D.W. (1976c) Efferents from medial basal forebrain and hypothalamus in the rat. II. An autoradiographic study of the anterior hypothalamus. *J. comp. Neurol.*, 169: 221–262.

Cross, B.A. and Dyball, R.E.J. (1974) Central pathways for neurohypophysial hormone release. In E.L. Knobil and W.H. Sawyer (Eds.), *Handbook of Physiology, Endocrinology IV, Part 1*, American Society for Physiology, Washington, DC, pp. 269–285.

Dubois, M.P. and Kolodziejczyk, E. (1975) Centres hypothalamiques du rat sécrétant la somatostatine; répartition des péricaryons en deux systèmes magno- et parvocellulaire (étude cytoimmunologique). *C.R. Acad. Sci. (Paris)*, 281(D): 1737–1740.

Dyball, R.E.J. and Prilusky, J. (1981) Responses of supraoptic neurones in the intact and deafferented rat hypothalamus to injections of hypertonic sodium chloride. *J. Physiol. (Lond.)*, 311: 443–452.

Dyball, R.E.J., Howard, M. and Kemplay, S.K. (1979) A Golgi study of the neurosecretory neurons in the supraoptic nucleus of the rat. *J. Anat.*, 128: 417.

Eng, R. and Miselis, R.R. (1981) Polydipsia and abolition of angiotensin-induced drinking after transections of subfornical organ efferent projections in the rat. *Brain Res.*, 225: 200–206.

Felten, D.L. and Cashner, K.A. (1979) Cytoarchitecture of the supraoptic nucleus. A Golgi study. *Neuroendocrinology*, 29: 221–230.

Freund-Mercier, M.J., Stoeckel, M.E., Moos, F., Porte, A. and Richard, Ph. (1981) Ultrastructural study of electrophysiologically identified neurones in the paraventricular nucleus of the rat. *Cell Tiss. Res.*, 216: 503–512.

Gash, D., Sladek, J.R. Jr. and Sladek, C.D. (1980) Functional development of grafted vasopressinergic neurons. *Science*, 210: 1379–1369.

Gregory, W.A., Tweedle, C.D. and Hatton, G.I. (1980) Ultrastructure of neurons in the paraventricular nucleus of normal, dehydrated, and rehydrated rats. *Brain Res. Bull.*, 5: 301–306.

Harris, M.C. (1978) The concept of the neuroendocrine reflex. In J.D. Vincent and C. Kordon (Eds.), *Cell Biology of Hypothalamic Neurosecretion*, CNRS, Paris, pp. 47–61.

Hartman, B.K., Swanson, L.W., Raichle, M.E., Preskorn, S.H. and Clark, H.B. (1980) Central adrenergic regulation of cerebral microvascular permeability and blood flow; anatomic and physiologic evidence. *Advanc. exp. Med. Biol.*, 131: 113–126.

Hatton, G.I. and Tweedle, C.D. (1982) Magnocellular neuropeptidergic neurons in hypothalamus: increases in membrane apposition and number of specialised synapses from pregnancy to lactation. *Brain Res. Bull.*, 8: 197–204.

Hayward, J.N. (1977) Functional and morphological aspects of hypothalamic neurons. *Physiol. Rev.*, 57: 574–658.

Hoover, D.B., Hancock, J.C. and Talley, N.S. (1981) Binding of ^{3}H-quinuclidinyl benzylate to regions of rat pituitary and hypothalamus. *Brain Res. Bull.*, 6: 209–211.

Iijima, K. and Ogawa, T. (1980a) An HRP study on cell types and their regional topography within the locus coeruleus innervating the supraoptic nucleus of the rat. *Acta histochem.*, 67: 127–138.

Iijima, K. and Ogawa, T. (1980b) Demonstration of projections from locus coeruleus to supraoptic nucleus by the HRP method with special reference to cell types in the rat. *Arch. Histol. Jap.*, 43: 411–421.

Johansson, O. and Hökfelt, T. (1980) Immunohistochemical distribution of thyrotropin-releasing hormone, somatostatin and enkephalin with special reference to the hypothalamus. In *Ferring Symposium on Brain and Pituitary Peptides*, Karger, Basel, pp. 202–212.

Jones, B.E. and Moore, R.Y. (1977) Ascending projections of the locus coeruleus of the rat — II. Autoradiographic study. *Brain Res.*, 127: 23–53.

Juss, T.S. and Wakerley, J.B. (1981) Mesencephalic areas controlling pulsatile oxytocin release in the suckled rat. *J. Endocr.*, 91: 233–244.

Kaelber, W.W. and Leeson, C.R. (1967) A degeneration and electron microscopic study of the nucleus hypothalamicus medialis of the cat. *J. Anat.*, 101: 209–221.

Kannan, H. and Koizumi, H. (1981) Pathways between the nucleus tractus solitarius and neurosecretory neurons of the supraoptic nucleus; electrophysiological studies. *Brain Res.*, 213: 17–28.

Kannan, H., Yagi, K. and Sawaki, Y. (1980) Pontine neurones mediate synaptic inputs from carotid baroreceptors to supraoptic neurosecretory neurons in rats. *Neurosci. Lett.*, Suppl. 4: S80.

Kaufman, S. (1981) Control of fluid intake in pregnant and lactating rats. *J. Physiol. (Lond.)*, 318: 9–16.

Koh, E.T. and Ricardo, J.A. (1980) Paraventricular nucleus of the hypothalamus: anatomical evidence of the functionally discrete subdivisions. *Soc. Neurosci. Abstr.*, 6: 521.

Lafarga, M., Palacios, G. and Perez, R. (1975) Morphological aspects of the functional synchronization of supraoptic nucleus neurons. *Experientia*, 31: 348–349.

Leibowitz, S.F., Hammer, N.J. and Chang, K. (1981) Hypothalamic paraventricular nucleus lesions produce overeating and obesity in the rat. *Physiol. Behav.*, 27: 1031–1040.

Leng, G. (1981a) The effects of neural stalk stimulation upon firing patterns in rat supraoptic neurones. *Exp. Brain Res.*, 41: 135–145.

Leng, G. (1981b) Phasically firing neurones in the lateral hypothalamus of anaesthetised rats. *Brain Res.*, 230: 390–393.

Leng, G. and Wiersma, J. (1981) Effects of neural stalk stimulation on phasic discharge of supraoptic neurones in Brattleboro rats devoid of vasopressin, *J. Endocr.*, 90: 211–220.

Leng, G., Mason, W.T. and Dyer, R.G. (1982) The supraoptic nucleus as an osmoreceptor. *Neuroendocrinology*, 34: 75–82.

Léránth, Cs., Záborsky, L., Marton, J. and Palkovits, M. (1975) Quantitative analysis on the supraoptic nucleus in the rat. I Synaptic organisation. *Exp. Brain. Res.*, 22: 509–523.

Lindvall, O. and Björklund, A. (1974) The organisation of the ascending catecholamine neurone system in the rat brain as revealed by the glyoxylic acid fluorescence method. *Acta physiol. scand.*, 92, Suppl. 412: 1–48.

Loewy, A.D., Wallach, J.H. and McKellar, S. (1981) Efferent connections of the ventral medulla. *Brain Res. Rev.*, 3: 63–80.

Luqui, I.J. and Fox, C.A. (1976) The supraoptic nucleus and the supraopticohypophysial tract in the monkey *(Macaca mulatta)*. *J. comp. Neurol.*, 168: 7–40.

Luttinger, D. and Seiden, L.S. (1981) Increased hypothalamic norepinephrine metabolism after water deprivation in the rat. *Brain Res.*, 208: 147–165.

McKellar, S. and Loewy, A.D. (1981) Organisation of some brain stem afferents to the paraventricular nucleus of the hypothalamus in the rat, *Brain Res.*, 217: 351–357.

McNeill, T.H. and Sladek, J.R., Jr. (1980a) Simultaneous monoamine histofluorescence and neuro-peptide immuno-cytochemistry· II Correlative distribution of catecholamine varicosities and magnocellular neurosecretory neurons in the rat supraoptic and paraventricular nuclei. *J. comp. Neurol.*, 193: 1023–1033.

McNeill, T.H. and Sladek, J.R., Jr. (1980b) Simultaneous monoamine histofluorescence and neuropeptide immuno-cytochemistry: V A methodology for examining correlative monoamine-neuropeptide neuroanatomy. *Brain Res. Bull.*, 5: 599–608.

Meibach, R.C. and Siegel, A. (1977a) Efferent connections of the septal area in the rat: an analysis utilizing retrograde and anterograde transport methods. *Brain Res.*, 119: 1–20.

Meibach, R.C. and Siegel, A. (1977b) Efferent connections of the hippocampal formation in the rat. *Brain Res.*, 124: 197–224.

Millhouse, O.E. (1980) A Golgi anatomy of the rodent hypothalamus. In P.J. Morgane and S. Panksepp (Eds.), *Handbook of Hypothalamus, Vol. 1*, Dekker, New York, pp. 221–265.

Miselis, R.R., Shapiro, R.E. and Hand, P.J. (1979) Subfornical organ efferents to neural systems for control of body water. *Science*, 205: 1022–1025.

Morris, J.F., Sokol, H.W. and Valtin, H. (1977) One neuron — one hormone? Recent evidence from Brattleboro rats. In A.M. Moses and L. Share (Eds.), *Neurohypophysis*, Karger, Basel.

Palkovits, M. (1981) Catecholamines in the hypothalamus: an anatomical review. *Neuroendocrinology*, 33: 123–128.

Palkovits, M. and Brownstein, M.J. (1978) Concentration of the neurotransmitters in the supraoptic and the paraventricular nuclei of the rat. In W. Bargmann, A. Oksche, A. Polenov and B. Scharrer (Eds.), *Neurosecretion and Neuroendocrine Activity*, Springer-Verlag, Berlin, pp. 250–255.

Palkovits, M. and Zaborsky, L. (1980) Neural connections of the hypothalamus. In P.J. Morgane and S. Panksapp (Eds.), *Handbook of Hypothalamus, Vol. 1*, Dekker, New York, pp. 379–509.

Poulain, D.A. and Wakerley, J.B. (1982) Electrophysiology of hypothalamic magnocellular neurones secreting oxytocin and vasopressin. *Neuroscience*, 7: 773–808.

Powell, E.W. and Rorie, D.K. (1967) Septal projections to nuclei functioning in oxytocin release. *Amer. J. Anat.*, 120: 605–610.

Rhodes, C.H. (1981) Distribution of estrogen-concentrating, neurophysin containing magnocellular neurons in the rat hypothalamus as demonstrated by a technique combining steroid autoradiography and immunohistology in the same tissue. *Neuroendocrinology*, 33: 18–23.

Ricardo, J.A. and Koh, E.H. (1978) Anatomical evidence of direct projections from the nucleus of the solitary tract to the hypothalamus, amygdala and other forebrain structures in the rat. *Brain Res.*, 153: 1–26.

Rogers, R.C., Talbot, K., Novin, D. and Butcher, L.L. (1979) Afferent projections to the supraoptic nucleus of the rat. *Soc. Neurosci. Abstr.*, 5: 233.

Saper, C.B., Swanson, L.W. and Cowan, W.M. (1976) The efferent connections of the ventromedial nucleus of the hypothalamus of the rat. *J. comp. Neurol.*, 169: 409–442.

Saper, C.B., Swanson, L.W. and Cowan, W.M. (1978) The efferent projections of the anterior hypothalamic area of the rat, cat and monkey. *J. comp. Neurol.*, 182: 575–600.

Saper, C.B., Swanson, L.W. and Cowan, W.M. (1979) An autoradiographic study of the efferent connections of the lateral hypothalamic area in the rat. *J. comp. Neurol.*, 183: 689–706.

18

Sar, M. and Stumpf, W.E. (1973) Autoradiographic localization of radioactivity in the rat brain after the injection of 1,2-^{3}H-testosterone. *Endocrinology*, 92: 251–256.

Sar, M. and Stumpf, W.E. (1980) Simultaneous localization of [^{3}H]estradiol and neurophysin I or arginine vasopressin in hypothalamic neurons demonstrated by a combined technique of dry-mount autoradiography and immunohistochemistry. *Neurosci. Lett.*, 17: 179–184.

Sawchenko, P.E. and Swanson, L.W. (1981) Central monoamine pathways for the integration of hypothalamic neuroendocrine and autonomic responses. *Science*, 214: 685–687.

Schmitt, F.O., Dev, P. and Smith, B.H. (1976) Electrotonic processing of information by brain cells. *Science*, 193: 114–120.

Scholer, J. and Sladek, J.R., Jr. (1981) Supraoptic nucleus of the Brattleboro rat has an altered noradrenergic input. *Science*, 214: 347–349.

Silverman, A.J., Hoffman, D.L. and Zimmerman, E.A. (1981) The descending afferent connections of the paraventricular nucleus of the hypothalamus, *Brain Res. Bull.*, 6: 47–61.

Sims, K., Hoffman, D.L., Said, S.I. and Zimmerman, E.A. (1980) Vasoactive intestinal polypeptide (VIP) in mouse and rat brain: an immunocytochemical study. *Brain Res.*, 186: 165–183.

Sladek, J.R., Jr. and McNeill, T.H. (1980) Simultaneous monoamine histofluorescence and neuropeptide immunochemistry. IV Verification of catecholamine-neurophysin interactions through single-section analysis. *Cell Tiss. Res.*, 210: 181–189.

Sofroniew, M.V. and Glassmann, W. (1981) Golgi-like immunoperoxidase staining of hypothalamic magnocellular neurons that contain vasopressin, oxytocin or neurophysin in the rat. *Neuroscience*, 6: 619–643.

Sofroniew, M.V., Eckenstein, F., Schrell, U. and Cuello, A.C. (1982) Evidence for colocalization of neuroactive substances in hypothalamic neurons. In V. Chan Palay and S. Palay (Eds.), *Coexistence of Neuroactive Substances*, John Wiley, New York, in press.

Streeten, D.H., Souma, M., Ross, G.S. and Miller, M. (1981) Action of cortisol introduced into the supraoptic nucleus on vasopressin release and antidiuresis during hypertonic saline infusion in conscious Rhesus monkeys. *Acta endocr.*, 98: 195–204.

Swanson, L.W. (1976) An autoradiographic study of the efferent connections of the preoptic region of the rat. *J. comp. Neurol.*, 167: 227–256.

Swanson, L.W. and Cowan, W.M. (1975a) Hippocampal–hypothalamic connections: origin in subicular cortex, not Ammon's horn. *Science*, 189: 303–304.

Swanson, L.W. and Cowan, W.M. (1975b) The efferent connections of the suprachiasmatic nucleus of the guinea pig. *J. comp. Neurol.*, 160: 1–12.

Swanson, L.W. and Hartman, B.K. (1980) Biochemical specificity in central pathways related to peripheral and intracerebral homeostatic functions. *Neurosci. Lett.*, 16: 55–60.

Swanson, L.W. and Kuypers, H.G.J.M. (1980) The paraventricular nucleus of the hypothalamus: cytoarchitectonic subdivisions and the organization of projections to the pituitary, dorsal vagal complex, and spinal cord as demonstrated by retrograde fluorescence double-labeling methods. *J. comp. Neurol.*, 194: 555–570.

Swanson, L.W. and Mogenson, G.J. (1981) Neural mechanisms for the functional coupling of autonomic, endocrine and somatomotor responses in adaptive behaviour. *Brain Res.*, 228: 1–34.

Swanson, L.W. and Sawchenko, P.E. (1980) Paraventricular nucleus: a site for the integration of neuroendocrine and autonomic mechanisms. *Neuroendocrinology*, 31: 410–417.

Swanson, L.W., Connelly, M.A. and Hartman, B.K. (1977) Ultrastructural evidence for central monoaminergic innervation of blood vessels in the paraventricular nucleus of the hypothalamus. *Brain Res.*, 136: 166–173.

Swanson, L.W., Connelly, M.A. and Hartman, B.K. (1978) Further studies on the fine structure of the adrenergic innervation of the hypothalamus. *Brain Res.*, 151: 165–174.

Swanson, L.W., Sawchenko, P.E., Wiegand, S.J. and Price, J.L. (1980) Separate neurons in the paraventricular nucleus project to the median eminence and to the medulla or spinal cord. *Brain Res.*, 198: 190–195.

Swanson, L.W., Sawchenko, P.E., Berod, A., Hartman, B.K., Helle, K.B. and Vanorden, D.E. (1981) An immunocytochemical study of the organisation of catecholaminergic cells and terminal fields in the paraventricular and supraoptic nuclei of the hypothalamus. *J. comp. Neurol.*, 196: 271–285.

Theodosis, D.T., Poulain, D.A. and Vincent, J.D. (1981) Possible morphological basis for synchronisation of neuronal firing in the rat supraoptic nucleus during lactation. *Neuroscience*, 6: 919–929.

Tribollet, E. and Dreifuss, J.J. (1981) Localization of neurones projecting to the hypothalamic paraventricular nucleus area of the rat: a horseradish peroxidase study. *Neuroscience*, 6: 1315–1328.

Van den Pol, A. (1982) The magnocellular and parvocellular nucleus of the rat: intrinsic organisation. *J. comp. Neurol.*, 206: 317–345.

Záborsky, L., Léránth, C.S., Makara, G.B. and Palkovits, M. (1975) Quantitative studies on the supraoptic nucleus in the rat. II. Afferent fiber connections. *Exp. Brain Res.*, 22: 525–540.

The Neurohypophysis: Structure, Function and Control, Progress in Brain Research, Vol. 60, edited by B.A. Cross and G. Leng

The Organization and Biochemical Specificity of Afferent Projections to the Paraventricular and Supraoptic Nuclei

P.E. SAWCHENKO* and L.W. SWANSON

The Salk Institute for Biological Studies and the Clayton Foundation for Research-California Division, La Jolla, CA 92037 (U.S.A.)

INTRODUCTION

The major stimuli that release oxytocin and vasopressin have been known for many years. Similarly, the final common path for hormone release, the paraventriculo-supraoptico-neuro-hypophysial system, is the most thoroughly characterized peptidergic system in the brain, both from the electrophysiological and the anatomical points of view. Until recently, however, little was known about the organization of the neural inputs which relay sensory information from the periphery to the paraventricular (PVN) and supraoptic (SON) nuclei, and which integrate activity in the magnocellular neurosecretory system with other, complementary, modes of neuroendocrine and autonomic regulation. In an insightful survey of the literature in 1974, Cross and Dyball concluded that no clearly defined system of afferent fibres to these nuclei had at that time been revealed by neuroanatomical methods. The development of sensitive tracing techniques based on the axonal transport of various marker molecules, and of immunohis-tochemical methods for localizing biochemically-defined neuronal systems have changed this situation dramatically, and it is now possible to outline the organization and biochemical specificity of inputs to the PVN and SON. Here we shall summarize the results of experiments carried out in the rat, and concentrate on systems that appear to influence the magnocellular system directly.

THE CYTOLOGICAL AND FUNCTIONAL ORGANIZATION OF THE PARAVENTRICULAR AND SUPRAOPTIC NUCLEI

To view the neural inputs to the PVN and SON in a functional context, it is necessary to begin with a summary of the cellular architecture of these nuclei (for more detailed treatment see Swanson and Sawchenko, 1983). The cells that project to the posterior pituitary are concentrated in the SON, and in the compact cell masses that form the magnocellular division of the PVN (Sherlock et al., 1975; Swanson and Kuypers, 1980). In the PVN, these cell groups are topographically segregated from populations of smaller, parvocellular neurones (some of which contain oxytocin and vasopressin; Sawchenko and Swanson, 1982a), that project to the external lamina of the median eminence or to autonomic centres in the brainstem and spinal

---

* Address for correspondence: The Salk Institute, P.O. Box 85800, San Diego, CA 92138, U.S.A.

cord (Swanson and Kuypers, 1980; Kelly and Swanson, 1980). In addition, smaller clusters of "accessory" magnocellular neurosecretory neurones, and cells scattered throughout the parvocellular division of the PVN and various basal forebrain nuclei, also project to the neural lobe (Sherlock et al., 1975; Swanson and Kuypers, 1980; Kelly and Swanson, 1980).

Both the SON and the magnocellular division of the PVN can be further subdivided on the basis of the distribution of oxytocin- and vasopressin-immunoreactive neurones. In the PVN, the anterior and medial parts of the magnocellular division (see Swanson and Kuypers, 1980) consist almost exclusively of oxytocin neurones; in the posterior magnocellular part, oxytocin cells are concentrated anteroventromedially, and vasopressin cells posterodorsolaterally, corresponding to the "medial" and "lateral" subdivisions recognized by Hatton et al. (1976) on cytoarchitectonic criteria alone (Rhodes et al., 1981; Sawchenko and Swanson, 1982a). In the SON oxytocin neurones are concentrated anterodorsally, while vasopressin cells are concentrated posteroventrally. This topographic arrangement has enabled us to suggest which cell type is associated with each particular afferent fibre system. Finally, recent Golgi studies have shown that the dendrites of cells within the PVN and SON are mainly confined within the morphological boundaries of the nuclei (e.g. van den Pol, 1982; Armstrong et al., 1982), thus facilitating the identification of projections that may influence the magnocellular neurones. The dendritic trees of neurones in the SON, and in both divisions of the PVN, are simple, and so we have attempted to draw functional inferences based on a light microscopic analysis of the distribution of fibre systems within each subdivision of the PVN and SON that has been recognized using cytoarchitectonic or immunohistochemical criteria.

AFFERENT CONTROL OF VASOPRESSIN SECRETION

Shortly after the advent of histofluorescence methods for the demonstration of catecholaminergic neurones, it was recognized that dense noradrenergic terminal fields lie within the PVN and SON (Carlsson et al., 1962). More recently, comparisons between the distribution of noradrenergic varicosities, stained with an antiserum against dopamine-β-hydroxylase (DBH; a marker for adrenergic and noradrenergic neurones), and the distribution of oxytocin- and vasopressin-immunoreactive cells in the PVN and SON established that DBH-stained fibres are concentrated in areas rich in vasopressin cell bodies (Swanson et al., 1981; see also McNeill and Sladek, 1980). Adrenergic fibres, demonstrated with an antiserum against phenylethanolamine-N-methyltransferase, are restricted almost entirely to the parvocellular division of the PVN (Swanson et al., 1981). To resolve a long-standing controversy as to which noradrenergic cells in the brainstem give rise to these inputs, we used a method that allows the concurrent localization within single cells of an antigen (DBH) and a retrogradely transported fluorescent dye (True Blue), after injections of the tracer in the PVN (Sawchenko and Swanson, 1981a). In these experiments (Sawchenko and Swanson, 1981b, 1982b) retrogradely labelled neurones were found to be associated with three noradrenergic cell groups (see Dahlström and Fuxe, 1964, for nomenclature). The greatest number (400–600 per brain) was found in the region of the A1 cell group in the ventrolateral medulla, while fewer (100–200 per brain) were found in the A2 cell group of the dorsal medulla, and in the locus coeruleus (30–60 per brain) or A6 cell group. The vast majority (over 80%) of retrogradely labelled cells were DBH-positive, indicating that the projection from each region is primarily noradrenergic.

We then injected [³H]amino acids into the A1, A2 and A6 regions (in separate experiments), and used the autoradiographic method to trace the course of each pathway to the PVN and SON as well as the distribution of labelled fibres in each nucleus. The results confirmed that the A1, A2 and A6 cell groups each project to the parvocellular division of the PVN, where each input ends preferentially in a different subset of the cytoarchitectonically- and functionally-defined parts of the nucleus (see also Jones and Moore, 1977; Ricardo and Koh, 1978; Loewy et al., 1981; McKellar and Loewy, 1981). Interestingly, only the A1 cell group was found to project substantially to the SON, and to the magnocellular division of the PVN. As with the distribution of noradrenergic varicosities observed immunohistochemically in the magnocellular system, the projection from the A1 region was concentrated over regions in which vasopressin cell bodies predominate (Fig. 1). The autoradiographic and retrograde transport-immunohistochemical experiments also suggested that a complex series of pathways interconnect the A1, A2 and A6 regions.

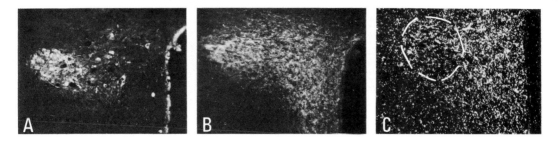

Fig. 1. These photomicrographs show sections through roughly the same level of the PVN and illustrate the distribution of cells stained with an antiserum against vasopressin (A), of fibres stained with an antiserum against dopamine-β-hydroxylase (B), and silver grains after an injection of [^{3}H]amino acids centred in the A1 catecholamine cell group of the ventral medulla (C). The magnocellular division of the PVN is outlined in C. Noradrenergic varicosities are concentrated in regions rich in vasopressin neurones, and the only noradrenergic neurones that appear to project to the magnocellular division of the PVN (and to the SON) are those of the A1 cell group. Original magnification $\times 100$.

The possible functional significance of these ascending noradrenergic pathways was brought into focus by the finding that the nucleus of the solitary tract (NTS) projects quite heavily to the A1 region (see also Norgren, 1978; Ricardo and Koh, 1978). Subsequent double-labelling experiments, in which True Blue was injected into the A1 region and the tissue was subsequently counterstained with an antiserum against DBH, indicated that this pathway is essentially non-noradrenergic. Important stimuli for vasopressin release are provided by sensory receptors that monitor the volume and composition of the blood. Atrial stretch receptors, carotid sinus baroreceptors, and carotid body chemoreceptors all influence the activity of neurones in the PVN and SON (e.g. Koizumi and Yamashita, 1978; Harris, 1979), and information supplied by these receptors is conveyed by the vagus and glossopharyngeal nerves to the nucleus of the solitary tract, the major central recipient of first-order visceral afferents. From the seminal experiments of Ricardo and Koh (1978), it has been generally assumed that cardiovascular stimuli influence the secretion of vasopressin by a direct projection from the nucleus of the solitary tract to the PVN, or by a disynaptic pathway involving the parabrachial nucleus, which receives an input from the nucleus of the solitary tract (Norgren, 1978) and projects to the PVN (Saper and Loewy, 1980). Careful analysis indicates, however, that neither input ends directly in the SON or in the magnocellular division of the PVN (McKellar and Loewy, 1981; Sawchenko and Swanson, 1981b, 1982b). The results suggest instead that visceral afferent information influences vasopressin secretion by way of the direct,

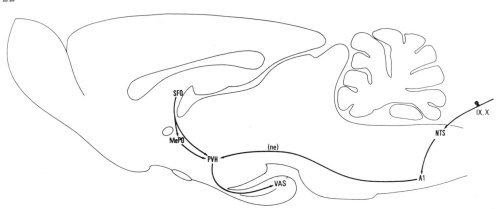

Fig. 2. A drawing of a sagittal section through the rat brain to show the organization of inputs to vasopressin cell groups in the PVN (PVH is the figure). The SON, which also receives inputs from each cell group indicated, is not shown for the sake of clarity. Sensory inputs from receptors in the cardiovascular system are conveyed by the vagus (X) and glossopharyngeal (IX) nerves to the nucleus of the solitary tract (NTS). Non-noradrenergic cells in the NTS project to the region of the A1 cell group which in turn projects selectively to vasopressin-containing parts of the magnocellular neurosecretory system. We have suggested this as a likely route by which visceral afferent inputs influence vasopressin (VAS) secretion. Other abbreviations: SFO, subfornical organ; MePO, median preoptic nucleus; ne, noradrenergic pathway.

primarily non-noradrenergic, pathway from the NTS to the A1 region, which in turn projects to vasopressin parts of the magnocellular neurosecretory system (Fig. 2). Although detailed ultrastructural studies are needed to confirm this suggestion, it is supported by functional evidence. For example, in the cat, single neurones in the region of the A1 cell group respond to stimulation of the carotid sinus nerve, and to selective baroreceptor or chemoreceptor activation (Ciriello and Calaresu, 1977; Thomas et al., 1977), while lesions of this region attenuate the pressor response to stimulation of the carotid sinus nerve (Ciriello and Calaresu, 1977). Thus, while it remains to be shown that noradrenergic cells of the A1 group receive viseroceptive inputs, at least some cells in this region do so, and are involved in the mediation of pressor responses. That vasopressin is involved in such responses is indicated by the recent demonstration that discrete lesions of the A1 cell group produce increases in blood pressure that are mediated predominantly by increased vasopressin release (Blessing et al., 1982).

Apart from the A1 cell group, the only additional sites that have been shown to project preferentially to vasopressin parts of the PVN and SON are the subfornical organ and the median preoptic nucleus. An input from the subfornical organ to the PVN and SON was first described by Miselis (1981), and we have confirmed this observation with both retrograde transport and autoradiographic techniques (Sawchenko and Swanson, 1983). The projection is distributed over all parts of the magnocellular neurosecretory system, but is considerably more dense over vasopressin regions. In agreement with this observation, Renaud et al. (1981) have provided electrophysiological evidence that stimulation of the subfornical organ most commonly excites phasically-firing (presumably vasopressin) cells in the SON. The pathway from the median preoptic nucleus, which receives an input from the subfornical organ (Miselis, 1981), also appears to reach both cell types, but its terminal distribution appears somewhat more uniform with respect to regions in which oxytocin- and vasopressin-neurones are located (Sawchenko and Swanson, 1983).

The subfornical organ is a richly vascularized circumventricular structure that lies outside the blood–brain barrier and is therefore well situated to monitor the concentration of substances in the blood, such as hormones and ions. It now seems likely that the subfornical organ contains receptors that mediate both the drinking and pressor responses to circulating angiotensin II (see Simpson, 1981, for a review). The projection from this region to the PVN and SON is, therefore, likely to play an important role in the integration of visceral responses that maintain fluid balance and blood pressure homeostasis.

PROJECTIONS TO OXYTOCIN CELL GROUPS

The best known stimulus for oxytocin release (in the female) is suckling, and until the function of oxytocin in the male is clarified, the milk ejection reflex will continue to provide the paradigm to study the sensory control of oxytocin secretion. Afferents from the mammary gland ascend in the spinal cord (Ingelbrecht, 1935), but the precise trajectories of relevant pathways, and their terminal distributions, remain poorly understood (see Cross and Dyball, 1974).

Studies of the afferent control of the PVN and SON that have utilized modern neuroanatomical techniques have provided few insights into what pathways relay primary afferent information from the spinal cord to magnocellular neurosecretory neurones. The only cell groups in the brainstem that have been shown to project to oxytocin parts of the PVN and SON are a number of serotonergic raphe nuclei.

Retrograde transport studies have suggested that cells in the dorsal and median raphe nuclei project to the PVN (Berk and Finkelstein, 1981; Tribollet and Dreifuss, 1981), and preliminary double-labelling studies (Sawchenko and Swanson, 1981c) with an antiserum against serotonin indicate that these neurones are primarily serotonergic and arise from the B7, B8 and B9 cell groups of Dahlström and Fuxe (1964). It was not possible to confirm (Loewy et al., 1981) that the ventral medullary (B1, B2, and B3) serotonergic cell groups also project to the PVN. These results must be viewed cautiously, however, because recent immunohistochemical studies (Steinbusch, 1981) have shown that the density of serotonergic varicosities in the neuropil surrounding the PVN and SON is greater than in the nuclei themselves, and markers injected in the region of the PVN may have been taken up primarily by nearby fibres-of-passage or terminals. Nevertheless, autoradiographic studies have shown light projections from the dorsal and median raphe nuclei to the PVN and SON in the rat (e.g. Azmitia and Segal, 1978; Moore et al., 1978).

A recent examination of the distribution of serotonin-immunoreactive varicosities in the PVN and SON (Sawchenko and Swanson, 1981c) indicates that the innervation of the magnocellular neurosecretory system is sparse, but is concentrated over regions containing oxytocin cell bodies. Based on their density alone, it would seem unlikely that serotonergic inputs are critically involved in the control of oxytocin secretion, a view that is supported by reports that microiontophoretic application of serotonin inconsistently affects (inhibits) the electrical activity of neurosecretory neurones (Barker et al., 1971; Moss et al., 1972).

Few other cell groups have been shown to project specifically to areas rich in oxytocin neurones (Fig. 3). A substantial projection to the PVN from a group of $ACTH_{1-39}$-stained neurones centred in the ventral part of the arcuate nucleus of the hypothalamus has been identified using the combined retrograde transport–immunofluorescence method, and while ACTH-stained varicosities in the PVN are concentrated in the parvocellular division of the nucleus, a clear and preferential input to oxytocin parts of the PVN and SON was identified (Sawchenko et al., 1982). ACTH has been shown to coexist with β-endorphin in single arcuate neurones (e.g. Bugnon et al., 1979), and thus β-endorphin and perhaps other pro-opiomelano-

24

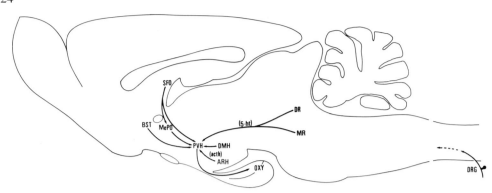

Fig. 3. A drawing to illustrate the organization of projections to oxytocin-containing parts of the magnocellular neurosecretory system. The best known peripheral stimulus for oxytocin (OXY) release is suckling, and sensory inputs from the mammary glands reach the spinal cord by way of the dorsal root ganglia (DRG). The course and terminal distribution of these pathways are poorly understood. A number of cell groups, located primarily in the forebrain, are now known to project to oxytocin-containing parts of the PVN (PVH in the figure) and the SON. What role, if any, these might play in the primary sensory control of oxytocin secretion remains to be determined. Other abbreviations: ARH, arcuate nucleus; BST, bed nucleus of the stria terminalis; DMH, dorsomedial nucleus of the hypothalamus; DR, dorsal raphe nucleus; MR, median raphe nucleus; 5-ht, serotonergic pathway; acth, $ACTH_{1-39}$-containing projection, and see Fig. 2.

cortin-derived peptides may be contained within the projections to magnocellular cell groups. The double-labelling experiments indicate that fewer than half of the retrogradely labelled neurones in the arcuate nucleus were also $ACTH_{1-39}$-positive, and this suggests that neurones in this region which contain other neuroactive substances, such as dopamine and acetylcholine (see Renaud, 1979, for a review), may also project to the PVN and SON. In view of the role of the arcuate nucleus in the control of anterior pituitary function, and of electrophysiological evidence indicating that some arcuate neurones project both to the median eminence and to the PVN (Renaud, 1979), this pathway is well situated to coordinate endocrine responses involving both the anterior and the posterior lobes of the pituitary.

Additional projections to oxytocin cell groups have been found to arise from the median preoptic nucleus, the subfornical organ (see above), and the dorsomedial nucleus of the hypothalamus (Sawchenko and Swanson, 1983). The functional importance of each of these is quite obscure. Finally, although we have emphasized that noradrenergic projections to the magnocellular neurosecretory system appear to mainly innervate the vasopressin cell groups, some DBH-stained varicosities are found within predominantly oxytocin parts of the PVN and SON (McNeill and Sladek, 1980; Swanson et al., 1981). As ventrally-directed dendrites of both oxytocin- and vasopressin-stained neurones aggregate along the ventral (pial) surface of the SON (Armstrong et al., 1982), a region replete with noradrenergic terminals, the distal dendrites of oxytocin cells in the PVN and SON may also receive an input from the A1 cell group.

LIMBIC REGION MODULATION OF NEUROSECRETORY NEURONS

There is little evidence for significant neocortical influences on oxytocin or vasopressin secretion. In contrast, it has been known for some time that the limbic region of the telencephalon can influence (generally by inhibition) the electrical activity of neurosecretory neurones (e.g. Pittman et al., 1981; Poulain et al., 1980), and hormone release (see Cross and

Dyball, 1974). Retrograde transport studies of the afferent connections of the PVN have found relatively large numbers of retrogradely labelled cells in parts of the septum, amygdala and hippocampal formation (specifically, the ventral part of the subiculum) (Berk and Finkelstein, 1981; Silverman et al., 1981; Tribollet and Dreifuss, 1981; Sawchenko and Swanson, 1983). These results, however, contrast sharply with autoradiographic studies of these regions, which have failed to document significant projections to either the PVN or the SON (Krettek and Price, 1978; Swanson and Cowan, 1977, 1979). We have re-examined much of this autoradiographic material and have found that while no inputs to either the PVN or the SON could be identified, projections from each of these regions either end in or traverse regions immediately adjacent to one or both magnocellular nuclei (Sawchenko and Swanson, 1983). For example, the ventral part of the subiculum projects heavily to the nucleus reuniens of the thalamus, and to (or through) the anterior hypothalamic area in a way that outlines (but does not end within) the morphological boundaries of the PVN. Fasciculated fibres from the ventral subiculum and caudal parts of the amygdala traverse the anterior parvocellular part of the PVN in the medial corticohypothalamic tract, however, and may give rise to synapses en passant in the PVN. Despite this possible exception it is clear that the amygdala, the septum and the hippocampal formation do not project in a substantial way to magnocellular cell groups. The results of the retrograde transport studies mentioned above are probably the result of uptake and transport of injected markers by nearby terminals, or by fibres-of-passage. How then, might limbic areas influence the PVN and SON?

The bed nucleus of the stria terminalis receives a massive input from the amygdala (Krettek and Price, 1978) and a smaller, but substantial, projection from the ventral subiculum (Swanson and Cowan, 1977). Autoradiographic experiments have shown that the bed nucleus projects heavily to all parts of the parvocellular division of the PVN, and moderately to the magnocellular division of the PVN and SON (Swanson and Cowan, 1977; Sawchenko and Swanson, 1983). Regions of the magnocellular system in which oxytocin cells predominate appear to be preferentially innervated. Thus, the bed nucleus of the stria terminalis provides a likely route through which information from the limbic system is funneled to reach the PVN and SON.

INTRANUCLEAR INTERACTIONS

As described above, only a handful of cell groups have been shown to project directly to the magnocellular neurosecretory system. However, retrograde transport studies (Berk and Finkelstein, 1981; Silverman et al., 1981; Tribollet and Dreifuss, 1981; Sawchenko and Swanson, 1982b, 1983) have suggested that many additional cell groups project to the PVN. A recent analysis of autoradiographic experiments has confirmed the existence of many of these projections and has shown that they end in various parts of the parvocellular division of the PVN (Sawchenko and Swanson, 1983). Among the structures that project primarily to the parvocellular division of the PVN are each recognized cell group (or area) in the hypothalamus and the preoptic region (with the exception of the SON, the mammillary nuclei and the magnocellular preoptic nucleus), the parabrachial nucleus, the locus coeruleus, and the nucleus of the solitary tract (Sawchenko and Swanson, 1981b, 1982b and c, 1983). A careful study of Golgi-impregnated neurones suggests that the axons of parvocellular neurones in the PVN ramify extensively in both the magnocellular and parvocellular parts of the nucleus (van den Pol, 1982). If this can be substantiated, it could broaden considerably the number of cell groups with the potential to influence the magnocellular neurones of the PVN.

It should be emphasized that, from a light microscopic analysis of autoradiographic material, we cannot exclude the possibility that the cell groups listed above may project, in a minor way, directly to magnocellular neurosecretory cell groups. Furthermore, while more massive pathways are likely to exert a greater influence on a target cell population, mounting evidence for labile ephaptic interactions between neurosecretory neurones (e.g. Andrew et al., 1981) suggests that under certain physiological conditions it may not be necessary to activate a large number of afferent fibres in order to influence the activity of entire clusters of neurosecretory neurones.

DISCUSSION AND CONCLUSIONS

The experimental results just described lead to several conclusions about the organization of central pathways that regulate the magnocellular neurosecretory system. First, while many cell groups project to the PVN, relatively few provide inputs that end in the magnocellular division, or in the SON, which does not contain a distinct parvocellular division. Pathways that do reach the magnocellular cell groups are summarized in Figs. 2 and 3. Second, with the possible exception of a projection from the median preoptic nucleus, inputs to the magnocellular neurosecretory system end preferentially, though not necessarily exclusively, in areas that are rich either in oxytocin- or in vasopressin-neurones. This is consistent with the view that secretion of the two hormones is largely independently controlled, although individual neurones may influence both cell types by way of axon collaterals or the diffusion of released neurotransmitter over relatively long distances through the extracellular fluid. Third, inputs that end in magnocellular cell groups display a similar distribution, with respect to regions in which oxytocin or vasopressin cells are concentrated, in both the SON and the magnocellular division of the PVN. This suggests that, regardless of their location within the hypothalamus, the magnocellular neurosecretory cells that produce oxytocin (or vasopressin) may be considered as a functional unit.

The major feature that distinguishes the PVN and SON is the association of an elaborately organized parvocellular division with the former, and recent evidence suggests that cells in the parvocellular division project to nearby magnocellular neurones (van den Pol, 1982). The most obvious functional role for such connections would be to integrate the activity of neurosecretory neurones in the PVN with the outputs of the parvocellular division that influence complementary neuroendocrine (by way of the anterior pituitary) and autonomic regulatory mechanisms. Clearly then, circuitry involved in the afferent control of hormone producing neurones in PVN is more complex than in the SON.

Even at the light microscopic level of analysis current knowledge of the origins of afferent projections to the magnocellular neurosecretory system is by no means complete. Projections from a number of cell groups to the PVN have been suggested on the basis of retrograde transport studies, and the relationship of projections from these regions to magnocellular cell groups await further analysis. The mesencephalic central grey is the most important example of this, as many functional studies suggest that it influences neurohypophysial hormone secretion (see Cross and Dyball, 1974).

A recent survey of the literature (Swanson and Sawchenko, 1983) indicates that over 30 possible neurotransmitters are found in the PVN and SON, and the functional significance of this diversity is only vaguely understood. Ten of these neuroactive substances have been described within cell bodies in the PVN, and there is now evidence that both oxytocin and corticotropin releasing factor are found in some magnocellular neurones, while vasopressin and dynorphin are found in others. Although the functional significance of the co-existence of peptides within neurosecretory neurones is not clear, it is tempting to speculate that inputs from different sources, which release different neuroactive substances, differentially affect the synthesis and (or) release of one or another of the peptides in a particular cell type in the PVN. Whether or not such mechanisms play a role in modulating the output of the PVN and SON, recent pharmacological studies indicate that multiple receptor subtypes for neuroactive substances exist and may mediate different responses (see Swanson and Sawchenko, 1983). Thus, it seems likely that new levels of complexity in the way in which the activity of the magnocellular neurosecretory system is controlled remain to be clarified.

ACKNOWLEDGEMENTS

The studies summarized here that were carried out in our laboratory were supported by Grant NS-16686 from the National Institutes of Health, a Grant-in-Aid from the American Heart Association — California Affiliate, and by the Clayton Foundation for Research-California Division. The authors are Clayton Foundation Investigators. We are grateful to Ms. Pat Thomas and Mr. Kris Trulock for assistance in the preparation of this manuscript.

REFERENCES

Andrew, R.D., MacVicar, B.A., Dudek, F.E. and Hatton, G.I. (1981) Dye transfer through gap junctions between neuroendocrine cells of rat hypothalamus. *Science*, 211: 1187–1189.

Armstrong, W.E., Schöler, J. and McNeill, T.H. (1982) Immunocytochemical, Golgi and electron microscopic characterization of putative dendrites in the ventral glial lamina of the rat supraoptic nucleus. *Neuroscience*, 7: 679–694.

Azmitia, E.C. and Segal, M. (1978) An autoradiographic analysis of the differential ascending projections of the dorsal and median raphe nuclei in the rat. *J. comp. Neurol.*, 179: 641–668.

Barker, J.L., Crayton, J.W. and Nicoll, R. (1971) Noradrenaline and acetylcholine responses of supra-optic neurosecretory cells. *J. Physiol. (Lond.)*, 218: 19–32.

Berk, M.L. and Finkelstein, J.A. (1981) Afferent projections to the preoptic area and hypothalamic regions in the rat brain. *Neuroscience*, 6: 1601–1624.

Blessing, W.W., Sved, A.F. and Reis, D.J. (1982) Destruction of noradrenergic neurons in rabbit brainstem elevates plasma vasopressin, causing hypertension. *Science*, 217: 661–663.

Bugnon, C., Bloch, B., Lenys, D., Gouget, A. and Fellman, D. (1979) Comparative study of the neuronal populations containing β-endorphin, corticotropin and dopamine in the arcuate nucleus of the rat hypothalamus. *Neurosci. Lett.*, 14: 43–48.

Carlsson, A., Falck, B. and Hillarp, N.-Å. (1962) Cellular localization of brain monoamines. *Acta physiol. scand.*, 56, Suppl. 196: 1–27.

Ciriello, J. and Calaresu, F.R. (1977) Lateral reticular nucleus: a site of somatic and cardiovascular integration in the cat. *Amer. J. Physiol.*, 233: R100–R109.

Cross, B.A. and Dyball, R.E.J. (1974) Central pathways for neurohypophysial hormone release. In *Handbook of Physiology*, Sect. 7, Vol. IV, American Physiological Society, Washington, DC, pp. 269–285.

Dahlström, A. and Fuxe, K. (1964) Evidence for the existence of monoamine-containing neurons in the central nervous system. I. Demonstration of monoamines in the cell bodies of brain stem neurons. *Acta physiol. scand.*, 62, suppl. 232: 1–80.

Harris, M.C. (1979) The effect of chemoreceptor and baroreceptor stimulation on the discharge of hypothalamic supraoptic neurones in rats. *J. Endocr.* 82: 115–125.

Hatton, G.I., Hutton, U.E., Hoblitzell, E.R. and Armstrong, W.E. (1976) Morphological evidence for two populations of magnocellular elements in the rat paraventricular nucleus. *Brain Res.*, 108: 187–193.

Ingelbrecht, P. (1935) Influence du système nerveux central sur la mammelle lactante chez le rat blanc. *C.R. Soc. Biol.*, 120: 1369–1371.

Jones, B.J. and Moore, R.Y. (1977) Ascending projections of the locus coeruleus in the rat. II. Autoradiographic study. *Brain Res.*, 127: 23–53.

28

Kelly, J. and Swanson, L.W. (1980) Additional forebrain regions projecting to the posterior pituitary: preoptic region, bed nucleus of the stria terminalis, and zona incerta. *Brain Res., 197*: 1–10.

Koizumi, K. and Yamashita, H. (1978) Influence of atrial stretch receptors on hypothalamic neurosecretory neurones. *J. Physiol. (Lond.), 285*: 341–358.

Krettek, J.E. and Price, J.L. (1978) Amygdaloid projections to subcortical structures within the basal forebrain and the brainstem in the rat and cat. *J. comp. Neurol., 178*: 255–280.

Loewy, A.D., Wallach, J.H. and McKellar, S. (1981) Efferent connections of the ventral medulla oblongata in the rat. *Brain Res. Rev., 3*: 63–80.

McKellar, S. and Loewy, A.D. (1981) Organization of some brain stem afferents to the paraventricular nucleus of the hypothalamus in the rat. *Brain Res., 217*: 351–357.

McNeill, T.H. and Sladek, J.R., Jr. (1980) Simultaneous monoamine histofluorescence and neuropeptide immunocytochemistry. II. Correlative distribution of catecholamine varicosities and magnocellular neurosecretory neurons in the rat supraoptic and paraventricular nuclei. *J. comp. Neurol., 193*: 1023–1033.

Miselis, R. (1981) The efferent projections of the subfornical organ of the rat: a circumventricular organ within a neural network subserving water balance. *Brain Res., 230*: 1–23.

Moore, R.Y., Halaris, A.E. and Jones, B.E. (1978) Serotonin neurons of the midbrain raphe: ascending projections. *J. comp. Neurol., 180*: 417–438.

Moss, R.L., Urban, I. and Cross, B.A. (1972) Microelectrophoresis of cholinergic and aminergic drugs on paraventricular neurons. *Amer. J. Physiol., 232*: 310–318.

Norgren, R. (1978) Projections from the nucleus of the solitary tract in the rat. *Neuroscience, 3*: 207–218.

Pittman, Q.J., Blume, H.W. and Renaud, L.P. (1981) Connections of the hypothalamic paraventricular nucleus with the neurohypophysis, median eminence amygdala, lateral septum and midbrain periaqueductal gray: an electrophysiological study in the rat. *Brain Res., 215*: 15–28.

Poulain, D.A., Ellendorf, F. and Vincent, J.D. (1980) Septal connections with identified oxytocin and vasopressin neurones of the rat. An electrophysiological investigation. *Neuroscience, 5*: 379–387.

Renaud, L.P. (1979) Neurophysiology and neuropharmacology of medial hypothalamic neurons and their extrahypothalamic connections. In P.J. Morgane and J. Panksepp (Eds.), *Handbook of the Hypothalamus, Vol. 1*, Dekker, New York, pp. 593–693.

Renaud, L.P., Arnauld, E., Cirino, M., Layton, B.S., Sgro, S. and Siatitsas, Y.W. (1981) Supraoptic neurosecretory neurons: modifications of excitabillity by electrical stimulation of limbic and subfornical organ afferents. *Soc. Neurosci. Abstr., 7*: 325.

Rhodes, C.H., Morrell, J.I. and Pfaff, D.W. (1981) Immunohistochemical analysis of magnocellular elements in rat hypothalamus: distribution and numbers of cells containing neurophysin, oxytocin, and vasopressin. *J. comp. Neurol., 198*: 45–64.

Ricardo, J.A. and Koh, E.T. (1978) Anatomical evidence of direct projections from the nucleus of the solitary tract to the hypothalamus, amygdala, and other forebrain structures in the rat. *Brain Res., 153*: 1–26.

Saper, C.B. and Loewy, A.D. (1980) Efferent connections of the parabrachial nucleus in the rat. *Brain Res., 197*: 291–317.

Sawchenko, P.E. and Swanson, L.W. (1981a) A method for tracing biochemically defined pathways in the central nervous system using combined fluorescence retrograde transport and immunohistochemical techniques. *Brain Res., 210*: 31–52.

Sawchenko, P.E. and Swanson, L.W. (1981b) Central noradrenergic pathways for the integration of hypothalamic neuroendocrine and autonomic responses. *Science, 214*: 685–687.

Sawchenko, P.E. and Swanson, L.W. (1981c) The distribution and cells of origin of some afferent projections to the paraventricular and supraoptic nuclei in the rat. *Soc. Neurosci. Abstr., 7*: 325.

Sawchenko, P.E. and Swanson, L.W. (1982a) Immunohistochemical identification of neurons in the paraventricular nucleus of the hypothalamus that project to the medulla or to the spinal cord in the rat. *J. comp. Neurol., 205*: 260–272.

Sawchenko, P.E. and Swanson, L.W. (1982b) The organization of noradrenergic pathways from the brainstem to the paraventricular and supraoptic nuclei in the rat. *Brain Res. Rev., 4*: 275–325.

Sawchenko, P.E. and Swanson, L.W. (1983) The organization of forebrain afferents to the paraventricular and supraoptic nuclei of the rat. *J. comp. Neurol.*, in press.

Sawchenko, P.E., Swanson, L.W. and Joseph, S.A. (1982) The distribution and cells of origin of ACTH(1−39)-stained varicosities in the paraventricular and supraoptic nuclei. *Brain Res., 232*: 365–374.

Sherlock, D.A., Field, P.M. and Raisman, G. (1975) Retrograde transport of horseradish peroxidase in the magnocellular neurosecretory system of the rat. *Brain Res., 88*: 403–414.

Silverman, A.J., Hoffman, D.L. and Zimmerman, E.A. (1981) The descending afferent connections of the paraventricular nucleus of the hypothalamus. *Brain Res. Bull., 6*: 47–61.

Simpson, J.B. (1981) The circumventricular organs and the central actions of angiotensin. *Neuroendocrinology, 33*: 248–256.

Steinbusch, H.W.M. (1981) Distribution of seotonin-immunoreactivity in the central nervous system of the rat — cell bodies and terminals. *Neuroscience,* 6: 557–618.

Swanson, L.W. and Cowan, W.M. (1977) An autoradiographic study of the organization of the efferent connections of the hippocampal formation in the rat. *J. comp. Neurol.,* 172: 49–84.

Swanson, L.W. and Cowan, W.M. (1979) The connections of the septal region in the rat. *J. comp. Neurol.,* 186: 621–656.

Swanson, L.W. and Kuypers, H.G.J.M. (1980) The paraventricular nucleus of the hypothalamus: cytoarchitectonic subdivisions and the organization of projections to the pituitary, dorsal vagal complex and spinal cord as demonstrated by retrograde fluorescence double-labeling methods. *J. comp. Neurol.,* 194: 555–570.

Swanson, L.W. and Sawchenko, P.E. (1983) Hypothalamic integration: organization of the paraventricular and supraoptic nuclei. *Ann. Rev. Neurosci.,* 6:269–324.

Swanson, L.W., Sawchenko, P.E., Berod, A., Hartman, B.K., Helle, K.B. and Van Orden, D.E. (1981) An immunohistochemical study of the organization of catecholaminergic cells and terminal fields in the paraventricular and supraoptic nuclei of the hypothalamus. *J. comp. Neurol.,* 196: 271–285.

Thomas, M.R., Ulrichsen, R.F. and Calaresu, F.R. (1977) Function of lateral reticular nucleus in central cardiovascular regulation in the cat. *Amer. J. Physiol.,* 232: H157–H166.

Tribollet, E. and Dreifuss, J.J. (1981) Localization of neurones projecting to the hypothalamic paraventricular nucleus area of the rat: a horseradish peroxidase study. *Neuroscience,* 6: 1315–1328.

Van den Pol, A.N. (1982) The magnocellular and parvocellular paraventricular nucleus of the rat; intrinsic organization. *J. comp. Neurol.,* 206: 317–345.

The Neurohypophysis: Structure, Function and Control, Progress in Brain Research, Vol. 60, edited by B.A. Cross and G. Leng

Combined Morphometric and Immunocytochemical Evidence That in the Paraventricular Nucleus of the Rat Oxytocin- but not Vasopressin-Neurones Respond to the Suckling Stimulus

J.A. RUSSELL

Department of Physiology, University Medical School, Edinburgh, EH8 9AG, Scotland (U.K.)

INTRODUCTION

The nuclear groups of magnocellular neurones that project to the posterior pituitary gland (Armstrong et al., 1980; Swanson and Kuypers, 1980) are a mixture of oxytocin (OXT)- and vasopressin (AVP)-containing neurones (Choy and Watkins, 1977); although other peptides, such as dynorphin and cholecystokinin, are present in some of these neurones (Vanderhaeghen et al., 1981; Watson et al., 1982) OXT and AVP are not found together in the same neurone (Vandesande and Dierickx, 1979). The proportions of OXT and AVP neurones vary between the nuclei, and more strikingly between their subdivisions, but none of the groups comprises only one type of peptidergic neurone (Choy and Watkins, 1977; Rhodes et al., 1981). Consequently it is not possible to study selectively the properties of OXT or AVP neurones using techniques in which only the location of the perikarya is identified. A range of techniques, from quantitative cytochemistry (Russell, 1980b) to electrophysiology (Poulain and Wakerley, 1982), has been used to compare the properties of neurones in the supraoptic nucleus (SON) with those in the paraventricular nucleus (PVN), and such studies have shown that neurones in these anatomically defined pools respond to the same stimuli.

Electrophysiological study of individual, antidromically identified neurones in the SON and PVN has revealed two major patterns of electrical activity in both nuclei; because only non-phasic neurones respond to the suckling stimulus they have been designated OXT-containing, and the phasic neurones AVP-containing (Dreifuss et al., 1981; Poulain and Wakerley, 1982). There is abundant evidence that OXT is secreted in response to suckling (Lincoln et al., 1973; Robinson et al., 1981) but the electrophysiological identification of OXT and AVP neurones depends crucially on whether only OXT and not AVP is secreted in response to suckling: this is difficult to establish. It has not been possible so far to identify with the immunocytochemical technique the peptide contained in mammalian neurones from which electrophysiological recordings are made in vivo.

An alternative approach is to measure morphological indicators of synthetic activity in neurones that have been identified immunocytochemically. This combination of techniques forms a tool to study the stimuli that activate pools of a particular type of neurone, given that a stimulus is sustained for long enough to lead to changes in protein synthesis. The nucleoli of neurosecretory neurones enlarge when they are stimulated in this way, indicating increased ribosome synthesis to provide more protein, some of which is secreted (Russell, 1980a). Nucleolar size was selected as an indicator of synthetic activity for the present study as it can be precisely measured and no additional preparation of tissue sections is required other than

[31]

immunocytochemistry to identify the type of neurone to be studied. Previously it has been shown with this combination of techniques that in the SON and PVN both OXT and AVP neurones respond to water deprivation (Russell, 1981, 1982a). In the present study the responses to the suckling stimulus of OXT and AVP neurones in the PVN were compared to answer the question of whether only OXT neurones and not AVP neurones respond.

METHODS

Animals

Rats that had suckled their young for nine days were compared with rats whose litters were removed at birth and thus had not received the suckling stimulus.

Twelve Sprague–Dawley rats were separated into two equal groups of similar body weight and range of litter size (14–18 pups). The litter size of the lactating rats was adjusted to ten pups within 24 h of birth; the litters of the non-suckled group were removed immediately after birth. The rats were killed on day 9 post partum (day 1 = day of parturition); the litters of the lactating group were weighed daily to check that lactation proceeded normally.

Procedures

Under ether anaesthesia blood was withdrawn by cardiac puncture for measurement of microhaematocrit and plasma osmolality (vapour pressure method, Wescor Inc. 5100B osmometer).

Histology

Each rat was perfused with 0.9% w/v saline via the left ventricle followed by Bouin's fluid for 15 min at 105 cm fluid pressure. The hypothalamus was removed, immersed in Bouin's fluid for 48 h followed by 70% ethyl alcohol for 48 h, dehydrated and embedded in paraffin wax below 60 °C. Serial transverse 7 μm sections were cut and mounted on gelatin-coated slides; every seventh section was mounted separately and stained with cresyl violet to locate appropriate regions of the PVN.

The anteroventromedial (medial) subnucleus of PVN comprises mainly OXT neurones, and the posterodorsolateral (lateral) subnucleus mainly AVP neurones, while the neurones in these two subnuclei project to the posterior pituitary gland (Armstrong et al., 1980; Swanson and Kuypers, 1980; Rhodes et al., 1981). Sections through the medial and lateral subnuclei were selected for immunocytochemical identification of OXT and AVP neurones respectively (Fig. 1).

Immunocytochemistry

OXT- and AVP-containing neurones were identified with the PAP technique described by Sternberger (1979) with minor modifications. The steps were as follows: (1) sections were dewaxed and incubated for 30 min with methanol containing 1% hydrogen peroxide (100 vol%) to inactivate endogenous peroxidase; (2) immersion for 30 min in phosphate-buffered saline (pH 7.35) containing 5% normal swine serum to block non-specific reactions — this buffer was used throughout except in step 5; (3) incubation with either purified anti-OXT serum or purified anti-AVP scrum, diluted 1:200, at 4 °C in a wet chamber for 20 h then at room temperature for 2 h — 3 drops of antiserum were placed on each section and 3 sections per slide were used; (4) incubation for 30 min with swine anti-rabbit immunoglobulin, diluted

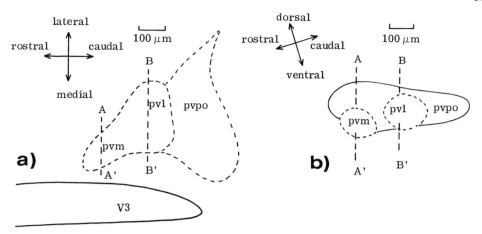

Fig. 1. Schematic drawings of sections through rat PVN to show subnuclei. a: horizontal section; b: sagittal section (after Armstrong et al., 1980; Swanson and Kuypers, 1980). pvm, anteroventromedial (medial) subnucleus; pvl, posterodorsolateral (lateral) subnucleus; pvpo, posterior subnucleus; V3, third ventricle; A, A' and B, B', planes of sections for immunocytochemical identification of OXT- and AVP-containing neurones, respectively

1:30 (Dako Products); (5) incubation for 30 min with rabbit PAP, diluted 1:100 (Dako Products); (6) incubation for 15 min at room temperature with diaminobenzidine hydrochloride (BDH Lot 1770600, 4 mg/ml Tris buffer, pH 7.6, with 2 drops 30 vol% hydrogen peroxide); (7) dehydration and mounting beneath a cover slip in Synthetic Neutral Mountant (n 1.515, GBI Labs. Ltd.) to give optimal contrast for phase contrast microscopy. Sections were washed with buffer between each step, except that distilled water was used after step 6.

Purification of antiserum. Both primary antisera were raised in rabbits. The use of the anti-AVP serum in immunocytochemistry has been described previously (Dierickx, 1980). The anti-OXT serum (IR-6) cross-reacts < 0.01 % with AVP in radioimmunoassay (I.C.A.F. Robinson, personal communication). To remove antibodies cross-reacting with OXT or AVP from the appropriate antiserum each antiserum was incubated with Sepharose 4-B beads covalently bound to either OXT or AVP. Samples of beads from each 25 mg lot were taken after sequential incubation with a 25 μl aliquot of antiserum and processed on slides with the PAP procedure (steps 4–6), purification was continued until a sample of beads failed to react with PAP (Swaab and Pool, 1975).

Specificity. Absorption of cross-reacting antibodies prior to incubation with tissue sections ensured that the anti-OXT serum did not react with AVP-containing neurones and that the anti-AVP serum did not react with OXT-containing neurones. Further specificity tests were used as follows: (1) omission of any of the steps 3–6 in the immunocytochemical procedure prevented staining of neurones; (2) absorption of anti-AVP serum with AVP bound to Sepharose 4-B beads and of anti-OXT serum with OXT bound to Sepharose 4-B beads prevented staining; (3) purified anti-AVP serum did not react with Sepharose 4-B beads bound to OXT and purified anti-OXT serum did not react with Sepharose 4-B beads bound to AVP when these beads were included, stuck to slides, in the immunocytochemical procedure (Swaab and Pool, 1975); (4) purified anti-AVP serum and purified anti-OXT serum reacted with neurones in different areas of the subnuclei of the PVN when used on adjacent sections; (5) purified anti-AVP serum did not react with neurones in the lateral subnucleus of the PVN of a homozygous Brattleboro rat, but purified anti-OXT serum reacted with neurones in the medial subnucleus of the PVN of this rat.

Microscopy

Sections were analyzed with a Vickers M17 microscope fitted with a green filter, a Microplan oil immersion phase contrast objective, magnification $100 \times$, numerical aperture 1.25, eyepiece magnification $10 \times$, additional magnification $1.6 \times$.

An OXT- or AVP-containing neurone was identified according to the following criteria: (1) brown reaction product was visible over the cytoplasm around a neuronal nucleus in the same focal plane; (2) brown colour was readily discerned from background in both positive phase contrast and normal transmitted illumination; (3) some neurones in the same subnucleus showed no colouration.

Measurement of nucleolar diameter. The image shearing method was used in which two images of the object are produced by moveable prisms; the images are then moved across one another from edge to edge by rotating the prisms and the displacement of the prisms is recorded (Dyson, 1960). A Vickers Instruments strain gauge image shearing device was fitted beneath the viewing head of the microscope and coupled to an electronic direct dimensional readout unit, calibrated at $10 \mu m$ against a stage micrometer. This is the most precise method of measuring linear dimensions of microscopic objects available; the theoretical setting accuracy of the shearing device is better than $0.02 \mu m$ and in practice measurements can be made with S.D. $\pm 0.009 \mu m$ (Dyson, 1960; Swyt and Rosberry, 1977).

Duplicate measurements were made for each nucleolus; if these differed by more than 2% the measurements were repeated. Measurements were made on the nucleoli of all immunocytochemically identified neurones in a section of the right or left PVN; if there were fewer than 20 neurones measurements were made on all the neurones in the contralateral PVN or in the next-but-one section.

Some neurones had two nucleoli; the diameter of each of these nucleoli (d_1, d_2) was measured and the diameter (deq) of a nucleolus of the same total volume was calculated from

$$deq = 2 \cdot \sqrt[3]{\frac{d_1^3 + d_2^3}{8}}$$

RESULTS

The nucleoli of OXT neurones in the medial subnucleus of the PVN were significantly larger in lactating rats than in post-partum rats deprived of their pups since birth with respect to both mean (Fig. 2a) and median values; the median nucleolar diameter of OXT neurones from lactating rats was $2.59 \mu m$, 99% confidence limits 2.51, 2.65 μm and for non-suckled rats 2.33 μm, 99% confidence limits 2.26, 2.39 μm.

In contrast, for nucleolar diameter of AVP neurones in the lateral subnucleus of the PVN there were no significant differences between lactating and non-suckled rats when either mean (Fig. 2b) or median values were compared; the median nucleolar diameter of AVP neurones from lactating rats was $2.48 \mu m$, 95% confidence limits 2.43, 2.54 μm and for non-suckled rats 2.40 μm, 95% confidence limits 2.35, 2.46 μm.

The proportion of nuclei with double nucleoli was similar in both groups: for OXT neurones the proportion was 1.5% in the non-suckled group and 1.1% in the lactating group; for AVP neurones the proportions were 1.6% and 1.7% respectively.

Microhaematocrit was significantly less in the lactating group; for lactating rats mean haematocrit $\pm$ S.E.M. was $41.1 \pm 1.36\%$, and for non-suckled rats $44.7 \pm 0.61\%$, $P < 0.05$ (Student's *t*-test).

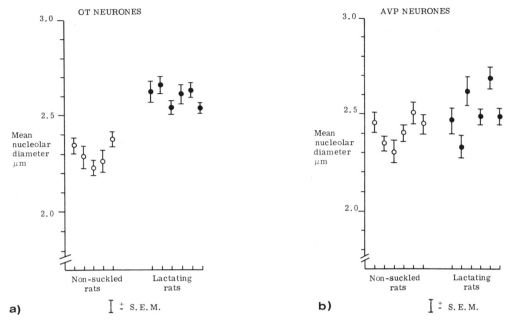

Fig. 2. Diameters of nucleoli from immunocytochemically identified neurones in the PVN of lactating and non-suc-kled rats. a: OXT (OT) neurones from the medial subnucleus. b: AVP neurones from the lateral subnucleus. Each point is the mean for 22–41 neurones per rat. Statistical comparisons (Student's t test, using group means based on animal means, $°F$ = number of animals − 1): lactating vs non-suckled, for OXT neurones $P < 0.001$, for AVP neurones $0.1 < P < 0.2$.

Plasma osmolality was not significantly different between the two groups; for lactating rats the mean ± S.E.M. was 291 ± 5.5 mOsm/kg and for non-suckled rats 289 ± 1.5 mOsm/kg.

DISCUSSION

Because cross-reacting antibodies in the primary antisera were specifically removed before use in the immunocytochemical procedures, and from the results of the specificity tests carried out, it can be stated that the anti-OXT serum demonstrated neurones containing OXT or a similar peptide other than AVP, and the anti-AVP serum similarly reacted with AVP neurones but not OXT neurones (Swaab et al., 1977). The relationship of increase in nucleolar size in neurosecretory neurones to increased synthetic and secretory activity has been discussed previously (Russell, 1980a, b); nucleolar enlargement indicates increased protein synthesis with or without increased peptide secretion.

The use of post-partum rats without litters as the control group ensured that the nucleolar changes measured in the lactating rats were not due to effects of the hormones of pregnancy, or to increased secretion of OXT or AVP during parturition (Russell, 1980a, 1982b) but must have been due to the suckling stimulus or the process of lactation. The possibility that increased secretion by OXT or AVP neurones during lactation might result from hypovolaemic or hyperosmotic stimuli arising from milk secretion seems unlikely as plasma osmolality was similar in the two groups of animals, as found previously (Russell, 1980b), and haematocrit was lower in the lactating group indicating increased blood volume; there was, anyway, no evidence that AVP neurones in the lateral subnucleus of the PVN were stimulated in the lactating rats. So the principal conclusion from the present study is that suckling stimulates synthetic activity in OXT neurones in the medial subnucleus of the PVN but does not stimulate AVP neurones in the lateral subnucleus. Nucleolar enlargement in OXT neurones reflects increased synthesis and secretion of OXT and neurophysin in lactation (Norström and Sjö-strand, 1972; Lincoln et al., 1973); in the absence of nucleolar changes it is unlikely that AVP secretion by neurones in the lateral subnucleus is increased in lactation. These findings contrast with the effects of water deprivation for five days which results in nucleolar enlargement in both OXT and AVP neurones in, respectively, the medial and lateral subnuclei of the PVN (Russell, 1981), accompanied by increased secretion of both hormones (Dogterom et al., 1977).

The results of the present study substantiate the premise of electrophysiological studies, that suckling selectively activates OXT neurones, while the previous studies of the effects of water deprivation on nucleolar size concur with the conclusion from electrophysiological investigations that both OXT and AVP neurones in the PVN are activated by hyperosmotic and hypovolaemic stimuli (Poulain and Wakerley, 1982). A simple model of the distribution of inputs to OXT and AVP neurones in the PVN is proposed (Fig. 3); it remains to be established whether this model applies to other magnocellular nuclei.

The combination of nucleolar size measurement and immunocytochemistry should be applicable to the study of the inputs that stimulate other types of peptidergic neurone.

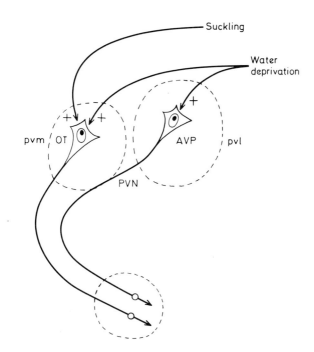

Fig. 3. Diagram of proposed distribution of stimuli that increase synthetic activity in OXT and AVP neurones in the PVN. OT, OXT-containing neurone; AVP, AVP-containing neurone; +, stimulatory input; other abbreviations as in Fig. 1.

SUMMARY

A method is described for measurement of nucleolar size by the image-shearing technique in immunocytochemically identified oxytocin- and vasopressin-containing neurones. Measurements were made on neurones in sections through the medial and lateral subnuclei of the paraventricular nucleus of 9-day lactating rats and a control group of post-partum rats deprived of their litters since birth. The nucleoli of oxytocin neurones but not vasopressin neurones were significantly enlarged in the lactating rats. It is concluded that the suckling stimulus activates oxytocin neurones but not vasopressin neurones in the paraventricular nucleus.

ACKNOWLEDGEMENTS

This work was supported by a grant from the Scottish Home and Health Department. Professor K. Dierickx and Dr. I.C.A.F. Robinson provided primary antisera and Dr. S. Gardner gave Brattleboro rat tissue. Technical assistance with histological procedures was given by Mrs. K. Johnston.

REFERENCES

Armstrong, W.E., Warach, S., Hatton, G.I. and McNeill, T.H. (1980) Subnuclei in the rat hypothalamic paraventricular nucleus: a cytoarchitectural, horseradish peroxidase and immunocytochemical analysis. *Neuroscience*, 5: 1931–1958.

Choy, V.J. and Watkins, W.B. (1977) Immunocytochemical study of the hypothalamo-neurohypophysial system. II. Distribution of neurophysin, vasopressin and oxytocin in the normal and osmotically stimulated rat. *Cell Tiss. Res.*, 180: 467–490.

Dierickx, K. (1980) Immunocytochemical localization of the vertebrate cyclic nonapeptide neurohypophyseal hormones and neurophysins. *Int. Rev. Cytol.*, 62: 119–185.

Dogterom, J., Van Rheenen-Verberg, C.M.F., Van Wimersma Greidanus, Tj.B. and Swaab, D.F. (1977) Vasopressin and oxytocin in cerebrospinal fluid of rats. *J. Endocr.*, 72: 74P–75P.

Dreifuss, J.J., Tribollet, E. and Mühlethaler, M. (1981) Temporal patterns of neural activity and their relation to the secretion of posterior pituitary hormones. *Biol. Reprod.*, 24: 51–72.

Dyson, J. (1960) Precise measurement by image-splitting. *J. opt. Soc. Amer.*, 50: 754–757.

Lincoln, D.W., Hill, A. and Wakerley, J.B. (1973) The milk ejection reflex of the rat: an intermittent function not abolished by surgical levels of anaesthesia. *J. Endocr.*, 57: 459–476.

Norström, A. and Sjöstrand, J. (1972) Effect of suckling and parturition on axonal transport and turnover of neurohypophysial proteins of the rat. *J. Endocr.*, 52: 107–117.

Poulain, D.A. and Wakerley, J.B. (1982) Electrophysiology of hypothalamic magnocellular neurones secreting oxytocin and vasopressin. *Neuroscience*, 7: 773–808.

Rhodes, C.H., Morrell, J.I. and Pfaff, D.W. (1981) Immunohistochemical analysis of magnocellular elements in rat hypothalamus: distribution and numbers of cells containing neurophysin, oxytocin and vasopressin. *J. comp. Neurol.*, 198: 45–64.

Robinson, I.C.A.F., Woolf, C.N. and Parsons, J.A. (1981) Suckling in the guinea-pig: the simultaneous release of oxytocin and neurophysin. *J. Endocr.*, 90: 227–236.

Russell, J.A. (1980a) Changes in nucleolar dry mass of neurones of the paraventricular and supraoptic nuclei in the rat during pregnancy and lactation. *Cell Tiss. Res.*, 208: 313–325.

Russell, J.A. (1980b) Water deprivation in lactating rats: changes in nucleolar dry mass of paraventricular and supraoptic neurones. *Cell Tiss. Res.*, 212: 315–331.

Russell, J.A. (1981) Synthetic responses of immunocytochemically identified oxytocin- and vasopressin-containing neurones of the paraventricular nucleus to water deprivation in the rat. *Acta endocr.*, Suppl., 243: 319.

Russell, J.A. (1982a) Synthetic activity in immunocytochemically identified neurons of the supraoptic nucleus during water deprivation in the rat. In D.S. Farner and K. Lederis (Eds.), *Neurosecretion: Molecules, Cells, Systems*. Plenum Press, New York, pp. 485–486.

Russell, J.A. (1982b) A study to compare the influence of suckling and hormones on nucleolar activity of supraoptic and paraventricular neurones of lactating rats. *Neuroendocrinology*, 35: 22–27.

Sternberger, L.A. (1979) *Immunocytochemistry*, 2nd edn., Wiley, New York, pp. 104–129.

Swaab, D.F. and Pool, C.W. (1975) Specificity of oxytocin and vasopressin immunofluorescence. *J. Endocr.*, 66: 263–275.

Swaab, D.F., Pool, C.W. and Van Leeuwen, F.W. (1977) Can specificity ever be proved in immunocytochemical staining? *J. Histochem. Cytochem.*, 25: 388–391.

Swanson, L.W. and Kuypers, H.G.J.M. (1980) The paraventricular nucleus of the hypothalamus: cytoarchitectonic subdivisions and organization of projections to the pituitary, dorsal vagal complex and spinal cord as demonstrated by retrograde fluorescence double-labeling methods. *J. comp. Neurol.*, 194: 555–570.

Swyt, D.A. and Rosberry, F.W. (1977) A comparison of some optical microscope measurements of photomask linewidths. *Solid State Technol.* August: 70–75.

Vanderhaegen, J.J. Lotstra, F., Vandesande, F. and Dierickx, K. (1981) Coexistence of cholecystokinin and oxytocin-neurophysin in some magnocellular hypothalamo-hypophyseal neurons. *Cell Tiss. Res.*, 221: 227–231.

Vandesande, F. and Dierickx, K. (1979) The activated hypothalamic magnocellular neurosecretory system and the one neuron–one neurohypophysial hormone concept. *Cell Tiss. Res.*, 200: 29–33.

Watson, S.J., Akil, H., Fischli, W., Goldstein, A., Zimmerman, E., Nilaver, G. and Van Wimersma Greidanus, Tj.B. (1982) Dynorphin and vasopressin: common localization in magnocellular neurons. *Science*, 216: 85–87.

The Neurohypophysis: Structure, Function and Control, Progress in Brain Research, Vol. 60, edited by B.A. Cross and G. Leng
© *1983 Elsevier Science Publishers B.V.*

Electrophysiology of the Afferent Input to Oxytocin- and Vasopressin-Secreting Neurones. Facts and Problems

D.A. POULAIN

Unité de Recherches de Neurobiologie des Comportements, I.N.S.E.R.M. U 176, Rue Camille Saint-Saens, 33077 Bordeaux Cedex (France)

INTRODUCTION

One of the main contributions of electrophysiology to the study of the hypothalamo-neurohypophysial systems has been to establish that hormone release is due to the electrical activity of magnocellular neurones. From an electrophysiological standpoint, then, to control hormone release is to control the electrical activity of the neurosecretory cells. It should be possible to determine how a stimulus which influences hormone release is transformed into a nervous signal, then processed at each synaptic relay so that it can modify the electrical activity of a neurosecretory cell.

The uncertainties about the neuroanatomical organization of the afferent pathways, and our lack of knowledge of many of the physiological aspects of hormone release, have motivated the use of widely differing electrophysiological approaches, and resulted in a bulk of observations at times difficult to reconcile. An exhaustive survey of the literature on this subject is beyond the scope of this paper (see also Cross and Dyball, 1974; Hayward, 1977). Nevertheless, from recent electrophysiological studies it has become clear that oxytocin- and vasopressin-secreting neurones show a complex organization of their electrical activity, both at the level of the individual neurone, and at the level of the whole neuronal population (see Poulain and Wakerley, 1982). In this chapter the afferent pathways will be considered from the point of view of the magnocellular neurone itself. We will raise questions concerning the mechanisms underlying each particular pattern of electrical activity, and discuss the relevance to these questions of the available electrophysiological information on the function of the afferent pathways.

AFFERENT CONTROL OF OXYTOCIN NEURONES

The electrical activity of oxytocin neurones during suckling-induced milk ejection offers the most dramatic example of a neuronal organization adapted to producing a pulsatile release of hormone. However, the activity of oxytocin neurones under other circumstances, during which hormone release is more graded, albeit enhanced, is completely different. Therefore the patterns of electrical activity of oxytocin neurones may depend largely on the organization of the afferent input, rather than on intrinsic properties of the neurones.

[39]

Suckling and the milk ejection reflex

In the lactating rat milk ejections occur intermittently and are induced by a pulsatile release of 0.5–1 mU oxytocin following a brief and synchronous activation of all the oxytocin neurones (Wakerley and Lincoln, 1973; Lincoln and Wakerley, 1974). The activation typically consists of a high frequency discharge of 70–80 action potentials lasting 3–4 sec. The functional organization of the pathways intervening in the milk ejection reflex is poorly understood. An excitatory input, provided by suckling, is necessary for the reflex, but the intermittent nature of the reflex suggests the participation of specific inhibitory mechanisms, the site and the nature of which are unknown.

Excitatory input

The pulsatile release of oxytocin does not appear to be exclusive to the rat. Recordings of intramammary pressure during reflex milk ejection show similar variations in the pig (Poulain et al., 1981b; Ellendorff et al., 1982). Moreover, electrical stimulation of the neurohypophysis, with parameters close to the high frequency discharge of oxytocin cells (i.e. 50 Hz, 5 sec) cause milk ejections similar to reflex milk ejections, in the rat, rabbit and pig (Harris et al., 1969; Wakerley and Lincoln, 1973; Ellendorff et al., 1982). It is therefore possible that the same intense neuronal activation underlies the release of hormone in other species. How the afferent pathway controls such a brief and intense activation of oxytocin cells remains to be established.

During suckling, afferent impulses from the nipples reach the spinal cord segmentally. Lesions of the lateral funiculi in the rat impair suckling induced milk ejections (Eayrs and Baddeley, 1956). Recently, we have seen that electrical stimulation of the lateral funiculi at 10–20 Hz for 15 sec can produce milk ejections similar to the natural ones. This is due to the release of oxytocin, since lesions of the neurohypophysis prevent the milk ejection caused by spinal cord stimulation (Dyer and Poulain, 1983). In the ewe, the dorsal tracts seem necessary for the milk ejection reflex, although their section does not interrupt the increased multiunit activity recorded in the hypothalamo-neurohypophysial tract in response to mammary gland stimulation (Richard, 1970; Richard et al., 1970).

The lateral tegmentum is also necessary for the reflex. Lesions of the lateral tegmentum have shown that the afferent pathway, at this level, is already crossed (Juss and Wakerley, 1981). Stimulation of the afferent pathway at this level induces milk ejections. However, repeated stimulation does not produce reproducible results (Tindal et al., 1967, 1968; Tindal and Knaggs, 1975). This may syggest that the pathway has a refractory period, which could be related to the intermittent nature of the reflex.

The morphological organization of the neurones of the magnocellular nuclei may facilitate the synchronous activation of the cells. In the lactating rat, the supraoptic nucleus possesses extensive neuronal surface membrane appositions and multiple synaptic contacts (one presynaptic element contacting two postsynaptic elements simultaneously) (Theodosis et al., 1981b; Hatton and Tweedle, 1982). In addition, gap junctions may exist between neurosecretory elements (Andrew et al., 1981; Mason, 1982). Whether electrical interaction of an ephaptic nature or direct electrotonic coupling (see Bennett, 1976) occurs between the oxytocin neurones awaits electrophysiological demonstration.

Iontophoretic studies have attempted to investigate the neurotransmitters involved, but the results so far obtained could apply to vasopressin neurones as well as to oxytocin neurones. Acetylcholine, which stimulates oxytocin release (Moos and Richard, 1975a; Yokoyama and Oba, 1971; Clarke et al., 1978), has excitatory effects (nicotinic) on the magnocellular neurones (Moss et al., 1971, 1972b; Dreifuss and Kelly, 1972). Dopamine, also excitatory for the reflex (Clarke et al., 1979a; Moos and Richard, 1979), activates about half of the neurosecretory cells (Moss et al., 1972a). It is also possible that oxytocin itself is a positive feed-back agent. Although oxytocin has no effect when injected systemically (Lincoln, 1974), when injected intraventricularly it enhances the firing rate within the high frequency discharges and reduces the delay between successive milk ejections (Freund-Mercier and Richard, 1981). The site of action of oxytocin thus injected remains to be established, but may be the secretory neurones themselves as iontophoretic applications of oxytocin increase the electrical activity of these neurones (Moss et al., 1972b).

Inhibitory pathways

In the rat, the intermittent character of milk ejections is particularly obvious because the young remain attached to the nipples through several successive milk ejections. A gating mechanism could therefore exist preventing a permanent excitatory input from reaching the neurosecretory cells, which, between two milk ejections, have an electrical activity similar to that seen in unsuckled animals. However, there is evidence in other species that milk ejections cannot occur repetitively without a delay. In the pig, suckling lasts for short periods (5–15 min), and the young are away from the sow for about 45–60 min after each suckling period. However, it takes 1–3 min from the onset of suckling to milk ejection, a delay much longer than the nervous transmission of impulses would suggest. Moreover, although the piglets may go on suckling for 5–10 min after the milk ejection, there is only one milk ejection per suckling episode. If the young suckle too soon after a milk ejection, no milk ejection occurs (Ellendorff et al., 1982). The intermittent nature of the reflex therefore seems to be the result of, first, a rather long period during which incoming stimuli are "summed up" before the activation of the cells occurs, and then, a refractory period after the activation.

A distinction should probably be made between those inhibitory mechanisms directly implicated in the functional organization of the reflex, and those intervening indirectly. Very little can be said about the direct mechanisms. Is the refractory period inherent to the mechanism (structure) that integrates the incoming stimuli, or is it the result of other structures that intervene as soon as the volley of excitatory input has been transmitted?
The only certain information we have is that there is no simple feed-back loop from the oxytocin cells themselves via a recurrent pathway: imposing extraneous activation on the cells by antidromic stimulation does not alter the rhythm of milk ejection (Wakerley and Deverson, 1975).

Under certain circumstances, such as stress or emotions, the milk ejection reflex can be inhibited through central mechanisms (Cross, 1955). As these circumstances are rather exceptional, the inhibitory pathways involved may not be an essential part of the functional organization of the reflex. In experiments to study the role of the septum on the milk ejection reflex, we have shown electrophysiologically that a number of septal neurones project directly to the supraoptic nucleus (SON), and that electrical stimulation of the septum inhibits the electrical activity of identified oxytocin cells (Poulain et al., 1980, 1981a). Massive septal lesions do not disrupt the reflex. Electrical stimulation of the septum at 5 Hz or more significantly increases the delay between milk ejections or, if prolonged, can interrupt the reflex altogether (Lebrun et al., 1983). These observations suggest that certain structures, such as the septum, although not essential to the reflex may inhibit the afferent pathway. In the case of the septum, this action could be related to the inhibition of the reflex by emotional disturbances.

If such inhibitory structures exist, then they should be inhibited at the time of milk ejection.

This may explain the importance of the state of vigilance at milk ejection. Sleep is probably not a prerequisite for the milk ejection reflex in general, for, although rats show an EEG pattern of slow-wave sleep at milk ejection (Voloschin and Tramezzani, 1979; Lincoln et al., 1980), behavioural observations suggest that this reflects a state of relaxation rather than sleep. In other species (rabbit: Neve et al., 1982; pig: Poulain et al., 1981b), the lactating mother shows cortical arousal, yet the animal is in a state of relaxation. In other words, it seems that only wakefulness associated with attention, noxious or emotional disturbances is inhibitory. It remains to be seen whether arousal inhibits the reflex, or is caused by the same factors that inhibit the reflex.

A very interesting suggestion has been made that a control occurs on the efferent side of the oxytocin system, by a presynaptic-like inhibition exerted at the level of the terminals (Clarke et al., 1979b; Moos and Richard, 1980). This contention is based upon the fact that oxytocin cells still display their high frequency discharges in response to suckling, while oxytocin release from the terminals is blocked by opioids or by β-adrenergic agonists (see Pittman et al., and Bicknell and Leng, this volume).

Parturition and related stimuli

Whether the release of oxytocin during labour is necessary for the onset of labour and for delivery of the conceptuses, or only a consequence of cervical and vaginal dilatation (Ferguson's reflex) is still a matter of controversy. In the non-anaesthetized rat, forceful abdominal contractions at parturition are followed by a brisk activation of magnocellular neurones. A few seconds before delivery of the foetuses, the same neurones also show high frequency discharges, which resemble those seen at milk ejection in the same neurones once the newborn start suckling (Summerlee, 1981). These observations suggest that oxytocin may be released both in response to cervical dilatation and, by another mechanism, to facilitate delivery.

In the case of Ferguson's reflex, the activation of receptors by vaginal distension causes a brisk acceleration of magnocellular neurones (Dreifuss et al., 1976b). The afferent pathway has been investigated to some extent in the sheep. Unlike the pathway for milk ejection, it seems that the dorsal columns are not necessary. Moreover, noradrenaline may intervene as an excitatory transmitter both through α and β receptors, whereas for the milk ejection pathway the beta component seems to be exclusively inhibitory (Richard, 1970; Richard et al., 1970; Moos and Richard, 1975a, b). The electrophysiological evidence suggests that the afferent pathway also influences vasopressin neurones. During parturition and vaginal distension, a number of neurones that did not subsequently react at milk ejection, or that were phasically firing (a mode of firing peculiar to vasopressin cells), were activated. However, this should not be surprising in view of the fact that cardiovascular changes are elicited by vaginal distension.

As to the excitation of the neurones before delivery, this seems to be an exclusive property of oxytocin cells (Summerlee, 1981). Whether the release of oxytocin in this case is a reflex response, or the result of more complex mechanisms intervening in parturition is not known.

In addition to the period of brisk activation at parturition, there is a more gradual increase in the general level of activity of the cells, first during gestation (Negoro, 1973a, b), and then a few minutes before parturition starts (Summerlee, 1981). It is therefore possible, that oxytocin is released not only in pulses at certain times of parturition, but also in a permanent, trickle-like manner. A sustained firing rate of 3–6 Hz should be sufficient for hormone release since long-term electrical stimulation of the neurohypophysis at 6 Hz does indeed release oxytocin (Boer et al., 1980).

Cardiovascular regulation and osmoregulation

Electrophysiological studies of the magnocellular neurones during cardiovascular and osmotic stimulation have shown that stimuli capable of releasing vasopressin also excite oxytocin cells identified by their high frequency discharges at milk ejection. The activation differs greatly from that observed at milk ejection, in that it consists of a gradual and sustained increase in the background activity. Such an activation has been reported during acute stimulation by haemorrhage or i.p. injection of hypertonic solutions, as well as during progressive dehydration, and corresponds to an increase in blood concentration of oxytocin (Poulain et al., 1977; Brimble and Dyball, 1977; Brimble et al., 1978; Wakerley et al., 1978). The activation of oxytocin cells by such stimuli cannot be discarded as a mere experimental artefact. Although haemorrhage may be an unphysiological stimulus, dehydration, up to a certain degree, is not an unlikely situation. The release of oxytocin under such conditions raises the question of a mutually synergistic or complementary role of the two populations of magnocellular neurones in the regulation of salt and water balance (Balment et al., 1980).

Do oxytocin cells receive afferents specifically implicated in such regulations, in addition to those implicated in milk ejection? Also, is the release of oxytocin due to the fact that the afferent input to the vasopressin neurones is distributed to the oxytocin cells as well? Experiments on the influence of peripheral cardiovascular receptors on the activity of vasopressin neurones point to a possible involvement of the oxytocin system. None of these experiments have been done on cells identified as vasopressin or oxytocin cells, so interpretation is difficult. However, insofar as a slow irregular pattern of firing is likely to identify oxytocin cells, stimulation of carotid receptors seems to affect a number of putative oxytocin cells (see section on vasopressin neurones).

AFFERENT CONTROL OF VASOPRESSIN NEURONES

A major physiological function of vasopressin is to control salt and water balance. We will therefore consider mainly the afferent input intervening in cardiovascular regulation and in osmoreception. The various patterns of electrical activity displayed by vasopressin neurones, under most experimental situations, will first be described briefly.

Patterns of electrical activity

Vasopressin neurones display three types of electrical activity: slow irregular activity, where action potentials occur occasionally, with a mean firing rate < 2.5 Hz; fast continuous activity, where the mean firing rate is > 2.5 Hz; and phasic activity, characterized by periodic bursts of action potentials, followed by periods of quiescence. The mean burst duration, and silence durations are usually between 5 and 25 sec but their range is quite wide (4–200 sec). The firing rates within the burst are between 4–15 Hz. The essential feature to emerge from recent electrophysiological studies is that the three patterns can occur within the same neurone, and depend on the functional state of activity of the cell (Brimble and Dyball, 1977; Poulain et al., 1977). Vasopressin neurones can thus be characterized by their lack of response to suckling, and their ability to evolve, under certain conditions, a phasic pattern of action potentials during stimulation of vasopressin release.

Two remarks

Although the phasic pattern can be considered as specific, among magnocellular cells, to the vasopressin neurones, it should nevertheless be kept in mind that: (1) under normal conditions most vasopressin neurones display a slow irregular pattern that is indistinguishable from the slow irregular activity seen in oxytocin cells, and (2) under stimulation, the recruitment of cells into phasic activity is progressive, i.e. for a given level of stimulation, not all of the cells are phasically firing (see Wakerley et al., 1978). Thus, although it seems reasonable to assume that phasic cells secrete vasopressin, it is not reasonable to assume that all non-phasic cells secrete oxytocin. At the moment, the only way to discriminate electrophysiologically between the two cell types is to study their reaction to suckling.

The second problem concerns the specificity of vasopressin-releasing stimuli. Under the experimental conditions used in electrophysiology, there is unambiguous evidence that oxytocin is released by osmotic or cardiovascular stimuli, and that such stimuli activitate oxytocin neurones (see Poulain et al., 1977; Brimble et al., 1978). The lack of specificity of these stimuli should not impair their interest for the study of their influence on the electrical activity of vasopressin neurones. However, it is dangerous to identify the nature of a non-phasic cell on the basis of its response to a vasopressin-releasing stimulus alone. First, the specificity being questionable, a participation of the oxytocin system may be wrongly assumed or denied; second, the excitability of a vasopressin neurone may differ according to its state of activity — for instance, a vasopressin neurone with a slow irregular pattern may be without reaction to a stimulus, but may become reactive when evolving a phasic pattern. The variability in the responses from one cell to another may thus be inherent to the organization of the vasopressin system, rather than due to experimental errors.

Cardiovascular regulation

The afferent pathways from cardiovascular receptors to the magnocellular neurones have been investigated using a variety of methods. It may be convenient to distinguish two types of experimental approach: (i) prolonged stimulation (lasting several minutes) inducing progressive changes in patterns of electrical activity, and (ii) acute and brief stimuli (lasting a few seconds), eliciting brief changes in the electrical activity of the cell.

Sustained stimulation by haemorrhage causes long-lasting modifications in the pattern of firing. Thus, a cell with a slow irregular pattern progressively evolves a phasic pattern (Poulain et al., 1977). The long delay required for such a change (10–20 min of sustained stimulation) suggests that prolonged excitation by afferent input induces not only postsynaptic potentials, but also changes in the membrane properties. This response appear specific to vasopressin cells, for it has never been observed in identified oxytocin neurones.

Acute stimuli have been used to study the role of the various peripheral receptors in the control of the activity of magnocellular cells, and to trace the pathways to the hypothalamus.

Baroreceptor input

At the level of the carotid sinus, excitation of baroreceptors (by increasing pressure at this level) inhibits vasopressin release. The electrophysiological data so far obtained are consistent with this observation. Stimulation of baroreceptors by increasing carotid sinus pressure in "isolated carotid sinus" preparations, by using inflated balloons (Yamashita, 1977; Kannan and Yagi, 1978; Kannan et al., 1981) or by increasing systemic blood pressure by i.v. injections of phenylephrine (Harris, 1979), inhibits the activity of SON neurones in cats and rats. In the rat, the effect was particularly evident on phasic neurones, since their bursts became shorter as the stimulus was applied (Harris, 1979).

Anatomical observations suggest that there is a fairly discrete pathway from the carotid sinus to the magnocellular nucleus, through the nucleus of the tractus solitarius (NTS), which projects in part to the nucleus of the locus coeruleus and the surrounding dorsal pontine region, where neurones in turn project to the magnocellular nuclei (Miura, 1975; Lipski et al., 1977; Cedarbaum and Aghajanian, 1978; Loizou, 1969; Iijima and Ogawa, 1980). Electrophysiological studies confirm such an organization of the pathway. Local anaesthesia of the carotid bifurcation abolishes the baroreceptor effect on magnocellular neurones (Harris, 1979). Neurones of the dorsal pontine region can be antidromically invaded from the SON (Kannan et al., 1981); neurones in the NTS can be antidromically invaded from the dorsal pontine region (Ward et al., 1977); and neurones in the NTS can be orthodromically activated by stimulation of the sinus nerve (Miura, 1975).

Carotid baroreceptors could influence the activity of vasopressin cells through two paths. (1) Activation of baroreceptors could activate an inhibitory noradrenergic pathway. Iontophoretic application of noradrenaline inhibits the majority of magnocellular neurones (Baker et al., 1971; Moss ct al., 1972b); the locus coeruleus contains noradrenergic fibres projecting directly to the SON (Loizou, 1969; Iijima and Ogawa, 1980), although other authors report that the catecholaminergic projections only correspond to the parvocellular part of the paraventricular nucleus (McKellar and Loewy, 1981; Sawchenko and Swanson, 1981). Electrolytic destruction of the locus coeruleus abolishes the inhibition of SON cells caused by baroreceptor stimulation (Banks and Harris, 1982); the two magnocellular nuclei also receive a major input from A1 noradrenergic neurones located in the caudal ventrolateral part of the medulla oblongata, which receives some input from the NTS (Sawchenko and Swanson, 1981). Destruction of this region releases vasopressin, possibly by suppressing a tonic inhibition exerted by A1 neurones on neurosecretory cells (Blessing et al., 1982). (2) Baroreceptor stimulation would also inhibit a non-adrenergic excitatory pathway to the magnocellular neurones: the existence of this pathway is substantiated by the observation that stimulation of the dorsal pontine region excites SON neurones. Increased pressure in the carotid sinus inhibits the dorsal pontine neurones which project to the SON (Kannan et al., 1981), and inhibits the activity of SON cells; conversely, inhibition of baroreceptors (by a fall in arterial blood pressure) excites NTS cells (Ward et al., 1980), dorsal pontine cells projecting to the SON (Kannan et al., 1981), and magnocellular neurones.

Stimulation of left atrial receptors is believed to inhibit the release of vasopressin. This hypothesis is supported by electrophysiological evidence. In cats and dogs, the electrical activity of SON neurones is inhibited by atrial stretching, and such an effect is abolished after section of the vagus nerve (Koizumi and Yamashita, 1978) — The afferent pathway may follow the same route as the pathway from the carotid sinus nerve.

Chemoreceptor input

Carotid occlusion stimulates the release of vasopressin, and excites magnocellular neurones (Dreifuss et al., 1976a; Kannan and Yagi, 1978; Koizumi and Yamashita, 1978; Harris, 1979). The effect was particularly evident on phasic neurones (Dreifuss et al., 1976a; Harris, 1979). As carotid occlusion activates chemoreceptors and depresses baroreceptors, the effect of activating chemoreceptors was looked at in more detail by using solutions saturated with CO_2. The stimulus systematically precipitated a burst of potentials in phasic cells, while anaesthesia of the carotid bifurcation depressed their activity. It seems therefore that vasopressin neurones receive a tonic excitatory input from chemoreceptors, via the carotid sinus nerve (Harris, 1979).

Conclusion

Electrophysiological evidence confirms that vasopressin neurones are involved in cardiovascular regulation. The same neurone appears to receive a tonic excitatory input from chemoreceptors, and an inhibitory input from baroreceptors. Whether this cardiovascular input reaches vasopressin cells exclusively is not clear since none of the short-term experiments that we have reported have been performed on identified vasopressin cells. The involvement of the oxytocin system remains to be determined since haemorrhage releases both oxytocin and vasopressin, and excites both types of cell.

Osmoregulation

Sustained stimulation by water deprivation or by i.p. injections or i.v. infusions of hypertonic solutions causes a progressive change in the pattern of electrical activity of vasopressin neurones from a slow irregular type to a phasic type (Arnauld et al., 1975; Brimble and Dyball, 1977; Wakerley et al., 1978; Jennings et al., 1978). When the effect is observed in the same cell, the phasic pattern occurs after about 10–20 min of continuous stimulation, as during haemorrage. Under water deprivation, the recruitment of the cells into phasic activity is progressive, from less than 10% of the neurones under normal conditions to 94% after 6 h of dehydration. Conversely, progressive rehydration produces a progressive decrease in the proportion of neurones firing phasically (Arnauld et al., 1975). I.v. infusions or i.p. injections of hypotonic solution decrease the firing rates of neurones with a progressive return from phasic activity to a slow irregular pattern (Brimble and Dyball, 1977; Brimble et al., 1978; Jennings et al., 1978).

Acute stimulation by intracarotid injection of a hypertonic solution causes a brief activation of neurosecretory cells, but this effect may not be specific for vasopressin cells (Hayward and Vincent, 1970; Dyball, 1971; Vincent et al., 1972; Hayward and Jennings, 1973). In monkeys submitted to water deprivation, water intake during a short period of time causes a brief inhibition of magnocellular neurones, including those firing phasically. This suggest that magnocellular neurones receive an inhibitory input of oro-pharyngeal origin (Vincent et al., 1972a; Arnauld and Du Pont, 1982).

Although there is good evidence that the osmoreceptors lie in the hypothalamus in a region close to or within the SON, it is unclear whether the vasopressin neurones themselves are osmoreceptors (for general discussion, see Fitzsimons, 1979; Andersson, 1978; Bie 1980). On the basis of their activation in response to intracarotid injection of hypertonic saline, non-neurosecretory cells in the periphery of the SON have been proposed as osmoreceptors (Hayward and Vincent, 1970; Vincent et al., 1972b; Hayward and Jennings, 1973). This suggestion clearly needs more experimental evidence. On the other hand, the reader will find an enthusiastic plea for considering the vasopressin cells themselves as osmoreceptors in Leng et al. (1982). A criticism of this idea, from an electrophysiological point of view, may be found in Poulain and Wakerley (1982). Some caution should be taken when equating osmosensitivity with osmoreception, particularly in view of the role of Na^+ in the maintenance of membrane potential and the generation of action potentials.

Finally, under osmotic stimulation, as under cardiovascular stimulation, it is clear that oxytocin neurones are activated (Brimble et al., 1978; Wakerley et al., 1978). The specificity of the afferent pathway has therefore, here also, to be questioned.

Control of phasic activity

The ability of vasopressin neurones to evolve a phasic activity raises numerous questions concerning the mechanisms involved. The phasic pattern may reflect an endogenous property of the membrane to generate bursts of action potentials; alternatively, the phasic activity could be entirely controlled by the afferent pathways to the vasopressin neurones.

The hypothesis of an endogenous bursting mechanism

In oxytocin neurones, the patterns of electrical activity differ greatly according to the physiological situation (for instance during suckling and haemorrhage). In vasopressin neurones submitted to a sustained stimulation, the phasic pattern seems to occur independently of the type of stimulus and, by extension, of the nature of the afferent pathway. This hypothesis is supported by experiments on hypothalamic slices or hypothalamic explants, which have shown that SON or paraventricular neurones disconnected from their afferent pathways are capable of displaying phasic activity, even when synaptic transmission is believed to be blocked (Haller et al., 1978; Haller and Wakerley, 1980; Mason, 1980; Hatton 1982; Armstrong and Sladek, 1982). The endogenous mechanism, if any, seems to be voltage-dependent. In vivo, vasopressin neurones display phasic activity only when the mean firing rate is > 2.5 Hz (Poulain and Wakerley, 1982). In vitro, depolarization by glutamate facilitates its occurrence (Haller and Wakerley, 1980; Noble and Wakerley, 1982).

To test this hypothesis, the best method would be to record vasopressin cells intracellularly during different states of activity. The technical difficulties encountered in vivo have prompted the development of various in vitro techniques (hypothalamic slices, explants, cell cultures). One possible mechanism for the generation of phasic activity could be similar to the bursting pacemaker potential described in invertebrates (see Gainer, 1972). Such a mechanism has been described in cells from hypothalamic explants (Gähwiler and Dreifuss, 1979, 1980). However, the data reported in intact animals are not fully compatible with this model. Bursting pacemaker potentials appear within a critical range of membrane potentials, and within this range the higher the level of depolarization, the more frequent the bursts. This does not seem to be the case in vivo, where bursts increase in duration at higher mean firing rates. Moreover, bursting pacemaker potentials result in fairly regular bursts, whereas in vivo a striking feature of the phasic pattern is the irregularity from one burst to the next.

Another mechanism could be that of a slow potential underlying the burst of action potentials, that would occur when the level of depolarization is in a critical range. Such slow regenerative potentials have been described in invertebrates as "driver" or "plateau" potentials. The main difference with the bursting pacemaker potentials is that they have no inherent periodicity. They occur when the level of depolarization is sufficient, and may be prematurely stopped by inhibitory influences; they start when the membrane is again depolarized (see Cooke, 1977). This results in bursts of variable duration, occurring in an irregular manner. In cultures of dissociated hypothalamic cells, putative vasopressin neurones (Theodosis et al., 1983) exhibit such slow regenerative potentials (Legendre et al., 1982). The fact that, in vivo, bursts of phasic activity can be triggered or interrupted prematurely by antidromic volleys (Dreifuss et al., 1976c; Leng, 1981) is also compatible with such a model.

Synaptic control

The role of synaptic influence in the generation of phasic activity is obvious since such activity is essentially caused by physiological stimuli. The afferent input may be necessary only to bring the membrane potential in the critical range for bursting activity. However, control by afferent pathways may alter the characteristics of phasic firing. For instance, carotid occlusion can briefly synchronize the activity of the cells (Dreifuss et al., 1976a), whereas usually there is no obvious synchrony. Septal stimulation at 1 Hz for a few minutes can disrupt an existing phasic pattern (Poulain et al., 1980). Stimulation of the amygdala can also modify the occurrence and duration of the bursts (Hamamura et al., 1982; Thomson, 1982). Assuming an important role for synaptic organization, the ability to observe a phasic pattern in hypothalamic slices suggests that intranuclear connectivity also plays a major part in controlling the number of cells firing phasically and the characteristics of firing within each cell. An endogenous mechanism may exist only in a few cells, which would be the pacemakers for the other cells in the nuclei (Gähwiler and Dreifuss, 1979). Alternatively, vasopressin cells may control their own activity by a short feed-back mechanism. However, evidence for a recurrent control is far from being convincing (for discussion, see Leng, 1981; Poulain and Wakerley, 1982). Vasopressin itself does not seem to be of major importance as phasic cells have been recorded in homozygous Brattleboro rats, which are genetically unable to synthesize vasopressin (Leng and Wiersma, 1981).

ACKNOWLEDGEMENTS

The author expresses his gratitude to Dr. D.T. Theodosis for her help in the preparation of this manuscript. The author's work referred to in this article was supported by grant INSERM C.R.L. 79.5372.6.

SUMMARY

It is now well established that a direct relationship exists between the level of electrical activity of magnocellular neurones and the rate of hormone they release. This relationship involves the development of patterns of action potentials characteristic of each type of cell: the phasic pattern for vasopressin-secreting neurones, the high frequency discharge for oxytocin cells during reflex milk ejections. As a corollary, it is now possible to discriminate in vivo the magnocellular neurones secreting vasopressin from those secreting oxytocin.

Electrophysiological techniques have yielded much information about the nature and the role of peripheral stimuli and receptors, about the connections and their function (excitatory or inhibitory) between several central structures and the magnocellular system, about the nature and the role of neurotransmitters acting in the pathways. This information, and future prospects, is discussed in terms of its relevance to what is known of the electrical behaviour of the two types of neurosecretory cell.

REFERENCES

Andersson, B. (1978) Regulation of water intake. *Physiol. Rev.,* 58: 582–603.
Andrew, R.D., MacVicar, B.A., Dudek, F.E. and Hatton, G.I. (1981) Dye transfer through gap junctions between neuroendocrine cells of rat hypothalamus. *Science,* 211: 1187–1189.
Armstrong, W.E. and Sladek, C.D. (1982) Spontaneous "phasic-firing" in supraoptic neurons recorded from hypothalamo-neurohypophysial explants in vitro. *Neuroendocrinology,* 34: 405–409.
Arnauld, E. and Du Pont, J. (1982) Vasopressin release and firing of supraoptic neurosecretory neurones during drinking in the dehydrated monkey. *Pflügers Arch.,* 394: 195–201.

Arnauld, E., Dufy, B. and Vincent, J.D. (1975) Hypothalamic supraoptic neurones: rates and patterns of action potential firing during water deprivation in the unanaesthetized monkey. *Brain Res.*, 100: 315–325.

Balment, R.J., Brimble, M.J. and Forsling, M.L. (1980) Release of oxytocin induced by salt loading and its influence on renal excretion in the male rat. *J. Physiol. (Lond.)*, 308: 439–449.

Banks, D. and Harris, M.C. (1982) Abolition of baroreceptor input to phasic supraoptic neurones following thermal or 6-hydroxydopamine lesions in the locus coeruleus of the rat. *J. Physiol. (Lond.)*, 327: 49 P.

Barker, J.L., Crayton, J.W. and Nicoll, R.A. (1971) Noradrenaline and acetylcholine responses of supraoptic neurosecretory cells. *J. Physiol. (Lond.)*, 218: 19–32.

Bennett, M.V.L. (1976) Electrical transmission: a functional analysis and comparison to chemical transmission. In E.R. Kandel (Ed.), *Handbook of Physiology, Cellular Biology of Neurons, Vol. 1, Section 1*. Amer. Physiol. Soc., Washington, DC, pp. 357–416.

Bie, P. (1980) Osmoreceptors, vasopressin, and control of renal water excretion. *Physiol. Rev.,* 60: 961–1048.

Blessing, W.W., Sved, A.F. and Reis, D.J. (1982) Destruction of noradrenergic neurons in rabbit brain stem elevates plasma vasopressin, causing hypertension. *Science,* 217: 661–663.

Boer, K., Cransberg, K. and Dogterom, J. (1980) Effect of low-frequency stimulation of the pituitary stalk on neurohypophysial hormone release in vivo. *Neuroendocrinology,* 30: 313–318.

Brimble, M.J. and Dyball, R.E.J. (1977) Characterization of the response of oxytocin- and vasopressin-secreting neurones in the supraoptic nucleus to osmotic stimulation. *J. Physiol. (Lond.)*, 271: 253–271.

Brimble, M.J., Dyball, R.E.J. and Forsling, M.L. (1978) Oxytocin release following osmotic activation of oxytocin neurones in the paraventricular and supraoptic nuclei. *J. Physiol. (Lond.)*, 278: 69–78.

Cedarbaum, J.M. and Aghajanian, G.K. (1978) Afferent projections to the rat locus coeruleus as determined by a retrograde tracing technique. *J. comp. Neurol.,* 178: 1–15.

Clarke, G., Fall, C.H.D., Lincoln, D.W. and Merrick, L.P. (1978). Effects of cholinoreceptor antagonists on the suckling-induced and experimentally evoked release of oxytocin. *Brit. J. Pharmacol.,* 63: 519–527.

Clarke, G., Lincoln, D.W. and Merrick, L.P. (1979a) Dopaminergic control of oxytocin release in lactating rats. *J. Endocr.,* 83: 409–420.

Clarke, G., Wood, P., Merrick, L. and Lincoln, D.W. (1979b) Opiate inhibition of peptide release from the neurohumoral terminals of hypothalamic neurones. *Nature (Lond.),* 282: 746–748.

Cooke, I.M. (1977) Electrical activity of neurosecretory terminals and control of peptide hormone release. In H. Gainer (Ed.), *Peptides in Neurobiology*. Plenum Press, New York, pp. 345–374.

Cross, B.A. (1955) Neurohormonal mechanisms in emotional inhibition of milk ejection. *J. Endocr.,* 12: 29–37.

Cross, B.A. and Dyball, R.E.J. (1974) Central pathways for neurohypophysial hormone release. In E.L. Knobil and W.H. Sawyer (Eds.), *Handbook of Physiology, Endocrinology IV, Part 1*. Amer. Physiol. Soc., Washington, DC, pp. 269–285.

Dreifuss, J.J. and Kelly, J.S. (1972) The activity of identified supraoptic neurones and their response to acetylcholine applied by iontophoresis. *J. Physiol. (Lond.)*, 220: 105–118.

Dreifuss, J.J., Harris, M.C. and Tribollet, E. (1976a) Excitation of phasically firing hypothalamic supraoptic neurones by carotid occlusion in rats. *J. Physiol. (Lond.)*, 257: 337–354.

Dreifuss, J.J., Tribollet, E. and Baertschi, A.J. (1976b) Excitation of supraoptic neurones by vaginal distension in lactating rats; correlation with neurohypophysial hormone release. *Brain Res.,* 113: 600–605.

Dreifuss, J.J., Tribollet, E., Baertschi, A.J. and Lincoln, D.W. (1976c) Mammalian endocrine neurones: control of phasic activity by antidromic action potentials. *Neurosci. Lett.,* 3: 281–286.

Dyball, R.E.J. (1971) Oxytocin and ADH secretion in relation to electrical activity in antidromically identified supraoptic and paraventricular units. *J. Physiol. (Lond.)*, 214: 245–256.

Dyer, R.G. and Poulais, D.A. (1983) Milk ejection in the lactating rat after spinal cord stimulation. *J. Physiol. (Lond.),* in press.

Eayrs, J.T. and Baddeley, R.M. (1956) Neural pathways in lactation. *J. Anat. (Lond.),* 90: 161–171.

Ellendorff, F., Forsling, M.L. and Poulain, D.A. (1982) The milk ejection reflex in the pig. *J. Physiol. (Lond.)*, 333: 577–594.

Fitzsimons, J.T. (1979) *The Physiology of Thirst and Sodium Appetite,* Cambridge University Press, Cambridge.

Freund-Mercier, M.J. and Richard, Ph. (1981) Excitatory effects of intraventricular injections of oxytocin on the milk ejection reflex in the rat. *Neurosci. Lett.,* 23: 193–198.

Gähwiler, B.H. and Dreifuss, J.J. (1979) Phasically firing neurons in long-term cultures of the rat hypothalamic supraoptic area: pacemaker and follower cells. *Brain Res.,* 177: 95–103.

Gähwiler, B.H. and Dreifuss, J.J. (1980) Transition from random to phasic firing induced in neurons cultured from the hypothalamic supraoptic area. *Brain Res.,* 193: 415–425.

Gainer, H. (1972) Electrophysiological behavior of an endogenously active neurosecretory cell. *Brain Res.,* 39: 403–418.

Haller, E.W. and Wakerley, J.B. (1980) Electrophysiological studies of paraventricular and supraoptic neurones recorded in vitro from slices of rat hypothalamus. *J. Physiol. (Lond.)*, 302: 347–362.

Haller, E.W., Brimble, M.J. and Wakerley, J.B. (1978) Phasic discharge in supraoptic neurones recorded from hypothalamic slices. *Exp. Brain Res.*, 33: 131–134.

Hamamura, M., Shibuki, K. and Yagi, K. (1982) Amygdalar inputs to ADH-secreting supraoptic neurones in rats. *Exp. Brain Res.*, 48: 420–428.

Harris, G.W., Manabe, Y. and Ruf, K.B. (1969) A study of the parameters of electrical stimulation of unmyelinated fibres in the pituitary stalk. *J. Physiol. (Lond.)*, 203: 67–81.

Harris, M.C. (1979) Effects of chemoreceptor and baroreceptor stimulation on the discharge of hypothalamic supraoptic neurones in rats. *J. Endocr.*, 82: 115–125.

Hatton G.I. (1982) Phasic bursting activity of rat paraventricular neurones in the absence of synaptic transmission. *J. Physiol. (Lond.)*, 327: 273–284.

Hatton, G.I. and Tweedle, C.D. (1982) Magnocellular neuropeptidergic neurones in hypothalamus: increases in membrane appositions and number of specialized synapses from pregnancy to lactation. *Brain Res. Bull.*, 8: 197–204.

Hayward, J.N. (1977) Functional and morphological aspects of hypothalamic neurons. *Physiol. Rev.*, 57, 574–658.

Hayward, J.N. and Jennings, D.P. (1973) Activity of magnocellular neuroendocrine cells in the hypothalamus of unanaesthetized monkeys. II. Osmosensitivity of functionnal cell types in the supraoptic nucleus and the internuclear zone. *J. Physiol. (Lond.)*, 232: 545–572.

Hayward, J.N. and Vincent, J.D. (1970) Osmosensitive single neurones in the hypothalamus of unanaesthetized monkeys. *J. Physiol. (Lond.)*, 210: 947–972.

Iijima, K. and Ogawa, T. (1980) An HRP study on cell types and their regional topography within the locus coeruleus innervating the supraoptic nucleus of the rat. *Acta histochem.*, 67: 127–138.

Jennings, D.P., Haskins, J.T. and Rodgers, J.M. (1978) Comparison of firing patterns and sensory responsiveness between supraoptic and other hypothalamic neurons in the unanaesthetized sheep. *Brain Res.*, 149: 347–364.

Juss, T.S. and Wakerley, J.B. (1981) Mesencephalic areas controlling pulsatile oxytocin release in the suckled rat. *J. Endocr.*, 91: 233–244.

Kannan, H. and Yagi, K. (1978) Supraoptic neurosecretory neurons: evidence for the existence of converging inputs both from carotid baroreceptors and osmoreceptors. *Brain Res.*, 145: 385–390.

Kannan, H., Yagi, K. and Sawaki, Y. (1981) Pontine neurones: electrophysiological evidence of mediating carotid baroreceptor inputs to supraoptic neurones in rats. *Exp. Brain Res.*, 42: 362–370.

Koizumi, K. and Yamashita, H. (1978) Influence of atrial stretch receptors on hypothalamic neurosecretory neurones. *J. Physiol. (Lond.)*, 285: 341–358.

Lebrun, C.J., Poulain, D.A. and Theodosis, D.T. (1983) The role of the septum in the control of the milk ejection reflex in the rat: effects of lesions and electrical stimulation. *J. Physiol. (Lond.)*, in press.

Legendre, P., Cooke, I. and Vincent, J.D. (1982) Regenerative responses of long duration recorded intracellularly from dispersed cell cultures of foetal mouse hypothalamus. *J. Neurophysiol.*, 48: 1121–1141.

Leng, G. (1981) The effect of neural stalk stimulation upon firing patterns in rat supraoptic neurones. *Exp. Brain Res.*, 41: 135–145.

Leng, G. and Wiersma, J. (1981) Effects of neural stalk stimulation on phasic discharge of supraoptic neurones in Brattleboro rats devoid of vasopressin. *J. Endocr.*, 90: 211–220.

Leng, G., Mason, W.T. and Dyer, R.G. (1982) The supraoptic nucleus as an osmoreceptor. *Neuroendocrinology*, 34: 75–82.

Lincoln, D.W. (1974) Does a mechanism of negative feedback determine the intermittent release of oxytocin during suckling? *J. Endocr.*, 60: 193–194.

Lincoln, D.W. and Wakerley, J.B. (1974) Electrophysiological evidence for the activation of supraoptic neurones during the release of oxytocin. *J. Physiol. (Lond.)*, 242: 533–554.

Lincoln, D.W., Hentzen, K., Hin, T., Van der Schoot, P., Clarke, G. and Summerlee, A.J.S. (1980) Sleep: a prerequisite for reflex milk ejection in the rat. *Exp. Brain Res.*, 38: 151–162.

Lipski, J., McAllen, R.M. and Spyer, K.M. (1977) The carotid chemoreceptor input to the respiratory neurones of the nucleus of tractus solitarius. *J. Physiol. (Lond.)*, 269: 797–810.

Loizou, L.A. (1969) Projections of the nucleus locus coeruleus in the albino rat. *Brain Res.*, 15: 563–566.

Mason, W.T. (1980) Supraoptic neurones of rat hypothalamus are osmosensitive. *Nature (Lond.)*, 287: 154–157.

Mason, W.T. (1982) Dye coupling, gap junction and synchronous unit activity in the rat supraoptic nucleus (SON). *J. Physiol. (Lond.)*, 327: 44 P.

McKellar, S. and Loewy, A.D. (1981) Organization of some brain stem afferents to the paraventricular nucleus of the hypothalamus in the rat. *Brain Res.*, 217: 351–357.

Miura, M. (1975) Postsynaptic potentials recorded from nucleus of the solitary tract and its subjacent reticular formation elicited by stimulation of the carotid sinus nerve. *Brain Res.*, 100: 437–440.

Moos, F. and Richard, Ph. (1975a) Role de la noradrenaline et de l'acetylcholine dans la libération d'ocytocine induite par des stimulations vaginale, vagale et mammaire. *J. Physiol. (Paris)*, 70: 315–332.

Moos, F. and Richard, Ph. (1975b) Importance de la libération d'ocytocine induite par la dilatation vaginale (reflexe de Fergusson) et la stimulation vagale (reflexe vago-pituitaire) chez la rate. *J. Physiol. (Paris)*, 70: 307–314.

Moos, F. and Richard, Ph. (1979) Effects of dopaminergic antagonist and agonist on oxytocin release induced by various stimuli. *Neuroendocrinology*, 28: 138–144.

Moos, F. and Richard, Ph. (1980) Double contrôle noradrenergique de la libération d'ocytocine pendant le reflexe d'éjection de lait chez la rate. *C.R. Acad. Sci. (Paris)*, 290 D: 1261–1264.

Moss, R.L., Dyball, R.E.J. and Cross, B.A. (1971) Responses of antidromically identified supraoptic and paraventricular units to acetylcholine, noradrenaline and glutamate applied iontophoretically. *Brain Res.*, 35: 573–575.

Moss, R.L., Dyball, R.E.J. and Cross, B.A. (1972a) Excitation of antidromically identified neurosecretory cells of the paraventricular nucleus by oxytocin applied iontophoretically. *Exp. Neurol.*, 34: 95–102.

Moss, R.L., Urban, I. and Cross, B.A. (1972b) Microelectrophoresis of cholinergic and aminergic drugs on paraventricular neurons. *Amer. J. Physiol.*, 233: 310–318.

Negoro, H., Visessuwan, S. and Holland, R.C. (1973a) Unit activity in the paraventricular nucleus of female rats at different stages of the reproductive cycle and after ovariectomy, with or without oestrogen or progesterone treatment. *J. Endocr.*, 59: 545–558.

Negoro, H., Visessuwan, S. and Holland, R.C. (1973b) Reflex activation of paraventricular nucleus units during the reproductive cycle and in ovariectomized rats treated with oestrogen or progesterone. *J. Endrocr.*, 59: 559–567.

Neve, H.A., Paisley, A.C. and Summerlee, A.J.S. (1982) Arousal. a prerequisite for suckling in the conscious rabbit. *Physiol. Behav.*, 28: 213–217.

Noble, R. and Wakerley, J.B. (1982) Behaviour of phasically active supraoptic neurones in vitro during osmotic challenge with sodium chloride or mannitol. *J. Physiol. (Lond.)*, 327: 41P.

Poulain, D.A. and Wakerley, J.B. (1982) Electrophysiology of hypothalamic magnocellular neurones secreting oxytocin and vasopressin. *Neuroscience*, 7: 773–808.

Poulain, D.A., Wakerley, J.B. and Dyball, R.E.J. (1977) Electrophysiological differentiation of oxytocin- and vasopressin-secreting neurones. *Proc. roy. Soc. B*, 196: 367–384.

Poulain, D.A., Ellendorff, F. and Vincent, J.D. (1980) Septal connections with identified oxytocin and vasopressin neurones in the supraoptic nucleus of the rat. An electrophysiological investigation. *Neuroscience*, 5: 379–387.

Poulain, D.A., Lebrun, C.J. and Vincent, J.D. (1981a) Electrophysiological evidence for connections between septal neurones and the supraoptic nucleus of the hypothalamus of the rat. *Exp. Brain Res.* 42: 260–268.

Poulain, D.A., Rodriguez, F. and Ellendorff, F. (1981b) Sleep is not a prerequisite for the milk ejection reflex in the pig. *Exp. Brain Res.*, 43: 107–110.

Richard, Ph. (1970) An electrophysiological study in the ewe of the tracts which transmit impulses from the mammary glands to the pituitary stalk. *J. Endocr.*, 47: 37–44.

Richard, Ph., Urban, I. and Denamur, R. (1970) The role of the dorsal tracts of the spinal cord and of the mesencephalic and thalamic lemniscal system in the milk ejection reflex during milking in the ewe. *J. Endocr.*, 47: 45–53.

Sawchenko, P.E. and Swanson, L.W. (1981) Central noradrenergic pathways for the integration of hypothalamic neuroendocrine and autonomic responses. *Science*, 214: 685–687.

Summerlee, A.J.S. (1981) Extracellular recordings from oxytocin neurones during the expulsive phase of birth in unanaesthetized rats. *J. Physiol. (Lond.)*, 321: 1–9.

Theodosis, D.T., Legendre, P., Cooke, I. and Vincent, J.D. (1983) Immunocytochemically identified vasopressin neurons in monolayer culture display slow calcium-dependent electrical responses. *Science*, in press.

Theodosis, D.T., Poulain, D.A. and Vincent, J.D. (1981b) Possible morphological bases for synchronisation of neuronal firing in the rat supraoptic nucleus during lactation. *Neuroscience*, 6: 919–929.

Thomson, A.M. (1982) Responses of supraoptic neurones to electrical stimulation of the medial amygdaloid nucleus. *Neuroscience*, 7: 2197–2205.

Tindal, J.S. and Knaggs, G.S. (1975) Further studies on the afferent path of the milk-ejection reflex in the brain stem of the rabbit *J. Endocr.*, 66: 107–113.

Tindal, J.S., Knaggs, G.S. and Turvey, A. (1967) The afferent path of the milk ejection reflex in the brain of the guinea pig. *J. Endocr.*, 38: 337–349.

Tindal, J.S., Knaggs, G.S. and Turvey, A. (1968) Preferential release of oxytocin from the neurohypophysis after electrical stimulation of the afferent path of the milk ejection reflex in the brain of the guinea pig. *J. Endocr.*, 40; 205–214.

52

Vincent, J.D., Arnauld, E. and Bioulac, B. (1972a) Activity of osmosensitive single cells in the hypothalamus of the behaving monkey during drinking. *Brain Res.*, 44: 371–384.

Vincent, J.D., Arnauld, E. and Nicolescu-Catargi, A. (1972b) Osmoreceptors and neurosecretory cells in the supraoptic complex of the unanaesthetized monkey. *Brain Res.*, 45: 278–281.

Voloschin, L.M. and Tramezzani, J.H. (1979) Milk ejection reflex linked to slow wave sleep in nursing rats. *Endocrinology*, 105: 1202–1207.

Wakerley, J.B. and Deverson, B.M. (1975) Stimulation of the supraopticohypophysial tract in the rat during suckling: failure to alter the inherent periodicity of reflex oxytocin release. *J. Endocr.*, 66: 439–440.

Wakerley, J.B. and Lincoln, D.W. (1973) The milk ejection reflex of the rat: a 20- to 40-fold acceleration in the firing of paraventricular neurones during oxytocin release. *J. Endocr.*, 57: 477–493.

Wakerley, J.B., Poulain, D.A. and Brown, D. (1978) Comparison of firing patterns in oxytocin- and vasopressin-releasing neurones during progressive dehydration. *Brain Res.*, 148: 425–440.

Ward, D.G., Baertschi, A.J. and Gann, D.S. (1977) Neurons in medullary areas controlling ACTH: atrial input and rostral projections. *Amer. J. Physiol.*, 233, R116-R126.

Ward, D.J., Lefcourt, A.M. and Gann, D.S. (1980) Neurons in the dorsal rostral pons process information about changes in venous return and in arterial pressure. *Brain Res.*, 181: 75–88.

Yamashita, H. (1977) Effect of baro- and chemoreceptor activation on supraoptic nuclei neurons in the hypothalamus. *Brain Res.*, 126: 551–556.

Yokoyama, A. and Oba, T. (1971) Participation of the cholinergic mechanisms in regulation of the release of oxytocin in response to the suckling stimulus in the rat. *Med. J. Osaka Univ.*, 21: 137–149.

The Neurohypophysis: Structure, Function and Control, Progress in Brain Research, Vol. 60, edited by B.A. Cross and G. Leng

In Vitro Studies of the Control of Phasic Discharge in Neurosecretory Cells of the Supraoptic Nucleus

J.B. WAKERLEY, R. NOBLE and G. CLARKE

University of Bristol, Department of Anatomy, The Medical School, Bristol BS8 1TD (U.K.)

INTRODUCTION

Early electrophysiological studies of the paraventricular and supraoptic nuclei revealed that some of the neurosecretory cells projecting to the neurohypophysis displayed a characteristic phasic discharge, with intermittent bursts of action potentials separated by periods of quiescence (Wakerley and Lincoln, 1971; Dreifuss and Kelly, 1972). Subsequent electrical recordings during the application of stimuli for oxytocin (Lincoln and Wakerley, 1974) or vasopressin (Dreifuss et al., 1976; Poulain et al., 1977) secretion showed that phasic discharge was encountered almost exclusively in vasopressin neurones; oxytocin neurones rarely fired phasically. Hence phasic discharge can be used as an "electrophysiological marker" of vasopressin neurones and this is of considerable value in interpreting recordings from the supraoptic and paraventricular nuclei which, inevitably, involve mixed populations of oxytocin and vasopressin cells.

The occurrence of phasic activity in vasopressin neurones correlates with elevated levels of vasopressin in the bloodstream (Poulain et al., 1977), and it has been suggested that the phasic pattern of firing facilitates vasopressin release from the neurosecretory terminals (Dutton and Dyball, 1979). Phasic firing is not disrupted by synaptic decoupling and seems to be an intrinsic property of the vasopressin cells (Hatton, 1982). However, the phasic activity of vasopressin cells is not completely autonomous, for the expression of this innate firing pattern depends upon the cell membrane being depolarized to within a critical range. Hence the appearance of phasic discharge is governed by extrinsic excitatory or inhibitory influences inpinging upon the vasopressin cells by way of their blood supply or synaptic contacts. The current paper reviews our recent investigations of some of these extrinsic factors regulating phasic discharge.

All of the studies were performed on phasic supraoptic neurones recorded from hypothalamic slices in vitro (for details see Haller and Wakerley, 1980), as this preparation enabled us to manipulate the extracellular environment and to apply neuroactive substances via the incubation medium. Antidromic identification was precluded in this preparation as the supraoptic cell axons were severed, but the recording electrode could be placed into the supraoptic nucleus under visual control. Using NaCl-filled extracellular electrodes the spontaneous activity of supraoptic neurones was low (Haller and Wakerley, 1980) and, with extracellular recording, this presented something of a problem: cell identification based on firing pattern was impossible and inhibitory or subthreshold excitatory effects would be undetectable. To avoid this problem we used glutamate to raise the level of excitation above the threshold for phasic discharge. The glass microelectrodes (10–40 MΩ) were filled with 0.5 M sodium glutamate and diffusion from the tip controlled by a retaining current (0.5–5 nA) from a bridge-balanced preamplifier. With glutamate, the firing rate of the cells increased from the range 0.01–0.5 Hz to 4–12 Hz and a phasic firing pattern (Figs. 1–3) occurred in about 40 % of the neurones. This phasic pattern was rarely apparent at the start of recording; most cells showed 10–20 min of continuous firing, which was subsequently interrupted by silent periods of increasing duration (see also in vivo recordings of Poulain et al., 1977 and Brimble and Dyball, 1977). A regular phasic pattern was usually established within a few cycles, but sometimes the silent periods continued to lengthen until the cell became virtually quiescent, despite continued glutamate application.

The remaining 60 % of the glutamate-stimulated supraoptic cells (hereafter referred to as "non-phasic") had either a persistent continuous discharge or fluctuating activity but without characteristic phasic bursts. Overall, the proportion of phasic cells was slightly lower than the 46 % reported from in vivo studies (Wakerley et al., 1978) which may indicate that for some vasopressin cells, the incubation conditions or level of glutamate excitation were inappropriate for the expression of phasic activity.

PHASIC ACTIVITY IN VITRO DURING CHANGES IN EXTRACELLULAR OSMOTIC PRESSURE

The most effective way of exciting vasopressin neurones of the supraoptic nucleus in vivo is to administer hypertonic NaCl, either into the peritoneum (Brimble and Dyball, 1977) or the lateral cerebral ventricle (G. Clarke, unpublished). This causes quiescent vasopressin neurones to fire phasically and phasic neurones to increase burst duration and intraburst firing rate. The question of whether vasopressin cells are directly osmosensitive has been extensively studied, especially using in vitro methods, since this deceptively simple point (for discussion see Leng et al., 1982) is crucial to our understanding of the osmoreceptor mechanism.

Phasic cells in vitro were excited by a physiological (25 mOsm/kg) increase in their extracellular osmotic pressure induced by adding NaCl to the incubation medium (Fig. 1). Notwithstanding the negative findings of earlier preliminary studies on phasic cells (Haller and Wakerley, 1980) this positive result is compatible with the observation of Leng (1980) that phasic cells in vivo were excited by local application of NaCl. As the phasic cells in our experiments were driven by glutamate, an excitatory effect of NaCl could relate to the possible involvement of sodium currents in glutamate depolarization (Engberg et al., 1979). It would seem reasonable that any excitatory input to phasic cells involving sodium currents would be potentiated by increasing extracellular sodium chloride concentration: thus phasic cells could act as sodium receptors. Without an excitatory input the response to NaCl would not be fully expressed, and this might explain the failure to observe NaCl responses in the deafferented nucleus (Dyball and Prilusky, 1981) and in the in vitro hypothalamic slice in the absence of glutamate (Haller and Wakerley, 1980).

As would be expected from classical descriptions of the osmoreceptor mechanism, systemic osmotic stimulation with non-ionic solutes, such as mannitol, also excites phasic cells (Brimble et al., 1978). Intracellular recording studies in vitro have suggested that non-ionic solutes directly depolarize supraoptic cells and increase the frequency of excitatory postsynaptic potentials (Mason, 1980; Abe and Ogata, 1982). However, we did not observe excitation of phasic cells in the isolated slice when we employed a non-ionic solute (mannitol) (Fig. 1). Hence our experiments suggest that the modulation of phasic activity by purely osmotic stimuli

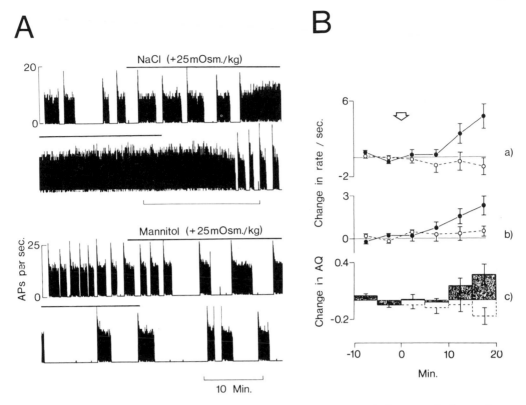

Fig. 1. Effects of osmotic challenge on glutamate-induced phasic activity in vitro. A: the upper pair of traces show a continuous integrator record of a phasic supraoptic cell challenged with a 25 mOsm/kg increase in the incubation medium using NaCl, and the lower traces show another cell tested with mannitol. Note the different time scale for the two sets of records. The neurone tested with NaCl showed an increase in firing (with a latency corresponding approximately to the turn-over time of the incubation chamber) whereas no such effect was observed with mannitol. B: composite data for nine phasic cells tested with NaCl and seven cells tested with mannitol showing the mean change (± S.E.) in: a, overall firing rate; b, intraburst firing rate; and c, activity quotient (AQ, equals proportion of time active) following the switch to test medium (arrowed).

depends more upon an increased excitatory drive from a separate osmoreceptor (or osmoreceptor complex) rather than a direct, osmotically-induced depolarization of the cell membrane. The rapid (within 30 sec) release of vasopressin from intraventricular injection of mannitol (G. Clarke, unpublished) might support a role for periventricular structures in osmoregulation.

ARE ENDOGENOUS OPIOID PEPTIDES INVOLVED IN PHASIC ACTIVITY?

Immunocytochemical studies indicate that opioid peptides are located within neurones of the supraoptic nucleus (Martin and Voigt, 1981; Weber et al., 1982). Intraventricular morphine inhibited vasopressin release (Aziz et al., 1981) and suppressed the discharge of phasically active neurones (Clarke et al., 1980). In view of these in vivo effects we examined the actions of both morphine and a synthetic enkephalin analogue, D-Ala, D-Leu-enkephalin (DADLE), on phasic discharge in hypothalamic slices. However we could detect no significant effect of either morphine or DADLE (10 μM) (Fig. 2) on the phasic cells and, in a small

56

number of experiments, we observed no effect of the opiate antagonist, naloxone ($10\,\mu$M), on phasic activity. Hence it seems that the action of opioid peptides on the firing of the phasically active vasopressin cells in vivo is indirect, and this contrasts with the direct action on vasopressin release at the level of the neurohypophysis (Iversen et al., 1980). It is possible that opioid peptides induce phasic activity, as observed in long-term cultures of supraoptic neurones (Gahwiler and Dreifuss, 1980), but this aspect has yet to be examined in detail.

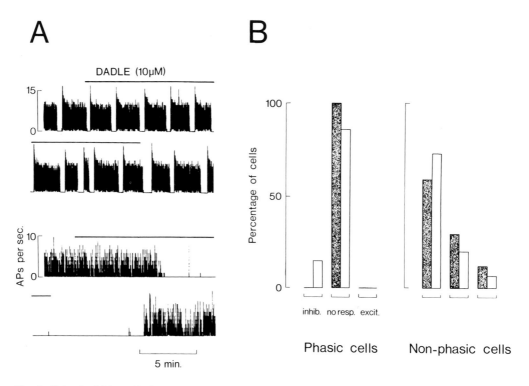

Fig. 2. Role of opioid peptides in the regulation of phasic and non-phasic cells in vitro. A: upper pair of traces show a continuous integrator record of a phasic cell tested with the opioid peptide analogue, D-Ala, D-Leu-enkephalin (DADLE). Note the absence of effect, contrasting with the profound inhibition observed in the non-phasic cell (lower traces). B: histograms giving the percentage of phasic and non-phasic cells showing inhibition, no response or excitation to $10\,\mu$M morphine (shaded) or $10\,\mu$M DADLE (open). The data is based on 23 (6 phasic, 17 non-phasic) supraoptic cells tested with morphine and 22 (7 phasic, 15 non-phasic) cells tested with DADLE.

Although there was no effect on phasically active neurones, a large proportion of the non-phasic supraoptic cells recorded from the hypothalamic slices were powerfully inhibited (Fig. 2). Inhibitory effects of morphine and opioid peptides have also been reported in in vitro experiments on the PV nucleus (Muehlethaler et al., 1980; Pittman et al., 1980). It is probable that a substantial number of the non-phasic cells in our experiments were oxytocin cells, and our results therefore suggest a role for opioid peptides in the control of oxytocin release at the level of hypothalamus. This inhibitory role would complement the action of opioid peptides in suppressing the release of oxytocin from the neurohypophysis (Clarke et al., 1979; see also Pittman et al., this volume).

NORADRENERGIC CONTROL OF PHASIC ACTIVITY

Histochemical studies have revealed a noradrenergic input to the supraoptic nucleus which probably originates from the brainstem and appears to preferentially contact vasopressin cells (McNeill and Sladek, 1980; Swanson et al., 1981). The precise role of this input in the control of vasopressin release is unclear. Bridges and Thorn (1970) showed that α-adrenoceptor antagonism prevented osmotically-stimulated vasopressin release and later it was found that intraventricular injection of noradrenaline released vasopressin by an α-adrenoceptor mechanism (Kuhn, 1974; Bridges et al., 1976). Whereas these experiments suggest an excitatory role for noradrenaline in vasopressin secretion, electrophysiological studies of supraoptic neurones have reported predominantly inhibitory effects, mediated by β-adrenoceptors (Barker et al., 1971; Sakai et al., 1974). However, neither of these electrophysiological studies attempted to discriminate the different cell types of the supraoptic nucleus.

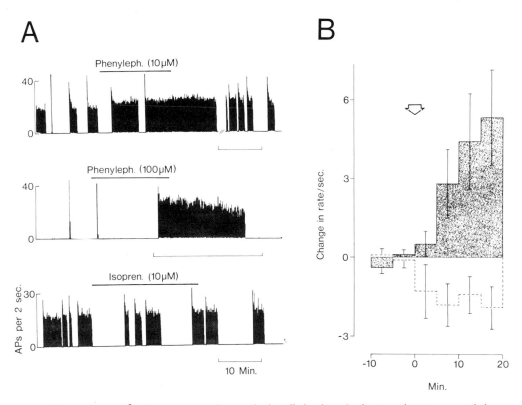

Fig. 3. Effect of α- and β-adrenoceptor agonists on phasic cells in vitro. A: the upper integrator record shows excitation of a phasic cell with the α-agonist phenylephrine (10 μM). The middle record (with a faster time scale) shows another neurone which fired phasically earlier in the recording (not illustrated) but subsequently fell silent. In this quiescent cell, 100 μM phenylephrine evoked a prolonged burst of activity, corresponding in time with passage of the agonist through the incubation chamber. The lower record shows the absence of excitation in a phasic cell tested with the β-agonist, isoprenaline (100 μM). B: composite data showing the mean change ($\pm$ S.E.) in firing rate of phasic cells perifused with 10 or 100 μM phenylephrine (shaded, n = 10), or with 10 or 100 μM isoprenaline (open, n = 5). The arrow marks the switch to test medium. Note the potent excitation with phenylephrine, contrasting with the slight inhibitory effect of isoprenaline.

In experiments on phasic supraoptic cells in vitro we found that the α-adrenoceptor agonist, phenylephrine (10–100 μM), was a potent excitant and caused an increase in the burst duration and intraburst firing rate (Fig. 3). Phasic cells which had become quiescent were also excited and showed a prolonged burst of activity which correlated with the presence of phenylephrine in the incubation medium. In contrast the β-adrenoceptor agonist, isoprenaline (10–100 μM) did not excite the phasic cells, but instead caused a slight suppression of activity (Fig. 3). Noradrenaline would be expected to activate both α- and β-adrenoceptors, and indeed, we have found that the responses to similar doses of noradrenaline are more complex, with mixed inhibitory and excitatory effects. Further work is necessary to characterize the responses to noradrenaline and its agonists but the results to date suggest a noradrenergic control of phasic cells which may be excitatory or inhibitory, depending upon which receptor populations are activated. The existence of functionally antagonistic α- and β-adrenoceptors on the same neurone, as has been suggested for several other areas of the brain (Szabadi, 1979), might explain the conflicting results obtained in previous studies of the role of noradrenaline in the nucleus.

SUMMARY

A substantial proportion of supraoptic neurones in hypothalamic slices display phasic discharge during glutamate excitation. As phasic discharge is characteristic of vasopressin neurones, this provides a means of discriminating the cell types of the nucleus in vitro. Phasic cells in vitro are excited by increasing extracellular NaCl concentration, but not by pure osmotic stimulation (mannitol), and this is incompatible with the idea that phasic cells are osmoreceptors. Opiates do not seem to influence phasic activity, contrasting with the potent inhibitory effects on the non-phasic supraoptic cells. Phasic cells in vitro are powerfully excited by phenylephrine, suggesting a role for excitatory α-adrenoceptors in governing phasic discharge. However, the β-adrenoceptor agonist, isoprenalin, produces a slight suppression of phasic activity and the possible involvement of dual receptor types in the noradrenergic control of phasic cells cannot be excluded.

ACKNOWLEDGEMENTS

This work was supported by a grant from the Medical Research Council.

REFERENCES

Abe, T. and Ogata, N. (1982) Ionic mechanism for the osmotically-induced depolarization in neurones of the guinea-pig supraoptic nucleus in vitro. *J. Physiol. (Lond.)*, 327: 157–172.

Aziz, L.A., Forsling, M.L. and Woolf, C.J. (1981) The effect of intracerebroventricular injections or morphine on vasopressin secretion in the rat. *J. Physiol. (Lond.)*, 311: 401–409.

Barker, T.L., Crayton, T.W. and Nicoll, R.A. (1971) Noradrenaline and acetylcholine responses of supraoptic neurosecretory cells. *J. Physiol. (Lond.)*, 218: 19–32.

Bridges, T.E., Hillhouse, E.W. and Jones, M.T. (1976) The effect of dopamine on neurohypophysial hormone release in vivo and from the rat neural lobe and hypothalamus in vitro. *J. Physiol. (Lond.)*, 260: 647–666.

Bridges, T.E. and Thorn, N.A. (1970) The effect of autonomic blocking agents on vasopressin release in vivo by osmoreceptor stimulation. *J. Endocr.*, 48: 265–276.

Brimble, M.J. and Dyball, R.E.J. (1977) Characterization of the responses of oxytocin and vasopressin-secreting neurones in the supraoptic nucleus to osmotic stimulation. *J. Physiol. (Lond.)*, 271: 253–271.

Brimble, M.J., Dyball, R.E.J. and Forsling, M.L. (1978) Oxytocin release following osmotic activation of oxytocin neurones in the paraventricular and supraoptic nuclei. *J. Physiol. (Lond.)*, 278: 69–78.

Clarke, G., Wood, P., Merrick, L. and Lincoln, D.W. (1979) Opiate inhibition of peptide release from the neurohumoral terminals of hypothalamic neurones. *Nature (Lond.)*, 282: 746–748.

Clarke, G., Lincoln, D.W. and Wood, P. (1980) Inhibition of vasopressin neurones by intraventricular morphine. *J. Physiol. (Lond.)*, 303: 59P.

Dreifuss, J.J., Harris, M.C. and Tribollet, E. (1976) Excitation of phasically firing hypothalamic supraoptic neurones by carotid occlusion in rats. *J. Physiol. (Lond.)*, 257: 337–354.

Dreifuss, J.J. and Kelly, J.S. (1972) The activity of identified supraoptic neurones and their response to acetylcholine applied by iontophoresis. *J. Physiol. (Lond.)*, 220: 105–118.

Dutton, A. and Dyball, R.E.J. (1979) Phasic firing enhances vasopressin release from the rat neurohypophysis. *J. Physiol. (Lond.)*, 290: 433–440.

Dyball, R.E.J. and Prilusky, J. (1981) Responses of supraoptic neurones in the intact and deafferented rat hypothalamus to injections of hypertonic sodium chloride. *J. Physiol. (Lond.)*, 311: 443–452.

Engberg, I., Flatman, J.A. and Lambert, J.D.C. (1979) The actions of excitatory amino acids on motoneurones in the feline spinal cord. *J. Physiol. (Lond.)*, 288: 227–262.

Gahwiler, B.H. and Dreifuss, J.J. (1980) Transition from random to phasic firing induced in neurons cultured from the hypothalamic supraoptic area. *Brain Res.*, 193: 415–425.

Haller, E.W. and Wakerley, J.B. (1980) Electrophysiological studies of paraventricular and supraoptic neurones recorded in vitro from slices of rat hypothalamus. *J. Physiol. (Lond.)*, 302: 347–362.

Hatton, G.I. (1982) Phasic bursting activity of rat paraventricular neurones in the absence of synaptic transmission. *J. Physiol. (Lond.)*, 327: 273–284.

Iversen, L.L., Iversen, S.D. and Bloom, F.E. (1980) Opiate receptors influence vasopressin release from nerve terminals in rat neurohypophysis. *Nature (Lond.)*, 284: 350–351.

Kuhn, E.R. (1974) Cholinergic and adrenergic release mechanisms for vasopressin in the male rat: a study with injections of neurotransmitters and blocking agents into the third ventricle. *Neuroendocrinology*, 16: 255–264.

Leng, G. (1980) Rat supraoptic neurones: the effects of locally applied hypertonic saline. *J. Physiol. (Lond.)*, 304: 405–414.

Leng, G., Mason, W.T. and Dyer, R.G. (1982) The supraoptic nucleus as an osmoreceptor. *Neuroendocrinology*, 34: 75–82.

Lincoln, D.W. and Wakerley, J.B. (1974) Electrophysiological evidence for the activation of supraoptic neurones during the release of oxytocin. *J. Physiol. (Lond.)*, 242: 533–554.

Martin, R. and Voigt, K.H. (1981) Enkephalins co-exist with oxytocin and vasopressin in nerve terminals of rat neurohypophysis. *Nature (Lond.)*, 289: 502–504.

Mason, W.T. (1980) Supraoptic neurones of rat hypothalamus are osmosensitive. *Nature (Lond.)*, 287: 154–157.

McNeill, T.H. and Sladek, J.R. (1980) Simultaneous monamine histofluorescence and neuropeptide immunocytochemistry: II. Correlative distribution of catecholamine varicosities and magnocellular neurosecretory neurons in the rat supraoptic and paraventricular nuclei. *J. comp. Neurol.*, 193: 1023–1033.

Muehlethaler, M., Gahwiler, B.H. and Dreifuss, J.J. (1980) Enkephalin-induced inhibition of hypothalamic paraventricular neurons. *Brain Res.*, 197: 264–268.

Pittman, Q.J., Hatton, J.D. and Bloom, F.E. (1980) Morphine and opioid peptides reduce paraventricular neuronal activity: studies on the rat hypothalamic slice preparation. *Proc. nat. Acad. Sci. U.S.A.*, 77: 5527–5531.

Poulain, D.A., Wakerley, J.B. and Dyball, R.E.J. (1977) Electrophysiological differentiation of oxytocin- and vasopressin-secreting neurones. *Proc. roy. Soc. Lond. B*, 196: 367–384.

Sakai, K.K., Marks, B.H., George, J.M. and Koestler, A. (1974) The isolated organ-cultured supraoptic nucleus as a neuropharmacological test system. *J. Pharmacol. exp. Ther.*, 190: 482–491.

Swanson, L.E., Sawchenko, P.E., Berod, A., Hartman, B.K., Helle, K.B. and Vanorden, D.E. (1981) An immunohistochemical study of the organization of catecholaminergic cells and terminal fields in the paraventricular and supraoptic nuclei of the hypothalamus. *J. comp. Neurol.*, 196: 271–285.

Szabodi, E. (1979) Adrenoceptors on central neurones: microelectrophoretic studies. *Neuropharmacology*, 18: 831–843.

Wakerley, J.B. and Lincoln, D.W. (1971). Phasic discharge of antidromically identified units in the paraventricular nucleus of the hypothalamus. *Brain Res.*, 25: 192–194.

Wakerley, J.B., Poulain, D.A. and Brown, D. (1978). Comparison of firing patterns in oxytocin- and vasopressin-releasing neurones during progressive dehydration. *Brain Res.*, 148: 425–440.

Weber, E., Roth, K.A. and Barchas, J.D. (1982) Immunohistochemical distribution of α-neo-endorphin/dynorphin neuronal systems in rat brain: evidence for colocalization. *Proc. nat. Acad. Sci. U.S.A.*, 79: 3062–3066.

The Neurohypophysis: Structure, Function and Control, Progress in Brain Research, Vol. 60, edited by B.A. Cross and G. Leng

Control of Neurosecretory Cell Activity in the Hypothalamic Slice Preparation

W.T. MASON

A.R.C. Institute of Animal Physiology, Babraham, Cambridge CB2 4AT (U.K.)

INTRODUCTION

Analysis of the control of hypothalamic neuronal activity has been greatly assisted by the development of in vitro techniques, principally the slice preparation. This technique allows the maintenance for many hours of 300–500 μm slices of any desired orientation, and allows both extra- and intracellular recordings to be made while substances of interest are applied. As the preparation is largely deafferented with many inputs to the magnocellular neurones severed as well as their axons projecting to the neural lobe, effects of test substances can be presumed to be local actions on cells and/or synaptic terminals in the area studied. Furthermore, access of test substances to neurones is not retarded by the blood–brain barrier.

In the last few years, the slice preparation has been used to examine control of magnocellular neuronal activity by a variety of substances, including those which are osmotically active, e.g. NaCl and mannitol, as well as neuroactive substances.

EFFECTS OF OSMOTICALLY ACTIVE SUBSTANCES

These studies were begun to examine the proposition of Jewell and Verney (1957), that the osmoreceptors for vasopressin secretion lie near the supraoptic nucleus. Much work since 1957 has been interpreted to suggest that neurosecretory cells in the supraoptic nucleus are not osmoreceptors. These arguments have been discussed recently in two reviews (Leng et al., 1982; Poulain and Wakerley, 1982). Evidence for the hypothesis of Jewell and Verney has come from the work of Brimble and Dyball (1977), who showed that the firing rate of putative vasopressin- and oxytocin-secreting neurones in the urethane-anaesthesized rat increased in response to systemic osmotic stimulation. More directly, Leng (1980), using a similar in vivo preparation, showed that application of NaCl by a microtap technique onto supraoptic neu-rones increased the activity of more than 95% of the cells studied. Both pieces of evidence could not, however, rule out the possibility that NaCl was acting at a site other than directly on supraoptic neurones.

I have examined local actions of ionic and non-ionic solutes directly on supraoptic neurones in the in vitro slice preparation. Intracellular recording techniques, difficult in the in vivo preparation, have been used to examine both pre- and postsynaptic actions of these solutes (Mason, 1980; Abe and Ogata, 1982). Magnocellular neurones of both the supraoptic and paraventricular nuclei in the slice fire spontaneously when recorded from either extra- or intracellularly (Hatton et al., 1978; Mason, 1980, 1982; Abe and Ogata, 1982) and application of excitatory substances such as glutamate, as suggested by Wakerley and coworkers (Haller and Wakerley, 1980 and Wakerley et al., this volume), is not required to bring about this firing.

Approximately 90% of spontaneously active supraoptic neurones recorded in the slice increase their firing rate in response to NaCl. With intracellular recording, this response has been shown to involve both an increase in synaptic input (in the form of excitatory postsynaptic potentials (e.p.s.ps) and possibly inhibitory postsynaptic potentials), as well as a direct depolarization of the postsynaptic cell membrane. Depolarization of the neuronal membrane by NaCl is not synaptically- or spike-mediated as it occurs in the presence of synaptic blocking agents such as 2–4 mM Mn^{2+} or Co^{2+}, or 10^{-6} M tetrodotoxin. Thus, steady depolarization of the cell by NaCl takes the membrane potential closer to spike threshold and increases neuronal excitability, while transient synaptic events trigger action potentials (Fig. 1). Therefore, despite early reports to the contrary (Haller and Wakerley, 1980), supraoptic and paraventricular magnocellular neurones are osmosensitive, an observation now confirmed by a number of workers (Hatton et al., 1978; Mason, 1980; Abe and Ogata, 1982; Noble and Wakerley, 1982; Yamashita, unpublished observations).

A question of interest is whether the osmoreceptor is purely a sodium receptor or a "true" osmoreceptor. Earlier in vivo experiments suggested that solutes such as mannitol, as well as NaCl or LiCl, applied intraperitoneally increase the firing rate of oxytocin and vasopressin neurones and lead to elevated plasma levels of hormone (Brimble et al., 1978). However, such solutes do not cross the blood–brain barrier, and therefore raise the Na concentration within the brain following osmotic withdrawal of water from the cerebrospinal fluid (see Ramsey et al., this volume). Thus it is not clear whether vasopressin release is controlled by sodium receptors (on the brain side of the blood–brain barrier) or by "osmoreceptors" (on the blood side of the blood–brain barrier). In the slice preparation supraoptic nucleus neurones respond to a small increase in extracellular osmolarity, brought about by mannitol or sucrose applied in the perifusion medium, with an increase in firing rate similar to that described above (Mason, 1980). Using larger concentrations of these non-ionic stimuli, Abe and Ogata (1982) reported identical results in the guinea pig supraoptic nucleus slice preparation. I found that 60–70% of supraoptic neurones respond to mannitol or sucrose, though this is a lower percentage than would have been expected from an equiosmolar solution of NaCl. The reason for this is not clear and the observation by Wakerley et al. (this volume) that mannitol is not stimulatory for supraoptic neurones also questions whether these neurones are osmosensitive, or merely Na sensitive. However, the data of Wakerley et al. are difficult to evaluate as the neurones were persistently stimulated by glutamate.

Experiments to date have thus confirmed that many magnocellular neurones in supraoptic and paraventricular nuclei are osmosensitive. In the isolated preparation as well as the intact animal, these neurones probably form part of an osmoreceptive complex, responding to changes in osmolality and altering hormone release from the terminals. This complex may also include osmosensitive inputs to supraoptic cells which have been lost in the slice. The preservation of an intact excitatory input, possibly cholinergic, is suggested by work on the slice to date and by the results obtained by Sladek and coworkers on the hypothalamo-neurohypophysial explant (Sladek and Knigge, 1977, and Sladek, this volume). Their results have shown that a rise in extracellular osmolality with NaCl or mannitol releases vasopressin, and that this release depends on an intervening chemical synapse (see *Note added in proof* on p. 70).

For the magnocellular neurones to be claimed as "true" osmoreceptors, it is necessary to

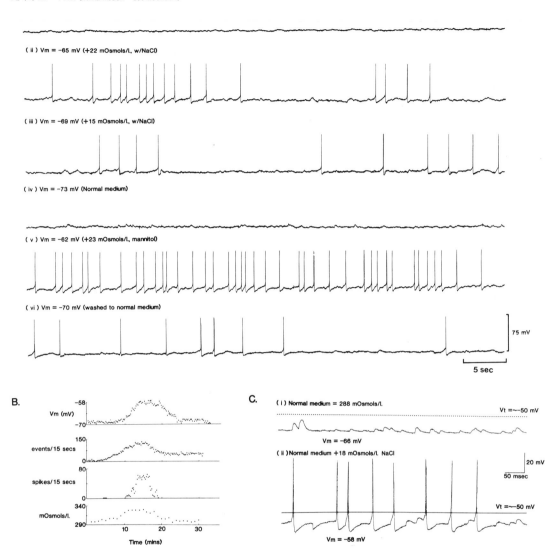

A. (i) Vm = −74 mV (Normal medium = 286 mOsmols/L.)

(ii) Vm = −65 mV (+22 mOsmols/L, w/NaCl)

(iii) Vm = −69 mV (+15 mOsmols/L, w/NaCl)

(iv) Vm = −73 mV (Normal medium)

(v) Vm = −62 mV (+23 mOsmols/L, mannitol)

(vi) Vm = −70 mV (washed to normal medium)

75 mV

5 sec

B.

Vm (mV) −58 / −70

events/15 secs 150 / 0

spikes/15 secs 80 / 0

mOsmols/L. 340 / 290

Time (mins) 10 20 30

C. (i) Normal medium = 288 mOsmols/L.

Vt = ~−50 mV

Vm = −66 mV

(ii) Normal medium +18 mOsmols/L. NaCl

20 mV

50 msec

Vt = ~−50 mV

Vm = −58 mV

Fig. 1. A: intracellular recordings from a supraoptic neurone, showing the progressive responses to variation in osmolarity brought about by addition of NaCl or mannitol. The resting membrane potential (Vm) is indicated for each trace, as well as the measured osmolarity in the bath at the time of each measurement, and how this change was brought about. The normal medium referred to is a modified Yamamoto's medium. With increase in osmolarity brought about by either NaCl or mannitol, progressive depolarization of the membrane is observed along with an increase in e.p.s.p. frequency leading to increased spike frequency. B: measurements from another intracellular recording from a supraoptic neurone, showing the relationship between membrane potential, synaptic events (e.p.s.ps), occurence of spikes, and osmolarity. C: intracellular recording from a supraoptic neurone at higher gain, illustrating the occurrence of spontaneous e.p.s.ps in normal medium of the indicated osmolarity, where the e.p.s.ps do not exceed spike threshold, indicated by Vt. In medium of increased osmolarity, the membrane is depolarized so that e.p.s.ps now exceed threshold for spike activation, leading to cell firing. Membrane potential is indicated for each record.

know that the magnocellular neurones are more exposed to, or more sensitive to osmotic stimuli than other areas of the brain, and whether they have a degree of specialization which allows them to function as physiological osmoreceptors.

The first question must await direct measurement of local rises in osmolality or ionic activity in the magnocellular nuclei and comparison of these changes with those which occur in other areas. These nuclei are perhaps the most highly vascularized of any brain region, and it is possible that in the magnocellular nuclei the blood–brain barrier may not be impervious to small solutes, although it is able to exclude large proteins such as horseradish peroxidase. The heavy vascularization of the magnocellular nuclei certainly makes them likely candidates to receive a blood-borne stimulus quickly and efficiently.

As regards the specialized osmosensitivity of the magnocellular neurones, we know now that the supraoptic neurones in the rat (Mason, 1982) and guinea pig (Abe and Ogata, 1982) have input resistances that are approximately 5 to 10 times greater (approximately 150–200 MΩ) than neurones recorded from other areas of the brain such as hippocampus (Schwartzkroin, 1975, 1977; Langmoen and Andersen, 1981; Abe and Ogata, 1982), locus coeruleus and mesencephalic nucleus of the trigeminal nerve (Henderson et al., 1982), olfactory cortex (Scholfield, 1978) and anterior hypothalamus (Abe and Ogata, 1982). This in itself is good evidence for the greater sensitivity of magnocellular neurones to ionic stimuli compared to other central neurones, as small current flow across this large input resistance upon exposure to osmotic stimuli will result in a large displacement of membrane potential compared to neurones with correspondingly smaller input resistance. This supposition is borne out by recent work of Abe and Ogata (1982) which suggests that neurones of the hippocampus and anterior or ventromedial hypothalamus do not respond to osmotic stimuli in the range where supraoptic neurones respond efficiently with an increase in firing.

PUTATIVE NEUROTRANSMITTERS AND NEUROMODULATORS IN THE SUPRAOPTIC NUCLEUS

The complexity of transmitter interactions in the central nervous system is widely recognized, and it appears that magnocellular neurones of the paraventricular and supraoptic nuclei are no exception. The presence of a cholinergic synapse in the pathway for release of vasopressin has been demonstrated by Sladek and co-workers using a hypothalamo-neurohypophysial explant (see Sladek, this volume). Wakerley and colleagues, using the hypothalamic slice, have reported excitatory actions of α-adrenoceptor agonists and possible weak inhibitory actions of β-adrenoceptor agonists on phasic activity of putative vasopressin cells. Furthermore, opiates such as morphine and D-Ala, D-Leu-enkephalin, whilst having no effects on phasic cells, have potent inhibitory actions on continuous firing putative oxytocin cells. Recent work in this laboratory on the slice preparation suggests that dopamine, its agonists and antagonists act on continuously firing cells but not on phasic cells (Mason, 1983), suggesting that dopamine may be an excitatory transmitter for oxytocin release. Finally, studies with Leng (Leng and Mason, 1982) and those of Mühlethaler and Dreifuss (this volume) have suggested the importance of vasopressin as a potential neuromodulator, being inhibitory in supraoptic nucleus and excitatory in hippocampus, respectively.

The role of dopamine in the pathway for reflex milk ejection has been indicated by several experiments: (1) dopamine levels in the hypothalamus increase during suckling (Voogt and Carr, 1974); (2) dopamine injected into the cerebral ventricles enhances the suckling induced milk-ejection reflex (Clarke et al., 1979); (3) dopamine antagonists such as haloperidol block reflex milk ejection (Moos and Richard, 1982 and this volume). In the urethane-anaesthesized suckled rat injection of dopamine into the cerebral ventricles facilitates the milk-ejection reflex by increasing the burst frequency and amplitude of neurosecretory bursts of putative oxytocin cells without direct effects on spontaneous firing rates (Moos and Richard, 1982, and Freund-Mercier et al., this volume).

Experiments in this laboratory have applied dopamine, its agonist apomorphine and antagonists including haloperidol, spiperone, *cis*-flupenthixol and sulpiride onto the supraoptic nucleus in both the conventional slice preparation and a microdisssction from the slice containing only the supraoptic nucleus and a small piece of optic chiasm. Dopamine or apomorphine applied in the bath at 10–20 μM or pressure ejected onto the slice surface were found to be potent excitatory agents for continuously firing cells but not phasic cells (Fig. 2). In addition, the butyrophenone dopamine antagonists spiperone and haloperidol (1–5 μM) and the thioxanthine antagonist *cis*-flupenthixol inhibited both spontaneous and dopamine-induced firing of a majority (85%) of continuous firing cells (Fig. 3a and 3b). In this class of cells the D2 receptor antagonist sulpiride at concentrations up to 100 μM had no effect on firing. Surprisingly, a second class of continuously firing neurone was detected which was also excited by dopamine, but unresponsive to either the butyrophenones or *cis*-flupenthixol (Fig. 3c). It was possible to test seven such cells, four in the slice and three in the island-slice, with sulpiride as well as the above compounds. In each of these neurones, sulpiride was found to be a potent inhibitor at micromolar concentrations (Fig. 3c).

These results thus suggest that dopamine may play a potent role at the level of the supraoptic nucleus. They also suggest that two distinct classes of dopamine receptor may exist in the

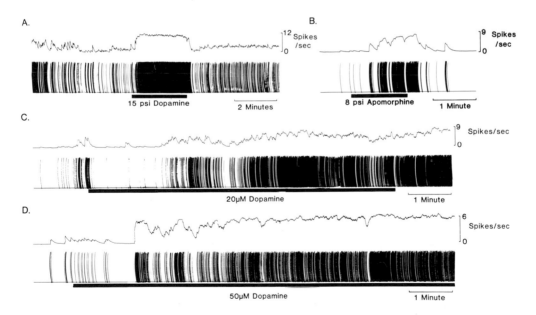

Fig. 2. Extracellular recordings of supraoptic neurones in the rat hypothalamic slice demonstrating the actions of dopamine and its agonist, apomorphine, on firing patterns of four continuously firing neurones. In A and B, dopamine was applied from a pressure ejection pipette into a microwell of perifusing medium surrounding the supraoptic nucleus. In C and D, dopamine at the indicated concentrations was applied in the perifusing medium. In all cases, dopamine and apomorphine activated continuously firing neurones. Integrated firing rate is indicated in the upper trace on each record.

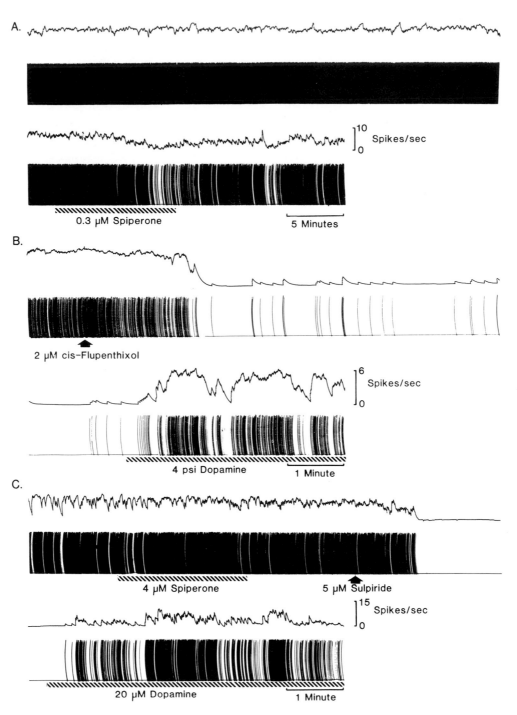

Fig. 3. Extracellular recordings from supraoptic neurones in the rat hypothalamic slice during application of dopamine and its antagonists. A: application of spiperone in the perifusion medium to a continuously and rapidly firing cell, showing inhibition of firing at low spiperone concentration. B: continuous application of *cis*-flupenthixol from the arrow, also in the perifusing medium, demonstrating the strong inhibition of cell firing obtained with this compound. Pressure ejection of dopamine to the region of the supraoptic nucleus in the presence of *cis*-flupenthixol transiently stimulated this neurone. C: this record illustrates the minority class of supraoptic neurone which was not affected by spiperone or haloperidol, but strongly inhibited by sulpiride (applied continuously from the arrow).

Dopamine subsequently added to the perifusing medium in addition to sulpiride excites the neurone.

supraoptic nucleus differentiating two populations of continuously firing cell. The majority of continuously firing neurones possess D1 receptors and the minority, the sulpiride-inhibited neurones, D2 class receptors. The functional significance of this is unclear but raises the possibility of subpopulations of continuously firing neurones not involved in the milk ejection reflex.

We have recently investigated the actions of vasopressin on phasic neurones in the supraoptic nucleus. Leng (1981) demonstrated that synaptic interaction between supraoptic neurones may modulate the discharge pattern of vasopressin cells. When all the neighbours of a phasic supraoptic neurone were stimulated to discharge by neural stalk stimulation, the phasic pattern of the recorded neurone changed dramatically. We wondered therefore whether vasopressin released locally in the supraoptic nucleus could influence the activity of phasic cells (Leng and Mason, 1982), particularly in the light of the inhibitory actions of vasopressin on invertebrate neurones (Barker and Gainer, 1975; Barker and Smith, 1976).

To test this, we perifused or pressure-ejected vasopressin onto the hypothalamic slice preparation while recording extracellularly from phasic and continuously firing cells. Vasopressin (10^{-7} M) dramatically inhibited firing of the majority of phasic cells but was without effect on continuously firing cells (Figs. 4 and 5A). In some cases, vasopressin shortened burst length of the phasic neurone and in other cases completely but reversibly inhibited firing. Vasopressin could also act to break up the phasic pattern of a cell into a slow continuous pattern of firing. We also tested the action of oxytocin on some phasic cells and found little effect. These data therefore suggest that vasopressin may be a neuromodulator of phasic neurones in the supraoptic nucleus. It is unlikely that vasopressin induces phasic firing as phasic neurones

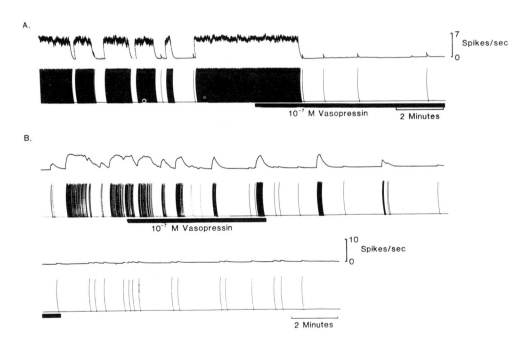

Fig. 4. Extracellular recordings from two supraoptic neurones in the rat hypothalamic slice, illustrating the inhibitory actions of vasopressin on phasic cells. In both examples, vasopressin was applied in the perifusing medium at the indicated concentration, and abolished firing.

68

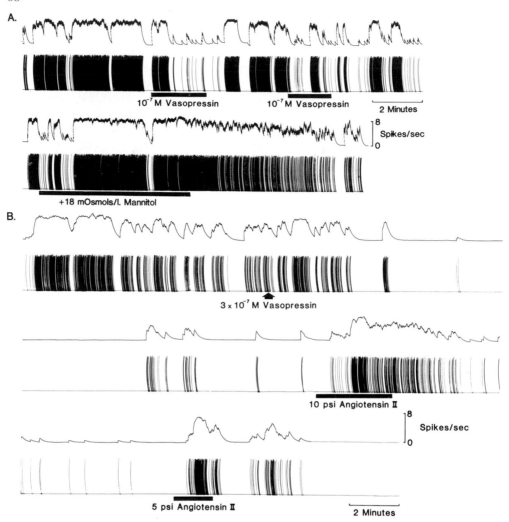

Fig. 5. Extracellular recordings from the supraoptic nucleus in the rat hypothalamic slice. A: the inhibitory action of vasopressin on a phasic neurone, where vasopressin was applied in the perifusing medium. Mannitol applied to this neurone brought about a strong and reversible excitation. B: vasopressin was continuously applied to this neurone from the arrow, causing a marked inhibition of firing. Pressure ejection of angiotensin II from a pipette close to the supraoptic nucleus caused a transient increase in firing rate, thus reversing the inhibitory actions of vasopressin.

occur in Brattleboro rats with diabetes insipidus (Dyball, 1974), but a local release of vasopressin within the supraoptic nucleus might assist in the development of efficient neuronal discharge (Bicknell and Leng, 1981).

Finally, previous work (Nicoll and Barker, 1971; Sladek and Joynt, 1979) has also suggested a role for angiotensin II in modulation of the electrical activity and hormone release of supraoptic neurones. In preliminary studies we found that angiotensin II applied to the supraoptic nucleus in a slice preparation is a potent excitant for phasic neurones, and is able to interact in a competitive manner to reverse the inhibitory action of vasopressin (Fig. 5B). The angiotensin II antagonist saralasin was also inhibitory for the majority of phasic cells tested.

SUMMARY

Intra- and extracellular recording from the supraoptic nucleus in the hypothalamic slice preparation has been used to study the role of osmotic solutes, neurotransmitters and neuromodulators on electrical activity of putative vasopressin- and oxytocin-containing neurones. These studies have revealed several substances which can modify spike patterning, firing rate and other parameters. The neurones respond efficiently to increased osmolality of their surrounding medium and appear for the most part to be sensitive to the osmotic nature of the stimulus rather than simply to specific ions such as Na^+ or Cl^-. In addition, neurotransmitters such as dopamine have a direct facilitatory effect on continuously firing neurones and possible subpopulations of continuously firing neurones have been delineated. Furthermore, vasopressin and angiotensin II have marked effects on neuronal discharge in supraoptic nucleus, possibly assisting in the evolution of firing patterns more efficient for neuronal discharge. Thus, the hypothalamic slice preparation, far from being a simplified model of hypothalamic function, is a system retaining complex afferents with the magnocellular neurones having a variety of receptors for neurotransmitters and neuromodulators.

REFERENCES

Abe, H. and Ogata, N. (1982) Ionic mechanism for the osmotically-induced depolarization in neurones of the guinea-pig supraoptic nucleus in vitro. *J. Physiol. (Lond.)*, 327: 157–172.

Barker, J.L. and Gainer, H. (1975) Studies on bursting pacemaker potential activity in molluscan neurones. I. Membrane properties and ionic contributions. *Brain Res.*, 84: 461–477.

Barker, J.L. and Smith, T.G. (1976) Peptide regulation of neuronal membrane properties. *Brain Res.*, 103: 167–170.

Bicknell, R.J. and Leng, G. (1981) Relative efficiency of neural firing patterns for vasopressin release in vitro. *Neuroendocrinology*, 33: 295–299.

Brimble, M.J. and Dyball, R.E.J. (1977) Characterization of the responses of oxytocin- and vasopressin-secreting neurones in the supraoptic nucleus to osmotic stimulation. *J. Physiol. (Lond.)*, 271: 253–271.

Brimble, M.J., Dyball, R.E.J. and Forsling, M.L. (1978) Oxytocin release following osmotic activation of oxytocin neurones in the paraventricular and supraoptic nuclei. *J. Physiol. (Lond.)*, 278: 69–78

Clarke, G., Lincoln, D.W. and Merrick, L.P. (1979) Dopaminergic control of oxytocin release in lactating rats. *J. Endocr.*, 83: 409–420.

Dyball, R.E.J. (1974) Single unit activity in the hypothalamo-neurohypophysial system of Brattleboro rats. *J. Endocr.*, 60: 135–143.

Haller, E.W. and Wakerley, J.B. (1980) Electrophysiological studies of paraventricular and supraoptic neurones recorded in vitro from slices of rat hypothalamus. *J. Physiol. (Lond.)*, 302: 347–362.

Hatton, G.I., Armstrong, W.E. and Gregory, W.A. (1978) Spontaneous and osmotically-stimulated activity in slices of rat hypothalamus. *Brain Res. Bull.*, 3: 497–508.

Henderson, G., Pepper, C.M. and Shefner, S.A. (1982) Electrophysiological properties of neurones contained in the locus coeruleus and mesencephalic nucleus of the trigeminal nerve in vitro. *Exp. Brain Res.*, 45: 29–37.

Jewell, P.A. and Verney, E.B. (1957) An experimental attempt to determine the site of the neurohypophyseal osmoreceptors in the dog. *Phil. Trans. roy. Soc. Lond. B*, 240: 197–324.

Langmoen, I.A. and Andersen, P. (1981) The hippocampal slice in vitro. A description of the technique and some examples of the opportunities it offers. In G.A. Kerkut and H.V. Wheal (Eds.), *Electrophysiology of Isolated Mammalian CNS Preparation*, Academic Press, London, pp. 51–106.

Leng, G. (1980) Rat supraoptic neurones: the effects of locally applied hypertonic saline. *J. Physiol. (Lond.)*, 304: 405–414.

Leng, G. (1981) The effects of neural stalk stimulation upon firing patterns in rat supraoptic neurones. *Exp. Brain Res.*, 41: 135–145.

Leng, G. and Mason, W.T. (1982) Influence of vasopressin upon firing patterns of supraoptic neurons. *Ann. N.Y. Acad. Sci.*, in press.

Leng, G., Mason, W.T. and Dyer, R.G. (1982) The supraoptic nucleus as an osmoreceptor. *Progr. Neuroendocr.*, 34: 75–82.

Mason, W.T. (1980) Supraoptic neurones of rat hypothalamus are osmosensitive. *Nature (Lond.)*, 242: 533–554.

Mason, W.T. (1982) Electrical properties of neurons recorded from the rat supraoptic nucleus in vitro. *Proc. roy. Soc. Lond. B*, 217: 141–161.

Mason, W.T. (1983) Excitation by dopamine of putative oxytocinergic neurones in the rat supraoptic nucleus in vitro: evidence for two classes of continuously firing neurones. *Brain Res.*, in press.

Moos, F. and Richard, Ph. (1982) Excitatory effect of dopamine on oxytocin and vasopressin reflex releases in the rat. *Brain Res.*, 241: 249–260.

Nicoll, R.A. and Barker, J.L. (1971) Excitation of supraoptic neurosecretory cells by angiotensin II. *Nature (Lond.)*, 233: 172–174.

Noble, R. and Wakerley, J.B. (1982) Behaviour of phasically active supraoptic neurones in vitro during osmotic challenge with sodium chloride or mannitol. *J. Physiol. (Lond.)*, 327: 41 P.

Poulain, D.A. and Wakerley, J.B. (1982) Electrophysiology of hypothalamic magnocellular neurones secreting oxytocin and vasopressin. *Neuroscience*, 7: 773–808.

Scholfield, C.N. (1978) A depolarizing inhibitory potential in neurons of the olfactory cortex in vitro. *J. Physiol. (Lond.)*, 275: 547–557.

Schwartzkroin, P.A. (1975) Characteristics of CA1 neurons recorded intracellularly in the hippocampal in vitro slice preparation. *Brain Res.*, 85: 423–436.

Schwartzkroin, P.A. (1977) Further characteristics of hippocampal CA1 cells in vitro. *Brain Res.*, 128: 53–68.

Sladek, C.D. and Joynt, R.J. (1979) Angiotensin stimulation of vasopressin release from the rat hypothalamo-neurohypophyseal system in organ culture. *Endocrinology*, 104: 148–158.

Sladek, C.D. and Knigge, K.M. (1977) Osmotic control of vasopressin release by rat hypothalamo-neurohypophyseal explants in organ culture. *Endocrinology*, 101: 1834–1838.

Voogt, J.L. and Carr, L.A. (1974) Plasma prolactin levels and hypothalamic catecholamine synthesis during suckling. *Neuroendocrinology*, 16: 108–118.

Note added in proof

We have recently discovered that cholinergic neurones presynaptic to the magnocellular supraoptic neurones exist in the dorsolateral hypothalamus close to the nucleus. Electrical stimulation of these dorsolateral neurones evokes e.p.s.ps in supraoptic neurones, and this transmission is blocked by the nicotinic antagonists hexamethonium and curare. These presynaptic, cholinergic cells appear to selectively innervate phasically active, putative vasopressin-secreting cells (Hatton, G.I., Ito, Y.W. and Mason, W.T. (1983) Synaptic activation of phasic bursting in rat supraoptic nucleus neurones recorded in hypothalamic slices. *J. Physiol. (Lond.)*, in press).

The Neurohypophysis : Structure, Function and Control, Progress in Brain Research, Vol. 60, edited by B.A. Cross and G. Leng

Regulation of Vasopressin Release by Neurotransmitters, Neuropeptides and Osmotic Stimuli

C.D. SLADEK

Departments of Neurology and Anatomy, University of Rochester School of Medicine and Dentistry, Rochester, New York, 14642 (U.S.A.)

INTRODUCTION

The involvement of vasopressin (AVP) in the maintenance of fluid and electrolyte balance has been recognized for decades (Verney, 1947), and its importance in the maintenance of cardiovascular homeostasis has become progressively better established (see Johnston et al., 1981). The signals regulating AVP release from the neurohypophysis for maintenance of these functions involve osmoreceptive mechanisms located primarily in the hypothalamus (Verney, 1947; see Bie, 1980) and signals relayed from the cardiovascular volume and baroreceptors. In addition, AVP release is altered by changes in emotional states, pain, exercise, and the act of drinking.

Knowledge of the morphology and chemical nature of the neural pathways utilized by these factors to alter AVP release is sparse. Only two neural pathways have been established which project directly to the supraoptic nucleus (SON): a large noradrenergic projection arising from the A1 neurones in the ventrolateral medulla (Sawchenko and Swanson, 1981), and a projection from the subfornical organ (SFO) (Miselis et al., 1979). The chemical nature of the SFO projection has not been identified. Other regions of the CNS which have been shown to alter activity of the SON, such as the hippocampus, amygdala, septum and lateral, ventromedial and preoptic hypothalamus, probably do not project directly to SON, but may project to adjacent areas. These areas were labelled in retrograde transport studies following horseradish peroxidase injections into SON (Miselis, 1982) or paraventricular nucleus (PVN) (Silverman et al., 1981a; Tribollet and Dreifuss, 1981; Berk and Finkelstein, 1981a, b), but were not confirmed by autoradiographic orthograde transport studies (Swanson and Cowan, 1977, 1979; Krettek and Price, 1978; Post and Mai, 1980). Thus, neither the specific pathways nor their chemical signals are known with certainty for input to the SON from the telencephalon and diencephalon and are only partially known from the mesencephalon.

In addition to the noradrenergic input, some of the other afferent connections to SON are recognized on the basis of the chemical content of the fibres, but their source remains to be established. Specifically, cholinergic (Meyer and Brownstein, 1980), histaminergic (Brownstein et al., 1974), and GABAergic (Meyer et al., 1980) inputs are suggested by several types of evidence, and immunocytochemical studies have described the presence of substance P (Ljungdahl et al., 1978; Haldar et al., 1979), angiotensin II (AII) (Fuxe et al., 1976), adrenocorticotrophic hormone (ACTH) (Sawchenko et al., 1982), β-endorphin (Bloom et al., 1978; Finley et al., 1981), and luteinizing hormone-releasing factor (LRF) (Hoffman, 1983) positive fibres in SON. Serotonin projections to SON have been described from dorsal raphe.

This is a sparse projection, but the surrounding neuropil contains a large number of serotonin fibres (Bobillier et al., 1976; Steinbusch, 1981). The β-endorphin, LRF and serotonin projections are located in the dorsal region of SON and therefore may preferentially innervate oxytocin neurones.

In addition, several peptides have been localized within neurones in SON including enkephalin, dynorphin, AII, cholecystokinin and glucagon (Sar et al., 1978; Finley et al., 1981b; Rossier et al., 1980; Watson et al., 1982; Weyhenmeyer and Phillips, 1979; Vanderhagen, 1980; Tager et al., 1980). The relevance of these peptides to the regulation of neurohypophysial hormone release is not understood, but they may modify hormone release by acting on the neurosecretory terminals or the pituicytes in the neural lobe.

The PVN is considerably more complex than the SON. It contains both parvocellular and magnocellular divisions, and the magnocellular division can be further subdivided on the basis of efferent projections to CNS areas other than the neural lobe (Armstrong and Hatton, 1980; Swanson and Kuypers, 1980; Koh and Ricardo, 1979). Functionally, PVN is more diversified than SON, participating in the regulation of food intake (see Leibowitz, 1980), ACTH release from the anterior pituitary (Zimmerman et al., 1977; Silverman et al., 1981b), and possibly modulation of cardiovascular reflexes (Matsuguchi et al., 1982) in addition to the functions regulated by the neurohypophysis. Correspondingly, the afferent projections to PVN are more complex. For example, projections from the nucleus tractus solitarius (NTS), locus coeruleus, suprachiasmatic nuclei and anterior, lateral, ventromedial and preoptic hypothalamus have been identified to PVN but not SON (Sawchenko and Swanson, 1981; Swanson and Cowan, 1975; Saper et al., 1976, 1978, 1979; Swanson, 1976). However, none of these projections appear to end in the magnocellular division of the PVN. Thus, as these areas do not project to SON or to the cells in PVN involved in neurohypophysial hormone release, it is possible that they mediate regulatory information for the other functions of PVN. Therefore, to focus attention on the regulation of AVP release from the neurohypophysis, the remainder of the review will discuss known effects of afferents to the SON. All known afferents to SON, including the pathways and chemically identified input, discussed above, are similarly represented in the magnocellular portion of PVN.

REGULATION OF AVP RELEASE BY NEUROTRANSMITTERS

Acetylcholine

Acetylcholine has been recognized as a stimulus for AVP release since the early studies of Pickford and co-workers (Pickford, 1939, 1947; Duke and Pickford, 1951; Duke et al., 1950). Subsequent studies using a wide variety of experimental designs have repeatedly demonstrated the effectiveness of cholinergic agents to stimulate AVP release (Dyball, 1968; Bhargava et al., 1972; Kuhn, 1974; Milton and Patterson, 1974; Sladek and Joynt, 1979a). Furthermore, repeated observations that SON and PVN neurones are stimulated by direct iontophoretic application of acetylcholine (Dreifuss and Kelly, 1970; Barker et al., 1971; Moss et al., 1971, 1972; Sakai et al., 1974a) suggest that the cholinergic receptor is located on the AVP neurone. This hypothesis is supported by autoradiographic experiments which demonstrated that [^{3}H]α-bungarotoxin, a cholinergic receptor ligand, was preferentially localized around the SON neurones (Silver and Billiar, 1976), and by the immunocytochemical studies of H. Kimura et al. (1981) which described punctate varicosities of choline acetyltransferase-positive material surrounding SON neurones. Choline acetyltransferase is a specific marker of cholinergic neurones and the punctate varicosities are believed to represent cholinergic nerve terminals.

The source of the cholinergic innervation is less clear. Studies on the ability of various lesions to alter the content of choline acetyltransferase in the SON suggest that the majority of the cholinergic input to SON arises from neurones either within or in the immediate vicinity of SON (Meyer and Brownstein, 1980). Choline acetyltransferase-positive neurones were not located in this region in the immunocytochemical study of Kimura et al. (1981) in cat; however in rat, Armstrong et al. (1983) observed choline acetyltransferase-labelled neurones lying dorsomedially adjacent to the SON, and occasionally processes from these labelled neurones could be traced into SON. Choline acetyltransferase-positive neurones also have been observed by Sofroniew (1983) in the hypothalamus adjacent to SON. Thus, it is possible that cholinergic neurones close to SON provide an excitatory input to AVP neurones which interact with cholinergic receptors on the perikarya. The receptors appear to be nicotinic, as the nicotinic blocking agents hexamethonium, tetraethylammonium chloride and trimethapan block acetylcholine-stimulated AVP release from explants of the hypothalamo-neurohypophysial system (HNS) in culture, whereas atropine, a predominantly muscarinic antagonist, does not interfere with the same response. Furthermore, nicotine itself is a potent stimulus for AVP release from HNS explants, while methacholine, a muscarinic agonist, is ineffective (Sladek and Joynt, 1979a). Electrophysiological studies on antidromically identified neurones of the hypothalamo-neurohypophysial tract provided evidence for the presence of muscarinic as well as nicotinic receptors (Barker et al., 1971; Moss et al., 1971, 1972), but as the recorded neurones were not characterized as AVP, oxytocin, or some other type, it is possible that the muscarinic receptors are located on non-AVP neurones.

Noradrenaline

The magnocellular nuclei receive a major projection from catecholamine neurones in the brainstem (Carlsson, 1962; Fuxe, 1965; Ungerstedt, 1971; Lindvall and Björklund, 1974) which is preferentially located in the same region of SON as the AVP neurones (McNeill and Sladek, 1980; Swanson et al., 1981). This input is predominantly noradrenergic (Palkovitz et al., 1974) and arises primarily from neurones in the ventrolateral medulla (Sawchenko and Swanson, 1981).

Numerous studies have been performed to evaluate the effect of noradrenaline on AVP release with contradictory results (Bhargava et al., 1972; Kuhn, 1974; Milton and Paterson, 1974; Barker et al., 1971; Urano and Kobayashi, 1978; Hoffman et al., 1977; Olssen, 1970; Vandeputte-Van Messon and Peters, 1975; Wolney et al., 1974; T. Kimura et al., 1981). The most recent of these reports that intraventricular (i.c.v.) application of noradrenaline decreases plasma AVP release in dogs, and discusses the discrepancies in the literature relative to the use of anaesthetics and whether blood pressure was altered by the administration of noradrenaline (T. Kimura et al., 1981). Inhibition of AVP release by centrally applied noradrenaline was confirmed in experiments with cultured HNS explants where noradrenaline significantly decreased basal AVP release at 10^{-5} M. Involvement of an α-adrenergic receptor was suggested by the ability of phentolamine and phenoxybenzamine, but not propranolol to block the effect. Noradrenaline also attenuated acetylcholine-stimulated AVP release in a concentration-dependent manner (Armstrong et al., 1982). The ability of noradrenaline to attenuate cholinergic stimulation of AVP release is consistent with the observation by Sakai et al. (1974a) that noradrenaline reduced the frequency of nicotinic-induced firing by cultured canine SON neurones. Inhibition of AVP release by noradrenaline is consistent with the alteration in AVP release observed following electrolytic lesion of the A1 neurones which give rise to the noradrenergic innervation. In rabbits, plasma AVP levels are markedly increased following bilateral electrolytic lesions which encompass the area where the A1 neurones are located (Blessing et al., 1982).

The role of this pathway remains to be established, but one possibility is that it participates in the cardiovascular control of AVP release. The morphological substrate exists which would allow the noradrenergic A1 fibres to transmit cardiovascular information. The signals from the carotid sinus baroreceptors and atrial volume receptors are transmitted to the NTS and dorsal motor nucleus of the vagus by the glossopharyngeal and vagus nerves. The NTS and dorsal motor nucleus in turn send afferents to the A1 neurones (Sawchenko and Swanson, 1981) which then project to the AVP neurones. The multisynaptic and inhibitory characteristics of this proposed pathway are consistent with established characteristics of the cardiovascular regulation of AVP release (see Share, 1974; Cross and Dyball, 1974).

Histamine

Histamine, administered through any of three routes (i.v., i.c.v. and microinjections into SON) decreases urine output (Itoh, 1974; Bennett and Pert, 1974); also, i.c.v. injection increases plasma AVP levels (Dogterom et al., 1976). Histamine is present in SON, is found in high concentrations in the median eminence, and is probably released by mast cells in the neural lobe (Brownstein et al., 1974; Taylor et al., 1972; Lederis, 1974). Microiontophoresis of histamine excites antidromically identified neurohypophysial neurones in the SON, and in one case the response to histamine was modified by prior exposure to an osmotic stimulus (Haas et al., 1975). These data suggest a role for histamine in the release of AVP and possibly more specifically in the osmotic regulation of AVP release.

GABA (γ-aminobutyric acid)

Considerable evidence suggests that GABA is an inhibitory transmitter in the HNS. GABA decreases the electrical activity of cultured canine SON neurones (Sakai et al., 1974a), decreases the amplitude of the compound action potential recorded in vitro from the pituitary stalk in response to electrical stimulation of the posterior pituitary (Zingg et al., 1979), and decreases electrically stimulated hormone release (milk ejecting activity) from isolated posterior pituitaries (Dyball and Shaw, 1979). GABA also decreases AVP release from HNS explants ($P < 0.05$, unpublished observation).

GABA may serve multiple roles in the regulation of neurohypophysial hormone release. GABA is localized in the SON (Tappaz et al., 1977). Approximately 60 % of this GABAergic input arises from neurones intrinsic or adjacent to the SON, and the remainder arises from the nucleus accumbens which is rostral to SON (Meyer et al., 1980). GABA is also present in pituicytes (Beart et al., 1974), but it may also be synthesized in nerve terminals (Minchen and Beart, 1975). Thus, GABAergic neurones may transmit inhibitory information from the nucleus accumbens, may serve as integrating elements within the SON, may transmit inhibitory signals to the neural lobe, and may mediate pituicyte interactions with the neurosecretory terminals in the neural lobe. Its action in the neural lobe has been extensively studied (see Mathison and Dreifuss, 1981) and is thought to involve activation of chloride conductance and possibly regulates a component of a metabolic exchange process.

SUBFORNICAL ORGAN

A direct projection from SFO to SON and magnocellular PVN (Miselis, 1981) appears to be concentrated in the region (Misalis et al., 1979) where the AVP neurones are located (McNeill and Sladek, 1980). The SFO is an important area for stimulation of drinking. Therefore, it is likely that the SFO projection to the AVP neurones represents a pathway integrating water intake and output. AVP release is stimulated by application of AII to the SFO (Simpson et al., 1979). The transmitter utilized by this pathway has not been identified.

REGULATION OF AVP RELEASE BY NEUROPEPTIDES

Substance P

The SON and PVN receive a dense projection of substance P fibres (Ljungdahl et al., 1978). The source of this input remains to be identified. Due to the presence of substance P-positive neurones in the septum, amygala, hypothalamus (including the preoptic area, suprachiasmatic nucleus, above the lateral optic chiasm, and ventromedial nucleus), locus coeruleus and NTS, substance P could represent input from any of these areas. Unger et al. (1981) observed only a small increase in plasma AVP following i.c.v. injection of $10\,\mu$g of substance P to unanaesthetized rats. In contrast, Haldar et al. (1979) reported a sustained antidiuresis when 0.2–$0.4\,\mu$g of substance P was administered i.c.v. to urethane anaesthetized rats, and Cantalamessa et al. (1981) observed a dose-dependent antidiuresis following i.c.v. administration of 5–$15\,\mu$g of substance P to conscious rats. This response was not observed in Brattleboro rats with diabetes insipidus. Substance P caused an increase in AVP release from HNS explants at 10^{-8} and 10^{-6} M ($P < 0.005$, Fig. 1). Drinking elicited by AII, carbachol, water deprivation or sodium load is inhibited by i.c.v. administration of substance P to rats (De Caro et al., 1978). Thus altered activity in pathways integrating drinking and AVP release may contribute to the AVP response following i.c.v. injection of substance P.

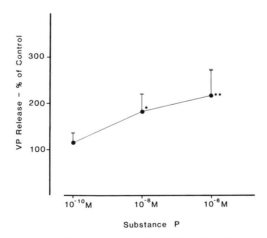

Fig. 1. Concentration-dependent stimulation by substance P of AVP release from 3-day cultured HNS explants. Explants were exposed to substance P during a 1 h test period and AVP release during that hour is expressed as a percentage of that observed during the preceding control hour. Values are mean ± S.E.M. *P < 0.001.

Angiotensin II

AII is a potent stimulus for AVP release (Bonjour and Malvin, 1970; Mouw et al., 1971; Keil et al., 1975; Uhlich et al., 1975) but the physiological significance of this effect has been a point of controversy (Cadnapaphornchai et al., 1975; Brooks and Malvin, 1979; Hammer et al., 1980; Reid, 1979; Cowley et al., 1979). Two questions are central to the controversy: (1) does AII generated in the blood as a result of renin release from the kidney regulate AVP release under physiological conditions? and (2) is AII generated in the CNS, and if so, does it regulate AVP release? Evidence supports a role for peripheral AII in the regulation of AVP release (Shimizu et al., 1973; Ramsay et al., 1978), however the site of action of blood-borne AII is likely not to be the AVP neurone itself, but rather a CNS site which is devoid of the blood—brain barrier and is connected to the SON. The SFO is an important site for the dipsogenic action of AII (Buggy et al., 1978) and application of AII to the SFO releases AVP (Simpson et al., 1979) presumably through activation of the pathway from SFO to SON described above. The organum vasculosum of the lamina terminalis (OVLT) also possesses receptors for AII (Stamler et al., 1980; Landas et al., 1980) and may be an important site for the interaction of peripheral AII and osmotic stimuli in the regulation of AVP release (see below).

The existence of a brain renin–angiotensin generating system has been extensively investigated and debated (see Ramsay, 1979, and Reid et al., this volume) and remains equivocal. AII immunoreactive material has been reported both in fibres terminating in SON (Fuxe et al., 1976) and in SON neurones (Changaris et al., 1978; Phillips et al., 1979; Kilcoyne et al., 1980), but this has not been consistently observed in other laboratories and remains controversial. Nevertheless, AII receptors have been identified in rat brain (Bennett and Snyder, 1976) and specifically in the hypothalamus (Sirett et al., 1977). Furthermore, AII excites cultured canine SON neurones (Sakai et al., 1974b) suggesting the presence of AII receptors on AVP neurones. Therefore, although it remains to be established whether AII is the endogenous ligand for these receptors and, if so, what the source of this ligand is in vivo, the presence of these receptors must be recognized when interpreting experimental effects of AII. Thus, in experiments with cultured HNS explants, it is likely that the stimulation of AVP release achieved by the addition of AII to the culture medium reflects the direct action of AII on the AVP neurone (Sladek and Joynt, 1979b). The inability of unilateral microinjections of AII into the SON to elevate plasma AVP levels (Simpson, 1979) could indicate that the AII receptors are on the AVP terminals. This is an attractive hypothesis, because it would place AII receptors on the portion of the AVP neurone which lies outside the blood–brain barrier and is therefore accessible to peripheral AII. Additionally, if AII is produced by SON neurones which terminate in the neural lobe, one potential role for this AII would be presynaptic regulation of hormone release. Unfortunately, attempts to demonstrate direct effects of AII on the neural lobe have yielded contradictory results. Ruoff et al. (1974) reported inhibition of AVP release when neural lobes were exposed to AII either in vitro or in vivo; Gagnon et al. (1975) reported stimulation of AVP release from isolated neural lobes incubated with AII; and Gregg and Malvin (1978) observed AII stimulation of AVP release from intact rat HNS tissue, but not from isolated neural lobes. However, another possible explanation for the absence of AVP release following microinjections of AII into the SON is that AII alters the release of regulatory transmitters in SON. AII may facilitate noradrenaline release (Taube et al., 1977; Garcia-Sevilla et al., 1979) which in turn inhibits AVP release (Armstrong et al., 1982). Thus, the effect of exposing the SON to AII in vivo with its noradrenergic innervation intact might be quite different to that obtained in culture systems where the noradrenergic input has degenerated.

Understanding the physiological relevance of these observations awaits conclusive evidence for AII fibres and/or production in the SON and ultrastructural evaluation of the morphological relationships between AII components, the AVP neurone, and other afferent components in the nucleus.

Opiate peptides

It has been recognized for decades that morphine alters neurohypophysial function (Feé, 1929; De Bodo, 1944). This, combined with the evidence for CNS opiate receptors and endogenous opiate ligands, initiated a surge of interest in the role of opiates in the regulation of the neurohypophysis. Immunocytochemical and radioimmunoassay studies indicate regional localization of opiate peptides within the HNS. As mentioned, β-endorphin is produced in arcuate neurones which project to the oxytocin-rich regions of SON (Bloom et al., 1978; Finley et al., 1981a; Sawchenko et al., 1982). In addition β-endorphin, produced by the intermediate lobe, is released from isolated neurointermediate pituitary preparations (Weitzman et al., 1977). Although most of the β-endorphin in the intermediate lobe is in the biologically inactive N-acetylated form (Akil et al., 1981), it is possible that the biologically active components institute some control over neural lobe function. Enkephalin and dynorphin have been localized in the SON and neural lobe (Micevych and Elde, 1980; Rossier et al., 1980; Martin and Voigt, 1981; Watson et al., 1982). Dynorphin coexists with AVP in neurones of the SON, and is present in the AVP-deficient neurones of Brattleboro rats with diabetes insipidus (Watson et al., 1982). Clarification is required as to whether enkephalin also is present in SON neurones or whether the reports of enkephalin-positive neurones reflect cross-reaction of the enkephalin antibodies with dynorphin.

Opiate receptors have been localized in the SON (Hillar et al., 1973) and neural lobe (Simanatov and Snyder, 1977). The receptors in the neural lobe appear to be concentrated on the pituicytes rather than on the neurosecretory terminals and therefore, at the level of the neural lobe, opiate-induced alterations in hormone release may be secondary to altered pituicyte function (Lightman et al., this volume).

Numerous studies have demonstrated alterations in neurohypophysial function as a result of administration of an opiate. However, the reported effects vary with the experimental paradigm employed and range from stimulation to inhibition of AVP release (Philbin et al., 1976; Mata et al., 1977; Bisset et al., 1978; Haldar and Sawyer, 1978; Philbin and Coggins, 1978; Van Wimersma Greidanus et al., 1978; Firemark and Weitzman, 1979; Brownell et al., 1980; Grossman et al., 1980; Lightman and Forsling, 1980a, b; Miller, 1980; Pittman et al., 1980; Vizi and Volbekas, 1980; Aziz et al., 1981a, b; Baertschi et al., 1981; Clarke et al., 1981; Ganten et al., 1981; Summy-Long et al., 1981; Van Wimersma Greidanus, 1981; Lightman et al., 1981). Two important considerations in evaluating these diverse observations are: (1) the opiates and their receptors are widely distributed in the CNS. Therefore, the site of action of the opiate can differ markedly depending on the route of administration; and (2) there are multiple opiate peptides and receptor types, and the affinity of the various peptides differs markedly from receptor to receptor (Martin, 1967; Lord et al., 1977). Therefore, the effect observed may depend on the specific opiate utilized.

The neural lobe represents one effector site for endogenous opiates. Opiate receptors are concentrated in the posterior pituitary and enkephalin and/or dynorphin fibres arising from the hypothalamus terminate in the neural lobe. Furthermore, D-Ala, D-Leu-enkephalin, β-endorphin and morphine inhibit electrically stimulated AVP release from isolated neural lobes

(Iversen et al., 1980) and i.c.v. application of morphine inhibits oxytocin release without altering the electrical activity of milk ejecting neurones in the SON, suggesting an inhibitory action of morphine on the oxytocin nerve terminal (Clarke et al., 1979). In addition, however, opiates may alter the activity of afferent pathways to the SON either by acting on the cell body of origin or presynaptically on the nerve terminal in the hypothalamus. Thus careful evaluation of the potential sites of action for opiates on neurohypophysial hormone release is required.

Furthermore, as the type of opiate receptors in regulation of neurohypophysial function may differ at various loci, the actions of endogenous opiates and their analogues may differ as a result of activation of predominantly different receptor populations. This has been demonstrated in cultured HNS explants where the effect of various opiates on AVP release have been studied (Sladek et al., 1982b). In confirmation of the observations of Iversen et al. (1980), D-Ala, D-Leu-enkephalin, the stable analogue of Leu-enkephalin, inhibited cholinergic and osmotically stimulated release from HNS explants, but this was not observed with either Leu-enkephalin itself or the stable Met-enkephalin analogue D-Ala, Met-enkephalinamide. In fact, both of the latter enkephalins stimulated AVP release, as did dynorphin. Thus, even in a relatively simple in vitro system, the opiate mechanisms regulating AVP release are quite complex which serves to emphasize that a complete understanding of the role of the opiates in the regulation of AVP release will require knowledge of the morphological and pharmacological interactions of specific opiate pathways with the HNS.

MECHANISMS OF OSMOTIC CONTROL

Since Verney's (1947) classical experiments, it has been recognized that the osmolality of the extracellular fluid (ECF) is an important determinant of AVP release. In spite of numerous studies on the osmotic control of AVP release (for review see Robertson et al., 1976; Bie, 1980), specific mechanisms underlying this important regulatory function remained controversial and poorly defined. The development of techniques for maintaining physiologically responsive AVP neurones in vitro has provided the means to study their electrophysiological and hormone release characteristics under conditions in which the osmotic environment can be selectively manipulated. Specifically, the effect of altering the osmolality of the incubation medium on the electrophysiological characteristics of SON neurones in hypothalamic slice preparations has been investigated with intracellular recording techniques (Mason, 1980), and the osmotic control of AVP release has been studied in organ-cultured explants of the HNS from rats (Sladek and Knigge, 1977) and guinea pigs (Ishikawa et al., 1980). These studies have provided evidence that the osmotic control of AVP release involves a complex system of multiple osmosensitive components (Leng et al., 1982; Sladek et al., 1983).

Location

Early observations which supported an anterior hypothalamic site for the osmoreceptive system (Jewell and Verney, 1957; Cross and Green, 1959; Woods and Bard, 1960; Sundsten and Sawyer, 1961), led investigators to hypothesize that the AVP neurones themselves may be osmoreceptive (see Joynt, 1966). However, subsequent experiments which demonstrated electrophysiologically the presence of multiple osmosensitive cell types in the region of the SON (see Hayward, 1975), and studies which indicated that cholinergic blocking agents blocked osmotically stimulated AVP release when applied in vivo in the CNS (De Wied and Laszlo, 1967; Bridges and Thorn, 1970; Morris et al., 1977) or in vitro to cultured HNS explants (Sladek and Joynt, 1979c) suggested that the osmosensitive mechanisms are close to, but separate from, the AVP neurones. Recent intracellular recordings from SON neurones in hypothalamic slices (Mason, 1980) suggest that the correct hypothesis is a combination of the two: the SON neurones are osmosensitive, but other elements located in the anterior hypothalamus which excite SON neurones also are osmosensitive and the input from these separate osmosensitive units is required to release AVP in response to an increase in osmolality.

The specific observations which gave rise to this hypothesis were that SON neurones in hypothalamic slices were depolarized in response to physiological increments in osmolality of the incubation medium. In addition, increasing the osmolality resulted in an increased frequency of excitatory postsynaptic potentials. These two responses summated to cause firing of the SON neurone. Under conditions in which synaptic excitation of the SON was prevented (i.e. high Mg^{2+}, low Ca^{2+} concentrations in the incubation medium), depolarization of the SON neurone was still observed but was not, by itself, capable of generating action potentials (Mason, 1980). These findings and the resultant hypothesis are consistent with observations that direct microtap application of hypertonic stimuli activated SON neurones in vivo (Leng, 1980) as well as with observations that pharmacologic blockers interfere with osmotically induced AVP release (Bridges and Thorn, 1980; Morris et al., 1977; Sladek and Joynt, 1979c).

One probable location of these separate osmoreceptive units is the region anterior and ventral to the third ventricle (AV3V) and specifically the OVLT. Electrolytic ablation of the medial preoptic area (Van Gemert et al., 1975) or AV3V region (Bealer et al., 1979) in rats results in attenuation of the antidiuretic responses to osmotic stimuli. Furthermore, HNS explants from rats previously prepared with AV3V lesions do not release AVP in response to increases in culture medium osmolality (Johnson and Sladek, 1979; Sladek and Johnson, 1983). The AV3V lesion encompasses the OVLT, and it has been shown that the relationship between plasma osmolality and plasma AVP concentration is ablated by OVLT lesions in dogs (Thrasher et al., 1982). These data are compatible with the hypothesis that osmoreceptive units are located in the OVLT.

Direct innervation of SON by OVLT has not been demonstrated. AV3V lesions result in degeneration of both axodendritic and axoaxonal synapses on SON neurones (Carithers et al., 1980), however these lesions interrupt the afferent connections from the SFO (Miselis, 1981) as well as possible innervation from the OVLT. Bilateral injections of horseradish peroxidase into SON resulted in retrograde labelling in the OVLT indicative of efferent projections (Miselis, 1982; Miselis et al., 1979), however these may represent projections to regions adjacent to SON rather than direct innervation of SON.

Role of acetylcholine

Acetylcholine is a potent stimulus for AVP release, and activates nicotinic receptors which are probably located on the AVP neurone. Nicotinic cholinergic blocking agents also block osmotically stimulated AVP release from cultured HNS explants (Sladek and Joynt, 1979c). These observations correspond to similar reports in vivo (De Wied and Laszlo, 1967; Bridges and Thorn, 1970; Morris et al., 1977), and suggest that a cholinergic synapse mediates the osmotic control of AVP release. As the majority of the cholinergic input to SON arises from neurones located in the immediate vicinity of SON it is possible that cholinergic neurones close to SON participate in the osmotic control of AVP release by transmitting information received from osmosensitive units in OVLT to SON.

Role of AII

In vivo and in vitro studies have suggested that AII is involved in the osmotic control of AVP release. Andersson and Westbye (1970) reported synergistic actions of i.c.v. infused AII and NaCl on antidiuresis in the goat, and in dogs intracarotid infusion of physiologically reasonable concentrations of AII potentiated AVP release in response to an i.v. infusion of hypertonic saline (Shimizu et al., 1973). AII also potentiates osmotic stimulation of AVP release from organ-cultured HNS explants (Fig. 2). Furthermore, addition of the AII antagonist saralasin or

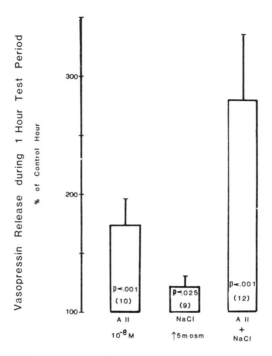

Fig. 2. AII potentiation of AVP release stimulated by a 5 mOsm increment in osmolality. Explants were exposed to AII, NaCl, or the two substances together during a 1 h period on day 3 of culture. All groups showed a significant increase in AVP release compared to the preceding control hour (*P* values). The response of the group exposed to the combined stimulus was greater than the summated responses of the groups exposed to AII and NaCl individually. Mean ± S.E.M. (n).

AII-antiserum to the culture medium blocks AVP release in response to osmotic stimuli (Sladek and Joynt, 1980a). The AII antagonists block AVP release stimulated by increasing the osmolality with either NaCl or mannitol (Sladek, 1980). Thus, the interaction is not limited to the ability of AII to alter sodium fluxes as has been shown in other tissues (Turker et al., 1967; Gutman et al., 1972).

The AII antagonists blocked osmotically stimulated AVP release from HNS explants without significantly altering basal release (Sladek et al., 1982b). This raises the issue of the ability of the CNS to generate AII. AII is continuously generated in the HNS culture system (i.e. medium plus explant), as captopril, the AII converting enzyme inhibitor, will block osmotically stimulated AVP release if explants are incubated with it prior to the osmotic stimulus (Sladek et al., 1982a). The physiological relevance of this production of AII remains to be assessed; it is not dependent on the presence of renin activity in the medium (Sladek et al., 1982a) as suggested previously (Sladek, 1980b). Of greater relevance to the role of AII in the osmotic control of AVP release is the observation that AII antagonists block osmotically stimulated AVP release without altering basal release. This also suggests the presence of multiple sites of action of AII in the HNS explant, because it indicates that concentrations of AII which are necessary for the osmotic response are insufficient to modify basal AVP release. As discussed previously, the AVP neurone is one site of action, and the stimulation of AVP release from HNS explants after the addition of AII to the culture medium may be a result of direct activation of receptors on the AVP neurone. This hypothesis is supported by the observations with HNS explants that AII-stimulated AVP release is not blocked by cholinergic antavonists (Sladek and Joynt, 1980a) or by AV3V lesions which destroy the elements required for osmotic response (Johnson and Sladek, 1979). Another site of action of AII may be the osmoreceptive element located in the OVLT. Thrasher et al. (1980, 1982) have shown that the OVLT is a likely site of reception for osmotic signals from the periphery. Therefore, it is also a likely site for potentiation of that response by peripheral AII (Shimizu et al., 1973). Further observations from HNS explant studies suggest that the role of AII in the osmotic control of AVP release is different from that of acetylcholine, and may represent a different site of action. As mentioned previously, AII potentiated the AVP response to osmotic stimulation by HNS explants. A similar potentiation was not observed with combined exposure to acetylcholine and NaCl or to acetylcholine and AII (Sladek et al., 1982a).

Interaction with noradrenaline

Noradrenaline inhibits basal AVP release from HNS explants and attenuates acetylcholine-stimulated AVP release in a concentration-dependent manner (Armstrong et al., 1982). As cholinergic mechanisms have been implicated in the osmotic control of AVP release, it was anticipated that noradrenaline would also attenuate osmotically stimulated AVP release from HNS explants. This was not observed. Stimulation of AVP release by a 20 mOsm increment in osmolality was comparable in the absence or presence of noradrenaline (10^{-9}, 10^{-7} or 10^{-5} M; Armstrong et al., 1982). The inability of noradrenaline to attenuate osmotically stimulated AVP release attests to the complexity of the osmoreceptive system and is consistent with the observation that SON neurones are depolarized by an increase in osmolality (Mason, 1980). Thus, under hypertonic conditions the noradrenergic-induced decreased responsiveness of SON neurones to acetylcholine would be offset by their increased sensitivity to excitatory input due to the depolarizing effect of osmotic stimulation.

SUMMARY

Fig. 3 presents a hypothetical osmoreceptive system which incorporates the observations described above. The AVP neurone itself is osmosensitive, in that increases in the osmolarity of the extracellular fluid cause depolarization of the membrane and a resulting sensitization of the neurone to other excitatory inputs (Mason, 1980). However, this inherent osmosensitivity is inadequate to generate firing of the neurone and subsequent AVP release by itself. Excitatory input from osmosensitive cells in the OVLT is also required to achieve an increase in AVP release. Cholinergic mechanisms mediate this information and therefore either the osmosensitive units themselves are cholinergic, or information from them is processed by cholinergic cells prior to transmittal to the AVP neurone. As the OVLT appears to project to the vicinity of

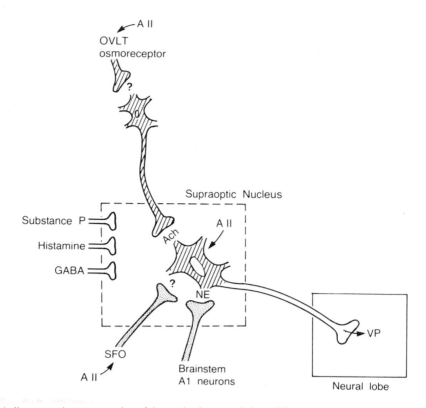

Fig. 3. A diagrammatic representation of the mechanisms regulating AVP neurones of the SON. The components involved in the osmotic regulation of AVP release are indicated with hatch markings. This includes the AVP neurone which is osmosensitive, but which requires excitatory input from an additional osmosensitive component located in the OVLT in order to generate action potentials and activate AVP release in response to an increase in osmolality. The information from the OVLT is mediated by cholinergic mechanisms. AII potentiates AVP release in response to an osmotic stimulus probably through an action on the osmosensitive cells in the OVLT, but it also stimulates release through a mechanism which is not dependent on cholinergic transmission and therefore, at higher concentrations, it may act directly on the AVP neurone to stimulate hormone release. The two afferent pathways whose origin is known are indicated with stipling. The noradrenergic pathway from the A1 neurones in the medulla may provide information from the cardiovascular volume and baroreceptors. This input is inhibitory to AVP release. The chemical nature of the SFO pathway has not been identified. Other afferent pathways are recognized by their chemical nature (i.e. substance P, histamine, GABA), but the location of the cells of origin of these fibres remains to be determined as well as their physiological role in the regulation of AVP release. Other chemically identified afferents to SON have been described (i.e. β-endorphin, ACTH, LRF and serotonin), but these are believed to project primarily to the oxytocin neurones.

SON, but direct connections to SON have not been demonstrated, the second possibility seems most likely. AII increases sensitivity of the osmoreceptor in the OVLT and thereby potentiates AVP release in response to an osmotic stimulus. In addition, AII can stimulate the AVP neurone directly, but the relevance of this action to the regulation of AVP release in vivo remains to be established. A third route for stimulation of AVP release by AII in vivo is through activation of afferents from the SFO.

The ability of osmotic stimulation to override noradrenergic inhibition emphasizes the prominent role of the osmotic control of AVP release, and is consistent with the postulated role for the noradrenergic innervation in conveying signals from the cardiovascular baro- and volume-receptors (Sawchenko and Swanson, 1980). In vivo, AVP release is extremely sensitive to small changes in osmolality of the extracellular fluid, but large changes in blood pressure or blood volume are required to achieve comparable plasma AVP concentrations (Robertson, 1976). Thus, interaction between noradrenaline and osmotic stimulation in determining AVP release would fit with a role for noradrenaline in transmitting cardiovascular information as the osmotic regulatory mechanisms can override the effects of noradrenaline.

The information conveyed by the other chemically identified afferents to the SON remain to be established. Furthermore, as discussed elsewhere (Pittman et al., this volume) afferents to the neural lobe probably represent another important source of information for regulation of AVP release. The mechanisms which integrate all of these signals to achieve a rate of hormone release appropriate to the physiological circumstances, remain to be elucidated.

ACKNOWLEDGEMENTS

This work was supported by grants from the National Institute of Health: AM-19761 and NS-00259.

REFERENCES

Akil, H., Young, E. and Watson, S.J. (1981) Opiate binding properties of naturally occurring N- and C-terminus modified β-endorphins. *Peptides*, 2: 289–292.

Andersson, B. and Westbye, O. (1970) Synergistic action of sodium and angiotensin on brain mechanisms controlling fluid balance. *Life Sci.*, 9: 601–608.

Armstrong, W. and Hatton, G.I. (1980) The localization of projection neurons in the rat hypothalamic paraventricular nucleus following vascular and neurohypophysial injections of HRP. *Brain Res. Bull.*, 5: 473–477.

Armstrong, D.M., Saper, C.B., Levey, A.I., Wainer, B.H. and Terry, R.D. (1983) Distribution of cholinergic neurons in rat brain demonstrated by immunocytochemical localization of choline acetyltransferase. *J. comp. Neurol.*, in press.

Armstrong, W.E., Sladek, C.D. and Sladek, J.R. (1983) Characterization of noradrenergic control of vasopressin release by the organ cultured rat hypothalamoneurohypophyseal system. *Endocrinology*, 111: 273–279.

Aziz, L.A., Forsling, J.L. and Woolf, C.J. (1981a) The effect of intracerebroventricular injections of morphine on vasopressin release in the rat. *J. Physiol. (Lond.)*, 311: 401–409.

Aziz, L.A., Forsling, M.L. and Woolf, C.J. (1981b) Does Met-enkephalin influence vasopressin release? *J. Physiol. (Lond.)*, 315: 7P.

Baertschi, A.J., Znigg, H.H. and Dreifuss, J.J. (1981) Enkephalins, substance P, bradykinin and angiotensin II: differential sites of action on the hypothalamoneurohypophysial system. *Brain Res.*, 220: 107–119.

Barker, J.L., Crayton, J.W. and Nicoll, R.A. (1971) Noradrenaline and acetylcholine responses of supraoptic neurosecretory cells. *J. Physiol. (Lond.)*, 218: 19–32.

Bealer, S.L., Phillips, M.I., Johnson, A.K. and Schmid, P.G. (1979) Effect of anteroventral third ventricular lesions on antidiuretic responses to central angiotensin II. *Amer. J. Physiol.*, 236: E610–615.

Beart, P.M., Kelly, J.S. and Schon, F. (1974) γ-Aminobutyric acid in the rat peripheral nervous system, pineal and posterior pituitary. *Biochem. Soc. Trans.*, 2: 266–268.

Bennett, C.T. and Pert, A. (1974) Antidiuresis produced by injections of histamine into the cat supraoptic nucleus. *Brain Res.*, 78: 151.

Bennett, J.P. and Snyder, S.H. (1976) Angiotensin II binding to mammalian brain membrane. *J. biol. Chem.*, 251: 7423–7430.

Berk, M.L. and Finkelstein, J.A. (1981a) Afferent projections to the preoptic area and hypothalamic regions in the rat brain. *Neuroscience*, 6: 1601–1624.

Berk, M.L. and Finkelstein, J.A. (1981b) An autoradiographic determination of the efferent projections of the suprachiasmatic nucleus of the hypothalamus. *Brain Res.*, 226: 1–13.

Bhargava, K.P., Kulshrestha, V.K. and Srivastava, Y.P. (1972) Central cholinergic and adrenergic mechanisms in the release of antidiuretic hormone. *Brit. J. Pharmacol.*, 44: 617–627.

Bie, P. (1980) Osmoreceptors, vasopressin and control of renal water excretion. *Physiol. Rev.*, 60: 961–1048.

84

Bisset, G.W., Chowdrey, H.S. and Feldberg, W. (1978) Release of vasopressin by enkephalin. *Brit. J. Pharmacol.*, 62: 370–371.

Blessing, W.W., Sved, A.F. and Reis, D.J. (1982) Destruction of noradrenergic neurons in rabbit brainstem elevates plasma vasopressin, causing hypertension. *Science*, 217: 661–663.

Bloom, F.E., Rossier, J., Battenberg, E.L.F., Bayon, A., French, E., Henriksen, S.J., Siggins, G.R., Segal, D., Browne, R., Ling, N. and Guillemin, R. (1978) β-Endorphin: cellular localization, electrophysiological and behavioral effects. *Biochem. Psychopharmacol.*, 18: 89–108.

Bobillier, P., Seguin, F., Petitjean, D., Sabiert, M., Touret, M. and Jouvet, M. (1976) The raphe nuclei of the cat brain stem: a topographic atlas of their efferent projections as revealed by autoradiography. *Brain Res.*, 113: 449–486.

Bonjour, J.P. and Malvin, R.L. (1970) Stimulation of ADH release by the renin–angiotensin system. *Amer. J. Physiol.*, 218: 1555–1559.

Bridges, T.E. and Thorn, N.A. (1970) The effect of autonomic blocking agents of vasopressin release in vivo induced by osmoreceptor stimulation. *J. Endocr.*, 48: 265.

Brooks, V.L. and Malvin, R.L. (1979) An intracerebral physiological role for angiotensin: effects of central blockade. *Fed. Proc.*, 38: 2272–2275.

Brownell, J., Del Pozo, E. and Donatsch, P. (1980) Inhibition of vasopressin secretion by a met-enkephalin (FK 33-824) in humans. *Acta endocr.*, 94: 304–308.

Brownstein, M.J., Saavedra, J.M., Palkovitz, M. and Axelrod, J. (1974) Histamine content of hypothalamic nuclei of the rat. *Brain Res.*, 77: 151.

Buggy, J., Fisher, A.E., Hoffmann, W.E., Johnson, A.K. and Phillips, M.I. (1978) Subfornical organ: a dipsogenic site of action of angiotensin II. *Science*, 201: 380–381.

Cadnapaphornchai, P., Boykin, J., Harbottle, J., McDonald, K. and Schrier, R. (1975) Effect of angiotensin II on renal water excretion. *Amer. J. Physiol.*, 228: 155–159.

Cantalamessa, F., De Caro, G., and Pefumi, M. (1981) Water intake inhibition and vasopressin release following intracerebroventricular administration of tachykinins to rats of the Wistar and Brattleboro strain. *Pharmacol. Res. Commun.*, 13: 641–655.

Carithers, J., Bealer, S.L., Brody, M.J. and Johnson, A.K. (1980) Fine structural evidence of degeneration in supraoptic nucleus and subfornical organ of rats with lesions in the anteroventral third ventricle. *Brain Res.*, 201: 1–12.

Carlsson, A. (1962) Cellular localization of brain monoamines. *Acta Physiol. Scand.*, Suppl. 196: 1.

Changaris, D.G., Severs, W.B. and Keil, L.C. (1978) Localization of angiotensin in rat brain. *J. Histochem. Cytochem.*, 26: 593–607.

Clarke, G., Wood, P., Merrick, L. and Lincoln, D.W. (1979) Opiate inhibition of peptide release from the neurohumoral terminals of hypothalamic neurones. *Nature (Lond.)*, 282: 746–748.

Clarke, G., Lincoln, D.W. and Wood, P. (1981) Inhibition of vasopressin neurones by intraventricular morphine. *J. Physiol. (Lond.)*, 303: 59P–60P.

Cowley, A.W., Jr., Quinn, M., Quillen, E.W. and Hockel, G.M. (1979) Vasopressin and thirst response to chronic i.v. angiotensin II infusion. *Fed. Proc.*, 38: 967.

Cross, B.A. and Green, J.D. (1959) Activity of single neurones in the hypothalamus: effect of osmotic and other stimuli. *J. Physiol. (Lond.)*, 148: 554–569.

Cross, B.A. and Dyball, R.E.J. (1974) Central pathways for neurohypophyseal hormone release. In E. Knobil and W.H. Sawyer (Eds.), *Handbook of Physiology. Endocrinology. Vol. IV*, Williams and Wilkins, 1974, pp. 269–286.

De Bodo, R.C. (1944) The antidiuretic action of morphine and its mechanism. *J. Pharmacol. exp. Ther.*, 82: 74.

De Caro, G., Massi, M. and Miscossi, L.G. (1978) Antidipsogenic effect of intracranial injections of substance P in rats. *J. Physiol. (Lond.)*, 279: 133–140.

De Wied, D. and Laszlo, F.A. (1967) Effect of autonomic blocking agents on ADH-release induced by hyperosmoticity. *J. Endocr.*, 37: xvi.

Dogterom, J., Van Wimersma Greidanus, Tj.B. and De Wied, D. (1976) Histamine as an extremely potent releaser of vasopressin in the rat. *Experientia*, 32: 659.

Dreifuss, J.J. and Kelly, J.S. (1970) Excitation of identified supraoptic neurones by the iontophoretic application of acetylcholine. *J. Physiol. (Lond.)*, 212: 170P–172P.

Duke, H.N. and Pickford, M. (1951) Observations on the action of acetylcholine and adrenaline on the hypothalamus. *J. Physiol. (Lond.)*, 114: 325–332.

Duke, H.N., Pickford, M. and Watt, J.A. (1950) The immediate and delayed effects of diisopropylflourophosphate injected into the supraoptic nuclei of dogs. *J. Physiol. (Lond.)*, 111: 81–88.

Dyball, R.E.J. (1968) The effects of drugs on the release of vasopressin. *Brit. J. Pharmacol. Chemother.*, 33: 329–341.

Dyball, R.E.J. and Shaw, F.D. (1979) Inhibition by GABA of hormone release from the neurohypophysis in the rat. *J. Physiol. (Lond.)*, 289: 78.

Fee, A.R. (1929) Studies on water diuresis. Part 1. The effect of decerebration, anesthesia and morphine upon water diuresis. *J. Physiol. (Lond.)*, 68: 39–44.

Finley, J.C.W., Lindstrom, P. and Petrusz, P. (1981a) Immunocytochemical localization of β-endorphin-containing neurons in the rat brain. *Neuroendocrinology*, 33: 28–42.

Finley, J.C.W., Maderdrut, J.L. and Petrusz, P. (1981b) The immunocytochemical localization of enkephalin in the central nervous system of the rat. *J. comp. Neurol.*, 198: 541–565.

Firemark, H.M. and Weitzman, R.E. (1979) Effects of β-endorphin, morphine and naloxone on AVP secretion and the electroencephalogram. *Neuroscience*, 4: 1895–1902.

Fuxe, K. (1965) Evidence for the existence of monoamine neurons in the central nervous system. IV. The distribution of monoamine nerve terminals in the central nervous system. *Acta physiol. scand.*, 64, Suppl. 247: 37–85.

Fuxe, K., Ganten, D., Hökfelt, T. and Bolme, P. (1976) Immunohistochemical evidence for the existence of angiotensin II containing nerve terminals in the brain and spinal cord in the rat. *Neurosci. Lett.*, 2: 229–234.

Gagnon, D.J., Sirois, P. and Boucher, P.J. (1975) Stimulation by angiotensin II of the release of vasopressin from incubated rat neurohypophyses-possible involvement of cyclic AMP. *Clin. exp. Pharm. Physiol.*, 2: 305–313.

Ganten, D., Unger, T., Simon, W., Schanz, K., Schölkens, B., Mann, J.F.E., Speck, G., Lang, R. and Rascher, W. (1981) Central peptidergic stimulation: Focus on cardiovascular actions of angiotensin and opioid peptides. In J.P. Buckley and C.M. Ferrario (Eds.), *Perspectives in Cardiovascular research, Vol. 6, Central Nervous System Mechanisms in Hypertension*, Raven, New York, pp. 265–282.

Garcia-Sevilla, J.A., Dubocovich, M.L. and Langer, S.Z. (1979) Angiotensin II facilitates the potassium-evoked release of ^{3}-H-noradenaline from the rabbit hypothalamus. *Europ. J. Pharmacol.*, 56: 173–176.

Gregg, C.M. and Malvin, R.L. (1978) Localization of central sites of action of angiotensin II on ADH release in vitro. *Amer. J. Physiol.*, 234: F135–F140.

Grossman, A., Besser, G.M., Milles, J.J. and Baylis, P.H. (1980) Inhibition of vasopressin release in man by an opiate peptide. *Lancet*, 1108.

Gutman, Y., Shamir, Y., Glushevitzky, D. and Hochman, S. (1972) Angiotensin increases microsomal (Na^+-K^+) ATPase activity in several tissues. *Biochim. biophys. Acta*, 273: 401–405.

Haas, H.L., Wolf, P. and Nussbaumer, J.C. (1975) Histamine: action on supraoptic and other hypothalamic neurons of the cat. *Brain Res.*, 88: 166.

Haldar, J. and Sawyer, W.H. (1978) Inhibition of oxytocin release by morphine and its analogs (40080). *Proc. Soc. exp. Biol. Med.*, 157: 476–480.

Haldar, J., Hoffman, D.L., Nilaver, G. and Zimmerman, E.A. (1979) Oxytocin and vasopressin release by substance P injected into the cerebral ventricles of rats. *Neuroendocrinology*, 1511: 447.

Hammer, M., Ølgaard, K. and Madsen, S. (1980) The inability of angiotensin II infusions to raise plasma vasopressin levels in haemodialysis patients. *Acta endocr.*, 95: 422–426.

Hayward, J.N. (1975) Neurol control of the posterior pituitary. *Ann. Rev. Physiol.*, 37: 191–210.

Hillar, J.M., Pearson, J. and Simon, E.J. (1973) Distribution of stereospecific binding of the potent narcotic analgesic etorphine in human brain: Predominance in the limbic system. *Pathol. Pharmacol.*, 6: 1052–1062.

Hoffman, G.E. (1983) LHRH neurons and their projections. In Y. Sano, Y. Ibata and E.A. Zimmerman (Eds.), *Structure and Function of Aminergic and Peptidergic Neurons*, Japan Sci. Soc. Press, in press.

Hoffman, W.E., Phillips, M.I. and Schmid, P. (1977) The role of catecholamines in central antidiuretic and pressor mechanisms. *Neuropharmacology*, 16: 563–569.

Ishikawa, S., Saito, T. and Yoshida, S. (1980) The effect of osmotic pressure and angiotensin II on arginine vasopressin release from guinea pig hypothalamo-neurohypophyseal complex in organ culture. *Endocrinology*, 106: 1571.

Itoh, K., Kamiya, T. and Hisada, S. (1974) Effects of histamine and related compounds on the release of antidiuretic hormone. *Jap. J. Pharmacol.*, 28: 128.

Iversen, L.L., Iversen, S.D. and Bloom, F.E. (1980) Opiate receptors influence vasopressin release from nerve terminals in rat neurohypophysis. *Nature (Lond.)*, 284: 350–351.

Jewell, P.A. and Verney, E.B. (1957) An experimental attempt to determine the site of neurohypophyseal osmoreceptors in the dog. *Phil. Trans. roy. Soc.*, 240: 197–324.

Johnson, A.K. and Sladek, C.D. (1979) The effect of anteroventral 3rd ventricle region lesions on osmotic stimulation of vasopressin release by the organ cultured rat hypothalamo-neurohypophyseal system. *Soc. Neurosci. Abstr.*, 5: 448.

Johnston, C.I., Newman, M. and Woods, R. (1981) Role of vasopressin in cardiovascular homeostasis and hypertension. *Clin. Sci.*, 61: 129s–139s.

Joynt, R.J. (1966) Verney's concept of the osmoreceptor. *Arch. Neurol.*, 14: 331–344.

Keil, L.C., Summy-Long, J. and Severs, W.B. (1975) Release of vasopressin by angiotensin II. *Endocrinology*, 96: 1063–1065.

Kilcoyne, M.M., Hoffman, D.L. and Zimmerman, E.A. (1980) Immunocytochemical localization of angiotensin II and vasopressin in rat hypothalamus: evidence for production in the same neuron. *Clin. Sci.*, 59: 57S–60S.

Kimura, H., McGeer, P.L., Peng, J.H. and McGeer, E.G. (1981) The central cholinergic system studied by choline acetyltransferase immunohistochemistry in the cat. *J. comp. Neurol.*, 200: 151–201.

Kimura, T., Share, L., Wang, B.C. and Crofton, J.T. (1981) The role of central adrenoreceptors in the control of vasopressin release and blood pressure. *Endocrinology*, 108: 1829–1836.

Koh, E.T. and Ricardo, J.A. (1979) Connections of hypothalamic neurosecretory nuclei with visceral sensory structures in the brainstem of the rat. *Soc. Neurosci. Abstr.*, 5: 450.

Krettek, J.E. and Price, J.L. (1978) Amygdaloid projections to subcortical structures within the basal forebrain of the brainstem in the rat and cat. *J. comp. Neurol.*, 178: 225–280.

Kuhn, E.R. (1974) Cholinergic and adrenergic release mechanism for vasopressin in the male rat: a study with injections of neurotransmitters and blocking agents into the third ventricle. *Neuroendocrinology*, 16: 255–264.

Landas, S., Phillips, M.I., Stamler, J.F. and Raizada, M.K. (1980) Visualization of specific angiotensin II binding sites in the brain by fluorescent microscopy. *Science*, 210: 791–793.

Lederis, K. (1974) Neurosecretion in the functional structure of the neurohypophysis. In *The Handbook of Physiology, Section 7, Endocrinology, Vol. 4*, Amer. Physiol. Soc., Washington, DC, pp. 81–102.

Leibowitz, S.F. (1980) Neurchemical systems of the hypothalamus in control of feeding and drinking behavior and water–electrolyte excretion. In P.J. Morgane and J. Panksepp (Eds.), *Handbook of the Hypothalamus, Vol. 3a*, Marcel Dekker, New York, pp. 299–437.

Leng, G. (1980) Rat supraoptic neurones: the effects of locally applied hypertonic saline. *J. Physiol. (Lond.)*, 304: 405–414.

Leng, G., Mason, W.T. and Dyer, R.G. (1982) The supraoptic nucleus as an osmoreceptor. *Neuroendocrinology*, 34: 75–82.

Lightman, S.L. and Forsling, M.L. (1980a) Evidence for endogenous opioid control of vasopressin release in man. *J. clin. Endocr. Metab.*, 50: 569–571.

Lightman, S.L. and Forsling, M.L. (1980b) The effects of the methionine enkephalin analogue DAMME on the vasopressin response to tilt in man. *Clin. Sci.*, 59: 501–503.

Lightman, S.L., Iversen, L.L. and Forsling, M.L. (1982) Dopamine and (D-Ala^2, D-Leu^5)-enkephalin inhibit the electrically stimulated neurohypophyseal release of vasopressin in vitro: evidence for calcium-dependent opiate action. *J. Neurosci.*, 2: 78–81.

Lindvall, O. and Björklund, A. (1974) The glyoxylic acid fluorescence histochemical method: A detailed account for the methodology for the visualization of central catecholamine neurons. *Histochemistry*, 39: 97–127.

Ljungdahl, A., Hökfelt, T. and Nilsson, G. (1978a) Distribution of substance P-like immunoreactivity in the central nervous system of the rat. I. Cell bodies and nerve terminals. *Neuroscience*, 3: 861–943.

Lord, J.A.H., Waterfield, A.A., Hughes, J. and Kosterlitz, H.W. (1977) Endogenous opioid peptides: multiple agonists and receptors. *Nature (Lond.)*, 267: 495–499.

Martin, R. and Voigt, K.H. (1981) Enkephalins co-exist with oxytocin and vasopressin in nerve terminals of rat neurohypophysis. *Nature (Lond.)*, 289: 502–504.

Martin, W.R. (1967) Opioid antagonists. *Pharmacol. Rev.*, 19: 463–522.

Mason, W.T. (1980) Supraoptic neurons of rat hypothalamus are osmosensitive. *Nature (Lond.)*, 287: 154–157.

Mata, M., Gainer, H. and Klee, W. (1977) Effect of dehydration on the endogenous opiate content of the rat neuro-intermediate lobe. *Life Sci.*, 21: 1159–1163.

Matsuguchi, H., Sharabi, F.M., Gordon, F.J., Johnson, A.K. and Schmid, P.G. (1982) Blood pressure and heart rate responses to vasopressin microinjection into the nucleus tractus solitarius region of the rat. *Neuropharmacol.*, 21: 687–693.

Mathison, R.D. and Dreifuss, J.J. (1981) The neurohypophysial GABA system. In F.V. DeFeudis and P. Mandel (Eds.), *Amino Acid Neurotransmitters*, Raven Press, New York.

McNeill, T.H. and Sladek, J.R., Jr. (1980) Simultaneous monamine histofluorescence and neuropeptide immunocytochemistry: II. Correlative distribution of catecholamine varicosities and magnocellular neurosecretory neurons in the rat supraoptic and paraventricular nuclei. *J. comp. Neurol.*, 193: 1023–1033.

Meyer, D.K. and Brownstein, M.J. (1980) Effect of surgical deafferentation of the supraoptic nucleus on its choline acetyltransferase content. *Brain Res.*, 193: 566–569.

Meyer, D.K., Oertel, W.H. and Brownstein, M.H. (1980) Deafferentation studies on the glutamic acid decarboxylase content of the supraoptic nucleus of the rat. *Brain Res.*, 200: 165–168.

Micevych, P. and Elde, R. (1980) The relationship between enkephalinergic neurons and the vasopressin-oxytocin neuroendocrine system of the cat. An immunohistochemical study. *J. comp. Neurol.*, 190: 135–146.

Miller, M. (1980) Role of endogenous opioids in neurohypophysial function in man. *J. clin. Endocr., Metab.*, 50: 1016–1020.

Milton, A.S. and Paterson, A.T. (1974) A microinjection study of the control of antidiuretic hormone release by the supraoptic nucleus of the hypothalamus in the cat. *J. Physiol. (Lond.)*, 241: 607–628.

Minchen, M.C.W. and Beart, P.M. (1975) Compartmentation of amino acid metabolism in the rat posterior pituitary. *J. Neurochem.*, 24: 881–884.

Miselis, R.R. (1981) The efferent projections of the subfornical organ of the rat: a circumventricular organ within a neural network subserving water balance. *Brain Res.*, 230: 1–23.

Miselis, R.R. (1982) Recent advances in subfornical organ morphology. *Front. Horm. Res.*, 9: 79–87.

Miselis, R.R., Shapiro, R.E. and Hand, P.J. (1979) Subfornical organ efferents to neural systems for control of body water. *Science*, 205: 1022–1025.

Morris, M., McCann, S.M. and Orias, R. (1977) Role of transmitters in mediating hypothalamic control of electrolyte excretion. *Cand. J. Physiol. Pharmacol.*, 55: 1143–1154.

Moss, R.L., Dyball, R.E. and Cross, B.A. (1971) Responses of antidromically identified supraoptic and paraventricular units to acetycholine, noradrenaline and glutamine applied iontophoretically. *Brain Res.*, 35: 573–575.

Moss, R.L., Urban, I. and Cross, B.A. (1972) Microelectrophoresis of cholinergic and aminergic drugs on paraventricular neurons. *Amer. J. Physiol.*, 223: 310–318.

Mouw, D., Bonjour, J.P., Malvin, R.L. and Vander, A. (1971) Central action of angiotensin in stimulating ADH release. *Amer. J. Physiol.*, 220: 239–242.

Nicoll, R.A. and Barker, J.L. (1971) Excitation of supraoptic neurosecretory cells by angiotensin II. *Nature New Biol.*, 233: 172–174.

Olssen, K. (1970) Effects on water diuresis of infusions of transmitter substances into the 3rd ventricle. *Acta physiol scand.*, 79: 133.

Palkovitz, M., Brownstein, M., Saavedra, J.M. and Axelrod, J. (1974) Norepinephrine and dopamine content of hypothalamic nuclei of the rat. *Brain Res.*, 77: 137–149.

Philbin, D.M. and Coggins, C.H. (1978) Plasma antidiuretic hormone levels in cardiac surgical patients during morphine and halothane anesthesia. *Anesthesiology*, 49: 95–98.

Philbin, D.M., Wilson, N.E., Sokoloski, J. and Coggins, C. (1976) Radioimmunoassay of antidiuretic hormone during morphine anaesthesia. *Canad. Anaesth. Soc. J.*, 23: 290–295.

Phillips, M.I., Weyhenmeyer, J., Felix, D., Ganten, D. and Hoffman, W.E. (1979) Evidence for an endogenous brain renin-angiotensin system. *Fed. Proc.*, 38: 2260–2266.

Pickford, M. (1939) The inhibitory effect of acetylcholine on water diuresis in the dog, and its pituitary transmission. *J. Physiol. (Lond.)*, 95: 226–238.

Pickford, M. (1947) The action of acetylcholine in the supraoptic nucleus of chloralosed dog. *J. Physiol. (Lond.)*, 106: 264–270.

Pittman, Q.J., Hatton, J.D. and Bloom, F.E. (1980) Morphine and opioid peptides reduce paraventricular neuronal activity: studies on the rat hypothalamic slice preparation. *Proc. nat. Acad. Sci. (U.S.A.)*, 77: 5527–5531.

Post, S. and Mai, J.K. (1980) Contribution to the amygdaloid projection field in the rat. A quantitative autoradiographic study. *J. Hirnforsch.*, 21: 199–225.

Ramsay, D.J. (1979) The brain renin angiotensin system: a re-evaluation. *Neuroscience*, 4: 313–321.

Ramsay, D.J., Keil, L.C., Sharpe, M.C. and Shinsako, J. (1978) Angiotensin II infusion increases vasopressin, ACTH and 11-hydroxycorticosteroid secretion. *Amer. J. Physiol.*, 234: R66–R71.

Reid, I.A. (1977) Is there a brain renin-angiotensin system? *Circulat. Res.*, 41: 147–153.

Reid, I.A. (1979) The brain renin–angiotensin system: a critical analysis. *Fed. Proc.*, 38: 2255–2259.

Robertson, G.L., Shelton, R.L. and Athar, S. (1976) The osmoregulation of vasopressin. *Kidney Int.*, 10: 25–37.

Rossier, J., Pittman, Q., Bloom, F. and Guillemin, R. (1980) Distribution of opioid peptides in the pituitary: a new hypothalamic-pars nervosa enkephalinergic pathway. *Fed. Proc.*, 39: 2555–2560.

Ruoff, J.J., Gosbee, J.L. and Lederis, K. (1974) Substances affecting the release of neurohypophyseal hormones. In K. Lederis and K.E. Cooper (Eds.), *Recent Studies Hypothalamic Function*, Karger, Basel, pp. 67–79.

Sakai, K.K., Marks, B.H., George, J.M. and Koestner, A. (1974a) The isolated organ cultured supraoptic nucleus as a neuropharmacological test system. *J. Pharmacol. exp. Ther.*, 190: 482–491.

Sakai, K.K., Marks, B.H., George, J. and Koostner, A. (1974b) Specific angiotensin II receptors in organ cultured canine supra-optic nucleus cells. *Life Sci.*, 14: 1337–1344.

Saper, C.B., Swanson, L.W. and Cowan, W.M. (1976) The efferent connections of the ventromedial nucleus of the rat. *J. comp. Neurol.*, 169: 409–442.

Saper, C.B., Swanson, L.W. and Cowan, W.M. (1978) The efferent connections of the anterior hypothalamic area of the rat, cat and monkey. *J. comp. Neurol.*, 182: 575–600.

Saper, C.B., Swanson, L.W. and Cowan, W.M. (1979) An autoradiographic study of the efferent connections of the lateral hypothalamic area. *J. comp. Neurol.*, 183: 689–706.

Sar, M., Stumpf, W.E., Miller, R.J., Chang, K.-J. and Cuatrecasas, P. (1978) Immunohistochemical localizations of enkephalin in rat brain and spinal cord. *J. comp. Neurol.*, 182: 17–38.

Sawchenko, P. and Swanson, L.W. (1981) Central noradrenergic pathways for the integration of hypothalamic neuroendocrine and autonomic responses. *Science*, 214: 685–687.

Sawchenko, P.E., Swanson, L.W. and Joseph, S.A. (1982) The distribution and cells of origin of $ACTH_{1-39}$-stained varicosities in the paraventricular and supraoptic nuclei. *Brain Res.*, 232: 365–374.

Share, L. (1974) Blood pressure, blood volume, and the release of vasopressin. In E. Knobil and W.H. Sawyer (Eds.), *Handbook of Physiology. Endocrinology, Vol. IV*, Williams and Wilkins, Baltimore, MD, pp. 243–256.

Shimizu, K., Share, L. and Claybaugh, J.R. (1973) Potentiation by angiotensin II of the vasopressin response to an increasing plasma osmolality. *Endocrinology*, 93: 42–50.

Silver, J. and Billiar, R.B. (1976) An autoradiographic analysis of $[^3H]\alpha$-bungarotoxin distribution in the rat brain after intraventricular injection. *J. Cell Biol.*, 71: 956–963.

Silverman, A.J., Hoffman, D.L. and Zimmerman, E.A. (1981a) The descending afferent connections of the paraventricular nucleus of the hypothalamus (PVN). *Brain Res. Bull.*, 6: 47–61.

Silverman, A.J., Hoffman, D., Gadde, C.A., Krey, L.C. and Zimmerman, E.A. (1981b) Adrenal steroid inhibition of the vasopressin-neurophysin neurosecretory system to the median eminence of the rat. *Neuroendocrinology*, 32: 129–133.

Simanotov, R. and Snyder, S.H. (1977) Opiate receptor binding in the pituitary gland. *Brain Res.*, 124: 178–184.

Simpson, J.B., Reed, M., Keil, L.C., Thrasher, T.N. and Ramsay, D.J. (1979) Forebrain analysis of vasopressin (AVP) secretion and water intake by angiotensin II (AII). *Fed. Proc.*, 38: 982.

Sirett, N.E., McClean, A.S., Bray, J.J. and Hubbard, J.I. (1977) Distribution of angiotensin II receptors in the rat brain. *Brain Res.*, 122: 299–312.

Sladek, C.D. (1980) Osmotic control of vasopressin release: role of acetylcholine and angiotensin. In S. Yoshida, L. Share and K. Yagi (Eds.), *Antidiuretic Hormone*, Univ. Park Press, Baltimore, pp. 117–132.

Sladek, C.D. and Johnson, A.K. (1982) The effect of anteroventral third ventricle lesions on vasopressin release by organ cultured hypothalamo-neurohypophyseal explants. *Neuroendocrinology*, in press.

Sladek, C.D. and Joynt, R.J. (1979a) Characterization of cholinergic control of vasopressin release by the organ cultured rat hypothalamo-neurohypophyseal system. *Endocrinology*, 104: 659–663.

Sladek, C.D. and Joynt, R.J. (1979b) Angiotensin stimulation of vasopressin release from the rat hypothalamo-neurohypophyseal system in organ culture. *Endocrinology*, 104: 148–153.

Sladek, C.D. and Joynt, R.J. (1979c) Cholinergic involvement in osmotic control of vasopressin release by the organ cultured rat hypothalamo-neurohypophyseal system. *Endocrinology*, 105: 367–371.

Sladek, C.D. and Joynt, R.J. (1980a) Role of angiotensin in the osmotic control of vasopressin release by the organ culture rat hypothalamo-neurohypophyseal system. *Endocrinology*, 106: 173–178.

Sladek, C.D. and Knigge, K.M. (1977) Osmotic control of vasopressin release by rat hypothalamo-neurohypophyseal explants in organ culture. *Endocrinology*, 101: 1834–1838.

Sladek, C.D., Blair, M.L. and Ramsay, D.J. (1982a) Further studies on the role of angiotensin in the osmotic control of vasopressin release by the organ cultured rat hypothalamo-neurohypophyseal system. *Endocrinology*, 111: 599–607.

Sladek, C.D., Gallagher, M. and Mudd, M. (1982b) The effects of opiate peptides on vasopressin release. *Soc. Neurosci., Abstr.*, 8: 223.

Sladek, C.D., Armstrong, W.E. and Sladek, J.R. (1983) Relationship between noradrenergic and osmotic control of vasopressin release. In Y. Sano, Y. Ibata and E.A. Zimmerman (Eds.), *Structure and Function of Aminergic and Peptidergic Neurons*, Japan Sci. Soc. Press, in press.

Sofroniew, M.V. (1983) *J. comp. Neurol.*, in press.

Stamler, J.F., Raizada, M.K., Fellows, R.E. and Phillips, M.I. (1980) Increased specific binding of Angiotensin II in the organum vasculosum of the laminae terminalis area of the spontaneously hypertensive rat brain. *Neurosci. Lett.*, 17: 173–177.

Steinbusch, H.W.M. (1981) Distribution of serotonin-immunoreactivity in the central nervous system of the rat-cell bodies and terminals. *Neuroscience*, 6: 557–618.

Summy-Long, J.Y., Rosella, L.M. and Keil, L.C. (1981) Effects of centrally administered endogenous opioid peptides on drinking behavior, increased plasma vasopressin concentration and pressor response to hypertonic sodium chloride. *Brain Res.*, 221: 343–357.

Sundsten, J.W. and Sawyer, C.H. (1961) Osmotic activation of neurohypophyseal hormone release in rabbits with hypothalamic islands. *Expl. Neurol.*, 4: 548–561.

Swanson, L.W. (1976) An autoradiographic study of the efferent connections of the preoptic region in the rat. *J. comp. Neurol.*, 167: 227–256.

Swanson, L.W. and Cowan, W.M. (1975) The efferent connections of the suprachiasmatic nucleus of the hypothalamus. *J. comp. Neurol.*, 160: 1–12.

Swanson, L.W. and Cowan, W.M. (1977) An autoradiographic study of the organization of the efferent connections of the hippocampal formation in the rat. *J. comp. Neurol.*, 172: 49–84.

Swanson, L.W. and Cowan, W.M. (1979) The connections of the septal region in the rat. *J. comp. Neurol.*, 186: 621–655.

Swanson, L.W. and Kuypers, H.G.J.M. (1980) The paraventricular nucleus of the hypothalamus: cytoarchitectonic subdivisions and the organization of projections to the pituitary, dorsal vagal complex and spinal cord as demonstrated by retrograde flourescence double-labeling methods. *J. comp. Neurol.*, 194: 555–570.

Swanson, L.W., Sawchenko, P.E., Bérod, A., Hartman, B.K., Helle, K.B. and Vanorden, D.E. (1981) An immunohistochemical study of the organization of catecholaminergic cells and terminal fields in the paraventricular and supraoptic nuclei of the hypothalamus. *J. comp. Neurol.*, 196: 271, 1981.

Tager, H., Hohenboken, M., Markese, J. and Dinerstein, R.J. (1980) Identification and localization of glucagon-related peptides in rat brain. *Proc. nat. Acad. Sci. U.S.A.*, 77: 6229–6233.

Tappaz, M., Brownstein, M.J. and Kopin, I. (1977) Glutamate decarboxylase (GAD) and γ-aminobutyric acid (GABA) in discrete nuclei of hypothalamus and substantia nigra. *Brain Res.*, 125: 109–121.

Taube, H.D., Starke, K. and Borowski, E. (1977) Presynaptic receptor systems on the noradrenergic neurones of rat brain. *Naunyn-Schmiedeberg's Arch. Pharmacol.*, 299: 123–141.

Taylor, K.M., Gfeller, E. and Snyder, S.H. (1972) Regional localization of histamine and histidine in the brain of the rhesus monkey. *Brain Res.*, 41: 171–176.

Thrasher, T.N., Brown, C.J., Keil, L.C. and Ramsay, D.J. (1980) Thirst and vasopressin release in the dog: an osmoreceptor or sodium receptor mechanism? *Amer. J. Physiol.*, 238: R333–R339.

Thrasher, T.N., Keil, L.C. and Ramsay, D.J. (1982) Lesions of the organum vasculosum of the lamina terminalis (OVLT) attenuate osmotically-induced drinking and vasopressin secretion in the dog. *Endocrinology*, 110: 1837–1839.

Tribollet, E. and Dreifuss, J.J. (1981) Localization of neurons projecting to the hypothalamic paraventricular nucleus area of the rat: a horseradish peroxidase study. *Neuroscience*, 6: 1315–1328.

Turker, R.K., Page, I.H. and Khairallah, P.A. (1967) Angiotensin alteration of sodium fluxes in smooth muscle. *Arch. int. Pharmacodyn.*, 165: 394–404.

Uhlich, E.P., Weber, P., Eigler, J. and Gröschel-Stewart, U. (1975) Angiotensin stimulated AVP-release in humans. *Klin. Wschr.*, 53: 177–180.

Unger, T., Rascher, W., Schuster, C., Pavlovitch, R., Schomig, A., Dietz, R. and Ganten, D. (1981) Central blood pressure effects of substance P and angiotensin II: role of the sympathetic nervous system and vasopressin. *Europ. J. Pharmacol.*, 71: 33–42.

Ungerstedt, J. (1971) Stereotaxic mapping of the monoamine pathways in the rat brain. *Acta physiol. scand.*, Suppl. 367: 1–48.

Urano, A. and Kobayashi, A. (1978) Effects of noradrenaline and dopamine injected into the supraoptic nucleus on urine flow rate in hydrated rats. *Exp. Neurol.*, 60: 140–150.

Vandeputte-Van Messon, G. and Peeters, G. (1975) Effect of intraventricular administration of noradrenaline on water diuresis in goats. *J. Endocr.*, 66: 375–383.

Vanderhaegen, J.J., Lotstra, F., Vierendulo, G., Gilles, C., Deschepper, C. and Verbanck, P. (1981) Cholecystokinins in the central nervous system and neurohypophysis. *Peptides*, 2, Suppl. 2: 81–88.

Van Gemert, M., Miller, M., Carey, R.J. and Moses, A.M. (1975) Polyuria and impaired ADH release following medial preoptic lesioning in the rat. *Amer. J. Physiol.*, 228: 1293.

Van Wimersma Greidanus, Tj.B., Thody, T.J., Verspaget, H., De Rotte, G.A., Goedemans, H.J.H., Croiset, G. and Van Ree, J.M. (1978) Effects of morphine and β-endorphin on basal and elevated plasma levels of α-MSH and vasopressin. *Life Sci.*, 24: 579–586.

Van Wimersma Greidanus, Tj.B., Van Ree, J.M., Goedemans, H.J.H., Van Dam, A.F., Andringa-Bakker, E.A.D. and De Wied, D. (1981) Effects of β-endorphin fragments on plasma levels of vasopressin. *Life Sci.*, 29: 783–788.

Verney, E.B. (1947) The antidiuretic hormone and the factors which determine its release. *Proc. roy. Soc. Lond. B.*, 135: 25–106.

Vizi, E.S. and Volbekas, V. (1980) Inhibition by dopamine of oxytocin release from isolated posterior lobe of the hypophysis of the rat; disinhibitory effect of β-endorphin/enkephalin. *Neuroendocrinology*, 31: 46–52.

Watson, S.J., Akil, H., Fischli, W., Goldstein, A., Zimmerman, E.A., Nilaver, G. and Van Wimersma Greidanus Tj.B. (1982) Dynorphin and vasopressin: Common localization in magnocellular neurons. *Science*, 216: 85–87.

Weitzman, R.E., Fisher, D.A., Minick, S., Ling, N. and Guillemin, R. (1977) β-Endorphin stimulates secretion of arginine vasopressin in vivo. *Endocrinology*, 101: 1643.

Weyhenmeyer, J.A. and Phillips, M.I. (1979) Immunocytochemical localization of angiotensin II in the CNS of Wistar Kyoto and spontaneously hypertensive rats. *Soc. Neurosci. Abstr.*, 5: 544.

Wolny, H.L., Plech, A. and Herman, Z.S. (1974) Diuretic effects of intraventricularly injected noradrenaline and dopamine in rats. *Experientia*, 30: 1062–1063.

Woods, J.W. and Bard, P. (1960) Antidiuretic hormone in the cat with a centrally denervated hypothalamus. *Acta endocr.*, Suppl. 51: 113.

Zimmerman, E.A., Stillman, M.A., Recht, L.D., Antunes, J.L., Carmel, P.W. and Goldsmith, P.C. (1977) Vasopressin and corticotropin-releasing factor: an axonal pathway to portal capillaries in the zona externa of the median eminence containing vasopressin and its interaction with adrenal corticoids. *Ann. N.Y. Acad. Sci.*, 297: 405–419.

Zingg, H.H., Baertschi, A.J. and Dreifuss, J.J. (1979) Action of γ-aminobutyric acid on hypothalamo-neurohypophysial axons. *Brain Res.*, 171: 453–459.

The Neurohypophysis: Structure, Function and Control, Progress in Brain Research, Vol. 60, edited by B.A. Cross and G. Leng
© *1983 Elsevier Science Publishers B.V.*

The Organum Vasculosum Laminae Terminalis: A Critical Area for Osmoreception

D.J. RAMSAY, T.N. THRASHER and L.C. KEIL[1]

Department of Physiology, University of California, San Francisco, San Francisco, CA 94143 and [1]Ames Research Center, Moffett Field, CA 94035 (U.S.A.)

INTRODUCTION

The volume and composition of the body fluids is maintained by coordinated control of water intake by thirst mechanisms and water output via vasopressin secretion. The knowledge that plasma osmolality has a major effect on drinking was firmly established by Gilman (1937). Ten years later, Verney established a link between plasma osmolality and vasopressin release and showed the location of these osmoreceptors to be in the area of perfusion of the carotid arteries (Verney, 1947). Since that time, relationships between plasma osmolality and drinking (Wood et al., 1977) and vasopressin secretion (Robertson et al., 1977) have been described in many species and in many laboratories. There is general agreement that if plasma osmolality is increased above a threshold, vasopressin secretion is stimulated (Wade et al., 1982). It is also clear that, as osmotic responses can be obtained when hyperosmotic solutions are infused via the carotids in doses which are ineffective given systematically, the osmoreceptors are located within the brain. The elegant experiments of Jewell and Verney (1957) localized the osmoreceptors to the anterior hypothalamus and concluded that they were in the vicinity and possibly even in the supraoptic nucleus.

THE NATURE AND LOCATION OF THE OSMORECEPTOR

The precise nature of the osmoreceptor as well as its location has also been the subject of debate. Andersson and his coworkers (1978) have postulated that the osmoreceptors are sensitive to sodium concentration rather than to osmolality. Moreover, from the results of infusion studies in goat, he argues that the sodium receptive elements are located in periventricular sites and are thus sensitive to changes in cerebrospinal fluid (CSF) sodium concentration rather than to plasma. The major evidence for this theory comes from the observation that intracerebroventricular (i.c.v.) infusions of hypertonic sodium solutions stimulate drinking and antidiuresis, whereas similarly hypertonic infusions of sucrose are without effect (Olsson, 1969). Moreover, i.c.v. injections of glycerol sufficient to decrease CSF sodium concentration by at least 25 mEq/l blocked drinking in dehydrated goats. Similarly, the drinking and antidiuresis produced by intracarotid infusions of hyperosmotic sodium chloride were blocked by simultaneous i.c.v. infusion of various saccharide solutions (Olsson, 1972, 1973).

In our laboratory using dogs as the experimental model, we can find no evidence in support of sodium receptors for CSF. I.c.v. infusions of sucrose and sodium chloride were equally

92

potent in the stimulation of vasopressin secretion and drinking (Thrasher et al., 1980b). In these experiments, similarly hypertonic solutions of glucose and urea were without effect on drinking and vasopressin release. Thus, it appears that to be effective a solute must be excluded by cell membranes and cause cell shrinkage, but that solute does not have to be sodium. These experiments also give some information about the location of the osmoreceptors if the size of the stimulus which has to be delivered is taken into account. To elicit increases in vasopressin secretion, the local osmolality in the third ventricle has to be increased by approximately 50 mOsm, that is, 18%. Calculations based on measurements of CSF sodium concentration made by McKinley et al. (1980) suggest that similar increases in osmolality are necessary in sheep to elicit osmotic responses (Thrasher, 1982). This contrasts sharply with the changes of 1–2% in plasma osmolality which are known to cause vasopressin secretion. Results from this type of study indicate that the osmoreceptors are likely to be located in an area of the brain influenced by plasma, rather than by CSF composition (McKinley et al., 1978).

Experiments involving peripheral infusion of solutes give further information about the location of osmoreceptors (Thrasher et al., 1980a). In these experiments, plasma osmolality was raised in conscious dogs by the infusion of hypertonic sodium chloride or sucrose, solutes which do not penetrate cells and thus cause osmotic extraction of water, and of glucose and urea, which do penetrate cells and thus would not cause withdrawal of cell water. Measurements of changes in plasma and CSF osmolality and sodium concentration were made, as well as plasma vasopressin concentration and drinking behaviour. In these experiments, dogs drank 14 ± 1 min after the beginning of infusion of sodium and 16 ± 1 min following the infusion of sucrose. No drinking was observed with hyperosmolar infusions of urea or glucose even though those infusions were continued for 45 min. At the point when drinking occurred in the case of sodium and sucrose infusions, marked elevation of plasma vasopressin concentration was noted. No increase in plasma vasopressin concentration was seen in the case of urea and glucose infusions. Similar results have been reported in sheep (McKinley et al., 1978).

The simultaneously measured changes in CSF sodium and osmolality are shown in Fig. 1. All hypertonic infusions cause similar elevation in CSF sodium and osmolality. This is presumably mainly due to withdrawal of water across the blood–CSF and blood–brain barriers.

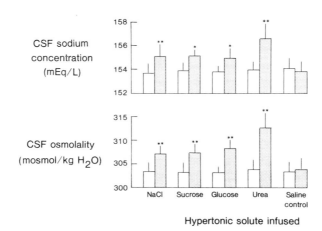

Fig. 1. Mean change in CSF sodium concentration and osmolality following intravenous infusion of 1.7 Osm solutions of NaCl, sucrose, glucose, urea or iso-osmotic saline in 5 dogs. Initial levels (open bars) and final levels (hatched bars) are shown. The final levels are either at the threshold of drinking (NaCl and sucrose) or after 45 min of infusion if no drinking occurred (glucose, urea, saline control). * $P < 0.05$, ** $P < 0.01$.

Although CSF sodium and osmolality were increased in all cases, drinking and vasopressin release was seen only in the case of sodium chloride and sucrose. The failure of glucose and urea to stimulate vasopressin secretion and drinking in the face of evidence of brain dehydration makes it unlikely that osmoreceptors can be sensitive to changes in CSF.

The significance of these findings is illustrated in Fig. 2. The figure represents two possible locations of osmoreceptors. The upper panel depicts the situation with osmoreceptors lying on the brain side of an intact blood–brain barrier. Thus, infusions of hyperosmotic sodium chloride and of urea would cause osmotic withdrawal of water across the interstitial fluid, raising the osmolality locally in this area causing osmotic extraction of water from cells. That the whole brain behaves in this way was shown from our peripheral infusion results in which intravenous urea infusion does cause increases in CSF sodium concentration and osmolality. If osmoreceptors were located on the brain side of the blood–brain barrier, then urea should have been as effective as sodium and sucrose in increasing vasopressin secretion.

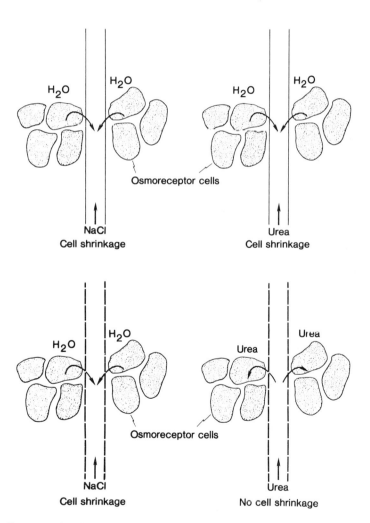

Fig. 2. Effect of hyperosmotic infusions of NaCl or urea on osmoreceptors lying inside (top) the blood–brain barrier, or where the blood–brain barrier is deficient (bottom).

The lower panel depicts the situation in which the blood supply to the area of brain containing osmoreceptors lacks a blood–brain barrier. Infusions of hypertonic sodium chloride would cause increases in interstitial fluid sodium concentration and osmotic extraction of cell water and the expected osmoreceptor response. However, the response to infusion of urea would be quite different. Infused urea could enter interstitial fluid due to the absence of a permeability barrier and then would be freely available to enter cells. Cell membranes — and brain cells are no exception — are freely permeable to urea. Therefore, there will be no osmotic extraction of water and no osmotic response. Similar arguments could be made for glucose and other solutes which can easily pass through cell membranes. Thus, the failure of infusion of such non-penetrating solutes in our experiments and in those of others to stimulate vasopressin secretion and drinking predicates that the osmoreceptors must be located in an area of brain lacking the blood–brain barrier. An obvious and likely site would seem to be one of the circumventricular organs.

An argument against this view has been put forth by Leng and his colleagues (1982). These authors have presented evidence largely based on electrophysiological experimentation in their and other laboratories that the osmoreceptors are within the supraoptic nucleus. Moreover, they argue that the high vascularity of the supraoptic nucleus makes it an ideal site for the location of such osmoreceptors. However, although the supraoptic nucleus is highly vascular, there is no evidence that there is an absence of the blood–brain barrier. Indeed, there is evidence to the contrary. Horseradish peroxidase, injected intravenously, readily penetrates circumventricular organs, but does not enter the supraoptic nucleus. Recently, it has been shown that ^{125}I-labelled angiotensin II following intravenous infusion is found in high concentrations in the subfornical organ (SFO) and organum vasculosum laminae terminalis (OVLT) but none is found in the supraoptic nucleus (van Houten, personal communication). There is no histological evidence for the presence of fenestrated capillaries as there is in circumventricular organs. As judged by these criteria, cells of the supraoptic nucleus lie on the brain side of an intact blood–brain barrier and should therefore respond to peripheral infusions of urea and of glucose (Fig. 2). It would seem that the circumventricular organ is a more likely site for such osmoreceptors.

Lesions of the anterior ventral region of the third ventricle (AV3V), which include the OVLT ventrally and extend to the anterior commissure dorsally, cause profound disturbances in both osmotic and volaemic regulation of water balance (Buggy and Johnson, 1977; Brody et al., 1978). Consequently, structures contained in this area of destruction which include the OVLT have been proposed as the critical area for this function (Phillips, 1978). The difficulty with the interpretation of these experiments in rats is the size of the lesion and the inclusion of many structures and the presumed destruction of many pathways. We therefore set out to examine this problem in dogs. Although the stereotaxic coordinates of brain structures are more variable and less known in the dog, the increased size of the brain makes it more feasible to carry out discrete lesions in this species. Moreover, the use of contrast X-ray techniques (Thrasher et al., 1980b) allow a precise localization of the electrode tip to be made before the lesion is made. Also, the advantage of being able to make multiple observations of vasopressin responses in an animal before and after lesioning make the dog an ideal experimental model.

EVIDENCE THAT THE OVLT CONTAINS THE OSMORECEPTORS

The OVLT is a likely candidate as the circumventricular organ containing the osmoreceptors for a number of reasons. This area is certainly contained in the AV3V lesions in rats. The result of intracarotid infusions localize the osmoreceptors to the forebrain. The subfornical organ would appear to be ruled out as the site of osmoreceptors in dogs as, judged by drinking data, lesions of this region cause a loss of sensitivity to angiotensin II but do not affect responses to hypertonic saline (Thrasher et al., 1982b). Furthermore, the experiments of Jewell and Verney (1957) localized the osmoreceptors to a region of the brain which included the OVLT. In experiments designed to evaluate the importance of the OVLT, a total of 17 dogs were employed. On separate occasions, the effect of infusions of hypertonic saline on plasma vasopressin concentration and on drinking were tested. This was necessary as we had previously shown that drinking acts as a potent inhibitory influence to vasopressin secretion (Thrasher et al., 1981). Lesions were made under sodium pentobarbital anaesthesia using full aseptic conditions. A third ventricular cannula was implanted and X-ray contrast medium (Iothalamate meglumine) was injected. Following a lateral view X-ray and knowing the position of the cannula in the ventricle, the longitudinal and the vertical coordinates of the optic recess were calculated. A second midline hole was then drilled in the midsagittal suture and the lesion electrode lowered to the calculated depth. Following a further X-ray to confirm accurate placement of the electrode, two anodal lesions, 0.5 mm apart on the vertical plane, were made, aimed at the dorsal and ventral margins of the optic recess.

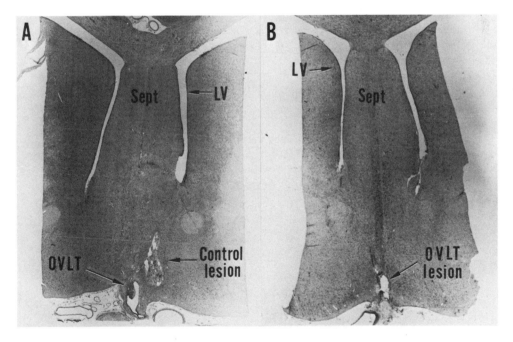

Fig. 3. A: coronal section at level of optic recess showing the OVLT. Lesion is lateral and dorsal to OVLT. B: coronal section showing complete lesion of OVLT.LV, lateral ventricle; Sept, septum. × 5. (From Thrasher et al., 1982a, with permission.)

A typical lesion is shown in Fig. 3. Six animals had lesions which destroyed more than 90 % of the OVLT. The lesion was centred on the midline and anterior tip of the optic recess showed heavy gliosis, but only slight damage to the anterior periventricular tissue. In 11 dogs, the lesion missed the OVLT and caused damage either unilaterally in the wall of the third ventricle or other surrounding tissues. However, the volume of tissue destroyed was similar to that in the OVLT-lesioned animals.

For seven days following the OVLT lesion, there was a significant elevation in plasma osmolality (Fig. 4). However, this was not accompanied by any increase in plasma vasopres-

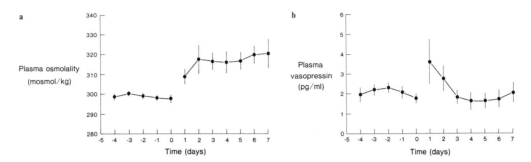

Fig. 4. The effect of OVLT lesions on plasma osmolality (a) and plasma vasopressin (b). The lesion was made on day 0. n = 6.

sin concentration. Moreover, there was no significant increase in daily water intake. One to six weeks following the OVLT lesion, plasma osmolality had returned to normal. At this point, the effect of hypertonic saline infusion on drinking and vasopressin release was repeated (Figs. 5 and 6). Before the lesion, there were significant relationships between plasma osmolality and both drinking and vasopressin secretion. In the OVLT-lesioned animals, however, the slopes of these relationships were significantly reduced. Thus, the lesioned animals were much less sensitive to osmotic stimulation.

This point may be further illustrated by a study of the increase in osmolality necessary to cause osmotic effects. Before lesioning, the increase in plasma osmolality that was necessary to stimulate drinking in all dogs was 9.0 ± 1.4 mOsm/kg H_2O. After lesioning, drinking began after an increase of 8.1 ± 0.9 mOsm/kg H_2O in the control group. In marked contrast, an increase of 24.1 ± 2.1 mOsm/kg H_2O was required to stimulate drinking in dogs with OVLT lesions. In normal dogs 24 h of water deprivation causes an increase in plasma osmolality of

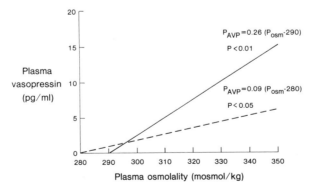

Fig. 5. The relationship between plasma osmolality and vasopressin concentration in 6 dogs following destruction of the OVLT. Solid line, before; broken line, after.

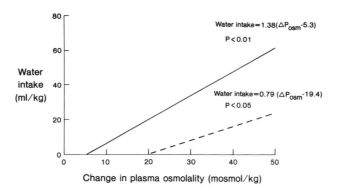

Fig. 6. The relationship between plasma osmolality and drinking in 6 dogs following destruction of the OVLT. Solid line, before; broken line, after.

approximately 10 mOsm/kg. This change in plasma osmolality represents the largest increase one might expect to occur under normal physiological circumstances. In the absence of an OVLT, dogs would be incapable of responding to such an osmotic challenge. It is of great interest that a recent report shows inhibition of osmotically induced water intake by OVLT lesions in sheep (McKinley et al., 1982).

A criticism of any lesion study may be made that a pathway is being destroyed. However, in our studies the OVLT lesions were small and confined mainly to the organ, its attachment to the lamina terminalis and to the ependyma of the optic recess. It would seem to be unlikely that bilateral destruction of periventricular pathways in this region occurred. Moreover, in animals where the OVLT was not destroyed, but where the lesions extended laterally, osmotic responses were similar to those in control animals. These results are not due to damage to the supraoptic nucleus, as in dogs the OVLT is approximately 3 mm anterior to this structure.

Unfortunately, studies aimed at elucidating the connections of the OVLT have not been carried out in the dog. However, there are projections from the OVLT to the supraoptic nucleus in rats. In this respect, the results of Dyball and Prilusky (1981) are intriguing. These authors report that anterior hypothalamic knife cuts inhibited the osmotic responsiveness of neurones in the supraoptic nucleus. Although the precise location of these knife cuts was unclear, they were certainly in the right area to have interrupted connections between the OVLT and the supraoptic nucleus. Further studies of this type are certainly warranted.

SUMMARY

Evidence from our laboratory and from others demonstrates that the osmoreceptors behave as if they were located in an area of the brain lacking the blood–brain barrier. Moreover, this area is likely to be in the anterior hypothalamus. Although there is electrophysiological evidence that cells elsewhere in the brain, such as the supraoptic nucleus, show osmosensitivity, their capacity to respond to reasonable osmotic challenges is in question. Animals with discrete lesions of the OVLT have greatly diminished responses to osmotic stimuli and abolition of these responses over reasonable physiological range (Thrasher et al., 1982a). Whereas the identity of the osmoreceptors remains elusive, their anatomical home, the OVLT, is more certain.

98

REFERENCES

Andersson, B. (1978) Regulation of water intake. *Physiol. Rev.*, 58: 582–603.

Broadwell, R.D. and Brightman, M.W. (1976) Entry of peroxidase into neurons of the central and peripheral nervous system from extracerebral and cerebral blood. *J. comp. Neurol.*, 166: 257–284.

Brody, M.J., Fink, G.D., Buggy, J., Haywood, J.R., Gordon, F.J. and Johnson, A.K. (1978) The role of the anteroventral third ventricle (AV3V) region in experimental hypertension. *Circulat. Res.*, 43: 12–18.

Buggy, J. and Johnson, A.K. (1977) Preoptic-hypothalamic periventricular lesions: thirst deficits and hypernatremia. *Amer. J. Physiol.*, 233 (Regulatory Integrative Comp. Physiol., 2): R44–R52.

Dyball, R.E.J. and Prilusky, J. (1981) Responses of supraoptic neurones in the intact and deafferented rat hypothalamus to injections of hypertonic NaCl. *J. Physiol. (Lond.)*, 311: 443–452.

Gilman, A. (1937) The relations between blood osmotic pressure, fluid distribution and voluntary water intake. *Amer. J. Physiol.*, 120: 323–328.

Leng, G., Mason, W.T. and Dyer, R.G. (1982) The supraoptic nucleus as an osmoreceptor. *Neuroendocrinology*, 34: 75–82.

Jewell, P.A. and Verney, E.B. (1957) An experimental attempt to determine the site of the neurohypophyseal osmoreceptors in the dog. *Phil. Trans. roy. Soc. Lond. B*, 240: 197–324.

McKinley, M.J., Denton, D.A. and Weisinger, R.S. (1978) Sensors for antidiuresis and thirst — osmoreceptors or CSF sodium detectors? *Brain Res.*, 141: 89–103.

Mc Kinley, M.J., Denton, D.A., Leksell, L., Tarjan, E. and Weisinger, R.W. (1980) Evidence for cerebral sodium sensors involved in water drinking in sheep. *Physiol. Behav.*, 25: 501–504.

McKinley, M.J., Denton, D.A., Leksell, L.C., Mouw, D.R., Scoggins, B.A., Smith, M.H., Weisinger, R.S. and Wright, R.D. (1982) Osmoregulatory thirst in sheep is disrupted by ablation of the anterior wall of the optic recess. *Brain Res.*, 236: 210–215.

Phillips, M.I. (1978) Angiotensin in the brain. *Neuroendocrinology*, 25: 354–377.

Olsson, K. (1969) Studies on central regulation of secretion of antidiuretic hormone (ADH) in the goat. *Acta physiol. scand.*, 77: 465–474.

Olsson, K. (1972) On the importance of CSF Na$^+$ concentrations in central control of fluid balance. *Life Sci.*, 11: 397–402.

Olsson, K. (1973) Further evidence for the importance of CSF Na$^+$ concentrations in central control of fluid balance. *Acta. physiol. scand.*, 88: 183–188.

Robertson, G.L., Athar, S. and Shelton, R.L. (1977) Osmotic control of vasopressin function. In T.E. Andreoli, J.J. Grantham and F.C. Rector, Jr. (Eds.), *Disturbances in Body Fluid Osmolality*, American Physiological Society, Bethesda, MD, pp. 125–148.

Thrasher, T.N. (1982) Osmoreceptor mediation of thirst and vasopressin secretion in the dog. *Fed. Proc.*, 41: 2528–2532.

Thrasher, T.N., Brown, C.J., Keil, L.C. and Ramsay, D.J. (1980a) Thirst and vasopressin release in the dog: an osmoreceptor or sodium receptor mechanism? *Amer. J. Physiol.*, 238 (Regulatory, Integrative Comp. Physiol., 7): R333–R339.

Thrasher, T.N., Jones, R.G., Keil, L.C., Brown, C.J. and Ramsay, D.J. (1980b) Drinking and vasopressin release during ventricular infusions of hypertonic solutions. *Amer. J. Physiol.*, 238 (Regulatory, Integrative Comp. Physiol., 7): R340–R345.

Thrasher, T.N., Nistal-Herrera, J.F., Keil, L.C. and Ramsay, D.J. (1981) Satiety and inhibition of vasopressin secretion after drinking in dehydrated dogs. *Amer. J. Physiol.*, 240 (Endocrinol. Metab., 3): E394–E401.

Thrasher, T.N., Keil, L.C. and Ramsay, D.J. (1982a) Lesions of the organum vasculosum of the lamina terminalis (OVLT) attenuate osmotically-induced drinking and vasopressin secretion in the dog. *Endocrinology*, 110: 1837–1841.

Thrasher, T.N., Simpson, J.B. and Ramsay, D.J. (1982b) Lesions of the subfornical organ block angiotensin-induced drinking in the dog. *Neuroendocrinology*, 35: 63–68.

Verney, E.B. (1947) The antidiuretic hormone and the factors which determine its release. *Proc. roy. Soc. Lond. B*, 135: 25–106.

Wade, C.E., Bie, P., Keil, L.C. and Ramsay, D.J. (1982) Osmotic control of vasopressin in the dog. *Amer. J. Physiol.*, in press.

Wood, R.J., Rolls, B.J. and Ramsay, D.J. (1977) Drinking following intracarotid infusions of hypertonic solutions in dogs. *Amer. J. Physiol.*, 232 (Regulatory, Integrative Comp. Physiol., 1): R88–R92.

Central Projections of the Magnocellular Neurosecretory Neurones

The Neurohypophysis: Structure, Function and Control, Progress in Brain Research, Vol. 60, edited by B.A. Cross and G. Leng

Morphology of Vasopressin and Oxytocin Neurones and Their Central and Vascular Projections

M.V. SOFRONIEW

Department of Human Anatomy, University of Oxford, South Parks Road, Oxford OX1 3QX (U.K.)

INTRODUCTION

The study of the morphology of the neurohypophysis and of the neurones which project to it has a long tradition using Golgi (Ramón y Cajal, 1911), silver (Romeis, 1940) and neurosecretory stains (Bargmann, 1949). During the past 10 years, immunohistochemical techniques have allowed identification of substances produced by individual neurones and visualization of different structures containing these substances.

Use of these techniques has not only answered a number of long standing questions, but has also greatly expanded concepts about the distribution, projections and functions of neurones producing vasopressin and oxytocin. There is increasing evidence that hypothalamo-neurohypophysial neurones produce peptides in addition to the two just mentioned. In this report, immunohistochemical studies on the distribution, morphology and projections of neurones producing classical neurohypophysial peptides will be reviewed. Evidence that neurones in this system may produce additional peptides will be discussed, and functional implications considered. Detailed descriptions of the principles underlying immunohistochemical studies and of the various techniques employed are widely available (see Cuello et al., 1983; Sternberger, 1979) and will not be described here.

BIOSYNTHESIS OF VASOPRESSIN, OXYTOCIN AND ASSOCIATED NEUROPHYSINS

Vasopressin and oxytocin are associated with a family of low molecular weight proteins, the neurophysins, also present in extracts of the neurohypophysis (Pickering, 1976). Gainer and co-workers (Gainer et al., 1977; Russell et al., 1980; Gainer, this volume) provided conclusive evidence that the neurophysins are portions of precursor proteins from which the peptides and the neurophysins are cleaved. Their findings indicate that there are separate precursors for vasopressin and its associated neurophysin and for oxytocin and its associated neurophysin. Recently, Land et al. (1982) derived the amino acid sequence for the bovine vasopressin precursor using cloned cDNA. This precursor contains one sequence of vasopressin, one sequence of vasopressin-associated neurophysin and a 39 amino acid glycoprotein, and contains no sequence for oxytocin or any other known peptide.

NEURONES PRODUCING VASOPRESSIN AND OXYTOCIN

One of the initial applications of immunohistochemical techniques to the study of the hypothalamo–neurohypophysial system was to investigate whether vasopressin and oxytocin were produced in the same or in separate neurones. Vandesande and co-workers (Vandesande and Dierickx, 1975; Vandesande et al., 1975a, b; Dierickx and Vandesande, 1979) showed in various mammals that neurones contain either vasopressin and its associated neurophysin, or oxytocin and its associated neurophysin. In view of the biochemical findings, it seems that these neurones express only one or the other of the two precursors. Immunohistochemical work from a number of laboratories has shown that both vasopressin and oxytocin neurones are present in each of the two principal hypothalamic magnocellular nuclei, the supraoptic and paraventricular nuclei (SON and PVN), and are not segregated into separate nuclei as some early studies had suggested. It is now clear that there are a large number of vasopressin and oxytocin neurones in various locations, and that these neurones are heterogeneous in morphology and probably in function as well.

Perhaps the most conspicuous of the newly identified locations is the suprachiasmatic nucleus, located bilaterally in the midline at the base of the third ventricle just dorsal to the optic chiasm. In this nucleus a portion of the neurones contain vasopressin (but not oxytocin) and its associated neurophysin and are parvocellular (10–15 μm in diameter). They have been found in all mammals investigated thus far including the human and other primates (Sofroniew and Weindl, 1980). In various mammals they constitute from 17 to 30% of the population of the suprachiasmatic nucleus. At present their function is unknown.

A large number of so-called accessory magnocellular vasopressin and oxytocin neurones have also been found scattered in various groups throughout the hypothalamus. Considerable species variation exists in their precise location, but several groups are present in most mammals including humans. As yet there is no accepted nomenclature for them. The most well represented groups in different mammals are: (1) a group in the dorsal anterior hypothalamus extending towards the stria terminalis; (2) diffuse cells and small groups in the anterior hypothalamus between the SON and PVN; (3) diffuse cells and small groups in the posterior hypothalamus; and (4) a group near the fornix in the posterior hypothalamus. Many species have other groups unique to themselves. For example, one prominent group in the rat, the anterior commissural nucleus, which is composed of oxytocin neurones projecting to the neurohypophysis, is not present in most other mammals, including other rodents such as the guinea pig (personal observation). Fig. 1 depicts the location of some of the larger groups in the rat, but it should be emphasized that this description cannot in all cases be extrapolated to other species. The function of these dispersed groups is not understood. Neurones in different groups appear in some cases to have differing projections. It also appears that different groups may be sensitive to different afferent stimuli. For example, neurones in some (but not other) accessory groups in the rat are contacted by somatostatin fibres and terminals as revealed by two-colour immunoperoxidase staining (see Fig. 6 in Sofroniew and Schrell, 1982).

We have recently found neurones containing neurophysin and vasopressin in several areas outside the hypothalamus (Fig. 1). These findings derive from normal and colchicine-treated Sprague–Dawley, Wistar and Brattleboro rats. Using a Bouin/sublimate (Sofroniew and Schrell, 1982) fixative and frozen or vibratome sections, the sensitivity of the immunoperoxidase staining surpassed that of our previous studies. In addition to revealing new fibre pathways, new locations of immunoreactive cell bodies have been found. These include perikarya in the medial amygdala (Fig. 2a) and bed nucleus of the stria terminalis (Fig. 2b) and ventral lateral septum. Neurones in these areas stain for neurophysin and vasopressin. The

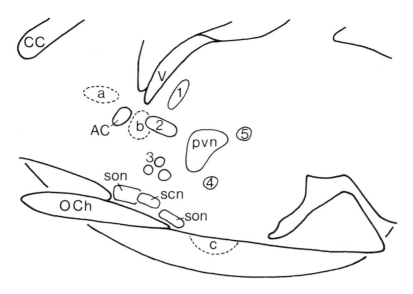

Fig. 1. Sagittal view of the rat diencephalon depicting the approximate topography of the more prominent groups of vasopressin and oxytocin neurones. The supraoptic (son) and paraventricular (pvn) nuclei contain both vasopressin and oxytocin neurones. The numbers 1–5 refer to large groups of so-called accessory magnocellular neurones for which there is no generally accepted nomenclature. The groups shown are: (1) a group extending towards the stria terminalis; (2) a group of oxytocin neurones just caudal to the anterior commissure sometimes referred to as the anterior commissural nucleus; (3) several groups in the rostral hypothalamus between the son and pvn; (4) groups in the posterior hypothalamus; (5) a group lateral to the fornix. The suprachiasmatic nucleus (scn) contains parvocellular vasopressin (but not oxytocin) neurones. The letters a, b and c refer to newly identified groups of neurophysin (and some vasopressin) parvocellular neurones such as those shown in Fig. 2 and found in the ventral lateral septum (a), bed nucleus of the stria terminalis (b) and medial amygdala (c). AC, anterior commissure; CC, corpus callosum; OCh, optic chiasm; V, ventricle.

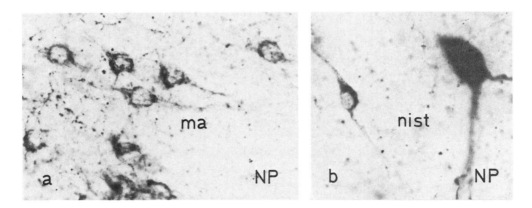

Fig. 2 a and b: parvocellular neurophysin (NP) immunoreactive neurones in (a) the medial amygdala (ma) and (b) the nucleus interstitialis (bed nucleus) stria terminalis (nist) in a normal rat. In b, compare the much smaller size and less intense staining of the parvocellular neurone on the left with the magnocellular neurone on the right.

staining is far weaker than that obtained for hypothalamic neurones but increases under colchicine treatment. The negative findings with staining for oxytocin are not conclusive as they may be due to the weaker affinity of the antiserum. Although more investigation is required to verify the specificity of the staining, the presence of these neurones could alter current concepts about the organization of the central projections of vasopressin and oxytocin neurones.

The immunohistochemical procedure can be used to achieve staining similar to Golgi impregnation, allowing a fairly detailed analysis of neuronal morphology. Hypothalamic vasopressin, oxytocin and neurophysin neurones examined in this way (Sofroniew and Glasmann, 1981) exhibit a heterogeneous morphology which varies according to location within the hypothalamus. Most neurones are simple in appearance, with one or several sparsely branching dendrites and one unbranching axon. The size and shape of perikarya varies considerably, ranging from 10 to 30 μm in diameter with some being round or oval and some having a spindle shape. Certain neurones also have different types of peptide-containing processes. Some groups consist of different shaped neurones, while others consist of similarly appearing neurones. The PVN is particularly heterogeneous, consisting of a number of differently appearing neurones which are in part intermingled and in part segregated into groups within the nucleus. In some areas, particularly the caudal PVN, a number of neurones have axons which give rise to short or long collateral branches. Thus some neurones may project to more than one area.

Similar findings have been observed in analysis of vasopressin and oxytocin neurones grown in tissue culture (Sofroniew et al., 1982b; Sofroniew, Gähwiler and Dreifuss, unpublished), which enables the detailed examination of single neurones and the full extent of their processes. A number of cultured PVN neurones have axons which give rise to long collaterals.

CO-LOCALIZATION OF DIFFERENT PEPTIDES AND ENZYMES IN VASOPRESSIN AND OXYTOCIN NEURONES

The concept that a neurone may release more than one active substance is expanding in all areas of the nervous system (see Chan-Palay and Palay, 1983). There is good evidence that in the SON some vasopressin neurones contain dynorphin (Watson et al., 1982) and some oxytocin neurones contain cholecystokinin (Vanderhaegen et al., 1981). These neurones also all contain acetylcholinesterase, and different subpopulations may contain other peptides and other enzymes as well (for review see Sofroniew et al., 1983). Space does not permit a detailed discussion of the methodological criteria for establishing co-localization; however, this is a critical issue since certain examples of immunohistochemical co-localization have been shown to be artifact (see Sofroniew et al., 1983). Nevertheless, the evidence in favour of some examples of co-localization is strong and this phenomenon will undoubtedly influence future functional concepts.

DISTRIBUTION OF VASOPRESSIN AND OXYTOCIN FIBRES AND TERMINALS

Immunohistochemical techniques were initially applied to studying neuroendocrine aspects of vasopressin and oxytocin neurones confirming their classical projection to the capillaries of the posterior pituitary. During these studies, a prominent vasopressin projection to the portal

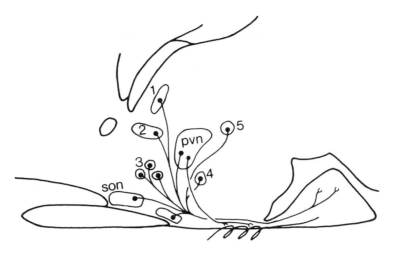

Fig. 3. Sagittal view of the rat hypothalamus and pituitary depicting the vascular projections of hypothalamic vasopressin and oxytocin neurones. Most vasopressin and oxytocin neurones in the supraoptic nucleus (son), rostral paraventricular nucleus (pvn) and various accessory nuclei (1–5, see Fig. 1) project to the posterior pituitary. In addition, some neurones in the pvn project to portal capillaries in the median eminence. No vascular projections have been found from the parvocellular vasopressin neurones of the suprachiasmatic nucleus.

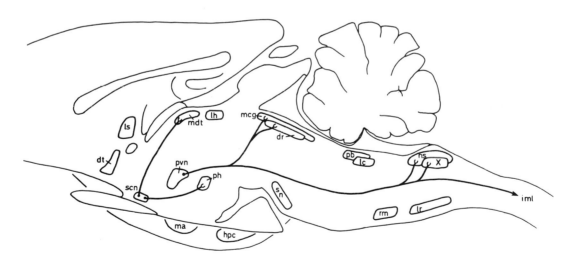

Fig. 4. Sagittal view of the rat brain depicting some of the major areas containing vasopressin and oxytocin fibres and terminals and showing some afferent pathways as established by experimental techniques. The abbreviations are: dr, dorsal raphe; dt, nucleus of the diagonal tract (Broca); hpc, hippocampus; iml, intermediolateral nucleus of the spinal cord; lc, locus coeruleus; lh, lateral habenula; lr, lateral reticular nucleus; ls, lateral septum; ma, medial amygdala; mcg, mesencephalic central grey; mdt, mediodorsal thalamus; ns, nucleus of the solitary tract; pb, parabrachial nuclei; ph, periventricular posterior hypothalamus; rm, raphe magnus; sn, substantia nigra; X, dorsal vagal nucleus. In some cases the projections derive from the paraventricular (pvn) or suprachiasmatic (scn) nuclei as shown. In the other cases the exact origin of the projections is not certain.

106

capillaries of the median eminence (Fig. 3) was noted, and evidence now suggests that this projection is involved in regulation of adenohypophysial ACTH release.

Subsequently, oxytocin and neurophysin fibres were found in areas not directly related to neuroendocrine pathways, leading to the discovery of an extensive network of such fibres throughout the central nervous system (Weindl and Sofroniew, 1976; Buijs, 1980; Sofroniew and Weindl, 1978; Nilaver et al., 1980). Although initial observations were made in rodents, the findings have largely been confirmed in other mammalian species including humans and other primates (Sofroniew, 1980; Sofroniew et al., 1981). Table I lists the major areas of the central nervous system containing fibres and (where known) the location of neurones giving rise to each projection. Fig. 4 depicts the location of some of the major target areas and known projections. Although species differences in the numbers of fibres in different areas have been observed, qualitatively the distribution of fibres appears to be similar in many mammals. The areas containing vasopressin and oxytocin fibres are diverse, ranging from autonomic centres in the brainstem and spinal cord, to limbic centres and even to neocortex (Fig. 5). However, the density of fibres or terminals varies dramatically from single isolated fibres, as in the neocortex, to dense innervation, as in the solitary nucleus and dorsal vagal nucleus in the medulla oblongata.

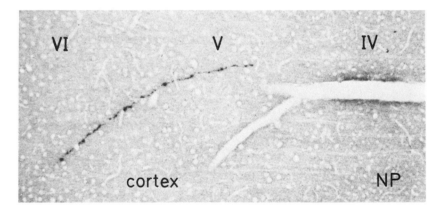

Fig. 5. Neurophysin (NP) fibre in layers V and VI of the frontal cortex of a Brattleboro (vasopressin deficient) rat.

NATURE OF TERMINALS IN VASCULAR AND NEURAL TARGET AREAS

In the neurohypophysis, terminals of neurosecretory axons have been studied at the ultrastructural level in connection with the mechanics of the secretory process (Theodosis et al., 1976; Morris and Nordmann, 1980). Due to the extreme density of terminals in the neurohypophysis it is difficult to visualize the extent of the terminals deriving from individual axons. In hypothalamic neurones grown in organotypic tissue culture (Sofroniew et al., 1982b) we noted cases of individual SON neurones reinnervating co-cultured neurohypophyses. In these cases single axons all gave rise to extensive plexuses of interconnected and highly arborized terminals, indicating that single neurosecretory neurones may give rise to many terminals in the neurohypophysis.

In neural target areas, fibres or terminals can often be seen contacting neuronal cell bodies (counterstained with a Nissl stain) or proximal processes. In fortunate preparations, terminals can be seen lining perikarya or dendrites (Fig. 6), even in human specimens (see Sofroniew,

TABLE I

DISTRIBUTION OF VASOPRESSIN AND OXYTOCIN FIBRES IN BRAIN AND SPINAL CORD

• Indicates regular presence of a few fibres and possibly terminals; + indicates regular presence of a number of fibres and/or terminals; ++ to ++++ indicate increasing density of fibres and/or terminals. The nucleus of origin is the nucleus giving rise to the vasopressin or oxytocin projections to the indicated area. pvn, paraventricular nucleus; scn, suprachiasmatic nucleus.

Area	Vasopressin	Oxytocin	Nucleus of origin
(I) Forebrain			
anterior hippocampus	•	•	
cerebral cortex (including frontal, piriform, cingulate and entorhinal cortex)	•	•	
n. accumbens	•	•	
n. tractus diagonalis Broca	++	•	
lateral septum	++++	•	
n. interstitialis stria terminalis	+	•	
central, anterior, basal, cortical and lateral amygdala	+	+	
medial amygdala	++	+	
ventral hippocampus	+	+	
mediodorsal thalamus	+++	•	scn[a]
lateral habenula	++++		
posterior periventricular hypothalamus	+++		scn
n. supramammillaris	•	+	
(II) Midbrain			
substantia nigra pars compacta	++	++++	
ventral tegmental area	+	++	
central grey	+	+	
n. raphe dorsalis	+	+	
n. interpeduncularis	•	+	
n. cuneiformis	•	+	
n. parabrachialis dorsalis	+	++	
n. parabrachialis ventralis	•	+	
locus coeruleus	+	+	
n. raphe pontis	•	•	
(III) Hindbrain			
n. raphe magnus	+	++	
n. raphe obscurus	•	•	
n. tractus solitarius	++	++++	pvn
n. dorsalis nervi vagus	++	++++	pvn
n. reticularis lateralis	+	++	
substantia gelatinosa trigemini	•	+	
(IV) Spinal cord			
laminae I–III	•	+	pvn
lamina X	+	++	pvn
n. intermediolateralis	•	+	pvn

[a] The scn gives rise only to vasopressin fibres.

1980, Figs. 4–7). The nature of the contacts is in most cases not certain since light microscopy does not provide adequate resolution. However, in some areas vasopressin and oxytocin have been identified in presynaptic structures using immunohistochemistry at the electron microscopic level (Buijs and Swaab, 1979). Fibre density generally increases in target areas over

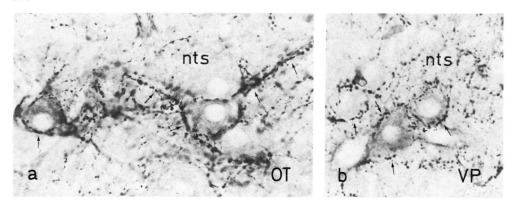

Fig. 6. a, oxytocin (OT) and b, vasopressin (VP) terminals (arrows) surrounding the somata and lining the dendrites of neurones in the nucleus of the solitary tract (nts). (From Sofroniew and Schrell, 1982.)

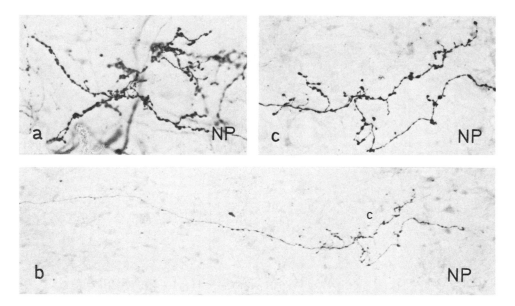

Fig. 7. a: neurophysin fibre in a 100 µm thick section through the bed nucleus of the stria terminalis. The fibre terminates within the section and gives rise to a large cluster of terminal branches. b: survey of a single axon deriving from a paraventricular neurone grown in culture. The axon ends in a cluster of terminal branches. c: detail of b showing the terminal branches. Note the similarity in appearance of the terminal branching exhibited by the in vivo (a) and cultured (b) axons. (From the unpublished work of M.V. Sofroniew, B. Gähwiler and J.J. Dreifuss.)

that seen in the afferent pathways suggesting some terminal arborization. Occasionally fibres can be seen branching in target areas (Fig. 7a). We have also examined axons of cultured PVN neurones and found many examples of single axons ending in highly branched terminal networks (Fig. 7b, c). These networks are similar to the examples of extensive terminal arborization observed in neural target areas in vivo.

ESTABLISHED PROJECTIONS

Given several types of vasopressin and oxytocin neurones in groups distributed in different locations, and an extensive network of vasopressin and oxytocin fibres in various vascular and neural target areas, an important question becomes whether different types of neurones and different groups have differing projections. Two approaches have been applied to answering this question. The first has been to lesion a group of neurones and test immunohistochemically for the loss of fibres. The second approach involves combined retrograde tracing and immunocytochemistry to establish that a group of neurones which produces a given peptide projects to a specific area. The first approach has been used to establish that the vasopressin terminals contacting the portal capillaries in the median eminence derive from the PVN (Antunes et al., 1977). These terminals, which may be involved in the regulation of ACTH secretion (Zimmerman et al., 1973; Yates and Maran, 1974; Dierickx et al., 1976; Stillman et al., 1977; Dornhost et al., 1978; Sofroniew, 1982), thus originate from the same nucleus in which separate neurones producing corticotropin releasing hormone are located (Bugnon et al., 1982). We have used the second approach to examine the distribution of vasopressin and oxytocin neurones projecting to the neurohypophysis or various areas in the central nervous system. In our procedure, tracer and peptide are both detected immunohistochemically in serial sections through the same neurone (Sofroniew and Schrell, 1981; Schrell and Sofroniew, 1982). Following injection of tracer into the posterior pituitary (Sofroniew et al., 1980), we found that all neurones in the SON which projected to the posterior pituitary also stained for neurophysin and for either vasopressin or oxytocin (Fig. 8). Conversely, virtually all vasopressin and oxytocin neurones in this nucleus project to the posterior pituitary (Fig. 8). In the PVN, vasopressin and oxytocin neurones primarily in the rostral and lateral parts of the nucleus project to the posterior pituitary, while relatively few neurones in the caudal part of the nucleus do so.

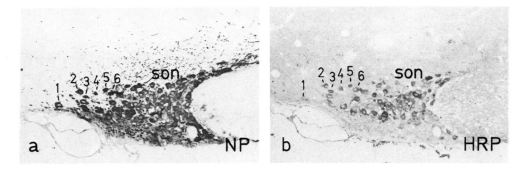

Fig. 8. Neighbouring serial 1.5 μm thick sections through the supraoptic nucleus (son) stained for (a) neurophysin (NP) and (b) horseradish peroxidase (HRP) from a rat injected with HRP into the posterior pituitary 48 h prior to fixation. All neurones in the son transporting HRP from the posterior pituitary also appear to contain NP. The numbers 1–6 indicate a few of the neurones identifiable on both sections. Neurones 2–6 stain positively for both NP and HRP while neurone 1 stains only for NP.

Some PVN neurones project to the posterior pituitary but do not contain vasopressin, oxytocin or neurophysin (see Sofroniew, 1982). Many magnocellular vasopressin and oxytocin neurones in accessory groups in various parts of the hypothalamus also project to the posterior pituitary. In particular these include all of the neurones in the anterior commissural nucleus (which are all oxytocin neurones), all the oxytocin and vasopressin neurones in the nucleus circularis, as well as those in the groups shown in Fig. 3 which summarizes the vascular projections of vasopressin and oxytocin neurones. In contrast, no vasopressin neurones in the suprachiasmatic nucleus project to the posterior pituitary. It seems likely that these neurones have no vascular projections since none of them are labelled following injection of the tracer horseradish peroxidase into the vascular system (Broadwell and Brightman, 1976).

The oxytocin and vasopressin terminals in the nucleus of the solitary tract and dorsal vagal nucleus derive from neurones in the caudal PVN (Sofroniew and Schrell, 1981; Sawchenko and Swanson, 1982). More recent experiments indicate that terminals in the spinal cord and mesencephalic central grey derive from the caudal PVN, while vasopressin terminals in the mediodorsal thalamus (Fig. 9) and periventricular posterior hypothalamus derive from the suprachiasmatic nucleus (Fig. 4). The origin of fibres in other areas is not certain, but it seems likely that fibres in the midbrain and brainstem derive largely from the PVN. However, if the preliminary observations of groups of neurophysin and vasopressin neurones outside the hypothalamus prove correct, these neurones may be responsible for the fibres observed in some areas.

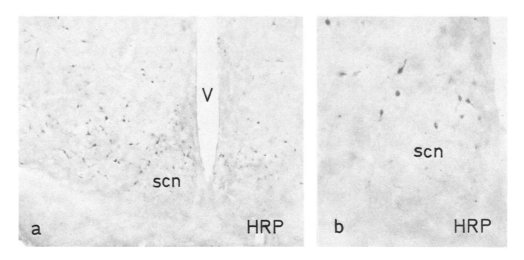

Fig. 9. Survey (a) and detail (b) of neurones in rat suprachiasmatic nucleus (scn) and surrounding hypothalamus, which have retrogradely transported horseradish peroxidase (HRP) from the mediodorsal thalamus. Note that there are a number of HRP-labelled neurones in the dorsal scn as well as in the hypothalamus dorsal and lateral to this. HRP was detected immunohistochemically. (From the unpublished work of U. Schrell and M.V. Sofroniew.)

Although much work remains to be done, a few basic tendencies regarding the projections of vasopressin and oxytocin neurones can be summarized. Vasopressin and oxytocin neurones in the SON project primarily if not exclusively to the posterior pituitary. The posterior pituitary also receives vasopressin and oxytocin projections from part of the PVN and from many accessory groups. The PVN also sends a vasopressin projection to the portal capillaries in the median eminence as well as oxytocin and vasopressin projections to various areas in the central nervous system. The vasopressin and oxytocin neurones with vascular or neural projections are located in different parts of the PVN. The parvocellular vasopressin neurones in the suprachiasmatic nucleus have no vascular projections, project to at least two neural targets, and may also make connections with other neurones within the suprachiasmatic nucleus. The exact origin of the vasopressin and oxytocin fibres in many areas is not yet certain. The tracing studies conducted so far have labelled comparatively few vasopressin or oxytocin neurones when contrasted with the density of innervation observed in neural target areas. Together with the observations of terminal arborization discussed above this suggests that a small number of neurones may give rise to a network of terminals and exert a fairly large influence.

FUNCTIONAL IMPLICATIONS

There is evidence that both vasopressin and oxytocin can alter the electrical activity of neurones in various parts of the central nervous system where fibres containing these peptides are present (Morris et al., 1980; Mühlethaler et al., 1982; Gilbey et al., 1982). These peptides might also influence other aspects of neuronal activity. Biochemical studies have shown that they can influence cAMP production (Schneider et al., 1982) or catecholamine turnover in specific brain areas (Versteeg et al., 1979). On a broader scale, much attention has been focused on the behavioural effects of vasopressin and oxytocin, particularly their effects on memory and learning (De Wied and Versteeg, 1979; Le Moal et al., 1981; Van Wimersma Greidanus et al., 1981) which have also been observed in clinical trials (Gold et al., 1979; Legros and Gilot, 1979). Vasopressin and oxytocin fibres are present in a number of areas thought to be involved in memory and other behavioural processes. These include the hippocampus; septum; nucleus of the diagonal tract (Broca), which contains cholinergic neurones (Sofroniew et al., 1982a) which probably innervate the hippocampus (Swanson and Cowan, 1979); amygdala; neocortex; and mediodorsal thalamus. In the hippocampus, which contains both oxytocin and vasopressin fibres, both peptides affect the firing rate of a particular class of neurone (Mühlethaler et al., 1982).

Vasopressin and oxytocin projections may be involved in the regulation of autonomic activity. The PVN sends vasopressin and oxytocin projections to various autonomic centres in the brainstem and spinal cord. Oxytocin and vasopressin terminals deriving from this nucleus contact preganglionic vagal neurones in the brainstem (Sofroniew and Schrell, 1981). The PVN also sends oxytocin and vasopressin projections to the sympathetic intermediolateral nucleus of the spinal cord (Sofroniew, 1980) where oxytocin, and to a lesser degree vasopressin, depresses the firing rate of neurones in a manner similar to the stimulation of the PVN (Gilbey et al., 1982). At present it is not clear which autonomic activities are affected, but both vasopressin and oxytocin have peripheral effects on blood pressure and the contractility of vascular smooth muscle. Recently, the possible involvement of vasopressin in certain forms of pathological hypertension has received much attention (Crofton et al., 1979; Möhring et al., 1981). As a large number of the areas thought to be involved in central cardiovascular regulation (Loewy and McKellar, 1980) receive vasopressin and oxytocin fibres, this may be an interesting area of future investigation. Vasopressin and oxytocin fibres are also present in brain areas thought to be involved in a variety of other functions ranging from nociception to general arousal.

SUMMARY

Vasopressin and oxytocin are present in fibres throughout the mammalian central nervous system. In target areas, fibres surround and contact neurones and in some cases these contacts have been identified as synaptic. In a number of these areas vasopressin and oxytocin have been shown to alter the electrical or biochemical activity of neurones, and may be involved in various centrally regulated functions. Thus these peptides, which were originally characterized as the circulating hormones released from the neurohypophysis, may have an additional important role in influencing the activity of central neurones through direct projections to these neurones.

ACKNOWLEDGEMENTS

The author wishes to thank B. Archer, A. Barclay and J. Lloyd for photographic and P. Campbell for editorial assistance. Grant support was provided by NINCDS (NRSA 1 F32 NS06959-01).

REFERENCES

Antunes, J.L., Carmel, P.W. and Zimmerman, E.A. (1977) Projections from the paraventricular nucleus to the zona externa of the median eminence of the rhesus monkey: an immunohistochemical study. *Brain Res.,* 173: 1–10.

Bargmann, W. (1949) Über die neurosekretorische Verknüpfung von Hypothalamus und Neurohypophyse. *Z. Zellforsch.,* 34: 610–634.

Broadwell, R.D. and Brightman, M.W. (1976) Entry of peroxidase into neurons of the central and peripheral nervous systems from extracerebral and cerebral blood. *J. comp. Neurol.,* 166: 257–284.

Bugnon, C., Fellmann, D., Gouget, A. and Cardot, J. (1982) Corticoliberin in rat brain: immunocytochemical identification and localization of a novel neuroglandular system. *Neurosci. Lett.,* 30: 25–30.

Buijs, R.M. (1980) Immunocytochemical demonstration of vasopressin and oxytocin in the rat brain by light and electron microscopy. *J. Histochem. Cytochem.,* 28: 357–360.

Buijs, R.M. and Swaab, D.F. (1979) Immuno-electron microscopical demonstration of vasopressin and oxytocin synapses in the limbic system of the rat. *Cell Tiss. Res.,* 204: 355–365.

Chan-Palay, V. and Palay, S.L. (Eds.) (1983) *Coexistence of Neuroactive Substances,* Wiley, New York.

Crofton, J.T., Share, L., Shade, R.E., Lee-Kwon, W.J., Manning, M. and Sawyer, W.H. (1979) The importance of vasopressin in the development and maintenance of DOC-salt hypertension in the rat. *Hypertension,* 1: 31–38.

Cuello, A.C., Milstein, C. and Galfre, G. (1983) Immunocytochemistry with monoclonal antibodies. In A.C. Cuello (Ed.), *Immunocytochemistry, IBRO Handbook Series, Methods in the Neurosciences,* John Wiley, Chichester, in press.

De Wied, D. and Versteeg, D.H.G. (1979) Neurohypophyseal principles and memory. *Fed. Proc.,* 38: 2348–2354.

Dierickx, K. and Vandesande, F. (1979) Immunocytochemical demonstration of separate vasopressin–neurophysin and oxytocin-neurophysin neurons in the human hypothalamus. *Cell Tiss. Res.,* 196: 203–212.

Dierickx, K., Vandesande, F. and De Mey, J. (1976) Identification, in the external region of the rat median eminence, of separate neurophysin-vasopressin and neurophysin-oxytocin-containing nerve fibres. *Cell Tiss. Res.* 168: 141–151.

Dornhorst, A., Carlson, D.E., Seif, S.M., Robinson, A.G., Zimmerman, E.A. and Gann, D.S. (1978) Control of release of adrenocorticotropin and vasopressin by the supraoptic and paraventricular nuclei. *Endocrinology,* 108: 1420–1424.

Gainer, H., Sarne, Y. and Brownstein, M.J. (1977) Biosynthesis and axonal transport of rat neurohypophysial proteins and peptides. *J. Cell Biol.,* 73: 366–381.

Gilbey, M.P., Coote, J.H., Fleetwood-Walker, S. and Peterson, D.F. (1982) The influence of the paraventriculo-spinal pathway, and oxytocin and vasopressin on sympathetic preganglionic neurones. *Brain Res.,* in press.

Gold, P.W., Weingartner, H., Ballenger, J.C., Goodwin, F.K. and Post, R.M. (1979) Effects of 1-desamino-8-D-arginine vasopressin on behaviour and cognition in primary affective disorder. *Lancet,* 992–994.

Land, H., Schütz, G., Schmale, H. and Richter, D. (1982) Nucleotide sequence of cloned cDNA encoding bovine arginine vasopressin-neurophysin II precursor. *Nature (Lond.),* 295: 299–303.

Legros, J.J. and Gilot, P. (1979) Vasopressin and memory in the human. In E.J. Peck, Jr. and A.E. Boyd, III (Eds.), *Brain Peptides: A New Endocrinology,* Elsevier/North-Holland, Amsterdam, pp. 347–364.

Le Moal, M., Koob, G.F., Koda, L.Y., Bloom, F.E., Manning, M., Sawyer, W.H. and Rivier, J. (1981) Vasopressor receptor antagonist prevents behavioral effects of vasopressin. *Nature (Lond.),* 291: 491–493.

Loewy, A.D. and McKellar, S. (1980) The neuroanatomical basis of central cardiovascular control. *Fed. Proc.*, 39: 2495–2503.

Möhring, J., Kintz, J., Schoun, J. and McNeill, J.R. (1981) Pressor responsiveness and cardiovascular reflex activity in spontaneously hypertensive and normotensive rats during vasopressin infusion. *J. Cardiovasc. Pharmacol.*, 3: 948–957.

Morris, J.F. and Nordmann, J.J. (1980) Membrane recapture after hormone release from nerve endings in the neural lobe of the rat pituitary gland. *Neuroscience*, 5: 639–650.

Morris, R., Salt, T., Sofroniew, M.V. and Hill, R.G. (1980) Actions of microiontophoretically applied oxytocin, and immunohistochemical localization of oxytocin, vasopressin and neurophysin in the rat caudal medulla. *Neurosci. Lett.*, 18: 163–168.

Mühlethaler, M., Dreifuss, J.J. and Gähwiler, B.H. (1982) Vasopressin excites hippocampal neurones. *Nature (Lond.)*, 296: 749–751.

Nilaver, G., Zimmerman, E.A., Wilkins, J., Michaels, J., Hoffman, D. and Silverman, A.J. (1980) Magnocellular hypothalamic projections to the lower brain stem and spinal cord of the rat. *Neuroendocrinology*, 30: 150–158.

Pickering, B.T. (1976) The molecules of neurosecretion: their formation, transport, and release. In M.A. Corner and D.F. Swaab (Eds.), *Perspectives in Brain Research, Progress in Brain Research, Vol. 45*, Elsevier North-Holland, Amsterdam, pp. 161–179.

Ramón y Cajal, S. (1911) *Histologie du Système Nerveux de l'Homme et des Vertébrés, Vol. 2*, A. Maloine, Paris, pp. 415–426.

Romeis, B. (1940) *Mikroskopische Technik*, Oldenbourg, München.

Russell, J.T., Brownstein, M.J. and Gainer, H. (1980) Biosynthesis of vasopressin, oxytocin, and neurophysins: isolation and characterization of two common precursors (propressophysin and prooxyphysin). *Endocrinology*, 107: 1880–1891.

Sawchenko, P.E. and Swanson, L.W. (1982) Immunohistochemical identification of neurons in the paraventricular nucleus of the hypothalamus that project to the medulla or to the spinal cord in the rat. *J. comp. Neurol.*, 205: 260–272.

Schneider, D.R., Felt, B.T. and Goldman, H. (1982) Desglycyl-8-arginine vasopressin affects regional mouse brain cyclic AMP content. *Pharmacol. Biochem. Behav.*, 16: 139–143.

Schrell, U. and Sofroniew, M.V. (1982) Use of serial 1–2 μm paraffin sections in neuropeptide immunocytochemistry for sequential analysis of different substances contained within the same neurons. *J. Histochem. Cytochem.*, 30: 512–516.

Sofroniew, M.V. (1980) Projections from vasopressin, oxytocin, and neurophysin neurons to neural targets in the rat and human. *J. Histochem. Cytochem.*, 28: 475–478.

Sofroniew, M.V. (1982) Vascular and neural projections of hypothalamic neurons producing neurohypophyseal or ACTH-related peptides. In A.J. Baertschi and J.J. Dreifuss (Eds.), *Vasopressin, Corticoliberin and ACTH-related Peptides*, Academic Press, New York, in press.

Sofroniew, M.V. and Glasmann, W. (1981) Golgi-like immunoperoxidase staining of hypothalamic magnocellular neurons that contain vasopressin, oxytocin or neurophysin in the rat. *Neuroscience*, 6: 619–643.

Sofroniew, M.V. and Schrell, U. (1981) Evidence for a direct projection from oxytocin and vasopressin neurons in the hypothalamic paraventricular nucleus to the medulla oblongata: immunohistochemical visualization of both the horseradish peroxidase transported and the peptide produced by the same neurons. *Neurosci. Lett.*, 22: 211–217.

Sofroniew, M.V. and Schrell, U. (1982) Long-term storage and regular repeated use of diluted antisera in glass staining jars for increased sensitivity, reproducibility, and convenience of single- and two-color light microscopic immunocytochemistry. *J. Histochem. Cytochem.*, 30: 504–511.

Sofroniew, M.V. and Weindl, A. (1978) Extrahypothalamic neurophysin-containing perikarya, fiber pathways and fiber clusters in the rat brain. *Endocrinology*, 102: 334–337.

Sofroniew, M.V. and Weindl, A. (1980) Identification of parvocellular vasopressin and neurophysin neurons in the suprachiasmatic nucleus of a variety of mammals including primates. *J. comp. Neurol.*, 193: 659–675.

Sofroniew, M.V., Schrell, Y., Glasmann, W., Weindl, A. and Wetzstein, R. (1980) Hypothalamic accessory magnocellular vasopressin, oxytocin and neurophysin neurons projecting to the neurohypophysis in the rat. *Soc. Neurosci. Abstr.*, 6: 456.

Sofroniew, M.V., Weindl, A., Schrell, U. and Wetzstein, R. (1981) Immunohistochemistry of vasopressin, oxytocin and neurophysin in the hypothalamus and extrahypothalamic regions of the human and primate brain. *Acta histochem.*, Suppl. 24: 79–95.

Sofroniew, M.V., Eckenstein, F., Thoenen, H. and Cuello, A.C. (1982a) Topography of choline acetyltransferase-containing neurons in the forebrain of the rat. *Neurosci. Lett.*, 33: 7–12.

Sofroniew, M.V., Gähwiler, B.H. and Dreifuss, J.J. (1982b) Cultured hypothalamic vasopressin (AVP), oxytocin

(OT) and neurophysin (NPH) neurons examined by Golgi-like immunoperoxidase staining. *Neuroscience, 7,* Suppl.: S198-199.

Sofroniew, M.V. Eckenstein, F., Schrell, U. and Cuello, A.C. (1983) Evidence for co-localization of neuroactive substances in hypothalamic neurons. In V. Chan-Palay and S.L. Palay (Eds.), *Coexistence of Neuroactive Substances,* John Wiley, New York, in press.

Sternberger, L.A. (1979) *Immunocytochemistry,* 2nd edn., John Wiley, New York.

Stillman, M.A., Recht, L.D., Rosario, S.L., Seif, S.M., Robinson, A.G. and Zimmerman, E.A. (1977) The effects of adrenalectomy and glucocorticoid replacement on vasopressin and vasopressin-neurophysin in the zona externa of the median eminence of the rat. *Endocrinology,* 101: 42–49.

Swanson, L.W. and Cowan, W.M. (1979) The connections of the septal region in the rat. *J. comp. Neurol.,* 186: 621–656.

Theodosis, D.T., Dreifuss, J.J., Harris, M.C. and Orci, L. (1976) Secretion-related uptake of horseradish peroxidase in neurohypophysial axons. *J. Cell Biol.,* 70: 294–303.

Vanderhaeghen, J.J., Lotstra, F., Vandesande, F. and Dierickx, K. (1981) Coexistence of cholecystokinin and oxytocin-neurophysin in some magnocellular hypothalamo-hypophyseal neurons. *Cell Tiss. Res.,* 211: 227–231.

Vandesande, F. and Dierickx, K. (1975) Identification of the vasopressin producing and of the oxytocin producing neurons in the hypothalamic magnocellular neurosecretory system of the rat. *Cell Tiss. Res.,* 164: 153–162.

Vandesande, F., Dierickx, K. and De Mey, J. (1975a) Identification of the vasopressin-neurophysin II and the oxytocin-neurophysin I producing neurons in the bovine hypothalamus. *Cell Tiss. Res.,* 156: 189–200.

Vandesande, F., Dierickx, K. and De Mey, J. (1975b) The origin of the vasopressinergic and oxytocinergic fibres of the external region of the median eminence of the rat hypophysis. *Cell Tiss. Res.,* 180: 443–452.

Van Leeuwen, F.W. and Caffe, R. (1982) A new locus in the rat brain containing immunoreactive vasopressin: the nucleus occultus. *Neurosci. Lett.,* Suppl. 10: S499–S500.

Van Wimersma Greidanus, Tj. B., Bohus, B. and De Wied, D. (1981) Vasopressin and oxytocin in learning and memory. In J.L. Martinez, Jr., R.A. Jensen, R.B. Messing, H. Rigter and J.L. McGaugh (Eds.), *Endogenous Peptides and Learning and Memory Processes,* Academic Press, New York, pp. 413–427.

Versteeg, D.H.G., De Kloet, E.R., Van Wimersma Greidanus, Tj. B. and De Wied, D. (1979) Vasopressin modulates the activity of catecholamine containing neurons in specific brain regions. *Neurosci. Lett.,* 11: 69–73.

Watson, S.J., Akil, H., Fischli, W., Goldstein, A., Zimmerman, E.A. and Nilaver, G. (1982) Dynorphin and vasopressin: common localization in magnocellular neurons. *Science,* 216: 85–87.

Weindl, A. and Sofroniew, M.V. (1976) Demonstration of extrahypothalamic peptide secreting neurons. *Pharmacopsychology,* 9: 226–234.

Yates, F.E. and Maran, J.W. (1974) Stimulation and inhibition of adrenocorticotropin release. In R.O. Greep and E.B. Astwood (Eds.), *Handbook of Physiology, Section 7: Endocrinology IV,* American Physiological Society, Washington, DC, pp. 367–404.

Zimmerman, E.A., Carmel, P.W., Husain, M.K., Ferin, M., Tannenbaum, M., Frantz, A.G. and Robinson, A.G. (1973) Vasopressin and neurophysin: High concentrations in monkey hypophyseal portal blood. *Science,* 182: 925–927.

The Neurohypophysis: Structure, Function and Control, Progress in Brain Research, Vol. 60, edited by B.A. Cross and G. Leng
© 1983 Elsevier Science Publishers B.V.

Vasopressin and Oxytocin: Distribution and Putative Functions in the Brain

R.M. BUIJS, G.J. DE VRIES, F.W. VAN LEEUWEN and D.F. SWAAB

Netherlands Institute for Brain Research, IJdijk 28, 1095 KJ Amsterdam (The Netherlands)

LOCALIZATION AND ORIGIN OF VASOPRESSIN AND OXYTOCIN FIBRES IN THE RAT BRAIN

Vasopressin (AVP)- and oxytocin (OXT)- containing fibres have been demonstrated by immunocytochemistry in a large number of rat brain regions from the olfactory bulb down to the spinal cord (Swanson, 1977; Sofroniew and Weindl, 1978; Buijs, 1978). The densest networks occur in subcortical brain structures, though in the cortex and cerebellum scattered — mostly AVP — fibres are found (Buijs, 1980). Limbic system structures, such as the lateral septum, the lateral habenular nucleus and the amygdala, are particularly heavily innervated by AVP fibres, while OXT fibres are predominant in the brainstem and spinal cord (Buijs, 1978; Swanson and McKellar, 1979). These extrahypothalamic fibres, which are already present at foetal day 17 (Buijs et al., 1980), innervate the lateral septum and lateral habenular nucleus from day 10 in a sexual dimorphic way (De Vries et al., 1981), viz. in male rats a much denser AVP innervation was found. This sex difference appears to depend on the presence of androgens in early postnatal development. In adulthood the female innervation pattern of the lateral septum can be changed to that of the male by the administration of a large dose of testosterone, which demonstrates the plasticity of the innervation of this area (De Vries et al., unpublished). The presence of AVP and OXT innervation of the brain has been demonstrated in various other mammalian species; for example, human subcortical brain structures are extensively innervated by AVP and OXT fibres which can already be found in the spinal cord of human foetuses 19 weeks after conception (Swaab and Ter Borg, 1981). Van den Dungen et al. (1982) demonstrated an even more widespread vasotocin and isotocin fibre system in the trout brain, while also the brains of lampreys were found to be densely innervated by vasotocin fibres. Consequently, the presence of neurohypophysial hormone-containing extrahypothalamic fibres is not a phenomenon acquired by higher vertebrates but is also present in species which are phylogenetically considered to be older.

The extrahypothalamic AVP and OXT fibres in the rat brain were thought to be derived from the paraventricular (PVN) and possibly also the supraoptic nuclei (SON), and from the parvocellular, AVP-containing, suprachiasmatic nucleus (SCN). Originally, the anatomy of the AVP and OXT fibre pathways was established mainly by following the fibres in serial sections (Buijs et al., 1978; Buijs, 1978; Sofroniew and Weindl, 1978). However, lesioning the SCN showed that its AVP fibre system is much less widespread than these earlier studies had suggested. The AVP fibres from the SCN appear to reach the organum vasculosum of the lamina terminalis (OVLT), the dorsomedial hypothalamic nucleus and the periventricular

116

nucleus (Hoorneman and Buijs, 1982) (Fig. 1). Apart from the AVP projections from the SCN, only the AVP projection from the PVN towards the nucleus of the solitary tract (NTS) has been demonstrated convincingly by means of retrograde transport of horseradish peroxidase (HRP) in combination with the immunocytochemical detection of the peptide content of the cell bodies (Sofroniew and Schrell, 1980; Sawchenko and Swanson, 1982). In a study by De Vries and Buijs (1983), lesioning of the PVN indeed resulted in the disappearance of AVP fibres in several regions of the brainstem. Surprisingly, it was not followed by a diminution of AVP fibres in the various other regions where the PVN was thought to project to, e.g. the amygdala, ventral hippocampus, dorsal raphe nucleus, etc.

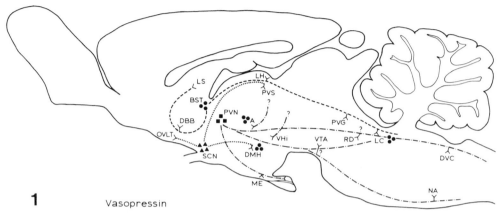

1 Vasopressin

Fig. 1. AVP pathways and possible sites of termination (——◁) in the rat brain projected in the sagittal plane. The pathways of the PVN (squares) are indicated by dashed-dotted lines (—·—·—·) and pathways of the SCN (triangles) are indicated by dotted lines (........). The AVP cell groups found only after colchicine treatment are indicated by large black dots, while the pathways of the bed nucleus of the stria terminalis (BST) are indicated by dashed lines (--------). A question mark indicates that the source of the AVP innervation in this area is still unknown. Abbreviations: A, amygdala; DBB, diagonal band of Broca; DMH, dorsomedial nucleus of the hypothalamus; DVC, dorsal vagal complex; LC, locus coeruleus; LH, lateral habenula; LS, lateral septum; ME, median eminence; OVLT, organum vasculosum of the laminae terminalis; PVG, periventricular grey; PVS, periventricular nucleus; RD, dorsal raphe nucleus; VHi, ventral hippocampus; VTA, ventral tegmental area.

Recently Van Leeuwen and Caffe (1983) demonstrated in rats which had been treated with colchicine, numerous AVP cell bodies in other brain regions outside the hypothalamus, i.e. in the bed nucleus of the stria terminalis, the amygdala, locus coeruleus, and in the dorsomedial nucleus of the hypothalamus (Fig. 2). This opens the possibility that these nuclei are the source of a substantial part of the vasopressin innervation of the brain. After lesioning the cell groups in the bed nucleus of the stria terminalis the AVP fibre innervation of the lateral septum decreased drastically. Furthermore, small cell bodies in the bed nucleus of the stria terminalis were found to be labelled after injection of HRP and fluorescent tracers in the lateral septum. Thus it is likely that the bed nucleus is the origin of the AVP fibres in the lateral septum. The AVP neurones of the bed nucleus of the stria terminalis probably also project to the lateral habenular nucleus, the periventricular grey and locus coeruleus (De Vries and Buijs, 1983) (Fig. 1). Because lesions might also have caused the destruction of passing AVP fibres, ultimate proof for these projections can only be obtained after retrograde tracing in combination with the demonstration of AVP in the labelled neurone.

Nevertheless, a new picture emerges with respect to the origin of the AVP fibres, viz. that the PVN and SCN contribute only for a minor part to these extrahypothalamic fibres. The

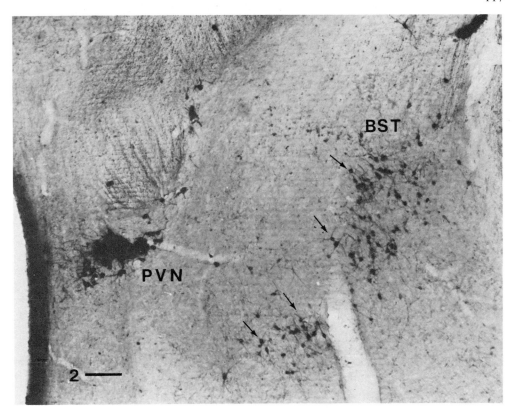

Fig. 2. Transversal section of AVP-positive cell bodies in the rat brain, demonstrated in the region of the bed nucleus of the stria terminalis (BST). PVN is the most rostral part of the paraventricular nucleus. The arrows point to the AVP cells in the BST, which are only visible after colchicine treatment. Bar = 100 μm.

origin of the major part must lie elsewhere, most probably in the AVP cell bodies that could be demonstrated only after colchicine treatment. Herewith AVP has lost one of its characteristics that had distinguished it so far from other peptides, in that its cell bodies were restricted to the hypothalamus and were readily visible without colchicine treatment. As it appears now, a combination of both cell types occurs, and the AVP cell bodies are much more widespread than has been assumed hitherto.

In contrast to AVP, practically all OXT fibres seem to be derived from the PVN, as lesioning of this nucleus results in an almost complete disappearance of the OXT innervation of the brain. Furthermore, in colchicine-treated rats no additional OXT neurones were detected, which reduces the probability of an alternative source. It appears, from its much more widespread sites of origin and terminal areas, that AVP is involved in the regulation of far more functions than OXT.

ELECTRON MICROSCOPIC LOCALIZATION

The assumption of Barry (1954) that neurosecretory fibres containing Gomori-positive material would terminate by means of "des synapses neurosecretoires" seemed to be plausible, as in many brain regions AVP- and OXT-containing fibres were found to form extensive ramification and perineuronal structures. Immunoelectron microscopy has been performed on regions in the limbic system and medulla that are densely innervated by AVP and OXT fibres, respectively. In these regions AVP and OXT have been localized within synapses mostly terminating on dendrites and less frequently on cell bodies. On no occasion were AVP- or OXT-containing structures found to be either pre- or postsynaptic to axonal processes (Buijs and Swaab, 1979; Voorn and Buijs, 1983). Therefore, results which suggest a "modulating" action of AVP on monoamine metabolism in terminal regions of monoaminergic and AVP fibres (Versteeg et al., 1979; Kovács et al., 1979) may be explained via an indirect mechanism and not via a direct presynaptic action of AVP on the monoamine-containing axon or terminal. In the same way, the absence of presynaptic terminals on AVP- and OXT-containing fibres suggests that presynaptic modulation of AVP and/or OXT release is not widespread, at least not in the areas investigated.

Although, for the visualization of these structures, it is necessary to use Triton X-100, which hampers the preservation of ultrastructure of the tissue, these synapses were found to contain clear vesicles and sometimes also 80–100 nm dense core vesicles (Buijs and Swaab, 1979). The presence of these dense core vesicles in extrahypothalamic brain regions suggests that the AVP and OXT fibres in these areas are derived from different neurones than those projecting to the neural lobe, where larger (140 nm) vesicles are found (Van Leeuwen et al., 1977). The presence of small vesicles might indicate a different processing mechanism for these peptides from that in the hypothalamo–neurohypophysial system. The fact that, in the brainstem, immunoreactive neurophysin is present predominantly as a high molecular weight precursor in contrast to the precursors found in the hypothalamo–neurohypophysial system (Sinding et al., 1982) supports this idea. Another possibility is that the release mechanism of these peptides in the brain is different from that in the pituitary, resulting in many more clear vesicles and fewer (and smaller) dense core vesicles.

In the human and in the trout and lamprey brain, the extrahypothalamic neurohypophysial hormone fibres form similar ramifications and boutons similar to those found in the rat, which suggests that these fibres also terminate synaptically, and indeed such synaptic terminations have recently been demonstrated in the human brain (Kerkhoven and Buijs, unpublished). Thus there seems little doubt that these neurohypophysial peptides influence neuronal structures via synaptic terminals in a wide variety of species. However, although the synaptic localization of AVP and OXT is established it remains an open question whether these peptides or other, unknown substances are released from these synapses.

CENTRAL RELEASE OF AVP AND OXT

To demonstrate that AVP- and OXT-containing synapses are able to release their peptide content upon depolarization, an in vitro release procedure was set up (Buijs and Van Heerikhuize, 1982). For this purpose various brain regions and the neurointermediate lobe were selected. Using high potassium or veratridine as the depolarizing stimulus, release from the septal area and NTS (areas where AVP and OXT fibres terminate) was compared with the release of these peptides from the neural lobe.

A calcium-dependent potassium- or veratridine-stimulated release of AVP and/or OXT could be demonstrated only for the brain regions where these fibres terminate synaptically on neuronal structures. The veratridine-stimulated release of OXT from the NTS ($6.1\% \pm 0.9\%$ of the tissue stores in 10 min) or the neural lobe ($7.7\% \pm 0.6\%$ in 10 min) is more pronounced than that of AVP from the septum (3.6 % ± 0.7 % in 10 min) or neural lobe (1.4 % ± 0.1 % in 10 min; values ± S.E.M.) (Buijs and Van Heerikhuize, 1982). This difference in sensitivity towards veratridine depolarization might point to different membrane properties for AVP and OXT neurones and a different release mechanism. As the AVP and OXT fibres between the PVN and SON are varicose and fail to evince synaptic specializations, this area was selected to study whether these peptides could also be released non-synaptically.

No potassium-stimulated release of AVP or OXT could be detected from these areas in spite of the large amounts of peptide. Taken together, the results suggest that AVP and OXT are released in the central nervous system and that this release occurs from synaptic terminals. That this release will also occur under physiological circumstances is demonstrated, for instance, by the experiments of Cooper et al. (1979), who found — by perfusion of the sheep septal area with a push–pull cannula — a release of AVP which was negatively correlated with a rise in body temperature.

Although research on the central action of AVP and OXT has gained momentum only recently, many pertinent neurotransmitter criteria have already been fulfilled. These criteria have been set up in relation to the action of acetylcholine on the neuromuscular junction. However, even acetylcholine cannot at present meet all neurotransmitter criteria in the brain fully satisfactorily.

THE POSSIBLE FUNCTIONS OF AVP AND OXT IN THE CENTRAL NERVOUS SYSTEM

Since the observation of Cushing (1932) that an injection of a posterior pituitary extract resulted in a drop in body temperature and in vasodilatation, various other putative central functions of AVP and OXT have been added. Recently the influence of AVP on thermoregulation (Cooper et al., 1979) and the involvement of AVP and OXT in the regulation of other autonomic functions has been documented in much more detail, both anatomically and physiologically (Bohus, 1980; Pittman et al., 1982; Swanson and Sawchenko, 1980; Sawchenko and Swanson, 1982). In addition, these peptides might be involved in learning processes (see De Wied, this volume). The question arises as to whether these various putative functions of AVP and OXT can be linked to what we have learned so far about the anatomical properties of peptidergic systems in the central nervous system.

From the present anatomical details a picture can be drawn of an extensive innervation of many areas in the CNS by AVP- and/or OXT-containing fibres. Moreover, retro- and anterograde tracing studies have revealed that most of these areas project directly to the PVN and SON. Depending on whether the PVN projects in turn with OXT or AVP fibres to such an area, a direct bidirectional pathway is established. The NTS and the dorsal nucleus of the vagus seem to fit this description. For example, it has been demonstrated that the PVN projects at least with AVP-, OXT-, enkephalin- and somatostatin-containing fibres to the dorsal vagus complex (Sawchenko and Swanson, 1982), while extensive projections from the NTS and dorsal nucleus of the vagus to the PVN have been described (Ricardo and Koh, 1978). The majority of the latter input to the PVN seems to be to the parvocellular part. As axons of the small medial cells of the PVN terminate on the dendrites of the larger lateral cells (Van den Pol, 1982), the incoming information on that part of the nucleus can be relayed throughout the PVN, thus enabling a direct feedback to the whole PVN. However, whether those neurones that project to the PVN are indeed also innervated by PVN fibres remains to be established. Anyhow, by this anatomical relationship the PVN seems to be able to modulate afferent and efferent autonomic information (cf. Swanson and Sawchenko, 1980). The role of AVP and OXT in the connection between the PVN and the hindbrain will probably lie in the regulation of processes in which these peptides are also involved in the periphery — such as the control of blood pressure and lactation. The fact that AVP concentrations are affected in brainstem and neural lobe in spontaneously hypertensive rats (Mohring et al., 1980), and that both AVP and OXT influence blood pressure, especially in caudal brain regions (Bohus, 1980; Pittman, 1982; Matsuguchi et al., 1982), supports this theory.

This coupling of central and peripheral action of AVP and OXT seems to be a general phenomenon of hypothalamic peptides (see Swaab, 1982). An example of such central and peripheral coupling might be found in the action of AVP in limbic brain areas such as the lateral septum and the amygdala. Both areas are densely innervated by AVP, fibres and project to the PVN and/or SON (Tribollet and Dreifuss, 1981; Silverman et al., 1981; Pittman et al., 1981a, b; Poulain et al., 1981), but it awaits elucidation whether the neurones that project to the PVN and SON are innervated by AVP fibres. The demonstration of a simultaneous AVP release following a hypertonic saline injection both in the periphery and in the septum and amygdala (Pittman, 1982) supports the idea that central and peripheral release of AVP are coupled. The possibility exists that, via the connections from the septum to the PVN and SON, central AVP might influence release of AVP into the periphery. Another possibility is that the simultaneous central and peripheral release will occur upon a specific stimulus and result in the initiation of processes, both centrally and peripherally, that help the animal adapt to this stimulus. The importance of such a coupled action might be found in the effect of AVP in temperature control. AVP release in the septal region of sheep measured by push–pull perfusion correlated negatively with a change in body temperature. That is, the release of AVP increases when body temperature falls, while by raising body temperature release of AVP decreases (Cooper et al., 1979; Kasting et al., 1982). The conclusion that this septal release has functional significance is warranted by the addition of AVP to the perfusate, which resulted in a drop in body temperature. In separate experiments it was demonstrated that peripheral AVP levels are enhanced when body temperature is elevated (Cooper et al., 1979). Thus AVP might exert an antipyretic effect in the CNS, while in the periphery it prevents the loss of water via the kidney to prevent dehydration by the perspiration induced by a rise in temperature. Thus central and peripheral actions of AVP may be coupled. Whether this will be a general rule for AVP and OXT or even for all hypothalamic releasing hormones will certainly be a point of future investigation.

REFERENCES

Barry, J. (1954) Neurocrinie et synapses "neurosecretoires", *Arch. Anat. Mikr.*, 43: 310–320.
Bohus, B. (1980) Effects of neuropeptides on adaptive autonomic processes. In D. de Wied and P.A. van Keep (Eds.), *Hormones and the Brain*, MTP Press Ltd., Lancaster.
Buijs, R.M. (1978) Intra- and extrahypothalamic vasopressin and oxytocin pathways in the rat. Pathways to the limbic system, medulla oblongata and spinal cord. *Cell Tiss. Res.*, 192: 423–435.
Buijs, R.M. (1980) *Vasopressin and Oxytocin Innervation of the Rat Brain. A Light- and Electronmicroscopical Study*. PhD Thesis, GU Amsterdam, The Netherlands.
Buijs, R.M. and Swaab, D.F. (1979) Immuno-electron microscopical demonstration of vasopressin and oxytocin in the limbic system of the rat. *Cell Tiss. Res.*, 204: 355–365.
Buijs, R.M. and Van Heerikhuize, J.J. (1982) Vasopressin and oxytocin release in the brain: a synaptic event. *Brain Res.*, 252: 71–76.
Buijs, R.M., Swaab, D.F., Dogterom, J. and Van Leeuwen, F.W. (1978) Intra- and extrahypothalamic vasopressin and oxytocin pathways in the rat. *Cell Tiss. Res.*, 186: 423–433.
Buijs, R.M., Velis, D.N. and Swaab, D.F. (1980) Ontogeny of vasopressin and oxytocin in the fetal rat: early vasopressinergic innervation of the fetal brain. *Peptides*, 1: 315–324.

Cooper, K.E., Kasting, N.W., Lederis, K. and Veale, W.L. (1979) Evidence supporting a role for endogenous vasopressin in natural suppression of fever in the sheep. *J. Physiol. (Lond.)*, 295: 33–45.

Cushing, H. (1932) Paper relating to the pituitary body. In C.C. Thomas (Ed.), *Hypothalamus and Parasympathetic Nervous System*. C.C. Thomas, Springfield, IL.

De Vries, G.J. and Buijs, R.M. (1983) The origin of the vasopressinergic and oxytocinergic innervation of the rat brain, with special reference to the lateral septum. *Brain Res.*, in press.

De Vries, G.J., Buijs, R.M. and Swaab, D.F. (1981) Ontogeny of the vasopressinergic neurons of the suprachiasmatic nucleus and their extrahypothalamic projections in the rat brain — presence of a sex difference in the lateral septum. *Brain Res.*, 218: 67–78.

Hoorneman, E.M.D. and Buijs, R.M. (1982) Vasopressin fiber pathways in the rat brain following suprachiasmatic nucleus lesioning. *Brain Res.*, 243: 235–241.

Kasting, N.W., Veale, W.L. and Cooper, K.E. (1982) Vasopressin: a homeostatic effector in the febrile process. *Neurosci. Biobehav. Rev.*, 6: 215–222.

Kovács, G.L., Bohus, B., Versteeg, D.H.G., De Kloet, E.R. and De Wied, D. (1979) Effect of oxytocin, and vasopressin on memory consolidation, sites of action and catecholaminergic correlates after local microinjection into limbic-midbrain structures. *Brain Res.*, 175: 303–314.

Matsuguchi, H., Sharabi, F.M. Gordon, F.J. and Johnsson, A.K. (1982) Blood pressure and heart rate responses to microinjection of vasopressin into the nucleus tractus solitarius region of the rat. *Neuropharmacology*, 21: 687–693.

Mohring, J., Schoun, J., Kintz, J. and McNeill, R. (1980) Decreased vasopressin content in brain stem of rats with spontaneous hypertension. *Arch. Pharmacol.*, 315: 83–84.

Pittman, Q.J., Blume, H.W. and Renaud, L.P. (1981a) Connections of the hypothalamic paraventricular nucleus with the neurohypophysis, median eminence, amygdala, lateral septum and midbrain periaqueductal gray: an electrophysiological study in the rat. *Brain Res.*, 215: 15–28.

Pittman, Q.J., Malkinson, T.J., Veale, W.L. and Lederis, K. (1981b) Central release of arginine vasopressin (AVP) in rabbit brain. *Soc. Neurosci. Abstr.*, 7: 506.

Pittman, Q.J., Lawrence, D. and McLean, L. (1982) Central effects of arginine vasopressin on blood pressure in rats. *Endocrinology*, 110: 1058.

Poulain, D.A., Lebrun, C.J. and Vincent, J.D. (1981) Electrophysiological evidence for connections between septal neurones and the supraoptic nucleus of the hypothalamus of the rat. *Exp. Brain Res.*, 42: 260–268.

Ricardo, J.A. and Koh, E.T. (1978) Anatomical evidence of direct projections from the nucleus of the solitary tract to the hypothalamus, amygdala, and other forebrain structures in the rat. *Brain Res.*, 153: 1–26.

Sawchenko, P.E. and Swanson, L.W. (1982) Immunohistochemical identification of neurons in the paraventricular nucleus of the hypothalamus that project to the medulla or to the spinal cord in the rat. *J. comp. Neurol.*, 205: 260–272.

Silverman, A.J., Hoffman, D.L. and Zimmerman, E.A. (1981) The descending afferent connections of the paraventricular nucleus of the hypothalamus (PVN), *Brain Res. Bull.*, 6: 47–61.

Sinding, C., Camier, M. and Cohen, P. (1982) Extra hypothalamo-neurohypophyseal immunoreactive neurophysin occurs predominantly as high M[r] forms in the rat brain stem. *FEBS Lett.*, 140: 124–126.

Sofroniew, M.V. and Schrell, U. (1980) Hypothalamic neurons projecting to the rat caudal medulla oblongata, examined by immunoperoxidase staining of retrogradely transported horseradish peroxidase. *Neurosci. Lett.*, 19: 257–263.

Sofroniew, M.V. and Weindl, A. (1978) Projections from the parvocellular vasopressin and neurophysin-containing neurons of the suprachiasmatic nucleus. *Amer. J. Anat.*, 153: 391–430.

Swaab, D.F. (1982) Neuropeptides and their distribution in the brain. The role of amines, aminoacids and peptides. In R.M. Buijs, P. Pevet and D.F. Swaab (Eds.), *Chemical Transmission in the Brain, Progress in Brain Research. Vol. 55*, Elsevier/North-Holland, Amsterdam, pp. 97–122.

Swaab, D.F. and Ter Borg, J.P. (1981) Development of peptidergic systems in the rat brain. In K. Elliott and J. Whelan (Eds.), *The Fetus and Independent Life, Ciba Foundation Symp. No. 86*, Pitman Medical, London, pp. 271–294.

Swanson, L.W. (1977) Immunohistochemical evidence for a neurophysin-containing autonomic pathway arising in the paraventricular nucleus of the hypothalamus. *Brain Res.*, 128: 346–353.

Swanson, L.W. and McKellar, S. (1979) The distribution of oxytocin- and neurophysin-stained fibers in the spinal cord of the rat and monkey. *J. comp. Neurol.*, 188: 87–106.

Swanson, L.W. and Sawchenko, P.E. (1980) Paraventricular nucleus: a site for the integration of neuroendocrine and autonomic mechanisms. *Neuroendocrinology*, 31: 410–417.

Tribollet, E. and Dreifuss, J.J. (1981) Localization of neurons projecting to the hypothalamic paraventricular nucleus area of the rat: a horseradish peroxidase study. *Neuroscience*, 6: 1315–1328.

Van den Pol, A.N. (1982) The magnocellular and parvocellular paraventricular nucleus of rat: intrinsic organization. *J. comp. Neurol.*, 206: 317–345.

Van den Dungen, H.M., Buijs, R.M., Pool, C.W. and Terlou, M. (1982) The distribution of vasotocin and isotocin in the brain of the rainbow trout. *J. comp. Neurol.*, 212: 146–157.

Van Leeuwen, F.W. and Caffe, R. (1983) Immunoreactive vasopressin cell bodies in the rat bed nucleus of the stria terminalis. *Cell Tiss. Res.*, 228: 525–534.

Van Leeuwen, F.W. and Swaab, D.F. (1977) Specific immunoelectronmicroscopic localization of vasopressin and oxytocin in the neurohypophysis of the rat. *Cell Tiss. Res.*, 177: 493–503.

Versteeg, D.M.G., De Kloet, R.E. and Van Wimersma Greidanus, Tj.B. (1979) Vasopressin modulates the activity of catecholamine containing neurons in specific brain regions. *Neurosci. Lett.*, 11: 69–73.

Voorn, P. and Buijs, R.M. (1983) An immuno-electronmicroscopical study comparing vasopressin, oxytocin, substance P and enkephalin containing nerve terminals in the nucleus of the solitary tract of the rat, *Brain Res.*, in press.

The Neurohypophysis: Structure, Function and Control, Progress in Brain Research, Vol. 60, edited by B.A. Cross and G. Leng
© *1983 Elsevier Science Publishers B.V.*

Quantitative Distribution of Neurohypophysial Hormones in Human Brain and Spinal Cord

J.S. JENKINS, V.T.Y. ANG, J. HAWTHORN and M.N. ROSSOR [1]

Department of Medicine, St. George's Hospital Medical School, London SW17 ORE, and [1]National Hospital for Nervous Diseases, Queen Square, London WC1 (U.K.)

INTRODUCTION

During the last few years immunocytochemical techniques have revealed that fibres containing vasopressin and oxytocin, as well as neurophysins, are present in many areas of the central nervous system other than the classical hypothalamic–hypophysial pathway (Buijs, 1978; Nilaver et al., 1980; Sofroniew et al., 1981). These studies have assumed special importance with the realization that the neurohypophysial peptides may have functions within the brain which are quite distinct from their well-established actions on the kidney and uterus. In particular, the extensive studies of De Wied (1980) in rats have indicated that these peptides may affect the memory process. However, while immunocytochemical methods have yielded considerable information about the pathways of peptides and their histological localization, there are limitations to their use. Accurate quantitation is not possible, and owing to technical difficulties when attempting to use antibodies to vasopressin and oxytocin, particularly in human tissues, several investigators have had recourse to the study of neurophysins as indirect markers of these hormones, with the result that the amounts of vasopressin and oxytocin specifically have not been firmly established. Much of the previous work has been carried out on the rat and lower primates, and in the case of the human brain information is much more restricted. We have therefore carried out an extensive survey of the human brain and the spinal cord, using specific radioimmunoassays to determine in a quantitative manner the distribution of both vasopressin and oxytocin. It is hoped that these observations, together with information already obtained by immunocytochemical studies, will lead to a greater understanding of the role of these neuropeptides within the central nervous system of man.

METHODS

Eight brains and four spinal cords were obtained at routine post-mortem and were stored, dissected, and prepared for assay according to methods previously described (Rosser et al., 1981). The relevant areas in the medulla and each segment of the spinal cord were removed at −10°C by a punch technique using 1 mm diameter capillary tubing. After extraction of the peptides from the tissue with octadecasilyl silica, arginine-vasopressin and oxytocin were measured by double antibody radioimmunoassays, using 1st International Standard arginine-vasopressin 77/501 and the 4th International Standard oxytocin 76/575. Antibodies to vasopressin and oxytocin conjugated with thyroglobulin were raised in rabbits. Each assay was

[123]

124

highly specific for the appropriate peptide, the cross-reactivity between oxytocin and vasopressin being < 0.01 %. The sensitivity was 0.6 pg per tube and the interassay coefficient of variation was 13 %.

RESULTS

The mean values for arginine-vasopressin and oxytocin in eight human brains are shown in Fig. 1. The whole hypothalamus contained about three times the amount of vasopressin as oxytocin. In the extrahypothalamic areas the greatest quantity of vasopressin was in the locus coeruleus, together with somewhat smaller amounts of oxytocin, and both peptides were also present in appreciable quantities in the periaqueductal grey matter. Vasopressin only was found in the substantia nigra and globus pallidus, but neither peptide was identified in the caudate nucleus and putamen. Other areas of the brain where these peptides were sometimes found are shown in Table I, and of these sites, the ventrolateral nucleus of the thalamus was most often positive for vasopressin and oxytocin.

In the medulla the proportion of the two peptides was reversed, so that oxytocin was more prominent than vasopressin in the dorsal nucleus of the vagus, the nucleus of the solitary tract and the nucleus of the spinal tract of the trigeminal nerve. An area within the lateral reticular formation was also found to contain both peptides.

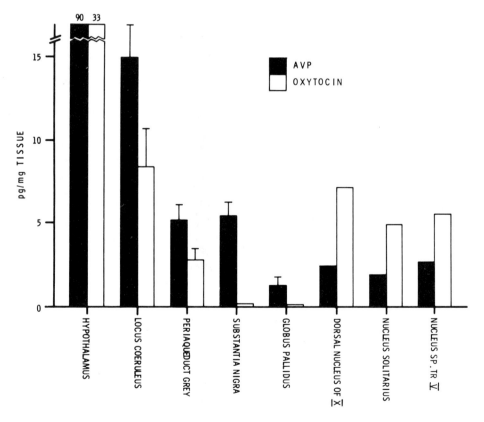

Fig. 1. Arginine-vasopressin and oxytocin (pg/mg tissue) in various sites within the human brain.

TABLE I

AREAS OF THE HUMAN BRAIN WHERE NEUROHYPOPHYSIAL PEPTIDES ARE SOMETIMES FOUND

(Total brains examined = 8)

Site	Arginine vasopressin		Oxytocin	
	No. of brains positive	Mean amount ± S.E.M. (pg/mg tissue)	No. of brains positive	Mean amount ± S.E.M. (pg/mg tissue)
Thalamus				
anteromedial nucleus	5	1.0 ± 0.2	4	1.2 ± 0.2
ventromedial nucleus	6	2.4 ± 1.0	6	2.8 ± 0.5
Amygdala	4	0.8 ± 0.2	3	0.9 ± 0.2
Hippocampus	5	0.5 ± 0.45	3	1.1 ± 0.2
Septal nuclei	5	0.8 ± 0.1	2	0.7

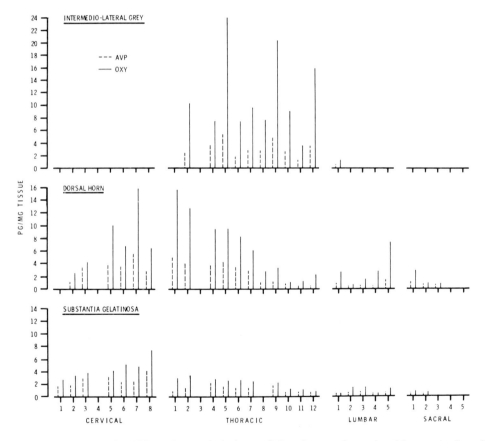

Fig. 2. Arginine-vasopressin (AVP) and oxytocin in intermediolateral grey column, dorsal horn and substantia gelatinosa of human spinal cord.

126

Throughout the spinal cord, oxytocin predominated over vasopressin and the greatest concentration of both peptides was within the intermediolateral grey column, where the ratio of oxytocin to vasopressin was about 4 : 1 (Fig. 2). The highest values were found in the lower thoracic segments. Large amounts of oxytocin, and smaller quantities of vasopressin, were also present in the dorsal horn as well as the substantia gelatinosa, especially in the lower cervical and upper seven thoracic segments. Smaller amounts were found throughout the central grey matter as well as the lateral white funiculus close to the ventral part of the dorsal horn. Other areas of white matter contained very little of either peptide.

Validation of the assays was carried out by demonstrating close immunological parallelism between material from tissue extracts and the authentic peptides, and by the use of high-performance liquid chromatography identical retention times were obtained (Fig. 3).

HPLC PROFILE

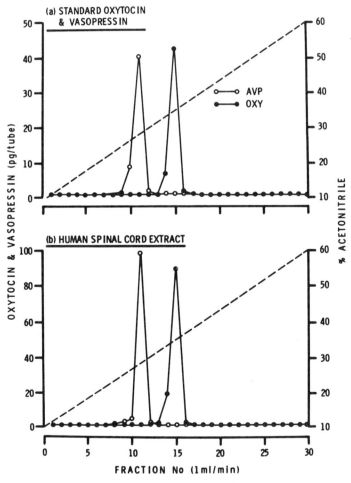

Fig. 3. Profiles of (a) standard oxytocin and arginine-vasopressin and (b) human spinal cord extract (intermediolateral grey column) in an HPLC system using a μ Bondapak C18 ODS column and elution with an increasing gradient of acetonitrile. Fractions were measured by radioimmunoassay.

DISCUSSION

These results extend our previous findings which were concerned with the distribution of vasopressin only in certain areas of the human and rat brains (Rosser et al., 1981; Hawthorn et al., 1980). The localization of both oxytocin and vasopressin in particular sites of the dorsal medulla and spinal cord, and the predominance of oxytocin which we observed, are in broad agreement with the immunocytochemical studies carried out in the rat by Buijs (1978), and in the monkey and limited areas of the human brainstem by Sofroniew et al. (1981), but are contrary to the results of Swanson and McKellar (1979) who could not identify vasopressin in the spinal cord of the rat and the monkey. However, in the human brain the greatest concentration of vasopressin and, to a lesser extent, oxytocin was found in the locus coeruleus and periaqueductal grey matter, which, together with their presence in the dorsal nucleus of the vagus and intermediolateral grey column of the cord, suggests that there is a close relationship with the ascending and descending noradrenergic pathways. There is now much evidence that the neurohypophysial peptides present in particular areas of the brainstem and spinal cord occur in fibres which are long projections from the paraventricular nucleus of the hypothalamus (Swanson and Sawchenko, 1980). It seems likely, therefore, that through these pathways the paraventricular nucleus can influence those centres in the brainstem and cord involved in the sympathetic and parasympathetic control of cardiovascular, respiratory and splanchnic function.

The effect of vasopressin on the memory process in the rat, extensively reported by De Wied and coworkers (1980), has also been related to the noradrenergic system. Thus, destruction of the noradrenergic pathways completely disrupted the effect of vasopressin on memory consolidation in rats (Kovács et al., 1980). In contradistinction to the facilitation of memory by vasopressin, it has been reported by Bohus et al. (1978) that oxytocin has the opposite effect, thereby attenuating the memory process. The differences in the proportion of the two peptides in various parts of the brain which we observed, may therefore be important in this respect.

The substantia nigra and globus pallidus contained vasopressin exclusively, and this finding would imply that vasopressin, in particular, may also be associated with the predominantly dopaminergic pathways of this region.

The presence of appreciable quantities of oxytocin, and smaller amounts of vasopressin in the dorsal horn of the cord, in the substantia gelatinosa, the nucleus of the spinal tract of the trigeminal nerve, as well as the solitary tract nucleus, suggests that these neurohypophysial peptides may have a role in modulating sensory afferents to the central nervous system. It is of interest that substance P and the enkephalins, which appear to be involved in pain perception, have also been found in very similar sites to those containing oxytocin and vasopressin (Douglas et al., 1982; Dupont et al., 1980). The possibility of interactions between these various peptides and the catecholaminergic pathways remains to be investigated.

SUMMARY

In extrahypothalamic areas of the human brain the largest amounts of vasopressin and oxytocin were consistently found in the locus coeruleus. Both peptides were present in the periaqueductal grey matter, but vasopressin only was found in the substantia nigra and globus pallidus. In the medulla oxytocin predominated over vasopressin in the dorsal nucleus of the vagus nerve, nucleus solitarius and nucleus of spinal tract of the trigeminal nerve. In the spinal cord the greatest concentration of the peptides was in the intermediolateral grey column, where the amount of oxytocin was four times that of vasopressin.

ACKNOWLEDGEMENT

This work was supported by a grant from the Wellcome Trust.

REFERENCES

Bohus, B., Kovács, G.L. and De Wied, D. (1978) Oxytocin, vasopressin and memory: opposite effects on consolidation and retrieval processes. *Brain Res.*, 157: 414–417.

Buijs, R.M. (1978) Intra- and extrahypothalamic vasopressin and oxytocin pathways in the rat. Pathways to the limbic system, medulla oblongata, and spinal cord. *Cell Tiss. Res.*, 186: 423–433.

De Wied, D. (1980) Behavioural actions of neurohypophyseal peptides. *Proc. roy. Soc. B*, 210: 183–195.

Douglas, F.L., Palkovits, M. and Brownstein, M.J. (1982) Regional distribution of substance P-like immunoreactivity in the lower brain stem of the rat. *Brain Res.*, 245: 376–378.

Dupont, A., Barden, N., Cusan, L., Merand, Y., Labrie, F. and Vaudry, H. (1980) β-Endorphin and met-enkephalins: their distribution, modulation by oestrogens and haloperidol and role in neuroendocrine control. *Fed. Proc.*, 39: 2544–2550.

Hawthorn, J., Ang, V.T.Y. and Jenkins, J.S. (1980) Localization of vasopressin in the rat brain. *Brain Res.*, 197: 75–81.

Kovács, G.L., Bohus, B. and Versteeg, D.H.G. (1980) The interaction of posterior pituitary neuropeptides with monoaminergic neurotransmission: significance in learning and memory processes. In P. McConnell, G.J. Boer, H.J. Romijn, N. van de Poll and M.A. Corner (Eds.), *Adaptive Capabilities of the Nervous System, Progress in Brain Research, Vol. 53*, Elsevier/North-Holland, Amsterdam, pp. 123–140.

Nilaver, G., Zimmerman, E.A., Wilkins, J., Michaels, J., Hoffman, D. and Silverman, A.J. (1980) Magnocellular hypothalamic projections to the lower brain stem and spinal cord of the rat. *Neuroendocrinology*, 30: 150–158.

Rosser, M.N., Iversen, L.L., Hawthorn, J., Ang, V.T.Y. and Jenkins, J.S. (1981) Extrahypothalamic vasopressin in human brain. *Brain Res.*, 214: 349–355.

Sofroniew, M.V., Weindl, A., Schrell, U. and Wetzstein, R. (1981) Immunohistochemistry of vasopressin, oxytocin, and neurophysin in the hypothalamus and extrahypothalamic regions of the human and primate brain. *Acta histochem.*, Suppl. xxiv: 79–95.

Swanson, L.W. and McKellar, S. (1979) The distribution of oxytocin- and neurophysin-stained fibers in the spinal cord of the rat and monkey. *J. comp. Neurol.*, 188: 87–106.

Swanson, L.W. and Sawchenko, P.E. (1980) Paraventricular nucleus: a site for the integration of neuroendocrine and autonomic mechanisms. *Neuroendocrinology*, 31: 410–417.

The Neurohypophysis: Structure, Function and Control, Progress in Brain Research, Vol. 60, edited by B.A. Cross and G. Leng

Neurohypophysial Peptides in Cerebrospinal Fluid

I.C.A.F. ROBINSON

Laboratory of Endocrine Physiology and Pharmacology, National Institute for Medical Research, Mill Hill, London NW7 1AA (U.K.)

"The object of this communication is to call attention to the presence of a substance in the cerebrospinal fluid which gives the same reaction as extracts of the pars nervosa itself, indicating in all probability that the active principle .... is actually secreted into the ventricular cavity." (Cushing and Goetsch, 1910)

INTRODUCTION

In the seventy or so years since these authors presented the first direct evidence of pressor and oxytocic substances in the cerebrospinal fluid (CSF), the notion that this fluid normally contains vasopressin (AVP) and oxytocin (OXT) has been pursued with varying degrees of enthusiasm (Heller, 1969). Numerous early reports suggested that CSF contained large amounts of OXT, but these findings were obtained using highly concentrated extracts of CSF which produced non-specific interference in the bioassays used at that time. When these problems were recognized (Van Dyke et al., 1929) and the bioassay methods improved somewhat (Friedman and Friedman, 1933), investigations of CSF for the presence of neurohypophysial hormones invariably proved negative, and interest in the subject disappeared until the late 1960s when Heller et al. (1968) and Vorherr et al. (1968) provided the first modern evidence for AVP in CSF. At that time, AVP levels were only detectable in CSF from anaesthetized animals subjected to haemorrhage or vagal stimulation. AVP levels in CSF from conscious, unstimulated animals lay below the detection limit of the bioassays. Since then, the presence of OXT, AVP and neurophysin (NP) in CSF has been firmly established for a number of species and there is now much current interest in the "cerebroventricular" physiology of these substances (Luerssen and Robertson, 1980; Post et al., 1982; Mens et al., 1982a).

Three main reasons can be advanced for this increased interest. Firstly, the realization that neurohypophysial peptides exert a wide variety of actions on the central nervous system (CNS), often following administration of exogenous peptides or their antisera into CSF. Secondly, the advent of elegant immunohistochemical methods which revealed the existence of pathways containing OXT, AVP or NP which do not project to the posterior pituitary, but rather to a number of extrahypothalamic sites within the CNS. Thirdly, the development of extremely sensitive radioimmunoassay (RIA) methods coupled with improved techniques for sampling from the CSF space in conscious laboratory animals (Bouman and Van Wimersma Greidanus, 1979; Jones and Robinson, 1981; Reppert et al., 1981). These techniques have now opened up a much wider range of experimental approaches to the study of neurohypophysial peptides in CSF.

BASAL LEVELS OF NEUROHYPOPHYSIAL PEPTIDES IN CSF

In common with measurements of most biologically active substances in body fluids, values for "basal levels" of OXT and AVP in mammalian CSF have tended to fall as the sensitivity of the assays used has gradually improved. Table I lists the range of values reported for a number of species in the last 15 years, converted to molar quantities for comparison. Values obtained in earlier studies are considerably higher and are listed in the comprehensive review by Rodriguez (1976). The peptides are relatively stable in CSF from most species tested and values are similar whether or not CSF is extracted before assay (Jenkins et al., 1980). Larger animals and man tend to have lower basal levels than smaller animals (Table I), perhaps due to their larger volume of bulk CSF, or to different CSF clearance rates. In man, there is little or no rostro-caudal gradient of AVP in CSF (Luerssen and Robertson, 1980; Hammer et al., 1982) and in fact basal levels of OXT, AVP and NP are very similar whether samples are taken from the lumbar, cisternal or ventricular spaces. Table I also shows that, whereas the nonapeptide levels are mostly in the low fmol/ml range, NP values are much higher, in the pmol/ml range.

TABLE I

BASAL LEVELS OF NEUROHYPOPHYSIAL PEPTIDES IN CSF

Species	OXT (fmol/ml)	AVP (fmol/ml)	NP (pmol/ml)	Anaes-thesia	Reference
Man	–	1.0	–	–	Luerssen and Robertson, 1980
	–	–	0.54	–	Robinson and Zimmerman, 1973
	–	2.4	–	–	Jenkins et al., 1980
	–	1.3	–	–	Hammer et al., 1982
	5–15	5	0.04[a], 0.45[b]	–	Robinson (unpublished)
	–	11	–	–	Dogterom et al., 1978b
	–	–	0.03[a], 0.3[b]	–	Born et al., 1981
Monkey	15	2.5	0.4[b]	–	Perlow et al., 1982
	8–50	–	–	–	Artman et al., 1982a
	–	–	0.2–0.7	–	Robinson and Zimmerman, 1973
Dog	–	6	–	+	Dogterom et al., 1978b
	–	6	–	+	Wang et al., 1981
Cat	–	2–15	–	–	Reppert et al., 1981
Rabbit	–	10	–	+	Vorherr et al., 1968
	–	8	–	–	Heller et al., 1968
	770	–	–	+	Schwarzberg et al., 1971
Guinea pig	5	15	1	–	Robinson and Jones, 1982a
Rat	–	< 0.8–8	–	–	Schwartz et al., 1982
	73	11.5	–	+	Dogterom et al., 1978b
	–	10–20	–	–	Mens et al., 1980
	50–70	10–20	0.8–1.2	–	Mens et al., 1982a
	10–20	–	–	–	Harris et al., 1981

[a] AVP-related NP; [b] OXT-related NP.

This large molar excess is found in all species examined and at first sight is at variance with the notion that neurophysins and the nonapeptides, being synthesized as part of a common precursor molecule (Land et al., 1982), should be stored and secreted in an equimolar ratio. The reasons for this curious excess of NP in CSF will be discussed later.

Pavel (1970, 1973) has suggested that mammalian CSF contains measurable amounts of another neurohypophysial peptide, arginine-vasotocin (AVT), secreted from the pineal gland (Pavel, 1971) or other circumventricular organs (Rosenbloom and Fisher, 1975). High levels of AVT have been reported in the CSF of newborn infants (Pavel, 1980), and in animals in response to injection of a wide variety of substances (Goldstein and Pavel, 1977; Pavel et al., 1977). However, Dogterom et al. (1980) could not detect AVT in the pineal or subcommissural organs of several mammalian species using specific and sensitive RIAs. As the identification of AVT in CSF has relied heavily on its hydroosmotic activity, it would seem desirable to confirm this activity as AVT by specific RIA and chromatographic characterization before accepting the presence of this peptide in mammalian CSF.

The evidence that AVP and OXT are present in CSF as the authentic neurohypophysial peptides is much firmer. In addition to recognition by a variety of bioassays, RIAs and parallel dilution studies, these peptides have been identified by destruction with trypsin or thioglycolate (Heller et al., 1968), reaction with pregnancy plasma oxytocinase and neutralization with specific antibodies (Vorherr et al., 1968), extraction by agarose-neurophysin (Robinson and Walker, 1979), and ion-exchange (Hammer et al., 1982) or high pressure liquid chromatography (HPLC, Reppert et al., 1981). Although NP-like material in CSF is much less well characterized, it does dilute in parallel with authentic NP in RIAs and co-chromatographs with pituitary NP in the monkey (Robinson and Zimmerman, 1973), guinea pig and human (Fig. 1, Robinson, unpublished).

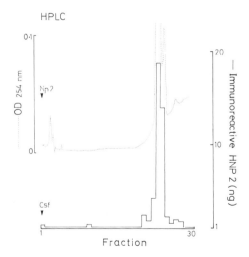

Fig. 1. High pressure liquid chromatography of NP in CSF. A 1 ml sample of human CSF was chromatographed on a reversed phase Nucleosil 5μ C18 column using a gradient of acetonitrile (9–27% in 30 min) in 0.2 M KH$_2$PO$_4$, pH 2.1. Solid line shows the NP immunoreactivity in 1.0 ml fractions; dotted line shows the elution profile of 12.5 μg purified human NPII (OXT-related) run under the same conditions.

WHAT IS THE SOURCE OF THESE PEPTIDES IN CSF?

Passage into CSF from the bloodstream

The question of a blood–brain barrier, or more properly a blood–CSF barrier, to neurohypophysial peptides has often been raised in attempts to determine to what extent the levels of these peptides in CSF merely reflect secretion from the posterior pituitary followed by transport or diffusion from the bloodstream into CSF.

Heller et al. (1968) were somewhat surprised to find AVP in CSF after i.v. injection in anaesthetized rabbits and suggested that the rise in systemic blood pressure produced by the relatively large bolus doses of AVP (50 mU/kg) may have altered the permeability of the blood–CSF barrier. In contrast, Vorherr et al. (1968) gave similar amounts by infusion to dogs and found no evidence for AVP crossing into CSF. Recently, Wang et al. (1981) showed that CSF levels in dogs remained unchanged ($\approx$ 3 μU/ml) during infusions of AVP which produced 100-fold greater levels in plasma. In man, peripheral administration of Pitressin had no effect on CSF levels of AVP (Luerssen et al., 1977; Jenkins et al., 1980), and in the syndrome of inappropriate secretion of antidiuretic hormone (SIADH), high plasma AVP levels were not accompanied by high CSF levels (Luerssen and Robertson, 1980), indicating that an effective blood–CSF barrier to AVP also exists in humans. Peripheral injections of [3H]LVP or [3H]OXT produced very small amounts of radioactivity in rabbit CSF (Zaidi and Heller, 1974), and even this small amount (1–2 % of injected dose) may not have represented intact peptide (Ang and Jenkins, 1982). In conscious guinea pigs (Jones and Robinson, 1982), CSF levels were unaffected by i.v. infusions of OXT which produced 450–1700 fmol/ml in plasma, although OXT was detected in CSF (2–3 % of plasma levels) when peripheral infusion rates were increased 10-fold.

Neurophysin is present in CSF in far higher concentrations than in plasma, so it is most unlikely that this protein reaches CSF by diffusion from the bloodstream. Robinson and Zimmerman (1973) injected bovine NPI into dogs and showed that it was undetectable (< 1 % plasma levels) in CSF. Using a similar approach, Jones and Robinson (1982) infused porcine NPIII into conscious guinea pigs and were unable to detect this protein crossing into CSF. In both these studies it was necessary to use species-specific RIAs to detect exogenous NP in the presence of the high levels of endogenous NP in CSF. It is therefore possible that the permeability of the blood–CSF barrier could be greater towards the endogenous protein.

One may conclude from these studies that there is an effective blood–CSF barrier to neurohypophysial peptides under normal physiological conditions. However, when very high plasma concentrations are produced by peripheral administration of large doses of exogenous peptides, significant amounts of these peptides or their metabolites (not necessarily inactive in the CNS) might reach CSF. Levels of AVP (Zimmerman et al., 1973; Recht et al., 1981) and OXT (Robinson and Fink, unpublished) can exceed 1 pmol/ml in the hypophysial portal circulation, and could well reach the surrounding CSF spaces. There are specialized areas (the circumventricular organs) which have little or no blood–brain barrier and contain large amounts of several neuropeptides (Kizer et al., 1976). Neurohypophysial peptides could gain restricted access to the CNS at these sites (Landgraf et al., 1979) without producing detectable changes in bulk CSF, and this could offer an explanation for CNS effects reported after peripheral administration of OXT and AVP. Nevertheless, the amounts usually employed produce plasma concentrations of OXT and AVP far outside the physiological range, and we may still conclude that under most circumstances plasma levels of endogenously released peptides make a negligible contribution to bulk CSF levels.

Direct secretion into CSF

Numerous studies have demonstrated neurosecretory material in fibres running close to or even penetrating the ependymal lining of the third ventricle (see Rodriguez, 1976) and there is recent immunohistochemical evidence for many OXT-, AVP- and NP-containing fibres at or near the ependymal lining of the cerebral ventricles and central canal of the spinal cord (Sofroniew and Weindl, 1981; Gibson et al., 1981). Release from these fibres would provide a simple explanation for the presence of OXT and AVP in CSF. However, morphological studies do not show whether these fibres actually release their contents into the ventricular system. Some of these structures might equally well be taking up material from CSF, just as specialized ependymal tanycytes in the third ventricle have long been implicated in the transport of neurohypophysial peptides to or from the CSF space (Robinson and Zimmerman, 1973).

Brownfield and Kozlowski (1977) reported the existence of an NP-containing hypothalamo-choroidal pathway, supporting the idea that neurohypophysial peptides might control the formation or absorption of CSF and be secreted into, or absorbed from, this fluid at the choroid plexus (Rodriguez, 1976). AVP-like material is present in extracts of choroid plexus (Rodriguez and Heller, 1970; Dogterom et al., 1978a) and central injections of AVP can alter brain water transport and capillary permeability (Raichle and Grubb, 1978; Noto et al., 1978). However, the immunohistochemical evidence for a choroidal projection has been questioned (Sofroniew and Weindl, 1981), and there is a large discrepancy ($> 10^4$-fold) between the CSF levels produced by intracerebroventricular (i.c.v.) injections and the normal levels of AVP in CSF. Abnormal CSF AVP levels may be involved in the pathology of cerebral oedema (Mather et al., 1981; Hammer et al., 1982), though whether as a cause or a result remains to be determined. Although the notion is teleologically attractive, one wonders whether the CSF side of the blood–CSF barrier is the most appropriate for an AVP-sensitive site?

Diffusion from brain extracellular fluid

It is not necessary to postulate direct secretion of neurohypophysial peptides into CSF from specialized neurones with terminals in the ventricular walls. There are many OXT- and AVP-containing neurones widely distributed throughout the CNS, whose terminal fields are close to ventricular spaces. If these terminals release their secretory products, they will diffuse through the extracellular fluid and they, or their metabolites, would enter bulk CSF without difficulty (Jackson, 1980). OXT and AVP are released from brain tissue depolarized in vitro (Buijs and Van Heerikhuize, 1982) or subjected to push–pull perfusion in vivo (Cooper et al., 1979; Pittman et al., 1981), and their levels in CSF rise after hypothalamic stimulation (Schwarzberg et al., 1971; Harris et al., 1981). Release within the brain followed by diffusion through brain extracellular fluid (ECF) probably represents the major source of neurohypophysial peptides in CSF.

It is difficult to distinguish direct secretion into CSF from secretion into brain ECF followed by passage into CSF, but the routes of entry have different implications for the presence of neurohypophysial peptides in CSF. If these peptides are secreted directly into CSF it is reasonable to suppose that the CSF may be transporting them to distant targets and that some central functions may be regulated by the normal levels of OXT or AVP in CSF. Such physiological roles should be demonstrable by administration of exogenous peptides in doses which produce CSF levels in the normal range. If, on the other hand, CSF levels reflect secretion into brain ECF, it is more likely that CSF is acting to remove the peptides from their central targets and disposing of the peptides or their metabolites as waste products. In this case, it would be necessary to administer large doses of exogenous peptides into CSF to enable sufficient peptide to achieve an effective concentration after penetration some distance into brain tissue.

WHAT STIMULI ALTER THE LEVELS OF NEUROHYPOPHYSIAL PEPTIDES IN CSF?

Several groups have applied physiological or pharmacological stimuli which activate the classical hypothalamo-neurohypophysial system to see if these stimuli also release OXT, AVP or NP into CSF. Haemorrhage is a convenient and powerful stimulus for pituitary AVP release. This stimulus also raises AVP levels in CSF (Vorherr et al., 1968; Schuart et al., 1981), although the rise is much smaller than that in plasma, and only occurs when the haemorrhage becomes severe (> 30 ml/kg, Wang et al., 1981). The disadvantage of haemorrhage is that it produces major cardiovascular changes and may alter the permeability of the blood–brain barrier at a time when plasma AVP levels are very high. Wang et al. (1981), using peripheral AVP infusions, showed that high levels of plasma AVP did not per se change CSF levels in their experiments. However, this control is not ideal since AVP infusions raise blood pressure, whereas haemorrhage lowers it. Subarachnoid haemorrhage in man is occasionally associated with slightly elevated CSF AVP levels (Mather et al., 1981), but the significance of this is unclear at present.

In a recent review, Luerssen and Robertson (1980) concluded that a major determinant of CSF AVP in normal man is the osmolality of body water since they found a correlation between plasma and CSF AVP levels in different states of water balance. However, the absolute levels of AVP in CSF were very similar in groups of patients with diabetes insipidus (DI) or SIADH, even though the corresponding plasma AVP values, as well as osmotic concentrations in both compartments, were widely different.

Dogterom et al. (1978b) found that 24-h water deprivation had no effect on CSF levels in the dog, although in this preliminary study plasma AVP levels were also unchanged. In later studies (Mens et al., 1980, 1982a) CSF levels of AVP in rats were unaffected by water deprivation or drinking 2% NaCl for 1–3 days, stimuli which produced 8–10-fold rises in plasma AVP. In anaesthetised dogs, i.v. infusion of 2.5 M saline for 3 h produced gradual rises in plasma AVP (up to 10-fold) without altering CSF AVP levels (Wang et al., 1982). However, a large hypertonic stimulus introduced into the lateral ventricle produced a different pattern of responses. Plasma AVP rose to a peak within 30 min and then fell to control levels even though the hypertonic infusion continued for 3 h. CSF levels rose slowly, reaching maximum values only after 2–3 h of i.c.v. infusion. Similarly, hyperosmotic solutions given by push–pull perfusion into the third ventricle of conscious rats (Barnard and Morris, 1982) produced a 4–5-fold increase in both OXT and AVP which returned towards control levels despite the continued infusion of hyperosmotic solution. The specificity of the response to such hyperosmotic solutions given directly into the ventricular system must be questioned. In the experiments of Wang et al. (1982), CSF osmolality rose further in response to the peripheral osmotic stimulus than it did during central infusions, without altering CSF AVP levels. There is a strong likelihood that central infusions of hyperosmotic solutions could produce non-specific excitation of many neurones (Leng et al., 1982), either generally, or locally at the ventricular walls, resulting in elevated levels of OXT and AVP in CSF. This author remains

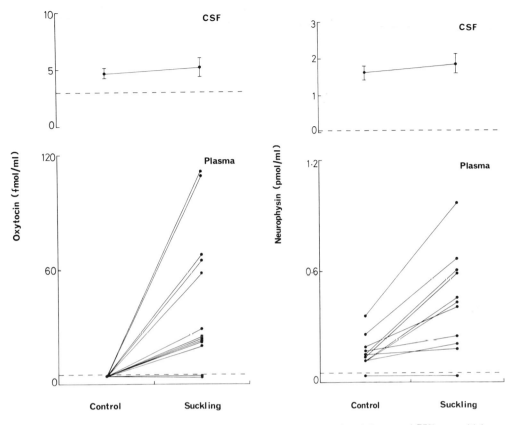

Fig. 2. OXT and NP in plasma and CSF during suckling. Simultaneous samples of plasma and CSF were withdrawn before and at milk-ejection in lactating guinea pigs and assayed for OXT or NP. Despite large rises in plasma, there were no significant changes in the CSF levels of either OXT or NP. Dotted lines show assay thresholds; CSF values are mean ± S.E.M. (Adapted from Robinson and Jones, 1982a.)

unconvinced that physiological osmotic stimuli play a major role in controlling levels of neurohypophysial peptides in CSF.

In looking for a specific stimulus for OXT release into CSF, Robinson and Jones (1982a) investigated suckling in conscious guinea pigs. Suckling produces large acute rises in plasma OXT and NP without altering CSF levels significantly (Fig. 2), and there are no differences in the levels of OXT, AVP or NP in CSF from lactating females compared to normal females or males. In a preliminary study, Pittman et al. (1982c) have found no evidence for activation of any centrally-projecting OXT neurones during suckling. These findings suggest that extrahypothalamic OXT terminals are not activated to release OXT during suckling, and do not support the notion that OXT in the brainstem or spinal cord is involved in the suckling reflex. However, Freund-Mercier and Richard (1981) have shown that the firing frequency of OXT neurones at milk-ejection can be increased by introducing OXT into CSF, and it is possible that small amounts of OXT could be released in the hypothalamus or spinal cord during suckling without producing much change in cisternal CSF OXT levels.

Other studies have used pharmacological stimuli to activate secretion from the neural lobe. Nicotine and histamine raise plasma AVP levels acutely in conscious rats without altering CSF

AVP levels (Mens et al., 1980). Higher doses of histamine will also release OXT in a similar fashion (Mens and Van Wimersma Greidanus, personal communication). Removal of the posterior pituitary gland abolishes the release of AVP into plasma, but, paradoxically, histamine is highly effective in elevating CSF levels in hypophysectomized rats (Mens et al., 1982b). Basal levels of OXT and AVP in CSF are raised following hypophysectomy (Dogterom et al., 1977), and in diabetes insipidus (DI) patients AVP levels in CSF are higher than in plasma, reversing the gradient normally found (Luerssen and Robertson, 1980). One possibility is that the structural re-organization which follows hypophysectomy may allow nerve endings, which in the normal animal only release into the bloodstream, to cause release into CSF. Cutting the pituitary stalk will drastically alter the flow and contact area of CSF in the third ventricle, and there may be release from resealed cut axons into an extracellular compartment which has little or no barrier to passage into bulk CSF.

Pentobarbitone releases AVP into blood and CSF in normal rats (Mens et al., 1982b); hypophysectomy abolishes the release into blood but CSF release is unchanged, suggesting that this barbiturate activates both pituitary and extrapituitary projections. This confirms the impression gained from earlier studies that plasma and CSF levels of neurohypophysial peptides are generally higher under barbiturate anaesthesia (Table I), and stresses the value of working with unanaesthetized animals. Angiotensin II (Artman et al., 1982a) and oestradiol (Perlow et al., 1982) cause no change in CSF levels of AVP or NP, respectively, even though both agents release these peptides into plasma. Clearly, further work is needed to establish whether the neuropharmacology of the classical hypothalamo-neurohypophysial system will apply to the central OXT and AVP systems.

Environmental cues may affect OXT and AVP levels in CSF. Many studies using central injections of OXT, AVP or their antisera directly into CSF have provided evidence implicating OXT or AVP in various aspects of behaviour or memory (De Wied, 1976; Van Wimersma Greidanus and De Wied, 1976), and there are several reports that CSF AVP levels in man may correlate with mental performance states (see Post et al., 1982). However, no differences were found in the levels of OXT, AVP or NP in the CSF of rats undergoing standardized tests involving the acquisition and retention of passive avoidance behaviour (Van Wimersma Greidanus et al., 1979; Mens et al., 1982a).

Reppert et al. (1981) were the first to report that CSF AVP levels show a diurnal rhythm. High concentrations of AVP in the CSF of cats occurred during daylight hours and the rhythm persisted despite placing the animals in constant light. Similar observations have since been made in the sheep, rat, monkey and guinea pig. In the latter two species, OXT and NP were assayed in addition to AVP. In the monkey (Perlow et al., 1982) the AVP rhythm was small, but a large rhythm of OXT concentrations (12-fold) was present. NP values varied throughout the day, but a diurnal rhythm was less apparent and bore no obvious relationship to the variation in OXT levels. In the guinea pig, there is a diurnal rhythm in AVP but not in OXT or NP (Jones et al., 1982). In the latter study, as in that of Perlow et al. (1982), the molar amounts of NP in CSF were far in excess of OXT or AVP (Fig. 3), so a diurnal rhythm of equimolar amounts of NP ($\pm$ 30 fmol/ml) might well accompany variations in AVP without significantly affecting the total amount of NP measured (1000 fmol/ml). In the cat and the guinea pig, neither of which show an OXT rhythm, the source of the diurnal variation of AVP may be the suprachiasmatic nucleus (Reppert et al., 1981; Robinson and Jones, 1982c). This nucleus contains a number of cells producing AVP, but not OXT, which project exclusively to sites other than the posterior pituitary (Vandesande et al., 1975; Sofroniew and Weindl, 1980; Hoorneman and Buijs, 1982). In contrast, the monkey shows a large diurnal rhythm in CSF OXT, normally synchronized with the phase of the light–dark cycle, but which persists

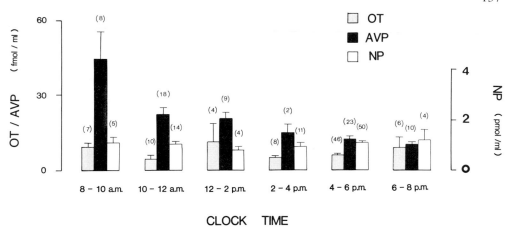

Fig. 3. Daily variation in CSF AVP levels in guinea pigs. CSF samples were withdrawn from conscious guinea pigs at various times and assayed either for OXT, AVP or NP. AVP levels varied markedly throughout the day, being highest in the morning. OXT and NP levels showed no significant change. (From Jones et al., 1982.)

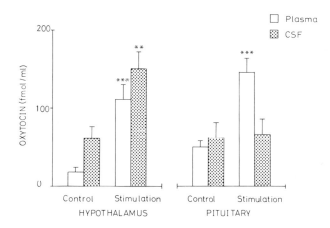

Fig. 4. OXT release into plasma and CSF by electrical stimulation. The figure shows the mean ($\pm$ S.E.M.) levels of OXT in plasma (open bars) and CSF (dotted bars) before and after electrical stimulation (75 HZ, 80–160 μA for 15 sec) of the paraventricular nucleus (hypothalamus) or the neural lobe (pituitary) in anaesthetized rats. (From Harris et al., 1981.) Hypothalamic stimulation raised OXT levels in both plasma and CSF, whereas pituitary stimulation released only into plasma. P vs control: ** < 0.01; *** < 0.001.

throughout 3–6 days of constant light or darkness (Artman et al., 1982b). Further studies are needed to establish which cell groups are responsible for the diurnal rhythm of OXT and AVP in different species, and whether such variation has any physiological significance.

Direct electrical stimulation can be used as a means of activating OXT-, or AVP-containing cells and thus releasing these peptides into CSF. Stimulation of the central end of a severed vagus nerve produced increases in AVP levels in rabbits (Heller et al., 1968), and Schwarzberg et al. (1971) found that a 15 min stimulation of the paraventricular, but not the supraoptic, nucleus increased OXT levels in rabbit CSF. There is also evidence that generalized activation of the CNS caused by seizures in man (Unger et al., 1971) or convulsions induced in animals

138

by pentylenetetrazol (Mens and Van Wimersma Greidanus, personal communication) are accompanied by increases in CSF levels of OXT or AVP. Brief stimuli (15 sec) applied to the paraventricular nucleus elicit reproducible increases in both plasma and CSF OXT levels in anaesthetized rats (Harris et al., 1981). Similar stimuli applied to the neural lobe produce plasma rises without altering CSF levels (Fig. 4), providing direct evidence against the existence of many bipolar neurones releasing OXT into blood and CSF. Although electrical stimulation is a relatively crude means of activating central OXT and AVP pathways, it is controllable and reproducible in its effects, and can be used (Fig. 5) to study the release of OXT, AVP or NP into perfusates of the cerebroventricular system or the spinal cord (Robinson and Jones, 1982b, c; Pittman et al., 1982b).

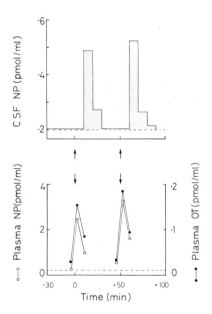

Fig. 5. NP release into cerebroventricular perfusates. In an anaesthetized guinea pig, the cerebroventricular system was perfused with artificial CSF (10 μl/min) from left lateral ventricle to cisterna magna and perfusate collected over 10 min periods. Two consecutive PVN stimulations (15 sec, arrow) released NP into the perfusate, although the rises were somewhat delayed compared with the rapid increases in plasma NP and OXT.

CLEARANCE OF NEUROHYPOPHYSIAL PEPTIDES FROM CSF

One area which has received surprisingly little attention is the fate of neurohypophysial peptides once they reach CSF. CSF is thought to be absorbed principally by bulk flow through arachnoid villi which act as valved passages providing a one-way connection between the CSF and plasma compartments (Pollay, 1977). The clearance of neurohypophysial peptides from CSF has recently been studied in conscious guinea pigs (Fig. 6). Whilst NP was cleared at a rate expected from bulk flow, the nonapeptides were cleared significantly faster, the half-times of clearance being 28 and 24 min for OXT and AVP, respectively, compared to 46 min for NP (Jones and Robinson, 1982). Infusion experiments showed that the available distribution space in equilibrium with bulk CSF was similar for both AVP and NP. Similar clearance rates for OXT and AVP have recently been reported in the rat (Mens et al., 1982c).

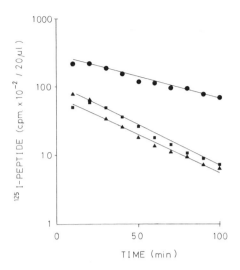

Fig. 6. Clearance of neurohypophysial peptides from CSF. CSF samples (20 μl) were withdrawn from the cisterna magna at 10 min intervals after i.c.v. injection of radioiodinated OXT (■), AVP (▲) or NP (●). The figure shows the clearance of each substance measured in three separate experiments using the same animal. Note that OXT and AVP disappear from cisternal CSF faster than does NP.

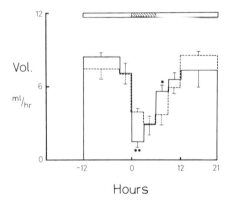

Fig. 7. Antidiuretic response to AVP infused i.v. and i.c.v. to Brattleboro rats. Homozygous Brattleboro rats were equipped with chronic indwelling cannulae in the jugular vein and lateral ventricle, housed individually in metabolic cages and given continuous infusions (horizontal bar) of saline (i.v.) or artificial CSF (i.c.v.). The figure shows two experiments on the same group of rats. AVP was infused for 6 h (hatched bar) at 3 ng/h i.c.v., and on the following day at 0.33 ng/h i.v. Urinary volume (Vol.) was markedly reduced during i.v. infusion (solid lines) but returned rapidly to normal when the AVP infusion ceased. Infusions of AVP i.c.v. (dashed lines) also produced antidiuresis, but the responses were delayed and prolonged compared to the i.v. route. * $P < 0.05$; ** $P < 0.01$.

Although it is not certain whether the nonapeptides are metabolized during their passage from CSF, several authors have invoked "leakage" of biologically active AVP from CSF into plasma to explain antidiuretic effects of large doses of AVP administered i.c.v. (Bhargava et al., 1977; Severs et al., 1978; Pittman et al., 1982a). We have investigated this by comparing the effects on urine flow of AVP administered i.v. or i.c.v. to chronically cannulated Brattleboro rats (Fig. 7). Clearly, there is a delayed response to AVP infused i.c.v. compared with i.v. infusion, but a significant amount of biologically active AVP does reach the kidney after i.c.v. infusion at relatively low rates. It is difficult to compare the renal responses quantitatively because of the difference in time-course, but results from a number of experiments of this type suggest that at least 10%, and possibly as much as 30%, of AVP infused centrally is cleared in an intact form. Whilst the amounts of AVP normally present in CSF make little or no contribution to plasma bioactivity under normal conditions, these findings should be borne in mind when exogenous peptides are administered into CSF. The same caution should also apply to the central administration of antisera or antagonists in attempts to neutralize OXT or AVP within the CNS. Anti-OXT antibodies are cleared efficiently from CSF and accumulate in the plasma where their half-life is long (≈ 7 days) compared to that in CSF (≈ 40 min, Jones and Robinson, 1982).

HOW CAN THE LARGE MOLAR EXCESS OF NP IN CSF BE EXPLAINED?

Although the apparent excess of NP in CSF has been noted previously (Luerssen and Robertson, 1980), it is only recently that this finding has been confirmed by simultaneous assays of NP and the nonapeptides in the same animal (Table II). In most cases, the assays have not been capable of distinguishing between OXT-related and AVP-related NPs. However, in man (Burford et al., 1981; Born et al., 1981) most of the NP excess can be attributed to the OXT-related protein (Table I) and in the guinea pig, where an OXT-related NP can be distinguished from the major AVP-related protein by HPLC (Robinson, unpublished), the CSF contains predominantly the minor, OXT-related NP. The most obvious explanation for excess NP in CSF would be that this 10,000 molecular weight protein is cleared more slowly than the nonapeptides, but direct measurements in the guinea pig show that the difference in clearance rates is nowhere near large enough to account for the amount of NP normally present in CSF (Jones and Robinson, 1982). Making several assumptions regarding available distribution volume, thorough mixing, and CSF production rate in the guinea pig, one can arrive at a figure of 3–4 fmol/min as the entry rate of NP into CSF compared to 0.1–0.2 fmol/min for OXT or AVP. Either NP and the nonapeptides are secreted in an equimolar ratio but are differentially degraded or taken up en route from secretion site to bulk CSF, or the total amount of NP released is far in excess over that of OXT or AVP.

TABLE II

CSF AND PITUITARY CONTENT OF OXT, AVP AND NP IN THE GUINEA PIG

In this experiment, all three neurohypophysial peptides were measured in the posterior pituitary gland and samples of CSF from the same male guinea pig. Note that whilst the NP:nonapeptide ratio is close to equimolar in the pituitary, there is a 50-fold NP excess in the CSF of this animal.

	Pituitary content (nmol/pit.)	CSF concentration (fmol/ml)
OXT	1.6	4.6
AVP	5.7	14.8
NP	6.2	1053
Ratio: $\frac{NP}{OXT+AVP}$	0.9	54

One possibility is that the substances present in CSF are not identical to those in the posterior pituitary and are thus misread by the assays. There is no reason to assume that the NP-nonapeptide precursors or their post-translational processing will be the same in centrally projecting neurones as in the neural lobe. Authentic NP could be secreted from some terminals with precursor-related peptides containing OXT-, or AVP-sequences, not detected by the specific RIAs used. Alternatively, the NP-like material in CSF, though chromatographically similar (Fig. 1), might be different from pituitary NP. Sinding et al. (1982) have reported that most of the NP-like material extractable from rat brain is chromatographically heterogeneous, and larger than 10,000 molecular weight, but this has not been confirmed by Lang et al. (1982) using specific RIAs and HPLC. The latter group also noted that OXT-NP predominated over AVP-NP in extracts of the brainstem, in line with immunohistochemical evidence that OXT or OXT-NP fibres in this area outnumber AVP or AVP-NP positive fibres (Nilaver et al., 1980). It seems reasonable to conclude that the excess of OXT-NP over AVP-NP in CSF may simply reflect the relative amounts of these proteins in central secretory stores. By the same argument, the large excess of NP over the nonapeptides in CSF might suggest that some central pathways store and secrete much more NP than the nonapeptides. Nilaver et al. (1980) noted that OXT-positive fibres are much more elusive than NP-positive fibres in the spinal cord, but suggested that this might be due to differential losses during tissue preparation. In preliminary studies using RIAs, we have found excess NP over OXT and AVP in many areas of the brain and spinal cord of animals whose pituitary NP:nonapeptide ratios, measured in the same assays, were close to equimolar.

There are dangers in extrapolating the release ratio from the tissue content of these peptides. It seems that the hormones must be contained in synaptic structures for normal release to occur; areas containing OXT and AVP in varicosities, but devoid of specialized synapses, do not release their content following depolarization in a Ca^{2+}-dependent manner (Buijs and Van Heerikhuize, 1982). OXT and AVP fibres differ widely in their distribution throughout the CNS and release from these different sites will give rise to varying amounts of OXT or AVP eventually appearing in lumbar or cisternal CSF. Localized perfusion of the lateral ventricle in guinea pigs showed that OXT, AVP and NP can all be released into this space following stimulation of the paraventricular nucleus (Robinson and Jones, 1982c), whereas this stimulus released far more OXT than AVP into perfusates of the spinal cord (Pittman et al., 1982b). Such perfusion techniques provide a convenient means of studying the release ratios from different brain regions under various physiological conditions, and should complement studies of granule content, biosynthetic processing and neuropharmacology of the central OXT and AVP systems.

CONCLUDING REMARKS

Virtually all the studies of neurohypophysial peptides in CSF assume that these substances function as neurotransmitters or neuromodulators within the CNS. For the most part, delivery of the peptides is achieved by neural projections which release locally at the sites of action, and it is difficult to see any role for the CSF other than in eliminating the peptides as waste products. Nevertheless, there are some areas of the CNS which are sensitive to OXT or AVP but which do not appear to receive a direct peptidergic innervation. Perhaps the peptides have more generalized actions, altering the electrophysiological, biochemical or morphological characteristics of some neurones over periods of hours, days or weeks. Since release into CSF is usually dissociated from release into the bloodstream, one may conclude that the central OXT and AVP pathways must be separate, functionally as well as morphologically (Sofroniew and Weindl, 1980, 1981; Armstrong et al., 1980; Swanson and Sawchenko, 1980), from the classical hypothalamo-neurohypophysial system, though why these central pathways should store and secrete excess NP is puzzling. Despite their limitations, CSF measurements still provide a convenient and relatively non-invasive way of studying the release of OXT, AVP and NP within the brain.

SUMMARY

Oxytocin (OXT), vasopressin (AVP) and neurophysin (NP) are found in many areas of the brain and spinal cord. Since there is a blood–CSF barrier to these peptides, CSF levels probably reflect release from central terminals rather than from the hypothalamo-neurohypophysial system.

The physiological stimuli which release these peptides into CSF are poorly understood. Endocrine stimuli (suckling, dehydration) causing release into plasma do not change CSF levels of OXT, AVP or NP, but central release of AVP does occur during haemorrhage. Electrical stimulation of the hypothalamus releases all three peptides into CSF and into perfusates of different parts of the ventricular system.

There is a marked diurnal rhythm of AVP in CSF and a large molar excess of NP over the nonapeptides. Although OXT and AVP are cleared somewhat faster than NP, this cannot explain the NP excess, which is mostly due to the OXT-related protein. Much of the AVP cleared from CSF reaches the bloodstream in a biologically active form.

It now seems likely that central OXT and AVP neurones are both morphologically and functionally separate from the neurohypophysial system. CSF measurements thus provide a useful, though indirect, means of studying these peptides within the central nervous system.

ACKNOWLEDGEMENTS

I am very grateful to R.M. Buijs, Q.J. Pittman, Tj.B. van Wimersma Greidanus and their co-workers for sending me advance copies of their most recent work, and to my own colleagues, R.G. Clark, P.M. Jones and M.C. Harris for unpublished data. In particular I would like to thank Peter Jones for his helpful and constructive criticisms of this manuscript.

REFERENCES

Ang, V.T.Y. and Jenkins, J.S. (1982) Blood–cerebrospinal fluid barrier to arginine-vasopressin, desmopressin and desglycinamide arginine-vasopressin in the dog. *J. Endocr.*, 93: 319–325.

Armstrong, W.E., Warach, S., Hatton, G.I. and McNeill, T.H. (1980) Subnuclei in the rat hypothalamic paraventricular nucleus: a cytoarchitectural, horseradish peroxidase and immunocytochemical analysis. *Neuroscience*, 5: 1931–1958.

Artman, H.G., Leake, R.D., Sawicki, G., Tarris, R., Oddie, T.H. and Fisher, D.A. (1982a) Separate control of vasopressin secretion into cerebrospinal fluid and blood. In *Abstracts, 64th Ann. Meeting Amer. Endocr. Soc.* Abstr. 167.

Artman, H.G., Reppert, S.M., Perlow, M.J., Swaminathan, S., Oddie, T.H. and Fisher, D.A. (1982b) Characterisation of the daily oxytocin rhythm in primate cerebrospinal fluid. *J. Neurosci.*, 2: 598–603.

Barnard, R.R., Jr. and Morris, M. (1982) Cerebrospinal fluid vasopressin and oxytocin: evidence for an osmotic response. *Neurosci. Lett.*, 29: 275–279.

Bhargava, K.P., Kulshrestha, V.K. and Srivastava, Y.P. (1977) Central mechanisms of vasopressin-induced changes in antidiuretic hormone release. *Brit. J. Pharmacol.*, 60: 77–81.

Born, J., Geenen, V. and Legros, J.J. (1981) Neurophysin II — but not neurophysin I — concentrations are higher in lumbar than in ventricular cerebrospinal fluid in neurological patients. *Neuroendocr. Lett.*, 4: 31–35.

Bouman, H.J. and Van Wimersma Greidanus, Tj.B. (1979) A rapid and simple cannulation technique for repeated sampling of cerebrospinal fluid in freely moving rats. *Brain Res. Bull.*, 4: 575–577.

Brownfield, M.S. and Kozlowski, G.P. (1977) The hypothalamochoroidal tract. I. Immunohistochemical demonstration of neurophysin pathways to telencephalic choroid plexuses and cerebrospinal fluid. *Cell Tiss. Res.*, 178: 111–127.

Buijs, R.M. and van Heerikhuize, J.J. (1982) Vasopressin and oxytocin release in the brain; a synaptic event. *Brain Res.*, in press.

Burford, G.D., Robinson, I.C.A.F. and Swann, R.W. (1981) Neurophysin and hormone levels in the hypothalamus, neurohypophysis and cerebrospinal fluid of the human fetus. *Acta endocr.*, 97, Suppl. 243: 317.

Cooper, K.E., Kasting, N.W., Lederis, K. and Veale, W.L. (1979) Evidence supporting a role for endogenous vasopressin in natural suppression of fever in the sheep. *J. Physiol. (Lond.)*, 295: 33–45.

Cushing, H. and Goetsch, E. (1910) Concerning the secretion of the infundibular lobe of the pituitary body and its presence in the cerebrospinal fluid. *Amer. J. Physiol.*, 27: 60–86.

De Wied, D. (1976) Behavioural effects of intraventricularly administered vasopressin and vasopressin fragments. *Life Sci.*, 19: 685–690.

Dogterom, J., Van Wimersma Greidanus, Tj.B. and Swaab, D.F. (1977) Evidence for the release of vasopressin and oxytocin into cerebrospinal fluid: measurements in plasma and CSF of intact and hypophysectomised rats. *Neuroendocrinology*, 24: 108–118.

Dogterom, J., Snijdewint, F.G.M. and Buijs, R.M. (1978a) The distribution of vasopressin and oxytocin in the rat brain. *Neurosci. Lett.*, 9: 341–346.

Dogterom, J., Van Wimersma Greidanus, Tj.B. and De Wied, D. (1978b) Vasopressin in cerebrospinal fluid and plasma of man, dog and rat. *Amer. J. Physiol.*, 234: E463–467.

Dogterom, J., Snijdewint, F.G.M., Pevet, P. and Swaab, D.F. (1980) Studies on the presence of vasopressin, oxytocin and vasotocin in the pineal gland, sub-commissural organ and fetal pituitary gland: failure to demonstrate vasotocin in mammals. *J. Endocr.*, 84: 115–123.

Freund-Mercier, M.J. and Richard, Ph. (1981) Excitatory effects of intraventricular injections of oxytocin on the milk-ejection reflex in the rat. *Neurosci. Lett.*, 23: 193–198.

Friedman, G.S. and Friedman, M.H. (1933) An examination of cerebrospinal fluid for oxytocic activity as tested by the rabbit uterine fistula preparation. *Amer. J. Physiol.*, 103: 244–254.

Gibson, S.J., Polak, J.M., Bloom, S.R. and Wall, P.D. (1981) The distribution of nine peptides in rat spinal cord with special emphasis on the substantia gelatinosa and on the area around the central canal (lamina X). *J. comp. Neurol.*, 201: 65–79.

Goldstein, R. and Pavel, S. (1977) Vasotocin release into the cerebrospinal fluid of cats induced by luteinizing hormone releasing hormone, thyrotrophin releasing hormone and growth hormone release-inhibiting hormone. *J. Endocr.*, 75: 175–176.

Hammer, M., Sorensen, P.S., Gjerris, F. and Larsen, K. (1982) Vasopressin in the cerebrospinal fluid of patients with normal pressure hydrocephalus and benign intracranial hypertension. *Acta endocr.*, 100: 211–215.

Harris, M.C., Jones, P.M. and Robinson, I.C.A.F. (1981) Differences in the release of oxytocin into blood and cerebrospinal fluid following hypothalamic and pituitary stimulation in rats. *J. Physiol. (Lond.)*, 320: 109–110P.

Heller, H. (1969) Neurohypophysial hormones in the cerebrospinal fluid. In G. Sterba (Ed.), *Zirkumventrikulare Organe und Liquor*, Fischer, Jena, pp. 235–242.

Heller, H., Hasan, S.H. and Saifi, A.Q. (1968) Antidiuretic activity in the cerebrospinal fluid. *J. Endocr.*, 41: 273–280.

Hoorneman, E.M.D. and Buijs, R.M. (1982) Vasopressin fibre pathways in the rat brain following suprachiasmatic nucleus lesioning. *Brain Res.*, 243: 235–241.

Jackson, I.M.D. (1980) Significance and function of neuropeptides in cerebrospinal fluid. In J.H. Woods (Ed.), *Neurobiology of the Cerebrospinal Fluid*, Plenum, New York, pp. 625–650.

Jenkins, J.S., Mather, H.M. and Ang, V. (1980) Vasopressin in human cerebrospinal fluid. *J. clin. Endocr. Metab.*, 50: 364–367.

Jones, P.M. and Robinson, I.C.A.F. (1981) A method for repeated sampling of cerebrospinal fluid from conscious guinea pigs. *J. Neurosci. Meth.*, 3: 295–300.

Jones, P.M. and Robinson, I.C.A.F. (1982) Differential clearance of neurophysin and neurohypophysial peptides from the cerebrospinal fluid in conscious guinea pigs. *Neuroendocrinology*, 34: 297–302.

Jones, P.M., Fairhall, K.M. and Robinson, I.C.A.F. (1982) Diurnal variations in vasopressin, oxytocin and neurophysin in guinea pig CSF. *J. Endocr.*, 94, Suppl.: 37P.

Kizer, J.S., Palkovits, M. and Brownstein, M.J. (1976) Releasing factors in the circumventricular organs of the rat brain. *Endocrinology*, 98: 311–317.

Land, H., Schutz, G., Schmale, H. and Richter, D. (1982) Nucleotide sequence of cloned cDNA encoding bovine arginine vasopressin-neurophysin II precursor. *Nature (Lond.)*, 295: 299–303.

144

Landgraf, R., Ermisch, A. and Hess, J. (1979) Indications for a brain uptake of labelled vasopressin and oxytocin and the problem of the blood–brain barrier. *Endokrinologie*, 73: 77–81.

Lang, R.E., Ganten, D., Herrman, R. and Unger, T. (1982) Distribution of neurophysins in rat brain: radioimmunological measurement and characterisation. *Neurosci. Lett.*, 30: 279–283.

Leng, G., Mason, W.T. and Dyer, R.G. (1982) The supra-optic nucleus as an osmoreceptor. *Neuroendocrinology*, 34: 75–82.

Luerssen, T.G. and Robertson, G.L. (1980) Cerebrospinal fluid vasopressin and vasotocin in health and disease. In J.H. Woods (Ed.), *Neurobiology of the Cerebrospinal Fluid*, Plenum, New York, pp. 613–623.

Luerssen, T.G., Shelton, R.L. and Robertson, G.L. (1977) Evidence for separate origin of plasma and cerebrospinal fluid vasopressin. *Clin. Res.*, 25: 14A.

Mather, H.M., Ang, V. and Jenkins, J.S. (1981) Vasopressin in plasma and CSF of patients with subarachnoid haemorrhage. *J. neurol. Neurosurg. Psychiat.*, 44: 216–219.

Mens, W.B., Bouman, H.J., Bakker, E.A. and Van Wimersma Greidanus, Tj.B. (1980) Differential effects of various stimuli on AVP levels in blood and cerebrospinal fluid. *Europ. J. Pharmacol.*, 68: 89–92.

Mens, W.B., Van Dam, A.F., van Egmond, M.A.H., Bakker, E.A.D., Legros, J.J. and Van Wimersma Greidanus, Tj.B. (1982a) Neurohypophyseal hormones in cerebrospinal fluid. *Front. Horm. Res.*, 9: 119–130.

Mens, W.B., Van Dam, A.F. and Van Wimersma Greidanus, Tj.B. (1982b) The influence of histamine and pentobarbitone on plasma and CSF vasopressin levels of hypophysectomised rats. *Brain Res. Bull.*, in press.

Mens, W.B., Witter, A. and Van Wimersma Greidanus, Tj.B. (1982c) Penetration of vasopressin and oxytocin from plasma into cerebrospinal fluid and clearance of the neuropeptides from CSF. *J. Endocr.*, 94, Suppl.: 30P.

Nilaver, G., Zimmerman, E.A., Wilkins, J., Michaels, J., Hoffman, D. and Silverman A.-J. (1980) Magnocellular hypothalamic projections to the lower brainstem and spinal cord of the rat. Immunocytochemical evidence for predominance of the oxytocin-neurophysin system compared to the vasopressin-neurophysin system. *Neuroendocrinology*, 30: 150–158.

Noto, T., Nakajima, T., Saji, Y. and Nagawa, Y. (1978) Effect of vasopressin on intracranial pressure of rabbit. *Endocr. jap.*, 25: 591–596.

Pavel, S. (1970) Tentative identification of arginine vasotocin in human cerebrospinal fluid. *J. clin. Endocr. Metab.*, 31: 369–371.

Pavel, S. (1971) Evidence for the ependymal origin of arginine vasotocin in the bovine pineal gland. *Endocrinology*, 89: 613–614.

Pavel, S. (1973) Arginine vasotocin release into cerebrospinal fluid of cats induced by melatonin. *Nature (Lond.)*, 246: 183–184.

Pavel, S. (1980) Presence of relatively high concentrations of arginine vasotocin in the cerebrospinal fluid of newborns and infants. *J. clin. Endocr. Metab.*, 50: 271–273.

Pavel, S., Goldstein, R., Gheorghui, C. and Calb, M. (1977) Pineal vasotocin: release into cat cerebrospinal fluid by melanocyte-stimulating hormone release-inhibiting factor. *Science*, 197: 179–180.

Perlow, M.J., Reppert, S.M., Artman, H.A., Fisher, D.A., Seif, S.M. and Robinson, A.G. (1982) Oxytocin vasopressin and estrogen-stimulated neurophysin: daily patterns of concentration in cerebrospinal fluid. *Science*, 216: 1416–1418.

Pittman, Q.J., Malkinson, T.J., Veale, W.L. and Lederis, K. (1981) Central release of arginine vasopressin (AVP) in rabbit brain. *Soc. Neurosci. Abstr.*, 7: 506.

Pittman, Q.J., Lawrence, D. and McLean, L. (1982a) Central effects of arginine vasopressin on blood pressure in rats. *Endocrinology*, 110: 1058–1060.

Pittman, Q.J., Simpson, J., Ko, D. and Lederis, K. (1982b) In vivo release of neurohypophysial peptides from rat spinal cord. *Soc. Neurosci. Abstr.*, 8: in press.

Pittman, Q.J. Veale, W.L. and Lederis, K. (1982c) Central neurohypophyseal peptide pathways — interactions with endocrine and other autonomic functions. *Peptides*, in press.

Pollay, M. (1977) Review of spinal fluid physiology: production and absorption in relation to pressure. *Clin. Neurosurg.*, 24: 254–269.

Post, R.M., Gold, P., Rubinow, D.R., Ballenger, J.C., Bunney, W.E., Jr. and Goodwin, F.K. (1982) Peptides in the cerebrospinal fluid of neuropsychiatric patients: an approach to central nervous sytem peptide function. *Life Sci.*, 31: 1–15.

Raichle, M.E. and Grubb, R.L., Jr. (1978) Regulation of brain water permeability by centrally-released vasopressin. *Brain Res.*, 143: 191–194.

Recht, L.D., Hoffman, D.L., Haldar, J., Silverman, A.-J. and Zimmerman, E.A. (1981) Vasopressin concentrations in hypophysial portal plasma: insignificant reductions following removal of the posterior pituitary gland. *Neuroendocrinology*, 33: 88–90.

Reppert, S.M., Artman, H.G., Swaminathan, S. and Fisher, D.A. (1981) Vasopressin exhibits a rhythmic daily pattern in cerebrospinal fluid but not in blood. *Science*, 213: 1256–1257.

Robinson, A.G. and Zimmerman, E.A. (1973) Cerebrospinal fluid and ependymal neurophysin. *J. clin. Invest.*, 52: 1260–1267.

Robinson, I.C.A.F. and Jones, P.M. (1982a) Oxytocin and neurophysin in plasma and CSF during suckling in the guinea pig. *Neuroendocrinology*, 34: 59–63.

Robinson, I.C.A.F. and Jones, P.M. (1982b) Release of neurophysin in CSF: local perfusion of cerebral ventricles in the guinea pig. *Neuroscience*, 7 Suppl.: S179.

Robinson, I.C.A.F. and Jones, P.M. (1982c) Neurohypophysial peptides in cerebrospinal fluid: recent studies. In A.J. Baertschi and J.J. Dreifuss (Eds.), *Vasopressin, Corticoliberin and Opiomelanocortins*, Academic Press, London, pp. 21–32.

Robinson, I.C.A.F. and Walker, J.M. (1979) Extraction of small amounts of oxytocin from biological fluids by means of agarose-bound neurophysin. *J. Endocr.*, 80: 191–202.

Rodriguez, E.M. (1976) The cerebrospinal fluid as a pathway in neuroendocrine integration. *J. Endocr.*, 71: 407–443.

Rodriguez, E.M. and Heller, H. (1970) Antidiuretic activity and ultrastructure of the toad choroid plexus. *J. Endocr.*, 46: 83–91.

Rosenbloom, A.A. and Fischer, D.A. (1975) Arginine vasotocin in the rabbit subcommissural organ. *Endocrinology*, 96: 1038–1039.

Schuart, J., Schellenberg, R. and Blume, M. (1981) Effect of discontinuous hemorrhage on plasma and cerebrospinal fluid vasopressin concentration in anaesthetised rabbits. *Acta biol. med. germ.*, 40: 201–207.

Schwartz, W.J., Coleman, R.J. and Reppert, S.M. (1982) Vasopressin exhibits a circadian rhythm in rat cerebrospinal fluid. In *Abstracts, 64th Ann. Meeting Amer. Endocr. Soc.*, Abstr. 167.

Schwarzberg, H., Schulz, H. and Unger, H. (1971) Oxytocin contents in the cerebrospinal fluid in awake rabbits following electric stimulation of nuclear areas near to the cerebrospinal fluid space. *Experientia*, 27: 1483–1484.

Severs, W.B., Keil, L.C. and Klase, P.A. (1978) Consummatory behaviour and urine production after cerebroventricular injection of vasopressin and vasopressin antiserum. *Europ. J. Pharmacol.*, 51: 389–396.

Sinding, C., Camier, M. and Cohen, P. (1982) Extrahypothalamo-neurohypophyseal immunoreactive neurophysin occurs predominantly as high M_r forms in the rat brain stem. *FEBS Lett.*, 140: 124–126.

Sofroniew, M.V. and Weindl, A. (1980) Identification of parvocellular vasopressin and neurophysin neurones in the suprachiasmatic nucleus of a variety of mammals including primates. *J. comp. Neurol.*, 193: 659–675.

Sofroniew, M.V. and Weindl, A. (1981) Central nervous system distribution of vasopressin, oxytocin and neurophysin. In J.L. Martinez, R.A. Jensen, R.B. Messing, H. Rigter and J.L. McGaugh (Eds.), *Endogenous Peptides and Learning and Memory Processes*, Academic Press, New York, pp. 327–369.

Swanson, L.W. and Sawchenko, P.E. (1980) Paraventricular nucleus: a site for the integration of neuroendocrine and autonomic mechanisms. *Neuroendocrinology*, 31: 410–417.

Unger, H., Pommrich, G. and Beck, R. (1971) Oxytocin contents in pathological cerebrospinal fluid in man. *Experientia*, 27: 1486.

Vandesande, F., Dierckx, K. and De Mey, J. (1975) Identification of the vasopressin-neurophysin producing neurons of the rat suprachiasmatic nuclei. *Cell Tiss. Res.*, 156: 377–380.

Van Dyke, H.B., Bailey, P. and Bucy, P.C. (1929) The oxytocic substance of cerebrospinal fluid. *J. Pharmacol. exp. Ther.*, 36: 595–610.

Van Wimersma Greidanus, Tj.B. and De Wied, D. (1976) Modulation of passive avoidance behaviour of rats by intracerebroventricular administration of anti-vasopressin serum. *Behav. Biol.*, 18: 325–333.

Van Wimersma Greidanus, Tj.B., Croiset, G., Goedemans, H. and Dogterom, J. (1979) Vasopressin levels in peripheral blood and in cerebrospinal fluid during passive and active avoidance behaviour in rats. *Horm. Behav.*, 12: 103–111.

Vorherr, H., Bradbury, M.W., Hoghoughi, M. and Kleeman, C.R. (1968) Antidiuretic hormone in cerebrospinal fluid during endogenous and exogenous changes in its blood level. *Endocrinology*, 83: 246–250.

Wang, B.C., Share, L., Crofton, J.T. and Kimura, T. (1981) Changes in vasopressin concentration in plasma and cerebrospinal fluid in response to haemorrhage in anaesthetised dogs. *Neuroendocrinology*, 33: 61–66.

Wang, B.C., Share, L., Crofton, J.T. and Kimura, T. (1982) Effect of intravenous and intracerebroventricular infusion of hypertonic solutions on plasma and cerebrospinal fluid vasopressin concentrations. *Neuroendocrinology*, 34: 215–221.

Zaidi, S.M. and Heller, H. (1974) Can neurohypophysial hormones cross the blood–cerebrospinal fluid barrier? *J. Endocr.*, 60: 195–196.

Zimmerman, E., Carmel, P.W., Hussain, M.K., Ferin, M., Tannenbaum, M., Frantz, A.G. and Robinson, A.G. (1973) Vasopressin and neurophysin: high concentrations in monkey hypophyseal portal blood. *Science*, 182: 925–927.

The Neurohypophysis: Structure, Function and Control, Progress in Brain Research, Vol. 60, edited by B.A. Cross and G. Leng

Excitation of Hippocampal Neurones by Posterior Pituitary Peptides: Vasopressin and Oxytocin Compared

M. MÜHLETHALER and J.J. DREIFUSS

Département de Physiologie, Centre Médical Universitaire, Rue Michel Servet, 1211 Geneva 4 (Switzerland)

INTRODUCTION

Oxytocin and vasopressin are synthesized in the hypothalamus and then either carried by axoplasmic transport to the neural lobe of the pituitary gland, or else transported to various areas within the central nervous system (for references, see Sofroniew and Weindl, 1981). A calcium-dependent, depolarization-induced release has been recently demonstrated (Buijs, 1982) from areas of the brain where vasopressin- and oxytocin-containing axons have been shown to terminate synaptically on neuronal elements (Buijs and Swaab, 1979). The view that oxytocin and vasopressin might exert neurotransmitter-like actions in these areas is supported by the observation that these peptides can influence the rate of firing of single neurones when applied iontophoretically (e.g. Olpe and Baltzer, 1981). Moreover, vasopressin and oxytocin have recently been found to excite mammalian neurones in brain slices in vitro (Mühlethaler et al., 1982). This communication reports ongoing studies using hippocampal slices.

METHODS

Male Sprague–Dawley rats ($\approx$ 250 g body weight) were decapitated and their brains quickly removed. Hippocampus or septum were carefully dissected and several 450 μm thick transverse slices cut with a tissue chopper and quickly transferred to an incubation chamber in which the upper surface of the slices were exposed to a humidified gas mixture (95 % O_2 : 5 % CO_2), while their undersurfaces were supported on a nylon grid and perifused with medium (Yamamoto and McIlwain, 1966) at a rate of 2.0 ml/min. Extracellular recordings from single neurones were obtained after letting the preparation "recover" for 1 h.

RESULTS AND DISCUSSION

Pilot studies, performed in slices that included the lateral septal area, a major recipient of extrahypothalamic vasopressin fibres, (Buijs, 1978; Sofroniew and Weindl, 1981) yielded negative results. Fig. 1 shows ratemeter records of the spontaneous firing of three neurones located in the lateral septum: none was affected when arginine-vasopressin, 10^{-6} M, was added to the perifusion medium. Similar results were found in seven additional septal neurones (but see Marchand and Hagino, 1981).

148

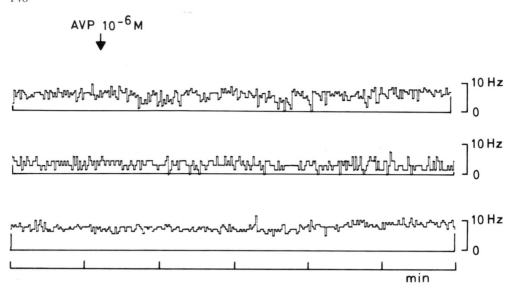

AVP 10⁻⁶M

10 Hz
0

10 Hz
0

10 Hz
0

min

Fig. 1. Lack of effect of arginine-vasopressin (AVP) on septal neurones. Ratemeter records of spontaneous firing from three single neurones, each from a separate slice. AVP was added to the perifusion medium at the time indicated by arrow to yield a concentration of 10^{-6} M. Duration of AVP application varied, but was always in excess of 3 min.

In contrast, vasopressin readily and reproducibly excited a class of spontaneously active hippocampal neurones which tended to fire in short intermittent bursts. Oxytocin, 10^{-6} M, also excited these neurones (Mühlethaler et al., 1982). We therefore systematically compared the potencies of oxytocin and vasopressin. Fig. 2 shows ratemeter records from a single neurone which was exposed to both substances: oxytocin produced a much quicker and

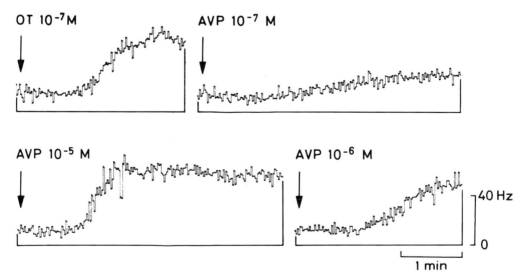

OT 10⁻⁷M   AVP 10⁻⁷ M

AVP 10⁻⁵ M   AVP 10⁻⁶ M

40 Hz
0

1 min

Fig. 2. Comparison of the effects of oxytocin (OT) and arginine-vasopressin (AVP) on a hippocampal neurone. The peptides were added to the perifusion medium (at the times indicated by the arrows) at the concentrations indicated.

stronger effect than vasopressin. To mimic the effect of 10^{-7} M oxytocin, vasopressin should have been applied at a concentration greater than 10^{-6} M. This experiment therefore suggested that oxytocin was at least ten times more powerful than arginine-vasopressin in the hippocampal slice.

In another group of experiments, arginine-vasopressin and oxytocin were bath-applied at concentrations ranging from 10^{-10} to 10^{-5} M. Each cell recorded was exposed to at least two different concentrations of both peptides. Results, plotted as the mean increase in firing rate at each concentration tested, fitted the Michaelis–Menten equation. The lowest effective concentration for oxytocin was 10^{-9} M and stimulation was maximal at approximately 10^{-7} M (Fig. 3). At all concentrations, except at 10^{-5} M, vasopressin consistently produced a smaller increase in firing than oxytocin, the activity ratio being approximately 20 (oxytocin: vasopressin). This ratio is similar to that of these two compounds acting as hormones on uterine and mammary gland cells. This result suggests that the hippocampal excitatory response might be purely oxytocic, since the effect of vasopressin can be entirely ascribed to its action on the postulated oxytocin receptors.

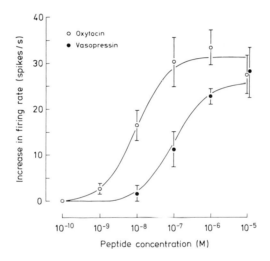

Fig. 3. Comparison of the effects of oxytocin and arginine-vasopressin on neuronal firing in hippocampal slices. Each point shows mean ($\pm$ S.E.M.) increase in firing induced at the concentration indicated. Background firing was 12.7 $\pm$ 0.9 Hz (n = 20). The two curves have been computer-drawn, using the Michaelis–Menten equation.

In our first report, we showed that a vasopressin (AVP) structural analogue, $d(CH_2)_5Tyr(Me)AVP$, antagonized the excitatory effects of vasopressin in the hippocampus (Mühlethaler et al., 1982). This finding was compatible with the view that the hippocampal effect was of the V_1-type (Michell et al., 1979). However, $d(CH_2)_5Tyr(Me)AVP$ is also a powerful oxytocin antagonist ($pA_2 = 7.24$, see Kruzynski et al., 1980); in view of the present results, we are led to believe that it acts as an oxytocin antagonist in the rat hippocampus.

Vasopressin fibres were previously reported in the ventral hippocampus (Buijs, 1978). Oxytocin fibres have recently been described in a similar distribution in the molecular layer and hilar area in the rat (Sofroniew, 1982). The specificity of this finding has been verified by the identification of neurophysin and oxytocin fibres in the hippocampus of homozygous Brattleboro rats which produce only oxytocin and no vasopressin.

Studies from several laboratories have shown that centrally acting neurohypophysial hormones can induce or modulate various behaviours. Vasopressin has received much attention, in particular with reference to tasks in which past experience plays an important role (De Wied, 1971; Koob et al., 1981; Weingartner et al., 1981). Oxytocin, however, may be equally important within the central nervous system. First, oxytocin is found in many areas throughout the brain and spinal cord and has been shown to modulate the rate of firing of neurones located in the hypothalamus (Moss et al., 1972), brainstem (Morris et al., 1980) and spinal cord (Gilbey et al., 1982) upon microiontophoretic application. In a study using the isolated rat spinal cord, both oxytocin and vasopressin depolarized motoneurones when applied to the bath at concentrations greater than 10^{-9} M (Suzue et al., 1981). Second, following intracerebroventricular injection, oxytocin can induce maternal behaviour (Pedersen and Prange, 1979; Pedersen et al., 1982) and has been shown to facilitate its own pulsatile release from the neural lobe during suckling (Freund-Mercier and Richard, 1981). We now report that hippocampal neurones are responsive to oxytocin. Further studies are in progress to ascertain whether the postulated hippocampal oxytocin receptors resemble the known uterotonic or galactobolic oxytocin receptors in structure–activity requirements (Sawyer et al., 1981) and binding characteristics (Soloff et al., 1977).

ACKNOWLEDGEMENTS

This work was supported in part by Swiss NSF Grant 3.875.081. We thank Professors M. Manning (Toledo, Ohio) and W.H. Sawyer (New York) for advice and for kindly supplying neurohypophysial peptides and structural analogues.

REFERENCES

Buijs, R.M. (1978) Intra- and extrahypothalamic vasopressin and oxytocin pathways in the rat. Pathways to the limbic system, medulla oblongata and spinal cord. *Cell Tiss. Res.,* 192: 423–435.

Buijs, R.M. (1982) Vasopressinergic and oxytocinergic pathways, synapses and central release. In A.J. Baertschi and J.J. Dreifuss (Eds.), *Neuroendocrinology of Vasopressin, Corticoliberin and Opiomelanocortins,* Academic Press, London, pp. 51–60.

Buijs, R.M. and Swaab, D.F. (1979) Immunoelectron microscopical demonstration of vasopressin and oxytocin synapses in the limbic system of the rat. *Cell Tiss. Res.,* 204: 335–365.

De Wied, D. (1971) Long term effect of vasopressin on the maintenance of a conditioned avoidance response in rats. *Nature (Lond.),* 232: 58–60.

Freund-Mercier, M.J. and Richard, Ph. (1981) Excitatory effects of intraventricular injections of oxytocin on the milk-ejection reflex in the rat. *Neurosci. Lett.,* 23: 193–198.

Gilbey, M.P., Coote, J.H., Fleetwood-Walker, S. and Peterson, D.F. (1982) The influence of the paraventriculo-spinal pathway, and oxytocin and vasopressin on sympathetic preganglionic neurones. *Brain Res.,* 251: 283–296.

Koob, C.F., Le Moal, M., Gaffori, O., Manning, M., Sawyer, W.H., Rivier, J. and Bloom, F.E. (1981) Arginine vasopressin and a vasopressin antagonist peptide: opposite effects on extinction of active avoidance in rats. *Regulat. Peptides,* 2: 153–163.

Kruszynski, M., Lammek, B., Manning, M., Seto, J., Haldar, J., and Sawyer, W.H. (1980) [1-(β-mercapto-β, β-cyclopentamethylenepropionic acid), 2-(O-methyl)tyrosine]arginine-vasopressin and [1-(β-mercapto-β, β-cyclopentamethylenepropionic acid]-arginine-vasopressin, two highly potent antagonists of the vasopressor response to arginine-vasopressin. *J. Med. Chem.,* 23: 364–368.

Marchand, J.E. and Hagino, N. (1981) The effect of iontophoretically applied vasopressin upon lateral septal neurones. *Soc. Neurosc. Abstr.* 7 (1981) 288. 22.

Michell, R.H., Kirk, C.J. and Billah, M.M. (1979). Hormonal stimulation of phosphatidyl inositol breakdown with particular reference to the hepatic effects of vasopressin. *Biochem. Soc. Trans.,* 7: 861–865.

Morris, R., Salt, T.E., Sofroniew, M.V. and Hill, R.G. (1980) Actions of microiontophoretically applied oxytocin, and immunohistochemical localization of oxytocin, vasopressin and neurophysin in the rat caudal medulla. *Neurosci. Lett.*, 18: 163–168.

Moss, R.L., Dyball, R.E.J. and Cross, B.A. (1972) Excitation of antidromically identified neurosecretory cells of the paraventricular nucleus by oxytocin applied iontophoretically. *Exp. Neurol.*, 34: 95–102.

Mühlethaler, M., Dreifuss, J.J. and Gähwiler, B.H. (1982) Vasopressin excites hippocampal neurones. *Nature (Lond.)*, 296: 749–751.

Olpe, H.-R. and Baltzer, V. (1981) Vasopressin activates noradrenergic neurones in the rat locus coeruleus: a microiontophoretic investigation. *Europ. J. Pharmacol.*, 77: 377–378.

Pedersen, C.A. and Prange, A.J. (1979) Induction of maternal behavior in virgin rats after intracerebroventricular administration of oxytocin. *Proc. nat. Acad. Sci.*, 76: 6661–6665.

Pedersen, C.A., Ascher, J.A., Monroe, Y.L. and Prange, A.J., Jr. (1982) Oxytocin induced maternal behaviour in virgin female rats. *Science*, 216: 648–650.

Sawyer, W.H., Grzonka, Z. and Manning, M. (1981) Neurohypophysial peptides. Design of tissue specific agonists and antagonists. *Molec. cell. Endocr.*, 22: 117–134.

Sofroniew, M.V. (1982) Vascular and neural projections of hypothalamic neurones producing neurohypophysial or ACTH-related peptides. In A.J. Baertschi and J.J. Dreifuss (Eds.), *Neuroendocrinology of Vasopressin Corticoliberin and Opiomelanocortins*, Academic Press, London, pp. 73–86.

Sofroniew, M.V. and Weindl, A. (1981) Central nervous system distribution of vasopressin, oxytocin and neurophysin. In J.L. Martinez et al. (Eds), *Endogenous Peptides and Learning and Memory Processes*, Academic Press, London, pp. 327–369.

Soloff, M.S., Schroeder, B.T., Chakraborthy, J. and Pearlmutter, A.F. (1977) Characterization of oxytocin receptors in the uterus and mammary gland. *Fed. Proc.*, 36: 1861–1866.

Suzue, T., Yanaihara, N. and Otsuka, M. (1981) Actions of vasopressin, gastrin releasing peptide and other peptides on neurons of newborn rat spinal cord in vitro. *Neurosci. Lett.*, 26: 137–142.

Weingartner, H., Gold, Ph., Ballenger, T.C., Smallberg, S.A., Summers, R., Rubinow, D.R., Post, R.M. and Goodwin, F.K. (1981) Effects of vasopressin on human memory functions. *Science*, 211: 601–603.

Yamamoto, C. and McIlwain, H. (1966) Electrical activity in thin sections from the mammalian brain maintained in chemically-defined media in vitro. *J. Neurochem.*, 13: 1333–1343.

Central Actions of Neurohypophysial Hormones

The Neurohypophysis: Structure, Function and Control, Progress in Brain Research, Vol. 60, edited by B.A. Cross and G. Leng
© 1983 Elsevier Science Publishers B.V.

Central Actions of Neurohypophysial Hormones

D. DE WIED

Rudolf Magnus Institute for Pharmacology, Medical Faculty, University of Utrecht, Vondellaan 6, 3521 GD Utrecht, (The Netherlands)

MODULATION OF MEMORY PROCESSES BY NEUROHYPOPHYSIAL HORMONES

Numerous experiments have shown that neurohypophysial hormones are involved in learning and memory processes. Removal of the neurointermediate lobe of the pituitary in rats interferes with the maintenance of shuttle box avoidance behaviour (De Wied, 1965). Rapid extinction of the response which is found in posterior lobectomized rats can be amended by treatment with Pitressin or Lys^8-vasopressin (LVP). In intact rats, Pitressin administered during either the acquisition or the extinction period of shuttle box avoidance behaviour results in a long-lasting resistance to extinction (De Wied and Bohus, 1966). LVP has a similar effect on extinction of pole-jumping avoidance behaviour (De Wied, 1971). Although attempts to replicate these effects have met with mixed success, Le Moal et al. (1981) successfully reproduced and extended these findings. Studies in which LVP was administered at different times during extinction of pole-jumping avoidance behaviour favoured the hypothesis that vasopressin facilitates memory consolidation. To be completely active, vasopressin has to be administered within 1 h before or after the first extinction session.

The consolidation hypothesis has been corroborated by studies on passive avoidance behaviour. By means of a one-trial passive avoidance paradigm, it has been shown that post-trial injection of vasopressin induces a long-term facilitation of passive avoidance behaviour (Bohus et al., 1978a). Intracerebroventricular (i.c.v.) administration of [Arg^8]vasopressin (AVP) at various times after the single learning trial indicated that vasopressin facilitates consolidation as well as retrieval processes. Treatment given immediately after the learning trial is most effective, and if postponed for 3 or 6 h the effect is greatly reduced or absent. Treatment given 23 h after the learning trial (i.e. 1 h prior to the retention test) is as effective as i.c.v. administration of AVP immediately after the learning trial. Vasopressin also facilitates passive avoidance behaviour where the aversive stimulus is attack by a trained fighter used as a more natural behaviour (Leshner and Roche, 1977). In addition, vasopressin increases resistance to extinction of sexually motivated approach behaviour (Bohus, 1977) and a positively awarded discrimination task (Hostetter et al., 1977). Vasopressin and related peptides prevent or reverse retrograde amnesia for a passive avoidance response in rats induced by CO_2 inhalation or electroconvulsive shock (Rigter et al., 1974, 1975), or by pentylenetetrazol (Bookin and Pfeiffer, 1977; Bohus et al., 1982) as well as puromycin-induced retrograde amnesia for a maze-learning task in mice (Flexner et al., 1977, 1978; Walter et al., 1975). The ability of vasopressin to reverse retrograde amnesia also suggests a retrieval hypothesis.

[155]

Oxytocin has an effect on memory processes opposite to that of vasopressin (Schulz et al., 1976; Bohus et al., 1978b). Attenuation of passive avoidance behaviour by oxytocin is also a time-dependent process (Bohus et al., 1978a).

The influence of oxytocin appears to be on consolidation as well as retrieval processes. In view of this it has been suggested that oxytocin is a naturally occurring amnesic neuropeptide.

PHYSIOLOGICAL IMPLICATION OF VASOPRESSIN IN MEMORY PROCESSES

Several approaches have been used to determine the physiological significance of the neurohypophysial hormones in memory processes. As most studies were performed with vasopressin, emphasis in this discussion will be focussed on this hormone. The various approaches include animals with a vasopressin deficiency as induced by removal of the neurointermediate lobe of the pituitary; rats of the Brattleboro strain which have a genetic disturbance in the synthesis of vasopressin; and rats with a temporary deficit in brain vasopressin produced by i.c.v. injection of specific vasopressin antiserum. Another approach has been the measurement of vasopressin levels in blood, CSF and various brain regions in relation to avoidance performance.

POSTERIOR LOBECTOMY

The suggestion that neurohypophysial hormones are involved in learning and memory came from studies on acquisition and maintenance of avoidance behaviour in posterior lobectomized rats (De Wied, 1965). These studies showed that acquisition of shuttle box avoidance behaviour was not materially affected by the removal of the neurointermediate lobe. Escape behaviour was not affected in posterior lobectomized rats indicating that neither sensory nor motor capacities were affected. However, extinction of shuttle box avoidance behaviour was markedly facilitated. This abnormal behaviour could be corrected by treatment with Pitressin given as a long-acting preparation, or with long-acting purified LVP. To be effective the treatment could be given either during acquisition or during extinction (De Wied, 1969). Such studies showed that Pitressin had a long-term effect on avoidance behaviour in hypophysec-tomized (Bohus et al., 1973) and in intact rats (De Wied and Bohus, 1966; De Wied, 1971).

In retrospect these studies are difficult to interpret, as extrahypothalamic neurohypophysial hormone-containing networks have since been demonstrated in a variety of limbic and midbrain structures such as hippocampus, septum, amygdala, medullary areas and the vicinity of the ventricular systems (Sterba, 1974; Buijs, 1978; Buijs et al., 1980). Unless the release of neurohypophysial hormones from these networks is disturbed due to the increased synthesis of vasopressin as a result of the mild diabetes insipidus of posterior lobectomized rats, an explanation for the memory dysfunction of these animals cannot be given. The existence of a strain of rats with hereditary diabetes insipidus provided a better animal model because this strain is totally deprived of vasopressin.

HOMOZYGOUS DIABETES INSIPIDUS (DI) RATS

A homozygous variant of the Brattleboro strain (DI rats) lacks the ability to synthesize vasopressin due to a mutation of a single pair of autosomal loci (Valtin and Schroeder, 1964).

Memory function of DI rats appeared to be severely impaired as assessed in a one-trial passive avoidance situation compared to heterozygous control animals when tested 24 h after the learning trial (De Wied et al., 1975). AVP or desglycinamide-LVP (DGLVP) given immediately after the learning trial restored passive avoidance behaviour of DI rats. The fact that DGLVP was as active as AVP suggested that the effect of vasopressin could not be ascribed to an influence on water metabolism: DGLVP is nearly devoid of antidiuretic activity (De Wied et al., 1972). Because the DI rat shows avoidance comparable to that of heterozygotous littermates immediately after the learning trial but not 24 h later, it was concluded that memory rather than learning is disturbed in the absence of vasopressin. If a multiple trial paradigm is used, such as shuttle box or pole-jumping avoidance behaviour, DI rats show nearly normal acquisition, but the behaviour is extinguished at a more rapid rate than that of heterozygotes or Wistar rats (Bohus et al., 1975). Celestian et al. (1975) reported that DI rats are inferior in acquiring shuttle box avoidance behaviour as only 30% of their animals reached the learning criterion. However, those rats that achieved the criterion maintained the response much better than control animals. Bailey and Weiss (1979) reported that passive avoidance behaviour of DI rats is inferior to that of heterozygous controls but the absence of vasopressin does not cause total impairment of passive avoidance behaviour. The absence of vasopressin in DI rats is associated with an increase in oxytocin synthesis (Valtin et al., 1965; Dogterom et al., 1977) and marked disturbances in other endocrine systems. There may also be variations in the Brattleboro strain due to local breeding influences which may explain the discrepancies in results. Recent experiments by us (Láczi et al., 1983) again demonstrated the markedly disturbed passive avoidance behaviour of the DI rat.

DI rats are unable to maintain copulatory behaviour after castration. Intromission and ejaculatory pattern disappear almost immediately after castration, while normal rats show a gradual decline of copulatory behaviour. This can be prevented by the administration of DGLVP to DI rats (Bohus, 1977). Brito et al. (1981) showed that DI rats adapt more slowly than normal animals in a T-maze and make fewer correct responses when learning a visual and olfactory discrimination task. In other tasks the DI rat is not always inferior. Brito et al. suggest that not all aspects of learning and memory are equally disturbed in DI rats.

BIOINACTIVATION OF BRAIN VASOPRESSIN

Reasoning that specific vasopressin antiserum would temporarily bind and therefore inactivate brain vasopressin, the i.c.v. administration of vasopressin antiserum was used to study the role of vasopressin in memory processes. The administration of vasopressin antiserum via one of the lateral ventricles interferes with active and passive avoidance behaviour (Van Wimersma Greidanus et al., 1975a; Van Wimersma Greidanus and De Wied, 1976). A marked deficit in passive avoidance behaviour is found if the antiserum is givzn immediately after the learning trial and rats are tested for retention between 6 and 24 h later. This is not the case if the retention test is run immediately or within 2 h after the learning trial. I.v. injection of vasopressin antiserum in an amount one hundred times as much as that used in the lateral ventricle does not affect passive avoidance behaviour although it effectively blocks the biological effects of circulating vasopressin as assessed by urine production and excretion of vasopressin in the urine. These results point to the importance of brain versus peripheral vasopressin in memory processes. The critical period for the antiserum to be active is approximately 2 h, which corroborates observations on the time-dependent influence of vasopressin in active avoidance behaviour (De Wied, 1971). These and later observations indicate that vasopressin is involved in memory consolidation. As the antiserum also attenuates passive avoidance behaviour when administered 1 h prior to the retention test, vasopressin also facilitates retrieval processes. This is in agreement with time-dependent studies with vasopressin on passive avoidance behaviour (Bohus et al., 1978a). Interestingly, if vasopressin antiserum is given 1 h prior to the 24 h retention test which causes attenuation of passive avoidance behaviour, rats thus treated but tested at a second retention test 24 h later show avoidance again. Van Wimersma Greidanus (1982) further showed that passive avoidance performance of rats treated 1 h before the retention test can be restored by co-administration of $ACTH_{4-10}$, but not if the antiserum is given immediately after the learning trial. This latter procedure interferes with the consolidation of memory. Vasopressin antiserum also affects one-way active avoidance behaviour. Although acquisition of the behaviour is somewhat delayed, extinction of the response of rats treated with the antiserum during acquisition is markedly facilitated (Van Wimersma Greidanus et al., 1975a).

VASOPRESSIN LEVELS IN BLOOD AND CSF DURING AVOIDANCE BEHAVIOUR

Vasopressin levels (AD activity) in eye plexus blood were measured by bioassay during retention of passive avoidance behaviour (Thompson and De Wied, 1973). Eye plexus blood contains much higher AD activity than peripheral trunk blood. A good correlation was found between shock intensity during the learning trial, avoidance latency at the 24 h retention test and the AD activity in eye plexus blood. This finding was interpreted as indicating an association between AD activity and memory formation. However, these studies measured blood levels of vasopressin. The existence of extrahypothalamic vasopressin-containing networks, and lack of knowledge on the regulation of the release of vasopressin from these networks, require the direct measurement of vasopressin in the brain either in the CSF or at the site of release.

Subsequent studies by our group uspng a radioimmunoassay (RIA) for vasopressin extracted from peripheral trunk blood could not corroborate the studies by Thompson and De Wied (1973). No change in immunoreactive AVP (IR-AVP) was found during passive avoidance retention as measured 24 h after the learning trial. Only with a high shock intensity which caused maximal avoidance latencies, was a slight increase in IR-AVP found (Van Wimersma Greidanus et al., 1979a). Neither acquisition nor extinction of pole-jumping avoidance behaviour were associated with a significant elevation of circulating IR-AVP levels.

Recent experiments to replicate and extend the findings by Thompson and De Wied (1973), however, again pointed to a relation between passive avoidance retention and AD activity and IR-AVP levels in eye plexus blood. Both assays were used. A good relation was found between plasma AD activity and IR-AVP levels (Láczi et al., 1983). The levels in eye plexus blood are high and can be determined without an extraction procedure. Levels were also determined immediately after the learning trial. AD activity and IR-AVP levels were high in eye plexus blood of non-shocked rats, probably because of the stress of handling and exposure to the test box. In fact, the levels in rats which received footshock of various intensities were not significantly higher whether determined immediately, 10 or 30 min after the learning trial. The avoidance latencies at the 24 h retention test, however, were related to the intensity of the electric footshock at the learning trial.

DI rats did not display passive avoidance behaviour at the 24 h retention test even when subjected to the highest shock intensity of 1 mA for 2 sec. The level of IR-AVP in eye plexus blood of these rats was below the limit of detection. Heterozygotous control rats showed maximal avoidance latency at the retention test, although IR-AVP in eye plexus blood was much lower than that found in Wistar animals and not significantly different from that of non-shocked heterozygote controls.

Finally, the i.c.v. administration of vasopressin antiserum to Wistar rats 30 min before the learning trial which attenuated passive avoidance behaviour, hardly affected IR-AVP levels of eye plexus blood immediately after the learning trial. However, if given 30 min before the retention test, attenuation of passive avoidance behaviour and a markedly reduced IR-AVP in eye plexus blood were found.

The augmented release of vasopressin into the blood raises the issue of whether peripherally circulating hormone levels influence avoidance behaviour. The memory effect of vasopressin is probably a direct effect on limbic midbrain structures (Kovács et al., 1979a, b) as microinjection of picogram amounts of vasopressin facilitates passive avoidance behaviour. However, this view has been challenged. Le Moal et al. (1981) showed that pretreatment with an analogue of vasopressin which prevents vasopressin from elevating blood pressure also prevents the influence on memory. They concluded that the memory effect of vasopressin is mediated in part by changes in blood pressure. This is not in accord with our findings that fragments of vasopressin like DGLVP, which is almost devoid of pressor activity, retain their effect on avoidance behaviour (De Wied et al., 1972). Le Moal et al. (1981), however, should have performed an experiment in which the agonist and antagonist were administered intracranially to determine whether the blockade of the memory effect of vasopressin could take place in the absence of changes in blood pressure. Still, peripheral mechanisms may play a role in the memory effect of vasopressin. Borrell et al. (1981) found that adrenalectomy or adrenomedullectomy result in a retention deficit of passive avoidance behaviour which can be corrected by the administration of adrenaline but not by vasopressin. However, vasopressin potentiated the influence of high doses of adrenaline which in itself are not effective in restoring passive avoidance behaviour of adrenalectomized rats.

The existence of a relationship between vasopressin levels in eye plexus blood collected immediately after the retention test and passive avoidance latencies (Thompson and De Wied, 1973) was confirmed by Láczi et al. (1983). The augmented release of vasopressin under these conditions probably reflects the activity of the supraoptic neurohypophysial system associated with the memory of the fearful aversive stimulation experienced by the rat during the learning trial. This augmented release may be important for retrieval processes.

As a similar augmented release from the terminals of the extrahypothalamic vasopressin network may occur, it was deemed of interest to determine the concentration of vasopressin in the CSF during passive avoidance behaviour. Extensive studies on the relationship between behavioural performance during retention of a passive avoidance response and vasopressin levels in the CSF revealed no significant effect (Mens et al., 1982). However, a subsequent study in which IR-AVP in cisternal CSF was measured showed that the levels of rats exposed to a high footshock (1.0 mA) are markedly elevated immediately after the learning trial. Rats trained at a mild footshock of 0.25 mA have IR-AVP levels in the CSF only slightly above those of non-shocked animals. In general, the level of vasopressin in CSF immediately after the learning trial is related to the intensity of the footshock (Láczi et al., in preparation). At the 24 h retention test IR-AVP levels in CSF of rats exposed to mild footshock are elevated. Surprisingly the levels of rats subjected to the highest shock intensity at the learning trial are under the limit of detection. An explanation may be that exposure to this high shock level releases the readily releasable pool of vasopressin from the terminals of the vasopressin neurones, thus preventing spill-over in the CSF. Although Dogterom and Buijs (1980), did not find a change in vasopressin concentration in various brain regions during passive avoidance behaviour, Láczi et al. (unpublished) detected a marked depletion of IR-AVP in various limbic structures 24 h after exposure of rats to the high shock intensity. In addition, the levels of IR-AVP in the CSF are markedly elevated when tested for avoidance performance at 5 days after the learning trial. This suggests that repletion of AVP in the terminals of the extrahypothalamic network has taken place.

In conclusion, passive avoidance behaviour in rats is accompanied by the release of IR-AVP into the CSF and the levels are related to the intensity of the aversive stimulus and avoidance latencies. It is conceivable that AVP is released during passive avoidance learning and retained at the sites of the memory effect. This local release may be reflected in changes in the CSF, but the measurement of AVP in brain nuclei involved in the CNS effect of vasopressin might provide additional evidence for a role of vasopressin in memory processes.

Of course other hormones may be released during passive avoidance behaviour as well. Pituitary–adrenal activity, as assessed by plasma corticosterone levels, is also related to passive avoidance behaviour (De Wied et al., 1975). At 15 min after the retention test, plasma corticosterone levels are markedly elevated when DI and heterozygote control rats are tested for retention immediately after the learning trial when avoidance latencies are also high. However, 24 h after the learning trial plasma corticosterone levels are low in DI rats which do not show avoidance, while those of heterozygotous control rats which avoid maximally are high. Treatment with AVP or DGLVP restores passive avoidance behaviour of DI rats but not the pituitary–adrenal response at the retention test. It is possible that other pituitary, i.e. brain-borne, hormones are released during acquisition and retention of passive avoidance behaviour which may all play a part in the complex adaptive process which is essential for the formation and maintenance of new behaviour patterns.

SITE OF ACTION OF VASOPRESSIN ON MEMORY PROCESSES

Destruction of the rostral septal region and the anterodorsal hippocampus prevent the effect of vasopressin on extinction of pole-jumping avoidance behaviour (Van Wimersma Greidanus et al., 1975b; Van Wimersma Greidanus and De Wied, 1976). Lesions of the thalamic parafascicular area only partially prevent the influence of vasopressin, while transection of the fornix and stria terminalis do not block vasopressin-induced resistance to extinction of pole-jumping avoidance behaviour (Van Wimersma Greidanus et al., 1979b).

Microinjection of picogram amounts of vasopressin in various limbic-midbrain nuclei has been used to further explore the site of action of this peptide. These studies used passive avoidance behaviour as the paradigm. Treatments were given immediately after the learning trial and thus were indicative for consolidation processes (Kovács et al., 1979a, b, 1980). Local microinjection into the dorsal septal area, the hippocampal dentate gyrus or the dorsal raphe nucleus facilitated passive avoidance behaviour, while microinjections into the central amygdaloid nucleus or the hippocampal subiculum were without effect. Thus, the hippocampus, septum and raphe regions are sensitive to the memory consolidating effect of vasopressin. Administration of vasopressin antiserum into the dorsal raphe nucleus or the hippocampal dentate gyrus had an opposite effect and attenuated passive avoidance performance (Kovács et al., 1980, 1982). Microinjection of vasopressin into the amygdala, however, partially reversed pentylenetetrazol-induced amnesia, but only if the peptide was given shortly before the retention test (Bohus et al., 1982). Microinjection into the dorsal raphe nucleus or dorsal septal area was without effect. Thus, the neuroanatomical substrate for the memory effect of vasopressin seems to be different for consolidation and retrieval processes.

Neurohypophysial hormones may modulate monoaminergic neurotransmission. Catecholamine metabolism in DI rats differs from that of homozygous normal controls (Versteeg et al., 1978). In many brain regions the differences in catecholamine turnover are opposite in vasopressin-deficient and vasopressin-treated normal animals. The same is found between vasopressin antiserum and vasopressin treatment (D.H.G. Versteeg et al., 1979). In addition, destruction of the catecholamine terminals of the dorsal noradrenergic bundle by local injection of 6-hydroxydopamine prevents the effect of vasopressin on memory consolidation but not on retrieval (Kovács et al., 1979a). As microinjections into the locus coeruleus, which contains the cell bodies of the dorsal noradrenergic bundle, do not interfere with the memory consolidating effect of vasopressin, the terminal regions of these neurones rather than cell bodies are regarded as the sites of catecholamine modulation by vasopressin.

STRUCTURE–ACTIVITY STUDIES

AVP is the most potent peptide which increases resistance to extinction of pole-jumping avoidance behaviour following subcutaneous administration (Table I). Removal of the C-terminal amino acid residue glycinamide yields a peptide with a somewhat reduced behavioural potency (De Wied et al., 1972). However, DGLVP has lost almost all peripheral endocrine effects. Thus, the removal of the C-terminal glycinamide dissociates the behavioural influence of vasopressin from the classical endocrine effects. Further studies with fragments of AVP indicate that the behavioural activity is located in the covalent ring structure, although a second activity site may be present in the linear part of the molecule (De Wied, 1976). Substitution in the amino acid residues of the covalent ring structure of AVP by different amino acids generally reduces the behavioural effect. Alterations in the linear part of the molecule are less damaging (Walter et al., 1978). Nevertheless, behavioural activities are more tolerant than endocrine activities to modification of the various amino acid residues in the vasopressin molecule.

TABLE I

AMINO ACID SEQUENCES OF VARIOUS NEUROHYPOPHYSIAL HORMONES
AND RELATED FRAGMENTS

Arg^8-vasopressin (AVP$_{1-9}$)	H–Cys–Tyr–Phe–Gln–Asn–Cys–Pro–Arg–Gly–NH$_2$
des-glycinamide^9-Arg^8-vasopressin (AVP$_{1-8}$)	H–Cys–Tyr–Phe–Gln–Asn–Cys–Pro–Arg–OH
pressinamide (AVP$_{1-6}$)	H–Cys–Tyr–Phe–Gln–Asn–Cys–NH$_2$
prolyl-arginyl-glycinamide (AVP$_{7-9}$)	H–Pro–Arg–Gly–NH$_2$
oxytocin (OXT$_{1-9}$)	H–Cys–Tyr–Ile–Gln–Asn–Cys–Pro–Leu–Gly–NH$_2$
tocinamide (OXT$_{1-6}$)	H–Cys–Tyr–Ile–Gln–Asn–Cys–NH$_2$
prolyl-leucyl-glycinamide (OXT$_{7-9}$)	H–Cys–Tyr–Ile–Gln–Asn–Cys–Pro–Arg–Gly–NH$_2$
Arg^8-oxytocin (vasotocin; AVT$_{1-9}$)	

Attenuation of retrograde amnesia has also been used to determine the active core of the vasopressin molecule on memory processes. DGLVP either before or after training attenuates puromycin-induced retrograde amnesia in mice (Lande et al., 1972). This peptide also counteracts CO_2-induced amnesia for a passive avoidance response in rats (Rigter et al., 1974). Interestingly, the C-terminal tripeptide of oxytocin is more active than that of vasopressin.

Moreover, the covalent ring structures of vasopressin or oxytocin are inactive (Walter et al., 1975). Although oxytocin slightly affects retrograde amnesia, Gly–Gly–Gly–oxytocin is fully active in this respect. The dipeptide Leu–Gly–NH_2 also is very active in this test. As attenuation of retrograde amnesia measures retrieval processes, the conclusion that the active sequence for these processes are mainly present in the C-terminal part of the neurohypophysial hormones seems justified.

Passive avoidance behaviour can be used to determine influences of neuropeptides on consolidation as well as retrieval processes. Peptides are considered to influence consolidation processes if passive avoidance latency measured 24 h after the learning trial is affected following the administration immediately after the learning trial. Effects on retrieval processes are assessed by the administration of the material 1 h prior to the 24 h retention test. Consolidation was facilitated by i.c.v. administered AVP_{1-9}, AVP_{1-8}, AVP_{1-7} and AVP_{1-6}. Interestingly, OXT_{1-7} and OXT_{1-6} facilitated avoidance latency following post-learning administration as well. Linear parts of both vasopressin and oxytocin also facilitated consolidation but were less active (Kovács et al., 1982).

Facilitation of retrieval was found with AVP_{1-9} and was less pronounced with AVP_{1-8}, AVP_{1-7}, OXT_{1-6}, OXT_{7-9} and OXT_{8-9}. Inhibition of consolidation was induced by OXT_{1-9}, OXT_{1-8} and AVT_{1-9}, while retrieval was attenuated by OXT_{1-9}, OXT_{1-8}, AVT_{1-9} and AVT_{1-8}. Thus, the covalent ring structures of both vasopressin and oxytocin facilitate consolidation of passive avoidance behaviour. The linear part of oxytocin is important for stimulation of retrieval processes. The requirement for the amnesic effect of oxytocin on consolidation concerns practically the whole molecule. Only the C-terminal amino acid residue glycinamide can be removed without appreciable loss of activity or reversal of the effect. To attenuate retrieval the covalent ringstructure of oxytocin plus the proline[7] residue is needed. AVT_{1-8} attenuates retrieval rather selectively. These studies suggest that consolidation and retrieval are separately located in the neurohypophysial hormones, but they fail to provide a clear answer regarding the active loci in this respect.

CONVERSION OF NEUROHYPOPHYSIAL HORMONES

Two main routes for the conversion of neurohypophysial hormones in the brain have been identified. Aminopeptidase action cleaving the Cys^1–Tyr^2 bond of LVP was found by Pliška et al. (1971) using minced cerebral cortex tissue. Further evidence for an aminopeptidase-mediated pathway was provided by Marks et al. (1973) who showed release of the Tyr^2 and Ile^3 residues from oxytocin and the release of Tyr^2 and Phe^3 from vasopressin by purified brain aminopeptidases. C-terminal cleaving enzymes produced Leu–Gly–NH_2 and glycinamide from oxytocin.

Burbach et al. (1980a, b) found evidence for the presence of aminopeptidase and C-terminal cleaving peptidase activities in synaptosomal plasma membrane (SPM) preparations of rat limbic brain tissue. Quantification of these activities utilizing differentially ^{14}C-labelled oxytocin preparations showed that the aminopeptidase pathway strongly prevails in SPM fractions. Other subcellular preparations which contain high aminopeptidase activity are the synaptosomal and microsomal fractions. Although C-terminal cleaving peptidase is low in SPM preparations, release of glycinamide and formation of minor amounts of Leu–Gly–NH_2 were detected. Formation of this dipeptide in the brain at synaptosomal plasma membranes may be of physiological signicance in view of the specific influence of Leu–Gly–NH_2 on memory retrieval (Kovács et al., 1982; Walter et al., 1975).

The two types of oxytocin-converting peptidase activities show some regional differentiation in the brain (Burbach et al., 1980a, b). Compared to the activity in parietal cortex, the aminopeptidase activities in SPM fractions of the medial basal hypothalamus, the nigrostriatal area, and the region of the dorsal raphe area are highest. These regions are densely innervated by neurohypophysial hormone-containing fibres. Neurohypophysial hormone-converting peptidase activities have also been detected in the cortex, which has a low density of vasopressin fibres. The activity of enzymes in that region is also the lowest of all areas tested.

In the course of experiments on SPM-mediated conversion of oxytocin, accumulation of an oxytocin fraction was observed, which did not co-migrate with known oxytocin fragments. This material contained the C-terminal glycinamide, but it was devoid of the tyrosine residue. The accumulation of this fraction resembled aminopeptidase action on oxytocin with respect to pH dependency, subcellular and regional distribution. In an attempt to identify the material from digests of oxytocin with SPM, the fraction was resolved into two components by high-pressure liquid chromatography (HPLC). Subsequently, the peptides were isolated and characterized by chemical analyses as the 4–9 and 1,4–9 sequences of oxytocin (Burbach and Lebouille, 1983). The structures of these fragments suggests that the peptides are formed by the action of aminopeptidases. This would be in agreement with the predominant presence of aminopeptidase activity in SPM fractions and the data showing similarities between accumulation of the products and aminopeptidase action on oxytocin. It is not known whether the 4–9 and 1, 4–9 fragments of oxytocin are centrally active, but studies with related synthetic peptide fragments suggest that they may possess memory effects.

OTHER CENTRAL EFFECTS MODULATED BY NEUROHYPOPHYSIAL HORMONES AND RELATED PEPTIDES

In addition to their role on memory processes, vasopressin and oxytocin and related peptides are implicated in several other centrally mediated responses such as tolerance development to and physical dependence on opiate, heroin and ethanol, addiction (Van Ree et al., 1978; Hoffman et al., 1978), rewarded behaviour (Schwarzberg et al., 1976), neuroendocrine and cardiovascular regulation (C.A.M. Versteeg et al., 1979), induction of maternal behaviour (Pedersen et al., 1982), control of body temperature (Cooper et al., 1979) and brain development (Boer et al., 1980).

DGLVP facilitates the development of resistance to the antinociceptive action of morphine in mice (Krivoy et al., 1974). The linear tripeptide of oxytocin OXT_{7-9} (PLG) facilitates the development of tolerance to the antinociceptive action of i.c.v. administered β-endorphin in rats (Van Ree et al., 1976) as well as the development of morphine tolerance in both mice and rats (Contreras and Takemori, 1980; Székely et al., 1979). Physical dependence on opiates as assessed by body weight loss and hypothermia is also affected by fragments of neurohypophysial hormones. The linear tripeptides of vasopressin and oxytocin both facilitate the development of physical dependence on morphine (Van Ree et al., 1978). However, the data on physical dependence are conflicting, possibly because of different test procedures and amounts of peptides used in the respective studies (Van Ree and De Wied, 1981). Various fragments of vasopressin and oxytocin modulate physical dependence on ethanol. Treatment with AVP attenuates the disappearance rate of tolerance to ethanol in mice (Hoffman et al., 1978). In mice continuously exposed to ethanol, DGAVP enhances residual tolerance to the hypothermic effect of ethanol (Rigter et al., 1983). Withdrawal convulsions are exacerbated in mice treated with DGAVP (Rigter and Crabbe, 1980). Thus, DGAVP facilitates development of tolerance to and physical dependence on opioids as well as ethanol. Acquisition of heroin self-administration of rats is reduced by the covalent ring structure of vasopressin and facilitated by PLG (Van Ree and De Wied, 1977). The same is found on electrical self-stimulation. Oxytocin and PLG facilitate while vasopressin and DGAVP have a suppressive effect (Schwarzberg et al., 1976; Dorsa and Van Ree, 1979).

Cardiovascular regulatory processes may also be modulated by neurohypophysial hormones (C.A.M. Versteeg et al., 1979). A centrally evoked pressor response following electrical stimulation of the mesencephalic reticular formation was found to be attenuated by peripherally injected LVP (Bohus, 1974). The same was observed for i.c.v. administered AVP, DGLVP, the covalent ring structure of AVP, and the linear part of vasopressin, AVP_{7-9} (C.A.M. Versteeg et al., 1979). OXT_{1-9} and PLG are also effective but the covalent ring structure is inactive. In fact, PLG is more effective in this respect than the other peptides.

When i.c.v. oxytocin is administered to virgin rats full maternal behaviour is displayed towards foster pups. This effect, which is dependent on the oestrogen level, is also produced by fragments of both oxytocin and vasopressin (Pedersen et al., 1982). In primed ovariectomized rats OXT_{1-6} appeared to be as active as oxytocin, while PLG had a relatively weak activity (Pedersen et al., 1982).

Effects of vasopressin on body temperature have as yet not been studied with fragments of the neurohypophysial hormones. The same holds for the implication of these hormones in brain development.

SUMMARY

The first evidence that the neurohypophysial hormones have central actions came from studies which demonstrated that these hormones modulate memory processes. Vasopressin facilitates memory consolidation and retrieval, while oxytocin may be regarded as an amnesic neuropeptide.

The CNS effects of these hormones are of central origin, as appeared from lesion studies, experiments in diabetes insipidus rats, studies from i.c.v. administered peptides and specific antisera in particular brain areas, and studies on the vasopressin levels in blood and CSF during memory consolidation and retrieval. Neurochemical experiments suggest that the memory effects of the neurohypophysial hormones are mediated by modulation of catecholamine transmission in restricted areas in the brain.

The effects of the neurohypophysial hormones on memory processes and other CNS effects are dissociated from their classical endocrine functions and are probably caused by neuropeptides generated from these hormones. Structure–activity and biotransformation studies corroborate the hypothesis that vasopressin and oxytocin are precursor molecules of the second order of neuropeptides with specific effects on memory processes.

The neurohypophysial hormones have a variety of CNS effects: they modulate drug-seeking behaviour, electrical self-stimulation and tolerance development to and physical dependence on opiates. In addition, effects of vasopressin on temperature regulation, cardiovascular control and brain development, and of oxytocin on maternal behaviour, have been found.

REFERENCES

Bailey, W.H. and Weiss, J.M. (1979) Evaluation of a "memory deficit" in vasopressin-deficient rats. *Brain Res.*, 162: 174–178.

Boer, G.J., Swaab, D.F., Uylings, H.B.M., Boer, K., Buijs, R.M. and Velis, D.N. (1980) Neuropeptides in rat brain development. In P.S. McConnell, C.J. Boer, H.J. Romijn, N.E. van de Poll and M.A. Corner (Eds.), *Adaptive Capabilities of the Nervous System, Progress in Brain Research, Vol. 53,* Elsevier/North-Holland, pp. 202–227.

Bohus, B. (1974) The influence of pituitary peptides on brain centers controlling autonomic responses. In D.F. Swaab and J.P. Schadé (Eds.), *Integrative Hypothalamic Activites, Progress in Brain Res., Vol. 41,* Elsevier, Amsterdam, pp. 175–183.

Bohus, B. (1977) Effect of desglycinamide-lysine vasopressin (DG-LVP) on sexually motivated T-maze behavior in the male rat. *Horm. Behav.,* 8: 52–61.

Bohus, B., Gispen, W.H. and De Wied, D. (1973) Effect of lysine vasopressin and $ACTH_{4-10}$ on conditioned avoidance behavior of hypophysectomized rats. *Neuroendocrinology,* 11: 137–143.

Bohus, B., Van Wimersma Greidanus, Tj. B. and De Wied, D. (1975) Behavioral and endocrine responses of rat with hereditary hypothalamic diabetes insipidus (Brattleboro strain). *Physiol. Behav.,* 14: 609–615.

Bohus, B., Kovács, G.L. and De Wied, D. (1978a) Oxytocin, vasopressin and memory: opposite effects on consolidation and retrieval processes. *Brain Res.,* 157: 414–417.

Bohus, B., Urban, I., Van Wimersma Greidanus, Tj. B. and De Wied, D., (1978b) Opposite effects of oxytocin and vasopressin on avoidance behavior and hippocampal theta rhytm in the rat. *Neuropharmacology,* 17: 239–247.

Bohus, B., Conti, L., Kovács, G.L. and Versteeg, D.H.G. (1982) Modulation of memory processes by neuropeptides: Interaction with neurotransmitter systems. In A. Marsan and H. Matthies (Eds.), *Neuronal Plasticity and Memory Formation,* Raven Press, New York, pp. 75–87.

Bookin, H.B. and Pfeiffer, W.D. (1977) Effect of lysine vasopressin on pentylenetetrazol-induced retrograde amnesia in rats. *Pharmacol. Biochem. Behav.,* 7: 51–54.

Borrell, J., Bohus, B., De Kloet, E.R., Versteeg, D.H.G. and De Wied, D. (1981) Passive avoidance retention deficit following short term adrenalectomy: the effects of post-learning arginine[8]-vasopressin on adrenaline. *Neurosci. Lett.,* 7: 265.

Brito, G.N., Thomas, G.J., Gingold, S.I. and Gash, D.M. (1981) Behavioral characteristics of vasopressin-deficient rats (Brattleboro strain). *Brain Res. Bull.,* 6: 71–75.

Buijs, R.M. (1978) Intra- and extrahypothalamic vasopressin and oxytocin pathways in the rat: pathways to the limbic system, medulla oblongata and spinal cord. *Cell Tiss. Res.,* 192: 423–435.

Buijs, R.M., Velis, D.N. and Swaab, D.F. (1980) Extrahypothalamic vasopressin and oxytocin innervation of fetal and adult rat brain. In P.S. McConnell, C.J. Boer, H.J Romijn, N.E. van de Poll and M.A. Corner (Eds.), *Adaptive Capabilities of the Nervous System. Progress in Brain Research Vol. 53,* Elsevier/North Holland, Amsterdam pp. 159–168.

Burbach, J.P.H. and Lebouille, J.L.M. (1983) Proteolytic conversion of arginine-vasopressin and oxytocin by brain synaptic membranes *J. biol. Chem.,* 258: 1487–1494.

Burbach, J.P.H., De Kloet, E.R. and De Wied, D. (1980a) Oxytocin biotransformation in the rat limbic brain: characterization of peptidase activities and significance in the formation of oxytocin fragments. *Brain Res.,* 202: 401–414.

Burbach, J.P.H., Schotman, P. and De Kloet, E.R., (1980b) Oxytocin biotransformation in the rat limbic brain: chemical characterization of two oxytocin fragments and proposed pathway for oxytocin conversion. *Biochem. Biophys. Res. Commun.,* 97: 1005–1013.

Celestian, F.F., Carey, R.J. and Miller, M. (1975) Unimpaired maintenance of a conditioned avoidance response in the rat with diabetes insipidus. *Physiol. Behav.,* 15: 707–711.

Contreras, P.C. and Takemori, A.E. (1980) The effects of prolyl-leucyl-glycinamide on morphine tolerance and dependence. *Fed. Proc.,* 39: 845.

Cooper, K.E., Kasting, N.W., Lederis, K. and Veale, W.L. (1979) Evidence supporting a role for endogenous vasopressin in natural suppression of fever in the sheep. *J. Physiol. (Lond.),* 295: 33–45.

De Wied, D. (1965) The influence of the posterior and intermediate lobe of the pituitary and pituitary peptides on the maintenance of a conditioned avoidance response in rats. *Int. J. Neuropharmacol.,* 4: 157–167.

De Wied, D. (1969) Effects of peptide hormones on behavior. In W.F. Ganong and L. Martini (Eds.), *Frontiers in Neuroendocrinology,* Oxford University Press, London, pp. 97–140.

De Wied, D. (1971) Long-term effect of vasopressin on the maintenance of a conditioned avoidance response in rats. *Nature (Lond.),* 232: 58–60.

De Wied, D. (1976) Behavioral effects of intraventricularly administered vasopressin and vasopressin fragments. *Life Sci.,* 19: 685–690.

De Wied, D. and Bohus, B. (1966) Long-term and short-term effects on retention of a conditioned avoidance response in rats by treatment with long acting pitressin and α-MSH. *Nature (Lond.),* 212: 1484–1486.

166

De Wied, D., Greven, H.M., Lande S. and Witter, A. (1972) Dissociation of the behavioral and endocrine effects of lysine vasopressin by tryptic digestion. *Brit. J. Pharmacol.*, 45: 118–122.

De Wied, D., Bohus, B. and Van Wimersma Greidanus, Tj. B. (1975) Memory deficit in rats with hereditary diabetes insipidus. *Brain Res.*, 85: 152–156.

Dogterom, J. and Buijs, R.M. (1980) Vasopressin and oxytocin distribution in rat brain: radioimmunoassay and immunocytochemical studies. In C. Ajmone Marsan and W.Z. Traczyk (Eds.), *Neuropeptides and Neural Transmission*, Raven Press, New York, pp. 307–314.

Dogterom, J., Van Wimersma Greidanus, Tj. B. and Swaab, D.F. (1977) Evidence for the release of vasopressin and oxytocin into cerebrospinal fluid: measurements in plasma and CSF of intact and hypophysectomized rats. *Neuroendocrinology*, 24: 108–118.

Dorsa, D.M. and Van Ree, J.M. (1979) Modulation of substantia nigra self-stimulation by neuropeptides related to neurohypophyseal hormones. *Brain Res.*, 172: 367–371.

Flexner, J.B., Flexner, L.B., Hoffman, P.L. and Walter, R. (1977) Dose–response relationships in attenuation of puromycin-induced amnesia by neurohypophyseal peptides. *Brain Res.*, 134: 139–144.

Flexner, J.B., Flexner, L.B., Walter, R. and Hoffman, P.L. (1978) ADH and related peptides: effect of pre- or post-training treatment on puromycin amnesia. *Pharmacol. Biochem. Behav.*, 8: 93–95.

Hoffman, P.L., Ritzmann, R.F., Walter, R. and Tabakoff, B. (1978) Arginine vasopressin maintains ethanol tolerance. *Nature (Lond.)*, 276: 614–616.

Hostetter, G., Jubb, S.L. and Kozlowski, G.P. (1977) Vasopressin affects the behavior of rats in a positively-rewarded discrimination task. *Life Sci.*, 21: 1323–1328.

Kovács, G.L., Bohus, B. and Versteeg, D.H.G. (1979a) The effect of vasopressin on memory processes: the role of noradrenergic neurotransmission. *Neuroscience*, 4: 1529–1537.

Kovács, G.L., Bohus, B., Versteeg, D.H.G., De Kloet, E.R. and De Wied, D. (1979b) Effect of oxytocin and vasopressin on memory consolidation: sites of action and catecholaminergic correlates after local microinjection into limbic midbrain structures. *Brain Res.*, 175: 303–314.

Kovács, G.L., Bohus, B. and Versteeg, D.H.G. (1980) The interaction of posterior pituitary neuropeptides with monoaminergic neurotransmission: significance in learning and memory processes. In P.S. McConnell, C.J. Boer, H.J. Romijn, N.E. van de Poll and M.A. Corner (Eds.), *Adaptive Capabilities of the Nervous System Progress in Brain Research, Vol. 53*, Elsevier/North-Holland, Amsterdam, pp. 123–140.

Kovács, G.L., Bohus, B., Versteeg, D.H.G., Telegdy, G. and De Wied, D. (1982) Neurohypophyseal hormones and memory. In H. Yoshida, Y. Hagihara and S. Ebashi (Eds.), *Advances in Pharmacology and Therapeutics II, Vol. 1, CNS Pharmacology, Neuropeptides*, Pergamon Press, Oxford, pp. 175–187.

Krivoy, W.A., Kroeger, D.G., Taylor, A.N. and Zimmermann, E. (1974) Antagonism of morphine by β-melanocyte stimulating hormone and by tetracosactin, *Europ. J. Pharmacol.*, 27: 339–345.

Láczi, F., Fekete, M. and De Wied, D. (1983) Antidiuretic activity and immunoreactive arginin-vasopressin levels in eye plexus blood during passive avoidance behavior in rats. *Life Sci.*, 32: 577–589.

Lande, S., Flexner, J.B. and Flexner, L.B. (1972) Effect of corticotropin and desglycinamide[9]-lysine vasopressin on suppression of memory by puromycin. *Proc. nat. Acad. Sci. U.S.A.*, 69: 558–560.

Le Moal, M., Koob, G.D. Koda, L.Y., Bloom, F.E., Manning, M., Sawyer, W.H. and Rivier, J. (1981) Vasopressor receptor antagonist prevents behavioral effects of vasopressin. *Nature (Lond.)*, 291: 491–493.

Leshner, A.I. and Roche, K.E. (1977) Comparison of the effects of ACTH and lysine vasopressin on avoidance-of-attack in mice. *Physiol. Behav.*, 18: 879–883.

Marks, N., Abrash, L. and Walter, R. (1973) Degradation of neurohypophyseal hormones by brain extracts and purified brain enzymes. *Proc. Soc. exp. Biol. Med.*, 142: 455–460.

Mens, W.B.J., Van Egmond, M.A.H., De Rotte, A.A., Van Wimersma Greidanus, Tj. B. (1982) Neurohypophyseal peptide levels in CSF and plasma during passive avoidance behavior in rats. *Horm. Behav.*, 16: 371–382.

Pedersen, C.A., Ascher, J.A., Monroe, Y.L. and Prange, A.J., Jr. (1982) Oxytocin induces maternal behavior in virgin female rats. *Science*, 216: 648–649.

Pliška, V., Thorn, N.A. and Vilhardt, H. (1971) In vitro uptake and breakdown of tritiated lysine-vasopressin by bovine neurohypophyseal and cortical tissue, *Acta endocr.*, 67: 12–22.

Rigter, H. and Crabbe, J.C. (1980) Neurohypophysial peptides and ethanol. In D. de Wied and P.A. van Keep (Eds.), *Hormones and the Brain*, MTP Press, Lancaster, pp. 263–275.

Rigter, H., Van Riezen, H. and De Wied, D. (1974) The effects of ACTH- and vasopressin-analogues on CO_2-induced retrograde amnesia in rats. *Physiol. Behav.*, 13: 381–388.

Rigter, H., Elbertse, R. and Van Riezen, H. (1975) Time-dependent anti-amnesic effect of $ACTH_{4-10}$ and desglycinamide-lysine vasopressin. In W.H. Gispen, Tj. B. van Wimersma Greidanus, B. Bohus and D. de Wied (Eds.), *Hormones, Homeostasis and the Brain, Progress in Brain Research, Vol. 42*, Elsevier, Amsterdam, pp. 163–171.

Rigter, H., Rijk, H. and Crabbe, J.C. (1983) Enhancement of tolerance to ethanol and severity of withdrawal in mice by a vasopressin fragment. Submitted.

Schulz, H., Kovács, G.L. and Telegdy, G. (1976) The effect of vasopressin and oxytocin on avoidance behavior in rats. In E. Endröczi (Ed.), *Cellular and Molecular Bases of Neuroendocrine Processes*, Akadémiai Kiadó, Budapest, pp. 555–564.

Schwarzberg, H., Hartmann, G., Kovács, G.L. and Telegdy, G. (1976) Effect of intraventricular oxytocin and vasopressin on self-stimulation in rats. *Acta physiol. Acad. Sci. hung.*, 47: 127–131.

Sterba, G. (1974) Ascending neurosecretory pathways of the peptidergic type. In F. Knowles and L. Vollrath (Eds.), *Neurosecretion — The Final Neuroendocrine Pathway*, Springer, Berlin, pp. 38–47.

Székely, J.I., Miglécz, E., Dunai-Kovácz, Z., Tarnawa, I., Ronai, A.Z., Gráf, L. and Bajusz, S. (1979) Attenuation of morphine tolerance and dependence by α-melanocyte stimulating hormone (α-MSH). Life Sci., 24: 1931–1938.

Thompson, E.A. and De Wied, D. (1973) The relationship between the antidiuretic activity of rat eye plexus blood and passive avoidance behavior. *Physiol. Behav.*, 11: 377–380.

Valtin, H. and Schroeder, H.A. (1964) Familial hypothalamic diabetes insipidus in rats (Brattleboro strain). *Amer. J. Physiol.*, 206: 425–530.

Valtin, H., Sawyer, W.H. and Sokol, H.W. (1965) Neurohypophysial principles in rats homozygous and heterozygous for hypothalamic diabetes insipidus (Brattleboro strain). *Endocrinology*, 77: 701–706.

Van Ree, J.M. and De Wied, D. (1977) Heroin selfadministration is under control of vasopressin. Life Sci., 21: 315–320.

Van Ree, J.M. and De Wied, D. (1981) Vasopressin, oxytocin and dependence on opiates. In J.L. Martinez, Jr., R.A. Jensen, R.B. Messing, H. Rigter and J.L. McGaugh (Eds.), *Endogenous Peptides and Learning and Memory Processes*, Academic Press, New York, pp. 397–411.

Van Ree, J.M., De Wied, D., Bradbury, A.F., Hulme, E.C., Smyth, D.G. and Snell, C.R. (1976) Induction of tolerance to the analgesic action of lipotropin C-fragment. *Nature (Lond.)*, 264: 792–794.

Van Ree, J.M., Bohus, B., Versteeg, D.H.G. and De Wied, D. (1978) Neurohypophyscal principles and memory processes. *Biochem. Pharmacol.*, 27: 1793–1800.

Van Wimersma Greidanus, Tj. B. (1982) MSH/ACTH$_{4-10}$: a tool to differentiate between the role of vasopressin in memory consolidation or retrieval processes. *Peptides*, 3: 7–11.

Van Wimersma Greidanus, Tj. B. and De Wied, D. (1976) Modulation of passive-avoidance behavior of rats by intracerebroventricular administration of antivasopressin serum. *Behav. Biol.*, 18: 325–333.

Van Wimersma Greidanus, Tj. B., Dogterom, J. and De Wied, D. (1975a) Intraventricular administration of antivasopressin serum inhibits memory consolidation in rats. *Life Sci.*, 16: 637–644.

Van Wimersma Greidanus, Tj. B., Bohus, B. and De Wied, D. (1975b) The role of vasopressin in memory processes. In W.H. Gispen, Tj. B. van Wimersma Greidanus, B. Bohus and D. de Wied (Eds.), *Hormones, Homeostasis and the Brain, Progress in Brain Research, Vol. 42*, Elsevier, Amsterdam, pp. 135–141.

Van Wimersma Greidanus, Tj. B., Croiset, G., Goedemans, H. and Dogterom J. (1979a) Vasopressin levels in peripheral blood and in cerebrospinal fluid during passive and active avoidance behavior in rats. *Horm. Behav.*, 12: 102–111.

Van Wimersma Greidanus, Tj. B., Croiset, G. and Schuiling, G. (1979b) Fornix transection: discrimination between neuropeptide effects on attention and memory. *Brain Res. Bull.*, 4: 625–629.

Versteeg, C.A.M., Bohus, B. and De Jong, W. (1979) Inhibitory effects of neuropeptides on centrally evoked pressor responses. In Y. Yamori, W. Lovenberg and E.D. Freis (Eds.), *Prophylactic Approach to Hypertensive Diseases*, Raven Press, New York, pp. 329–335.

Versteeg, D.H.G., Tanaka, M. and De Kloet, E.R. (1978) Catecholamine concentration and turnover in discrete regions of the brain of the homozygous Brattleboro rat deficient in vasopressin. *Endocrinology*, 103: 1654–1661.

Versteeg, D.H.G., De Kloet, E.R., Van Wimersma Greidanus, Tj. B. and De Wied, D. (1979) Vasopressin modulates the activity of catecholamine containing neurons in specific brain regions. *Neurosci. Lett.*, 11: 69–73.

Walter, R., Hoffman, P.L., Flexner, J.B. and Flexner, L.B. (1975) Neurohypophyseal hormones, analogs, and fragments; Their effect on puromycin-induced amnesia. *Proc. nat. Acad. Sci. U.S.A.*, 72: 4180–4184.

Walter, R., Van Ree, J.M. and De Wied, D. (1978) Modification of conditioned behavior of rats by neurohypophyseal hormones and analogues. *Proc. nat. Acad. Sci. U.S.A.*, 75: 2493–2496.

The Neurohypophysis: Structure, Function and Control, Progress in Brain Research, Vol. 60, edited by B.A. Cross and G. Leng

Vasopressin-like Peptides and the Treatment of Memory Disorders in Man

J. JOLLES *

Psychiatric University Clinic, and Rudolf Magnus Institute for Pharmacology, Medical Faculty; University of Utrecht (The Netherlands)

INTRODUCTION

Peptides related to vasopressin and oxytocin affect animal behaviour in a number of different test situations. The notion that these peptides are involved in memory processes and learning evolved from the pioneering work of De Wied and co-workers. Rats which lack vasopressin are impaired in the acquisition and retention of certain learned behaviours, and these behavioural deficits can be corrected by treatment with arginine[8]-vasopressin (AVP) or lysine[8]-vasopressin (LVP) (Table I) (De Wied, 1969 and this volume; Van Ree et al., 1978; Rigter and Crabbe, 1979). Similar behavioural activity has been found for fragments of vasopressin with virtually no vasopressor or antidiuretic activity, such as des-glycinamide-arginine[8]-vasopressin (DGAVP) and des-glycinamide-lysine[8]-vasopressin (DGLVP). These peptides also improved learning and retention in intact rats, and in rats with memory disturbances of other origin (e.g. puromycin or CO_2 treatment, or electroconvulsive shock).

The behavioural action of vasopressin and congeners has been interpreted in terms of an effect on "memory processes", and this has led to the suggestion that the peptides might have clinical application in the treatment of "memory disorders". An evaluation of the clinical efficiency of these peptides is difficult, for a number of reasons. Positive and negative results have been obtained, and it is clear that a number of parameters are important. This applies particularly to the questions: "what is a memory disorder", "what patient population do we test", and "what methodology do we use, to study the peptide effects on memory"? The present review gives a critical evaluation of the clinical studies reported to date. Relevant aspects of the neuropsychology of memory disorders are reviewed, and some emphasis given to the pharmacological methods used to study treatment effects, i.e. with the use of LVP, AVP, DGAVP or DDAVP (1-desamino-D-arginine[8]-vasopressin, which has weak behavioural and antidiuretic actions, but has no vasopressor activity, see Table I).

---

* Address for correspondence: Psychiatric University Clinic, Nicolaas Beetsstraat 24, 3511 HG Utrecht, The Netherlands

TABLE I

AMINOACID SEQUENCE OF SOME RELEVANT NEUROPEPTIDES

Arginine[8]-vasopressin (AVP)	H–Cys–Tyr–Phe–Gln–Asn–Cys–Pro–Arg–Gly–NH$_2$
Lysine[8]-vasopressin (LVP)	H–Cys–Tyr–Phe–Gln–Asn–Cys–Pro–Lys–Gly–NH$_2$
Desglycinamide[9]-arginine[8]-vasopressin (DGAVP)	H–Cys–Tyr–Phe–Gln–Asn–Cys–Pro–Arg–OH
Desglycinamide[9]-lysine[8]-vasopressin (DGLVP)	H–Cys–Tyr–Phe–Gln–Asn–Cys–Pro–Lys–OH
1-Desamino-D-arginine[8]-vasopressin (DDAVP)	(desamino)Cys–Tyr–Phe–Gln–Asn–Cys–Pro–Arg(D)–Gly–NH$_2$
Oxytocin	H–Cys–Tyr–Ile–Gln–Asn–Cys–Pro–Leu–Gly–NH$_2$
ACTH$_{4-10}$	H–Met–Glu–His–Phe–Arg–Trp–Gly–OH

CLINICAL TRIALS CONCERNING BEHAVIOURAL EFFECTS OF VASOPRESSIN-LIKE PEPTIDES

(1) Brain trauma patients (Table II)

The first clinical trial concerning the anti-amnesic effects of vasopressin was performed with patients that suffered from a post-traumatic amnesia (three patients) and chronic alcoholism (one patient) (Oliveros et al., 1978; Table I). LVP was administered by nasal spray. Cognitive functions were not measured systematically, but a clinical impression was that all patients improved after 3 to 9 days. In a study by Timsit-Berthier et al. (1980), five out of seven patients treated with LVP nasal spray improved on tests that are supposed to measure "attention" or "short-term visual retention". In addition, a clinical improvement was found in activity, motivation and social adjustment. The peptide effect developed in time, and was maximal after weeks or months. This study also found that the seven memory-disturbed patients had decreased levels of neurophysin-1, the vasopressin-transport protein. These levels increased to normal in four out of five patients that improved after treatment. Another treatment effect of LVP in a brain trauma patient was reported by Drago et al. (1981), and a study with memory-disturbed trauma patients has also been conducted in our Institute (Verhoeven, Verdonck and Van Ree, unpublished), where six brain trauma patients were treated with DGAVP nasal spray in a double-blind cross-over study. No effects were seen on the tests used to evaluate the treatment. However, five out of six patients reported a subjective improvement from the fourth day of treatment on. Basal levels of vasopressin and neurophysins in blood and cerebrospinal fluid were in the normal range for all patients, and did not change as a result of the peptide treatment.

No treatment effects were seen in patients with more serious head injuries. For instance, no effect was seen after treatment of such patients with low doses of DGAVP or LVP (Jenkins et al., 1979) and higher doses of DDAVP and DGAVP were also ineffective (Jenkins et al., 1981). Two other studies with patients treated with LVP were also negative (Koch-Henriksen et al., 1981; Fewtrell et al., 1982). Therapeutic efficiency may depend on the extent to which degenerative processes have taken place in the brain: relatively less serious defects may benefit more from peptide treatment.

TABLE II

STUDIES CONCERNING VASOPRESSIN EFFECTS IN BRAIN TRAUMA PATIENTS

The *Frequency* column gives the frequency of administration per day up to the total amount stated under *Dose*. If not stated otherwise, the frequency is once per day. For the *Design* column, A indicates a comparison between groups, and B indicates a comparison within groups or subjects. Several studies were performed on heterogenous patient groups and are therefore indicated in more than one table.

Reference	n	Peptide	Dose	Route	Frequency	Duration	Design
Oliveros et al., 1978	3	LVP	11–30 IU	i.n.	4–5	1–several weeks	Open
Jenkins et al., 1979	6	DDAVP	4 µg	i.m.		6 weeks	Open
Jenkins et al., 1981	5	DDAVP	160 µg	i.n.	4 ×	1 week	Open
		DGAVP	260 µg	i.n.	4 ×	2 weeks	Open
Timsit-Berthier et al., 1980	7	LVP	14 IU	i.n.	2 ×	15 days	Double blind, placebo controlled A
	7	LVP	14 IU	i.n.	2 ×	15–30 days	Open
Koch-Henriksen et al., 1981	5	LVP	22.5 IU	i.n.		2 weeks	Double blind, placebo controlled A
Drago et al., 1981	1	LVP	25 IU	i.n.		2 weeks	Double blind, cross-over
Fewtrell et al., 1982	6	LVP	16 IU	i.n.		2 weeks	Double blind, cross-over
Verhoeven, Verdonck and Van Ree (unpublished)	6	DGAVP	200 µg	i.n.	t.i.d.	2 weeks	Double blind, cross-over

(2) Alcoholic patients (Table III)

After the study mentioned above, in which one alcoholic patient seemed to benefit from treatment with LVP (Oliveros et al., 1978), another study reported a similar effect in an alcoholic with the amnesic syndrome. This patient remembered more, and had better concentration, attention and time orientation after intranasal application of LVP (Le Bœuf et al., 1978). A more recent study of two alcoholics treated according to a double-blind cross-over design with LVP also reported a treatment effect (Drago et al., 1981). However, Tinklenberg et al. (1981a, 1982), using better research methods, found no improvement in alcoholic patients treated with DGAVP or DDAVP. Apart from the fact that different peptides were used the duration of the treatment was also much shorter in this study. Another negative study was performed by Blake et al. (1978) who concluded that a serious amnesic syndrome induced by alcohol does not benefit from vasopressin treatment.

(3) Dementia patients (Table IV)

Twelve patients (aged 50–64 years) that were hospitalized with somatic complaints were treated with LVP applied intranasally (Legros et al., 1978). These patients performed better than control subjects on certain tests of attention and memory. The same investigators reported later that the scores of one of these "memory tests" correlate with levels of neurophysin-1 in the blood (Legros and Gilot, 1979). Effects of LVP were also found in senile dementia patients (average age 80 years, Delwaide et al., 1980): a single administration of LVP improved the performance of nine out of ten patients on a word list retention task, and these effects were still present after 48 h. Others have also found that a single administration of DDAVP can improve the memory for semantic structures (i.e. word memory) in patients suffering from progressive dementia (Weingartner et al., 1981b). Ferris and Reisberg (1982) treated 20 patients suffering from mild to moderate dementia with LVP for periods of seven days in a placebo controlled cross-over study. Consistent, but small improvements on memory tests were noted. However, in another study in which carefully diagnosed Alzheimer patients were treated with LVP, no effects were noted on tests of memory, learning and visual perception. The only measurable effect concerned an improved performance in a reaction time test. These authors concluded that vasopressin might have a "non-specific activating effect" (Durso et al., 1982). A similar suggestion was made by Tinklenberg et al. (1981a, 1982), who treated patients suffering from a primary degenerative disorder (Alzheimer). Neither DDAVP nor DGAVP had measurable effects on the tests used. An impression was that some patients might have more energy and less depression, and especially patients with comparatively mild dysfunctions. That may imply that patients in which more extensive degeneration has taken place in the brain cannot benefit from the peptide treatment.

(4) Other patients (Table V)

Several authors have claimed that the anti-amnesic action of vasopressin-like peptides is related to an anti-depressant effect. In a study in which patients with endogenous depression and cognitive disorders were treated with DDAVP (Weingartner et al., 1981a; Gold et al., 1979), three out of four patients manifested a significant improvement in the level of cognitive functioning. After four weeks they were back at their pretreatment level. In a follow-up study by the same researchers in two depressed patients, DDAVP appeared to counteract the amnesia which is a characteristic side-effect of electroconvulsive shock therapy. Others report that LVP improved memory processes in three depressed patients (Drago et al., 1981).

TABLE III

STUDIES CONCERNING VASOPRESSIN EFFECTS IN ALCOHOLIC PATIENTS

For legend, see Table II

Reference	n	Peptide	Dose	Route	Frequency	Duration	Design
Oliveros et al., 1978	1	LVP	11 IU	i.n.	4×	several weeks	Open
Blake et al., 1978	2	LVP	16 IU	i.n.	4×	15–21 days	Open
Le Bœuf et al., 1978	1	LVP	22.5 IU	i.n.	3×	14 days	Double blind, placebo controlled B
Drago et al., 1981	2	LVP	25 IU	i.n.		14 days	Double blind, cross-over
Tinklenberg et al., 1981a, 1982	2	DGAVP	200 µg	i.n.	t.i.d.	5 days	Double blind, placebo controlled A
	4	DDAVP	10–20 µg	i.n.	t.i.d.	3–8 days	Double blind, cross-over

TABLE IV

STUDIES CONCERNING VASOPRESSIN EFFECTS IN ELDERLY PEOPLE AND SENILE DEMENTIA PATIENTS

For legend, see Table II.

Reference	n	Peptide	Dose	Route	Frequency	Duration	Design
Legros et al., 1978	12	LVP	16 IU	i.n.	3×	3 days	Double blind, placebo controlled A
Delwaide et al., 1980	10	LVP	15 IU	i.n.		single adm.	Double blind, placebo controlled B
Durso et al., 1982	14	LVP	16 IU	i.n.	2×	10 days	Double blind, placebo controlled A
Weingartner et al., 1981b	7	DDAVP	30–60 µg	i.n.		several times	Double blind, placebo controlled B
Ferris et al., 1981	20	LVP	16 IU	i.n.	2×	7 days	Double blind, cross-over
Tinklenberg et al., 1981a, 1982	1	DGAVP	200 µg	i.n.	t.i.d.	5 days	Double blind, placebo controlled A
	2	DDAVP	10–20 µg	i.n.	t.i.d.	3–8 days	Double blind, cross-over

174

TABLE V

STUDIES CONCERNING VASOPRESSIN EFFECTS IN OTHER PATIENTS AND IN VOLUNTEERS

For legend, see Table II.

Reference	n	Peptide	Dose	Route	Frequency	Duration	Design
Depression							
Gold et al., 1979	4	DDAVP	60–160 µg	i.n.		3–7 weeks	Double blind, placebo controlled B
Weingartner et al., 1981a, b	2	DDAVP	40–60 µg	i.n.		3 days	Double blind, placebo controlled B
Drago et al., 1981	3	LVP	25 IU	i.n.		2 weeks	Double blind, cross-over
Diabetes insipidus							
Gilot et al., 1980	5	DDAVP	?	?		3 days	Open
Láczi et al., 1982	16	LVP	1.5, 10 IU	i.n., i.m.		single adm.; 7 days	Double blind, cross-over
Láczi et al., 1983	13	DDAVP	4,10 µg	i.n., i.m.		7 days	Double blind, cross-over
		DGAVP	3,30 µg	i.m.		3 days; 3 days	Double blind, placebo controlled B
		DGAVP	80 µg	i.n.	2×	7 days	Double blind, placebo controlled B
Waggoner et al., 1978	7	DDAVP		i.n.	2×	4 months	Open
Volunteers							
Weingartner et al., 1981a, b	6	DDAVP	30–60 µg	i.n.	t.i.d.	2–3 weeks	Double blind, placebo controlled A
Láczi et al., 1982	10	LVP	1.5,10 IU	i.n., i.m.		single adm.; 7 days	Double blind, cross-over
Láczi et al., 1983	9	DDAVP	4,10 µg	i.n., i.m.		7 days	Double blind, cross-over
		DGAVP	3,30 µg	i.m.		3 days; 3 days	Double blind, placebo controlled B
		DGAVP	80 µg	i.n.	2×	7 days	Double blind, placebo controlled B
Medvedev et al., 1981	20	AVP	25–35 µg	i.n.	2×	single adm.	Single blind, placebo controlled B
Psychosis							
Forisz, 1952a, b	80	Pitressin	10 IU	i.m.		several months	Open
Vranckx et al., 1979	16	LVP	7.5–45 IU	i.n.	1–6	4 weeks	Open
Korsgaard et al., 1981	16	LVP	22.5,67.5 IU	i.n.	t.i.d.	3 weeks	Single blind, cross-over
Encephalitis							
Koizumi et al., 1981	1	AVP	12 U.S.P.	i.n.	3×	2 weeks	Double blind, placebo controlled B
Hypothalamic disorders							
Calandra et al., 1980	1	AVP	5 IU	i.m.		2 weeks	Open

TABLE V. Continued

Reference	n	Peptide	Dose	Route	Frequency	Duration	Design
Brain hypoxia							
Verhoeven, Verdonck and Van Ree, unpublished	1	DGAVP		i.n.		2 weeks	Double blind, cross-over
Fewtrell et al., 1982	1	LVP	16 IU	i.n.		2 weeks	Double blind, cross-over
Lesch–Nyhan disease in children							
Anderson et al., 1979	3	DDAVP	40 µg	i.n.		single adm.	Single blind
Attention and learning disorders in children							
Eisenberg et al., 1982	5	DDAVP	20 µg	i.n.		3 days	Open
	7	DDAVP	20 µg	i.n.		10 days	Double blind, cross-over
Cerebral vascular insufficiency							
Verhoeven, Verdonck and Van Ree, unpublished	1	DGAVP	200 µg	i.n.	t.i.d.	2 weeks	Double blind, cross-over
Brain surgery							
Verhoeven, Verdonck and Van Ree, unpublished	1	DGAVP	200 µg	i.n.	t.i.d.	2 weeks	Double blind, cross-over

Memory complaints accompany many different diseases. For instance, memory processes are reported to be improved in diabetes insipidus patients, in open studies with DDAVP (Gilot et al., 1980; Waggoner et al., 1978), and in double-blind studies with LVP, DDAVP or DGAVP applied either intranasally or i.m. (Láczi et al., 1982, 1983). The latter authors claim that different aspects of memory (e.g. short-term or long-term memory) can be manipulated by the nature of the peptide and the route of administration.

Several studies have been performed with patients suffering from deep brain lesions of different etiology. Some reports indicate an effect of vasopressin on amnesia caused by herpes simplex encephalitis (Koizumi et al., 1981) and hypothalamic disorders (Calandra et al., 1980). On the other hand, no treatment effect was found in cases of brain hypoxia treated with LVP (Fewtrell et al., 1982) or DGAVP (Verhoeven, Verdonck and Van Ree, unpublished), or in a patient suffering from cerebral vascular insufficiency (Verhoeven et al., unpublished). A subjective improvement after treatment with DGAVP was found in one patient suffering from a disorder of semantic and episodic memory after left temporal brain surgery (Verhoeven et al., unpublished).

As early as 1937, Forisz treated chronic schizophrenic patients with i.m. Pitressin for prolonged periods (Forisz, 1952a, b). About 40 % of treated patients improved in that after an initial sedative effect lasting 1–2 weeks, positive symptoms of the psychosis reappeared, resulting eventually in a more social and interested attitude. A number of patients could leave the clinic. More recently, in a study of 16 chronic schizophrenic patients (Korsgaard et al., 1981), a decrease in thinking disorder was noted, accompanied by an increase in energy and activity (in six of the 16 patients). This increase in activity was not of therapeutic value in four patients because they were agitated/aggressive. In a similar study by Vrankx et al. (1979) these undesirable effects of disorientation and agitation occurred in only a few patients. These authors reported that fairly high doses of LVP (45 IU) have a beneficial effect on emotional withdrawal and blunted affect.

A beneficial effect of DDAVP has been reported in children suffering from Lesch–Nyhan disease. This desease is characterized by automutilation behaviour which has been interpreted as a disorder of passive avoidance behaviour (Anderson et al., 1979). Specific effects of DDAVP on "memory retrieval" were reported in a study on children suffering from attention and learning disorders (Eisenberg et al., 1982). Finally, volunteers without memory defects have also been found to benefit from peptide treatment. Six young, healthy, volunteers appeared to have improved memory and learning performance after treatment with DDAVP for 2–3 weeks (Weingartner et al., 1981a). Similarly, ten healthy young subjects improved on some tests thought to measure aspects of memory, after LVP or DDAVP (Láczi et al., 1982). Nine patients without a memory deficit also improved in these respects after DGAVP (Láczi et a., 1983). Medvedev et al. (1981) found that a single administration of AVP can be effective. This peptide was administered to 20 students, and the data were taken to indicate that vasopressin would specifically improve long-term memory and recall.

MEMORY COMPLAINTS AND MEMORY DISORDERS

Many different types of patients have been used in the study of the treatment effects of vasopressin-like peptides (Tables II–V). An implicit assumption seems to be that a peptide shown to affect memory processes in animals will also do so in any aspect or type of memory in humans. We feel that this is unlikely in view of present knowledge on the neuropsychology of memory (see Russell, 1981). Memory complaints accompany many types of disease, and the brain processes which underly these complaints may be very different. It is therefore necessary to discriminate relatively "true" memory disorders from those that are secondary to another disorder. For instance, memory complaints can be the result of a decrease in the rate of information processing. Such a patient may complain about his memory, but his true problem may be that things in everyday life happen too quickly for him. Another type of secondary complaint is due to a disorder in behavioural organization or planning such as frequently accompanies minor lesions in the frontal lobes. Such a patient "forgets" how to perform complex behavioural acts and does not evaluate his own performance. Other memory disturbances are associated with attention: when you cannot focus your attention on the things you have to learn, this may show itself as a memory deficit. Still other memory disorders are related to language disorders: the patient cannot find the words which are necessary to describe what he has in memory, a concentration deficit, etc. The importance of discriminating between types of memory disorder is demonstrated by neuropsychological data (Luria, 1976; Dimond, 1980). A relatively "true" memory deficit, which is specific for a particular type of material, is taken to be due to dysfunction of posterior neocortical structures (e.g. left temporal neocortex — memory for verbal material; right temporal parietal neocortex — memory for faces). The primary brain structure involved in retrieval deficits is the frontal cortex, and consolidation deficits seem to relate to dysfunction in deep brain structures, notably the thalamus. The hippocampus may be specifically involved in spatial/temporal memory (O'Keefe and Nadel, 1978) and brainstem structures including ascending fibres to the neocortex are involved in the rate of information processing.

This knowledge on the neuropsychology of memory is pertinent to our discussion of vasopressin effects in different kinds of patients in the light of animal experiments which show that vasopressin (DGAVP) may primarily affect the consolidation and retrieval of information or a process common to both (Bohus et al., 1978; Rigter and Crabbe, 1979). Another important finding from animal experiments is that vasopressin loses its behavioural effects when relevant limbic brain structures are lesioned (such as septum, amygdala and dorsal hippocampus; Van Wimersma Greidanus et al., 1976). It is therefore to be expected that the peptide will act on certain types of memory deficit and not on others. A number of clinical findings support this hypothesis. For instance, peptide effects were found in brain trauma patients with relatively mild deficits (Timsit-Berthier et al., 1980), but not in patients with more serious and complex deficits (Jenkins et al., 1979, 1981; Koch-Hendriksen et al., 1981; Fewtrell et al., 1982). The same applies to the studies with alcoholic patients and senile dementia patients; treatment effects were found in relatively mild cases (Oliveros et al., 1978; Le Bœuf et al., 1978; Drago et al., 1981 — alcoholics; Legros et al., 1978; Delwaide et al., 1980; Weingartner et al., 1981a, b — dementia cases), but not in older patients who had more serious, long-term defects (Blake et al., 1978; Tinklenberg et al., 1981a, b). The extent to which degenerative processes have taken place in the brain probably determines the effectiveness of the peptide.

Another relevant point concerns patients who are sometimes considered to be particularly suitable for anti-amnesic treatment. In some disorders the memory deficit is especially obvious, such as (pre)senile dementia or amnesic syndrome resulting from chronic alcohol consumption (Korsakoff syndrome) or herpes simplex encephalitis. A disadvantage of the study of peptide effects in these patients is that as a rule they have a more complex pattern of deficits, such as confabulation, disorders in the planning of the behaviour, language disorders, depression, etc. In the Korsakoff and encephalitis patients destruction of deep structures, such as those lining the third ventricle (see Newcombe, 1980), makes these patients unsuitable for peptide treatment, as is the case with (pre)senile patients who usually have extensive degeneration of both subcortical and cortical structures. This is of particular importance as the dorsal noradrenergic bundle seems to be involved in the effect of vasopressin (Kovács et al., 1982).

Other patient groups — which are etiologically homogeneous — may be very heterogenous with respect to the nature of the memory disorder. We have recently demonstrated that this is the case in brain trauma patients, and in senile dementia patients. New testing procedures based partly upon laboratory research have shown that the deficit(s) in brain trauma patients and also in senile dementia patients, differs widely (Jolles et al., 1983). Thus a patient group assembled on the basis of etiological factors alone may be very heterogenous, neuropsychologically, which may explain the variability in the results which is characteristic for most of the clinical studies. A final point with respect to the nature of the memory deficit concerns the methods of evaluation used.

Much information has been gathered on the nature of memory and of memory disorders, yet no adequate methods exist for use in the clinic (see Russell, 1981). The most widely used measures are the Wechsler Memory Scale, sub-tests from the Wechsler Adult Intelligence Scale and the Benton test: these tests measure only minor aspects of memory and do not exist in sufficiently parallel forms to enable repeated testing, which is essential for adequate evaluation of treatment. The best results can be expected from new research methods adopted from the psychological laboratory. Among the tests we have recently developed is a memory comparison task to assess aspects of the "rate of information processing" (Jolles et al., 1983). In two pilot studies this task seemed to be particularly sensitive to treatment effects of vasopressin. This may indicate that such an action on the rate at which the brain processes perceptual information may underly the memory effects induced by vasopressin. Furthermore, the only significant vasopressin effect found by Durso et al., (1982) in senile dementia patients was on a reaction time task (faster). Similarly, Verhoeven et al. (unpublished) found that intranasal vasopressin improved the speed of motor performance (tapping test) in brain trauma patients. The observations in schizophrenic patients also support the notion of an effect on the rate of working, thinking, etc., in that vasopressin had an activating effect (Forisz, 1952a, b; Vranckx et al., 1979; Korsgaard et al., 1981). The peptide effect reported in depressed patients (e.g. Gold et al., 1979; Weingartner et al., 1981a, b) may be based upon the same mode of action of the hormones as a decrease in the rate of thinking and working is a characteristic of depressed patients. Finally, some authors, on the basis of behavioural observations on patients, have suggested that vasopressin might have a general "non-specific" activating effect, which may mean the same thing as formulated above (e.g. Tinklenberg et al., 1981a, 1982). Bohus et al. (1978) suggested that vasopressin might act on consolidation and retrieval, or a process common to both. We hypothesize that this process is the "rate of information processing". Both neurochemical and pharmacological experiments on the mode of action of vasopressin (e.g. Tanaka et al., 1977; Versteeg et al., 1979), and neuropsychological evidence on the relevant brain structures underlying the rate of information processing (Luria, 1980), strengthen this suggestion. They emphasize the importance of brain structures, at the level of the lower brainstem, and ascending fibres to limbic-subcortical and fronto-cortical areas such as the dorsal noradrenergic bundle (Kovács et al., 1982). The finding that vasopressinergic nerve fibres project from hypothalamic nuclei to distant sites all over the brain, and especially to structures which are known to be crucial for memory (Buijs, 1978; Sofroniew and Weindl, 1981) also supports this view.

We feel that future studies should focus on the assembly of treatment groups based on homogeneity with respect to the neuropsychological profile and not (only) with respect to etiology. Better research methods should be used, preferably based on laboratory findings, and with a particular focus on the rate of working, thinking, information processing. Finally, those patients should be treated which have relatively mild (and not complex) deficits.

A CRITICAL EVALUATION OF VASOPRESSIN STUDIES: DIVERSE METHODOLOGICAL PROBLEMS

The vasopressin studies reviewed above differ in many respects, including the type of vasopressin used (AVP, LVP, DDAVP, DGAVP), the dose, route, frequency and duration of administration, and the type of experimental design used (open, blind, etc.) (Tables II–V). Some of these parameters are very important and the results of the different studies must be interpreted accordingly.

(1) The nature of the vasopressin-congener used

LVP has been the most "popular" type of vasopressin used (127 patients treated in 14 studies), followed by the more recently developed DDAVP (89 patients treated in 9 studies) and DGAVP (41 patients in 4 studies). AVP was used in 22 patients (3 studies) and Pitressin in one study. Both LVP and DDAVP have peripheral "side-effects" (antidiuretic/cardiovascular, and antidiuretic, respectively). Several authors have noted these changes in patients in which the anti-amnesic action of the peptides was used, after both intranasal and i.m. application of LVP (Forisz, 1952a, b; Timsit-Berthier et al., 1980; Láczi et al., 1982) and DDAVP (Tinklenberg et al., 1981a). A crucial point concerns the perception by the patient of changes taking place in his body. How do we exclude the possibility that the reported effects are secondary to a peripheral effect? This applies to studies in diabetes insipidus patients in particular (Gilot et al., 1979; Láczi et al., 1982, 1983), as cognitive functioning in such a patient may change as a result of normalized water retention. Furthermore, "double-blind" may not mean very much when the patient is able to discern placebo treatment from active treatment by his perception of bodily symptoms. Therefore, DGAVP, which has virtually no peripheral side-effects, is the agent of choice in studies on behavioural actions of vasopressin-like peptides.

(2) The route of administration

Intranasal application of the peptide is the most frequently used route, although some investigators have also used i.m. administration. The premise is that the peptide reaches its site of action in the CNS more efficiently via the intranasal route, but unfortunately there is no evidence that this is indeed the case. On the contrary, Ang and Jenkins (1982) have shown recently that there is a blood–brain barrier for AVP, DDAVP and DGAVP, and that intranasal administration provides no increased access to the CNS. This indicates that at present we are seriously restricted in the therapeutic use of vasopressin in humans. Animal work suggests that the amount of vasopressin needed to elicit behavioural effects is 20–40 times greater after intracerebro-ventricular administration than after application in specific brain nuclei, and another 100–1000 times more peptide is needed after peripheral administration (De Wied, 1976). Note the problem in clinical trials with vasopressin, which are very seriously handicapped as a large amount of vasopressin has to be administered peripherally to reach the CNS but the administration of large amounts of LVP or DDAVP is contraindicated due to peripheral side-effects.

(3) Duration of administration

Some reports suggest that a single administration of LVP, AVP or DDAVP can induce a measurable antiamnesic effect (Medvedev et al., 1981; Láczi et al., 1982; Anderson et al.,

1979; Delwaide et al., 1980), and that these effects are still present after 48 h (Delwaide et al., 1980). There is thus a parallel with the animal experiments in which acute effects of the peptide have been reported (De Wied, 1976). On the other hand, it is our impression that patients treated with DGAVP (intranasally) report a subjective improvement 4–5 days after the start of treatment (Verhoeven, Verdonck and Van Ree, unpublished). Others have similarly reported that effects of vasopressin develop in time (e.g. Timsit-Berthier et al., 1980) and can be manifested after the end of the period of active peptide treatment. This was one of the important findings in the animal research, in that the behavioural effects of LVP or DGAVP can be monitored for many days after administration. These findings imply several things: a serious question can be raised with respect to the use of cross-over studies without a washout period, as peptide effects may still be present in the post-vasopressin-placebo period. Secondly a treatment evaluation must be performed some time after treatment termination, to assess the effects of longer duration. Thirdly, brief treatment periods (e.g. less than a week) may be too short for a relevant effect to develop. It is likely that the effects which were seen after a single administration were dependent on the moment of assessment, as has been found in animal experiments (De Wied, 1971).

SUMMARY

Clinical trials with vasopressin-like peptides are difficult to evaluate, as there are many sources of difference and error. Nevertheless, it seems that these peptides do have behavioural effects in humans. This conclusion is based upon the fact that most studies find something, be it a clinical impression of improvement, or objective test results. Many studies in which the peptide was ineffective were performed on patients with a complex pattern of neuropsychological deficits or other symptoms of a profound brain degeneration. This should not be surprising, because degeneration of the relevant brain structures may well destroy the sites of action of the peptide.

The amount of active principle that can be used in humans is limited, due to peripheral side-effects, while high doses are necessary to enable sufficient vasopressin to pass the blood–brain barrier and reach the CNS. Vasopressin-congeners which are resistant to metabolic degradation would therefore be of value; in this respect, DDAVP may not be the peptide of choice because in animal studies it is much less active than AVP or DGAVP (Walter et al., 1978). The data obtained to date, coupled with knowledge on the neuropsychology of memory, make it clear that future studies on vasopressin should make use of patient groups which are more defined neuropsychologically, to assess specific influences on types or aspects of memory. We suggest that the rate of information-processing, or a process underlying both consolidation and retrieval may be the most relevant factor to study. Better, and more specific methods of treatment evaluation (including parallel test versions) should therefore be used. Another important methodological point concerns the nature of the active principle to be used; DGAVP is favoured above DDAVP, and especially LVP, because it lacks the peripheral endocrine effects which occur with AVP/LVP and partly with DDAVP. Finally, it may be necessary to treat for relatively prolonged periods of time (weeks) to enable a relevant treatment effect to develop.

Conclusions that can be drawn from the clinical studies performed to date are in line, generally, with those based upon animal experiments. Future patient studies may yield more relevant information when they make more use of the extensive knowledge collected for the last decade in animal experiments.

REFERENCES

Anderson, L.T., David, R., Bonnet, R. and Dancis, J. (1979) Passive avoidance learning in Lesch–Nyhan disease: effect of 1-desamino-8-arginine-vasopressin. *Life Sci.*, 24: 905–910.

Ang, V.T.Y. and Jenkins, J.S. (1982) Blood CSF barrier to arginine-vasopressin, desmopressin and desglycinamide arginine-vasopressin in the dog. *J. Endocr.*, 93: 319–325.

Blake, D.R., Dodd, M.J. and Grimley Evans, J. (1978) Vasopressin in amnesia. *Lancet*, I: 608.

Bohus, B., Kovács, G. and De Wied, D. (1978) Oxytocin, vasopressin and memory: opposite effects on consolidation and retrieval processes. *Brain Res.*, 157: 414–417.

Buijs, R.M. (1978) Intra- and extrahypothalamic vasopressin and oxytocin pathways in the rat: pathways to the limbic system, medulla oblongata and spinal cord. *Cell Tiss. Res.*, 192: 423–435.

Calandra, C., Drago, F. and Filetti, S. (1980) Su un caso con turbe mnestiche trattato con vasopressina. *Min. Psychiat.*, 21: 63–66.

Delwaide, P.J., Devoitille, J.M. and Ylieff, M. (1980) Acute effects of drugs upon memory of patients with senile dementia. *Acta psychiat. belg.*, 80: 748–754.

De Wied, D. (1969) Effects of peptide hormones on behavior. In W.F. Ganong and L. Martini (Eds.), *Frontiers in Neuroendocrinology*, Oxford Univ. Press, London, pp. 97–140.

De Wied, D. (1971) Longterm effect of vasopressin on the maintenance of a conditioned avoidance response in rats. *Nature (Lond.)*, 232: 58–60.

De Wied, D. (1976) Behavioral effects of intraventricularly administered vasopressin and vasopressin fragments. *Life Sci.*, 19: 685–690.

Dimond, S. (1980) *Neuropsychology*, Butterworths, London.

Drago, F., Rapisarda, V., Calandra, A., Filetti, S. and Scapagnini, U. (1981) A clinical evaluation of vasopressin effects on memory disorders. *Acta ther.*, 7: 345–352.

Durso, R., Fedio, P., Brouwers, P., Cox, C., Martin, A.J., Ruggieri, S.A., Tamminga, C.A. and Chase, T.N. (1982) Lysine vasopressin in Alzheimer's disease. *Neurology*, 32: 674–677.

Eisenberg, J., Greenberg, E., Greenberg, L.M., Mandel, B. and Belmaker, R.H. (1982) ADH derivatives in childhood attention and learning disorders: preliminary results of a controlled study. Submitted for publication.

Ferris, S.H., Reisberg, B. and Gershon, S. (1981) Neuropeptide modulation of cognition and memory in humans. In L. Poon (Ed.), *Aging in the 1980's: Selected Contemporary Issues in the Psychology of Aging*, Amer. Psychol. Ass., Washington, DC, pp. 212-220.

Fewtrell, W.D., House, A.O., Jamie, P.F., Oates, M.R. and Cooper, J.E. (1982) Effects of vasopressin on memory and new learning in a brain-injured population. *Psychol. Med.*, 12: 423–425.

Forisz, L. (1952a) Treatment of mental patients with antidiuretic hormone of the posterior pituitary. *Dis. Nerv. Syst.*, 13: 42–44.

Forisz, L. (1952b) The use of Pitressin in the treatment of schizophrenia with deterioration. *N. Carolina Med. J.*, 13: 76–80.

Gilot, P., Crabbe, J. and Legros, J.J. (1980) Bilan mnésique de cinq subjects présentent un diabète central idiopathique familial. *Acta psychiat. belg.*, 80: 755–761.

Gold, P.W., Ballenger, J.C., Weingartner, H., Goodwin, F.K. and Post, R.M. (1979) Effects of l-desamino-8-D-arginine vasopressin on behavior and cognition in primary affective disorders. *Lancet*, I: 992–994.

Jenkins, J.S., Mather, H.M., Coughlan, A.K. and Jenkins, D.G. (1979) Desmopressin in posttraumatic amnesia. *Lancet*, 1245–1246.

Jenkins, J.S., Mather, H.M., Coughlan, A.K. and Jenkins, D.G. (1981) Desmopressin and desglycinamide vasopressin in posttraumatic amnesia. *Lancet*, I: 39.

Jolles, J., Gaillard, A.W.K. and Hijman, R. (1983) Memory disorders and vasopressin. In E. Endröczi, D. De Wied, L. Angelucci and U. Scapagnini (Eds.), *Integrative Neurohumoral Mechanisms*, Elsevier Biomedical, Amsterdam, pp. 63–73.

Koch-Henriksen, N. and Nielsen, H. (1981) Vasopressin in post-traumatic amnesia. *Lancet*, I: 38–39.

Koizumi, H.M., Rowe, H. and Clark, R. (1981) Vasopressin (antidiuretic hormone) for postencephalitic memory loss: a pilot study. *J. clin. Psychiat.*, 42: 217.

Korsgaard, S., Casey, D.E., Damgaard Pedersen, N.E., Jørgensen, A. and Gerlach, J. (1981) Vasopressin in anergic schizophrenia. *Psychopharmacology*, 74: 379–382.

Kovács, G.L., Bohus, B., Versteeg, D.H.G., Telegdy, G. and De Wied, D. (1982) Neurohypophyseal hormones and memory. In H. Yoshida, Y. Hagihara and S. Ebashi (Eds.), *Advances in Pharmacology and Therapeutics II. Vol. 1, CNS Pharmacology, Neuropeptides*, Pergamon Press, Oxford, pp. 175–187.

Láczi, F., Valkusz, Zs., Laszlo, F.A., Wagner, A., Jardanhazy, T., Szasz, A., Szilard, J. and Telegdy, G. (1982)

Effects of lysine-vasopressin and l-desamino-8-D-arginine-vasopressin on the memory in healthy individuals and diabetes insipidus patients. *Psychoneuroendocrinology*, 7: 185–193.

Láczi, F., Van Ree, J.M., Wagner, A., Valkusz, Zs., Jardanhazy, T., Kovács, G.L., Telegdy, G., Szilard, J., Laszlo, F.A. and De Wied, D. (1983) Effects of desglycinamide-arginine-vasopressin (DGAVP) on memory processes in diabetes insipidus patients and in non-diabetic subjects. *Acta endocr.*, 102: 205–212.

Le Bœuf, A., Lodge, J. and Eames, P.G. (1978) Vasopressin and memory in Korsakoff syndrome. *Lancet*, II: 1370.

Legros, J.J. and Gilot, P. (1979) Vasopressin and memory in the human. In A.M. Gotto, Jr., E.J. Peck, Jr. and A.E. Boyd, III (Eds.), *Brain Peptides, a New Endocrinology*, Elsevier/North-Holland, Amsterdam, pp. 347–363.

Legros, J.J., Gilot, P., Seron, X., Claessens, J., Adam, A., Moeglen, J.M., Audibert, A. and Berchier, P. (1978) Influence of vasopressin on learning and memory. *Lancet*, I: 41–42.

Luria, A.R. (1976) *The Neuropsychology of Memory*, Winston, Washington, DC.

Luria, A.R. (1980) *Higher Cortical Functions in Man*, 2nd edn., Basic Books, New York.

Medvedev, V.I., Bakharev, V.D., Grechko, A.T. and Nezovibat'ko, V.N. (1981) Effect of vasopressin and adrenocorticotrophic hormone fragment $ACTH_{4-7}$ on human memory. *Hum. Physiol.*, 6: 307–310.

Newcombe, F. (1980) Memory: a neuropsychological approach. *Trends Neurosci.*, 3: 179–182.

O'Keefe, J. and Nadel, L. (1978) *The Hippocampus as a Cognitive Map*, Clarendon Press, Oxford.

Oliveros, J.C., Jandali, M.K., Timsit-Berthier, M., Remy, R., Beghezal, A., Audibert, A. and Moeglen, J.M. (1978) Vasopressin in amnesia. *Lancet*, I: 42.

Rigter, H. and Crabbe, J.C. (1979) Modulation of memory by pituitary hormones and related peptides. *Vitamins Hormones*, 37: 153–241.

Russell, E.W. (1981) The pathology and clinical examination of memory. In S.B. Filskov and T.J. Boll (Eds.), *Handbook of Clinical Neuropsychology*, Wiley, New York, pp. 287–319.

Sofroniew, M.W. and Weindl, A. (1981) Central nervous system distribution of vasopressin, oxytocin and neurophysin. In J.L. Martinez, Jr., R.A. Jensen, R.B. Messing, H. Rigter and J.L. McGaugh (Eds.), *Endogenous Peptides in Learning and Memory Processes*, Academic Press, New York, pp. 327–369.

Tanaka, M., De Kloet, E.R., De Wied, D. and Versteeg, D.H.G. (1977) Arginine-8-vasopressin affects catecholamine metabolism in specific brain nuclei. *Life Sci.*, 20: 1799–1808.

Timsit-Berthier, M., Mantanus, H., Jacques, M.C. and Legros, J.J. (1980) Utilité de la lysine-vasopressine dans le traitement de l'amnesie post-traumatique. *Acta psychiat. belg.*, 80: 728–747.

Tinklenberg, J.R., Pfefferbaum, A. and Berger, P.A. (1981a) 1-Desamino-D-arginine-vasopressin in cognitively impaired patients. *Psychopharmacol. Bull.*, 17: 206–207.

Tinklenberg, J.R., Peabody, C.A. and Berger, P.A. (1981b) Vasopressin effects on cognition and affect in the elderly. In J. Ordy, J.R. Sladek and B. Reisberg (Eds.), *Neuropeptide and Hormone Regulation of Brain Function and Homeostasis*, Raven, New York.

Tinklenberg, J.R., Pigache, R., Pfefferbaum, A. and Berger, P.A. (1982) Vasopressin peptides and dementia. In S. Corkin, K.I. Davis, J.H. Growdon, E. Usdin and R.J. Wurtman (Eds.), *Alzheimer's Disease, A Report of Progress in Research*, Raven Press, New York, pp. 463–469.

Van Ree, J.M., Bohus, B., Versteeg, D.G.H. and De Wied, D. (1978) Neurohypophyseal principles and memory processes. *Biochem. Pharmacol.*, 27: 1793–1800.

Van Wimersma Greidanus, Tj.B., Bohus, B. and De Wied, D. (1976) CNS sites of action of ACTH, MSH and vasopressin in relation to avoidance behavior. In W.E. Strumpf and L.D. Grant (Eds.), *Anatomical Neuroendocrinology*, Karger, Basel, pp. 284–289.

Versteeg, D.H.G., De Kloet, E.R., Van Wimersma Greidanus, Tj.B. and De Wied, D. (1979) Vasopressin modulates the activity of catecholamine containing neurones in specific brain regions. *Neurosci. Lett.*, 11: 69–73.

Vranckx, C.H., Minne, Ph., Benghezal, A., Moeglen, J.M. and Audibert, A. (1979) Vasopressin and schizophrenia. In J. Obiols, C. Ballus, E. Gonzales, E. Mondus and J. Pujol (Eds.), *Biological Psychiatry Today*, Elsevier/North-Holland, Amsterdam, pp. 735–758.

Waggoner, R.W., Jr., Slonim, A.E. and Armstrong, S.H. (1978) Improved psychological status of children under DDAVP therapy for central diabetes insipidus. *Amer. J. Psychiat.*, 135: 361–362.

Walter, R., Van Ree, J.M. and De Wied, D. (1978) Modification of conditioned behavior of rats by neurohypophyseal hormones and analogues. *Proc. nat. Acad. Sci. U.S.A.*, 75: 2493–2496.

Weingartner, H., Gold, P., Ballenger, J.C., Smallberg, S.A., Summers, R., Rubinow, D.R., Post, R.M. and Goodwin, F.K. (1981a) Effects of vasopressin on human memory functions. *Science*, 211: 601–603.

Weingartner, H., Kaye, W., Gold, P., Smallberg, S., Peterson, R., Gillin, J.C. and Ebert, M. (1981b) Vasopressin treatment of cognitive dysfunction in progressive dementia. *Life Sci.*, 29: 2721–2726.

The Neurohypophysis: Structure, Function and Control, Progress in Brain Research, Vol. 60, edited by B.A. Cross and G. Leng

A Comparison of the Learning Abilities of Brattleboro Rats with Hereditary Diabetes Insipidus and Long–Evans Rats Using Positively Reinforced Operant Conditioning

J.F. LAYCOCK, I.B. GARTSIDE and J.T. CHAPMAN

Department of Physiology, Charing Cross Hospital Medical School, London W6 8RF (U.K.)

INTRODUCTION

In 1966 De Wied and Bohus showed that the administration of Pitressin to normal rats improved their acquisition of a conditioned avoidance response. Since then, the active principle of Pitressin which is implicated in memory processes has been shown to be the antidiuretic hormone vasopressin (De Wied, 1971). One particularly useful experimental model for studies into the actions of vasopressin is the Brattleboro rat with hereditary diabetes insipidus (DI) which cannot synthesize vasopressin. Experiments comparing these animals with other rats which do not manifest the disease indicate that DI rats are inferior in acquiring conditioned avoidance behaviour (Bohus et al., 1975). However, this conclusion remains controversial since some investigators have been unable to confirm this behavioural defect in the DI rat (Celestian et al., 1975; Bailey and Weiss, 1979). In addition, most studies have been confined to trials involving active and/or passive avoidance tasks. The few positive reinforcement trials carried out so far have been difficult to interpret and inconclusive. For example one recent study included four different food-rewarded tasks, and in two of these the DI rats performed as well as control rats of the parent Long–Evans (LE) strain (Brito et al., 1981). These authors concluded that vasopressin cannot be involved to the same degree in all aspects of learning.

Learning is dependent on a number of factors which include motivation for the behaviour to be conditioned, as well as the neural mechanisms involved in the consolidation of memory. Therefore vasopressin need not be involved in the memory consolidation process to influence learning behaviour but instead could alter the motivation to learn. For example if LE rats are more fearful than DI rats, then the LE rats should be more strongly motivated to avoid footshock and will thus learn such a conditioned avoidance (negatively reinforced) task more readily. If vasopressin is involved in some aspect of fear-based motivation to learn rather than in memory consolidation, then there should be no difference in the learning abilities of LE and DI rats on a positively reinforced task. To test this hypothesis we have investigated the acquisition of a food-rewarded operant task and the learning of a discrimination procedure using the same operant task.

METHODS

Nine adult male LE rats and nine adult male DI rats matched for age were used in this study. The LE rats weighed between 208 and 277 g at the start of the study while the DI rats weighed between 184 and 247 g.

The experiments were performed using a Skinner box, $190 \times 240 \times 170$ mm deep, placed in a sound attenuating cabinet. To obtain a food reward (ca. 40 mg pellets of rat food, Campden Instruments), the rats had to push open the transparent door (hinged at the top) of the food dispenser. This was placed 30 mm above the floor in one of the 190 mm walls of the box. Water was available ad libitum from a spout on the wall at the opposite end of the box to the food dispenser.

Rats were deprived of food 24 h before the start of training and food, additional to that earned in the Skinner box, was given when necessary to maintain their body weight at 80 % of the initial weight. Daily water intake was recorded. On the first day of training rats were placed in the Skinner box, the door held open and four pellets of food placed in the food dispenser. Once the rats had eaten this food, the door was closed and food then supplied on a continuous reinforcement (CRF) schedule. After 20–30 presses on the CRF schedule, the animals were placed on a fixed ratio (FR) schedule where every second press was rewarded (FR2). The ratio was incremented in steps of 2 after 10–20 reinforcements until FR10 was reached. The rats spent 30 min per day in the box and once FR10 had been reached, were given an extra 30 min session at FR10, after which discrimination training began in the following session. The times taken to reach FR2 and FR10 were read from the cumulative recorder trace, along with the rate of responding at FR10 on the last day of initial training.

The discrimination learning consisted of seven daily sessions. Each session consisted of ten periods, each comprising 2 min of rewarded responding, signalled by a dim light in the food dispenser and no sound, followed by a 2 min period of unrewarded responding, signalled by no light and a 400 Hz tone at 72 dB. The number of presses under each condition (i.e. rewarded and unrewarded responding) was counted automatically. The ratio of unrewarded (Time out, T_o) to rewarded responding (Time in, T_i) was computed for each day. Mann–Whitney U tests were performed for all statistical comparisons unless stated otherwise.

RESULTS

The most striking difference between the two strains of rats was seen in the initial acquisition of operant behaviour. All the DI rats were responding by the end of the first session and 3 rats had reached FR10 on the first day. In contrast, only three LE rats responded in the first session and three rats took three or more sessions before responding. The DI rats when first placed in the Skinner box would rapidly find the food dispenser and free food and start to eat and then to respond on CRF. The LE rats, however, tended to freeze and exploration of the box developed only slowly. This is shown by the significant differences in the times taken to reach FR2 and FR10, and the total training time (see Table I). The body weights of LE and DI rats decreased at a similar rate during the study. Table I also gives a measure of "fear" (Broadhurst, 1958) in terms of the number of rats defaecating in the Skinner box on the first day of training. The significantly higher number of LE rats defaecating (χ^2 test, $P < 0.01$) agrees well with their freezing behaviour and suggests a greater fear of being placed in a novel environment than that shown by the DI rats.

TABLE I

MEANS AND RANGES FOR TOTAL TRAINING TIMES, LATENCIES TO FR2 AND FR10, PRESSING RATE
ON THE LAST DAY OF FR10 AND THE NUMBERS OF RATS DEFAECATING ON THE FIRST DAY IN THE
SKINNER BOX, FOR DI AND LE RATS

P = probability level for comparisons between the two groups.

		Brattleboro DI	Long–Evans	P
Total training time	mean	113	271	< 0.002
(min)	range	74–168	136–587	
Latency to FR2	mean	9	96	< 0.002
(min)	range	2–20	17–216	
Latency to FR10	mean	53	195	< 0.002
(min)	range	19–83	79–546	
Pressing rate on last day of FR10	mean	24	18	n.s.
(presses/min)	range	13–35	12–27	
Number of rats defaecating on day 1 in box		1	7	< 0.01

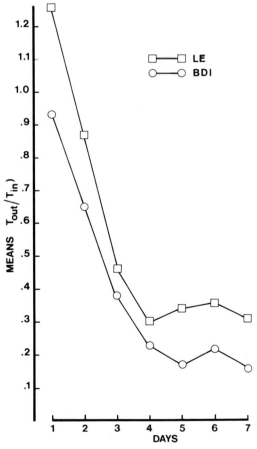

Fig. 1. The mean T_{out}/T_{in} ratios on the seven days of the discrimination task for DI rats (○) and LE rats (□).
Differences between the ratios of the two groups of rats were significant on days 1, 6 and 7 (see text).

Both groups of rats showed a similar learning curve on the discrimination task, although the curve for the LE rats was slightly above that for the DI rats (Fig. 1). Mann–Whitney U tests were performed on the ratio of presses during non-reward periods (T_o) and presses during reward periods (T_i) and significant differences were found on day (U = 15, P < 0.05), day 6 (U = 17, P < 0.05) and day 7 (U = 11, P < 0.02). The total numbers of presses on the first day of discrimination learning, during T_i were significantly higher in DI rats (U = 7, P < 0.002), than in LE rats. This was probably due to the fact that the T_o sound stimulus startled some of the LE rats and suppressed responding during both time in and time out periods for up to five periods.

DISCUSSION

Our results indicate that LE rats appear to learn a simple positively-reinforced task less well than DI rats during the initial training period. This difference in initial learning ability occurs despite both groups of animals being similarly motivated by hunger, as indicated by similar decreases in body weight.

In many earlier experiments involving conditioned avoidance responses to electrical shock stimuli, the motivation to avoid the shock due to fear may have differed between the groups of animals. This would then have influenced subsequent behaviour. When the rats in our study were each placed in the modified Skinner box for the first time the LE rats appeared more "fearful" than the DI rats, according to various criteria. Thus the "fear" of the novel situation conflicted with the hunger motivation and inhibited subsequent learning behaviour in the LE rats. On the other hand, in avoidance behaviour studies the more "fearful" LE rats would perhaps escape the shock stimulus faster than the less "fearful" DI rats because of the different degrees of motivation in the two groups of animals. This would account for the poor response of DI rats faced with avoidance tasks compared with normal rats, as observed by De Wied and his colleagues (Bohus et al., 1975).

In the present investigation, once both groups of rats were equally motivated and had been trained to work for reward at the same rate, the DI rats learnt the discrimination task at least as well as the LE rats. Therefore it is difficult to involve vasopressin in the actual process of memory consolidation. Instead, differences in response between DI and LE rats could be due to differences in motivation, particularly in negative reinforcement trials. Experiments involving the administration of vasopressin to hypophysectomized Wistar rats (Bohus et al., 1973) or DI rats (De Wied et al., 1975) and the intracerebroventricular administration of vasopressin antiserum to normal rats (Van Wimersma Greidanus et al., 1975) nevertheless implicate this hormone in the behavioural responses to avoidance-related tasks, but here also the involvement could be in the expression of fear motivated behaviour.

Adrenal weight in male rats may be positively correlated with measures of "emotionality" (Yaekel and Rhoades, 1941). As DI rats have smaller adrenals than other rats (Bohus et al., 1975) they might be expected to demonstrate a lesser degree of "emotionality" (e.g. fear). However there is some confusion about the relationship between adrenal weight and different measures of emotionality (for review, see Ader, 1969).

Other research groups have used positive reinforcement procedures to study the effect of vasopressin on learning. Garrud et al. (1974), using a food reward task, found no difference in the acquisition of food-rewarded behaviour in normal rats whether treated with vasopressin or not. However differences may not have been observed because the resting level of vasopressin in the untreated rats was already maximal for behavioural effects of the peptide. Hostetter et al.

(1977) also found no difference between normal untreated and vasopressin-treated rats in the acquisition of a food-rewarded black arm/white arm T-maze discrimination task. An interesting finding was that the vasopressin-treated rats trained to enter the black arm of the maze showed a significantly prolonged extinction of the learnt procedure compared with saline-treated rats trained to the black colour, or rats trained to the white colour and treated with either vasopressin or saline. This is consistent with an involvement of vasopressin in the expression of fear-motivated behaviour since the natural preference for the black (darker) arm of the maze would be strengthened.

In conclusion, our results suggest that vasopressin is not necessary for memory consolidation in general. The differences which have been observed between positive and negative reinforcement learning indicate either that the peptide is only necessary for memory consolidation in avoidance conditioning and not in food-rewarded conditioning, or that vasopressin influences certain learning and memory processes by altering the expression of fear motivation. One possible complication in the interpretation of behavioural, and other, studies using DI rats is that strain differences may have emerged between colonies of these animals in different laboratories. As different strains are well known to have different behavioural characteristics this possibility warrants further investigation.

REFERENCES

Ader, R. (1969) Adrenocortical function and the measurement of "emotionality". Ann. N.Y. Acad. Sci., 159: 791–805.
Bailey, W.H. and Weiss, J.M. (1979) Evaluation of a "memory deficit" in vasopressin-deficient rats. Brain Res., 162: 174–178.
Bohus, B., Gispen, W.H. and De Wied, D. (1973) Effect of lysine vasopressin and $ACTH_{4-10}$ on conditioned avoidance behavior of hypophysectomized rats. Neuroendocrinology, 11: 137–143.
Bohus, B., Van Wimersma Greidanus, Tj.B. and De Wied, D. (1975) Behavioral and endocrine responses of rats with hereditary hypothalamic diabetes insipidus (Brattleboro strain). Physiol. Behav., 14: 609–615.
Brito, G.N.O., Thomas, G.J., Gingold, S.I. and Gash, D.M. (1981) Behavioral characteristics of vasopressin-deficient rats (Brattleboro strain). Brain Res. Bull., 6: 71–75.
Broadhurst, P.L. (1958) Determinants of emotionality in the rat: III. Strain differences. J. comp. physiol. Psychol., 51: 55–59.
Celestian, J.F., Carey, R.J. and Miller, M. (1975) Unimpaired maintenance of a conditioned avoidance response in the rat with diabetes insipidus. Physiol. Behav., 15: 707–711.
De Wied, D. (1971) Long term effect of vasopressin on the maintenance of a conditioned avoidance response in rats. Nature (Lond.), 232: 58–60.
De Wied, D. and Bohus, B. (1966) Long term and short term effects on retention of a conditioned avoidance response in rats by treatment with long acting Pitressin and α-MSH. Nature (Lond.), 212: 1484–1486.
Garrud, P., Gray, J.A. and De Wied, D. (1974) Pituitary–adrenal hormones and extinction of rewarded behavior in the rat. Physiol. Behav., 12: 109–119.
Hostetter, G., Jubb, S.L. and Kozlowski, G.P. (1977) Vasopressin affects the behaviour of rats in a positively-rewarded discrimination task. Life Sci., 21: 1323–1328.
Van Wimersma Greidanus, Tj.B., Dogterom, J. and De Wied, D. (1975) Intraventricular administration of anti-vasopressin serum inhibits memory consolidation in rats. Life Sci., 16: 637–644.
Yaekel, E.H. and Rhoades, R.P. (1941) A comparison of the body and endocrine gland (adrenal, thyroid and pituitary) weights of emotional and nonemotional rats. Endocrinology, 28: 337–340.

The Neurohypophysis: Structure, Function and Control, Progress in Brain Research, Vol. 60, edited by B.A. Cross and G. Leng
© *1983 Elsevier·Science Publishers B.V.*

Transplanted Vasopressin Neurones and Central Nervous System Effects of Vasopressin

D.M. GASH, G.J. BOER&, M.F.D. NOTTER and J.R. SLADEK, Jr.

Department of Anatomy, Box 603, School of Medicine and Dentistry, University of Rochester, Rochester, NY 14642 (U.S.A.) and ¹Netherlands Institute for Brain Research, Amsterdam (The Netherlands)

INTRODUCTION

One of the major advances in neurobiology over the past decade has been the increasing realization that neural peptides are significantly involved in central nervous system (CNS) function. The pioneering studies of De Wied and his associates on vasopressin and behaviour (reviewed elsewhere in this volume) have, in no small measure, contributed to the current interest in brain–neuropeptide interactions. There are at least three potential anatomical routes by which vasopressin could influence the CNS; plasma-borne vasopressin in the brain vasculature, vasopressin in the cerebrospinal fluid (Reppert et al., 1981; Perlow et al., 1982), and the extensive vasopressin-containing projections to extra-hypothalamic regions of the brain (Armstrong et al., 1980; Buijs, 1978; Swanson and Sawchenko, 1983).

A variety of approaches have been employed to investigate the role of vasopressin in the CNS (for a review, see Rigter and Crabbe, 1979). Test animals have included hypophysectomized rats (De Wied, 1969), Brattleboro rats with a congenital absence of vasopressin (Bailey and Weiss, 1981), and normal rats of various strains (Le Moal et al., 1981). Early studies analyzed behaviour following systemic injections of vasopressin or vasopressin analogues (De Wied et al., 1975). More recent investigations have entailed microinjections of vasopressin and vasopressin analogues into the ventricular spaces and parenchyma of the brain (De Wied, 1976; Kovács et al., 1979; Le Moal et al., 1981). Vasopressin antisera have been injected into the same sites (Van Wimersma Greidanus et al., 1975; Kovács et al., 1982) on the assumption that the antisera would bind to endogenous vasopressin and significantly lower the titres available for functional activity. Studies using these techniques have yielded important information, but many questions remain about the extent and exact nature of vasopressin's involvement(s) in CNS function. Depending on the route of delivery (plasma, extracellular space or by synaptic contact), it is possible to envisage quite different actions for vasopressin. Indeed, it may be that vasopressin has multiple roles in the CNS with its specific effects depending not only on the route of administration, but also on the population of cells affected. In the present paper, we review our studies on transplants of foetal vasopressin neurones and discuss why such grafts, because of their ability to integrate with and functionally interact with the host nervous system, may prove useful in elucidating the roles and mechanisms of action of vasopressin in the brain.

NEURAL TRANSPLANTS

Experimental evidence, accumulated over the past six decades from a number of laboratories (Dunn, 1917; Das, 1971; Stenevi et al., 1976), has demonstrated that foetal and neonatal neurones can survive transplantation into a host brain. At least seven types of chemically identified neurones have been successfully transplanted (see Table I), including vasopressin neurones (Gash and Sladek, 1980). Within the host, grafted neural tissue often develops relatively normal cytoarchitectural features indicative of their site of origin in the donor brain (Das, 1974; Gash et al., 1980b; Jaeger and Lund, 1980). Tissue rejection has not been a problem in neural transplantation (Gash et al., 1980a; Freed et al., 1980; Stenevi et al., 1980). Stenevi et al. (1980), for example, have shown that foetal hypothalamic tissue, transplanted onto the choroidal pia overlying the superior colliculus in young adult female rats, can survive for periods up to at least 19 months, the longest time interval examined. The reasons for the apparent lack of graft rejection may relate to the foetal nature of the transplants as well as the status of the brain as an immunologically privileged site (Scheinberg et al., 1964; Barker and Billingham, 1977).

TABLE I

SUCCESSFUL GRAFTS OF CHEMICALLY IDENTIFIED NEURONES

Neuronal type	Reference
Cholinergic	Björklund and Stenevi, 1977 Lewis et al., 1979
Dopamine	Stenevi et al., 1976 Seiger and Olson, 1977 Perlow et al., 1979
Luteinizing hormone-releasing hormone	Stenevi et al., 1980 Krieger et al., 1982
Noradrenaline	Stenevi et al., 1976 Seiger and Olson, 1977
Serotonin	Seiger and Olson, 1977 Azmitia et al., 1981
Somatostatin	Stenevi et al., 1980
Vasopressin	Gash et al., 1980a, b Stenevi et al., 1980

Neural grafts exhibit a propensity toward establishing some afferent and/or efferent connections with the host brain (Lund and Harvey, 1981; Jaeger and Lund, 1980; Björklund and Stenevi, 1977). Thus, an anatomical pathway exists for transplanted neurones to interact with the host nervous sytem. Increasing evidence suggests that grafted neurones utilize these neural connections and are capable of providing appropriate and meaningful information to the host. Four different model systems have been described in which transplants of the appropriate neurones have ameliorated disease symptoms or altered behaviour in rodents with well-characterized behavioural patterns (see Table II).

TABLE II

MODEL SYSTEMS OF FUNCTIONAL GRAFT DEVELOPMENT

	Neural deficiency	Symptoms/Behaviour	Graft effectiveness	Reference
1. Nigrostriatal dopamine pathway	Dopamine neurones	Motor asymmetry	+	Perlow et al., 1979
		Choice behaviour	+	Freed et al., 1980
		Akinesia	+/−	
		Aphagia	+/−	Dunnett et al., 1981a–c
		Adipsia	−	
2. Hypothalamic neurosecretory system	Vasopressin neurones	Diabetes insipidus	+	
		Adaptability	not tested	Gash et al., 1980a, b
		Hyperresponsiveness	not tested	
		Memory consolidation	not tested	
3. Periventricular hypothalamus	Luteinizing hormone-releasing factor neurones	Hypotrophied gonads	+	Krieger et al., 1982
4. Medial preoptic area	Sexually dimorphic nucleus	Sexual behaviour	+	Arendash and Gorski, 1981

STRUCTURAL AND FUNCTIONAL CORRELATES OF TRANSPLANTED VASOPRESSIN NEURONES

We have developed a model system for analyzing both the development and function of neural transplants by using the Brattleboro rat with congenital diabetes insipidus (DI rat) as a graft recipient of normal vasopressin neurones (Gash et al., 1980a, b; Gash and Scott, 1980). In the homozygous condition, DI rats lack the capacity to synthesize vasopressin and vasopressin-associated neurophysin (Sokol et al., 1976; Vandesande and Dierickx, 1976). Thus transplanted vasopressin neurones can be identified by immunocytochemical staining for either vasopressin or vasopressin-specific neurophysin. Functional development of the transplant is evaluated as a correlate of increased antidiuretic activity as evidenced by decreased host water consumption and increased urine osmolality.

The structural development of normal 17- and 19-day foetal hypothalamic transplants into DI hosts has been evaluated by a variety of light and electron microscopic techniques. In host animals ranging from 5 days postnatal to 6 months old at the time of transplantation, foetal hypothalamic grafts can develop cytoarchitectural features of normal hypothalamic tissue and become structurally integrated into the host hypothalamus (Gash and Sladek, 1980; Gash et al., 1980b; Boer and Gash, unpublished data). Transplanted magnocellular neurones, which are positive for vasopressin and neurophysin by immunocytochemistry, send processes coursing through the graft–host interface into the host's median eminence. Catecholamine-containing fibres from the host similarly cross the graft–host interface into the transplants.

Transplants have also been conducted into 12- and 25-month old hosts (Gash and Sladek, unpublished data). Although the sample size of test animals in our initial study was small, the transplants in the aged rats exhibited a number of features common to neural grafts in younger animals. A significant number of foetal neurones, including a combination of approximately 690 vasopressin- and oxytocin-containing magnocellular neurones in one graft, survived and grew in the aged DI brain. The transplants were well-vascularized and were not separated from the host parenchyma by obvious scar or glial barriers. No clear evidence of appropriate transplant function was obtained in this study of grafts into older hosts. Although negative data must be viewed with caution, the failure of the grafts to exert an antidiuretic influence may reflect the importance of the target site for proper graft function. The major apparent difference between grafts in one- and two-year-old hosts and functional grafts in younger DI rats was the absence of efferent fibres from the transplant into the host median eminence in the older animals. The numerous beaded axonal and dendritic processes from the vasopressin neurones ramified extensively within the boundaries of the graft, but were only rarely seen to cross into the host brain in the older rats. Non-functional grafts in younger animals had a similar morphology. An essential correlate for function may be a requirement for transplanted vasopressin neurones to establish neurohaemal contacts on fenestrated capillaries in the host neurohypophysis in order to effectively release vasopressin into the systemic circulation.

Additional evidence that the site of transplantation is an important factor in transplant function comes from studies of grafts placed outside of the hypothalamus. When the anterior hypothalami from 19- and 21-day normal rat foetuses are grafted into the lateral ventricles of young adult (4–8-month-old) DI rats, no marked changes in the host's symptoms of diabetes insipidus are observed (Gash et al., 1982). The results from our studies are consistent with those of Dunnett et al. (1981a–c) on behavioural recovery in nigrostriatal-lesioned rats.

Innervation of the host brain by grafted neurones seems to be heaviest in the regions near the transplant and decreases rapidly with increasing distance from the graft (Björklund and Stenevi, 1977; Freed et al., 1980). The predilection of grafts to innervate adjacent areas may account, in part, for the importance of the transplantation site in behaviour recovery. In our studies on DI rats, the only transplants thus far which have alleviated the symptoms of diabetes insipidus have: (i) been located in the third ventricle juxtaposed to the median eminence, and (ii) have vasopressin-containing axons projecting from the graft into the well-vascularized median eminence/neurohypophysial region. Transplants in other sites, even grafts containing numerous vasopressin neurones, have not been found to affect drinking behaviour. The close relationship between site and effect seen thus far in functional transplants suggests the utilization of grafted vasopressin neurones to investigate the CNS effects of vasopressin. For example, using either animals with a congenital absence of vasopressin or with appropriate lesions, vasopressin neurones can be grafted into areas of the brain shown to receive extrahypothalamic vasopressin-containing fibres. By carefully analyzing the neuroanatomical pattern of graft development and correlative behavioural changes in the host, our understanding of vasopressin–brain interactions could advance.

SUMMARY

Our laboratory has developed a model system for investigating the development and function of transplanted vasopressin neurones. Vasopressin neurones derived from normal foetal donors can be identified unambiguously in the brain of the vasopressin-deficient DI host by immunocytochemical staining, and vasopressin-containing axons from the transplant traced to sites of termination in the host nervous system.

We have evidence that the neuroanatomical pattern of graft development correlates closely with the functional ability of the transplant as measured by amelioration of the hosts' symptoms of polydipsia and polyuria. The only transplants thus far which have been effective in alleviating the diabetes insipidus have: (i) been located in the third ventricle juxtaposed to the host median eminence, and (ii) have vasopressin-containing axons projecting from the graft into the well-vascularized median eminence/neurohypophysial region. Transplants in other sites, even grafts containing numerous vasopressin neurones, have not been found to effect drinking behaviour.

In addition to diabetes insipidus, DI rats exhibit a number of behavioural differences when compared to rats from which the mutation originated, the Long–Evans strain. We suggest that neural transplantation into various brain regions of DI rats, with correlated anatomical and functional analysis, may offer a valuable probe to analyze the CNS effects of vasopressin on these other behavioural patterns.

REFERENCES

Arendash, G.W. and Gorski, R.A. (1981) Transplantation of neonatal male preoptic tissue into the preoptic area of neonatal females increases masculine sexual behaviour. Soc. Neurosci. Abstr., 7: 287.

Armstrong, W.E., Warach, S., Hatton, G.I. and McNeill, T.H. (1980) Subnuclei in the rat hypothalamic paraventricular nucleus: a cytoarchitectural, horseradish peroxidase and immunocytochemical analysis. Neuroscience, 5: 1931–1958.

Azmitia, E.C., Perlow, M.J., Brennan, M.J. and Lauder, J.M. (1981) Fetal raphe and hippocampal transplants into adult and aged C57BL/6N mice: a preliminary immunocytochemical study. Brain Res. Bull., 7: 703–710.

Bailey, W.H. and Weiss, J.M. (1981) Avoidance conditioning and endocrine function in Brattleboro rats. In J.L. Martinez, Jr., R.A. Jensen, R.B. Messing, H. Rigter and J.L. McGaugh (Eds.), Endogenous Peptides and Learning and Memory Processes, Academic Press, New York, pp. 371–396.

Barker, C.F. and Billingham, R.E. (1977) Immunologically privileged sites. In H.G. Kunkel and F.J. Dixon (Eds.), Advances in Immunology, Academic Press, New York, pp. 1–54.

Björklund, A. and Stenevi, U. (1977) Reformation of the severed septohippocampal cholinergic pathway in the adult rat by transplanted septal neurons. *Cell Tiss. Res.*, 185: 289–302.

Buijs, R.M. (1978) Intra- and extrahypothalamic vasopressin and oxytocin pathways in the rat. Pathways to the limbic system, medulla oblongata and spinal cord. *Cell Tiss. Res.*, 192: 423–435.

Das, G.D. (1974) Transplantation of embryonic neural tissue in the mammalian brain. I. Growth and differentiation of neuroblasts from various regions of the embryonic brain in the cerebellum of neonate rats. *T.I.T.J. Life Sci.*, 4: 93–124.

Das, G.D. and Altman, J. (1971) Transplanted percursors of nerve cells: Their fate in the cerebellums of young rats. *Science*, 173: 637–638.

De Wied, D. (1969) Effects of peptide hormones on behaviour. In W.F. Ganong and L. Martini (Eds.), *Frontiers in Neuroendocrinology, 1969*, Oxford University Press, London, pp. 97–140.

De Wied, D. (1976) Behavioral effects of intraventricularly administered vasopressin and vasopressin fragments. *Life Sci.*, 19: 685–690.

De Wied, D., Bohus, B. and Van Wimersma Greidanus, Tj. B. (1975) Memory deficit in rats with hereditary diabetes insipidus. *Brain Res.*, 85: 152–156.

Dunn, E.H. (1917) Primary and secondary findings in a series of attempts to transplant cerebral cortex in the albino rat. *J. comp. Neurol.*, 27: 565–582.

Dunnett, S.B., Björklund, A., Stenevi, U. and Iversen, S.D. (1981a) Behavioral recovery following transplantation of substantia nigra in rats subjected to 6-OHDA lesions of the nigrostriatal pathway. I. Unilateral lesions. *Brain Res.*, 215: 147–161.

Dunnett, S.B., Björklund, A., Stenevi, U. and Iversen, S.D. (1981b) Grafts of embryonic substantia nigra reinnervating the ventrolateral striatum ameliorate sensormotor impairments and akinesia in rats with 6-OHDA lesions of the nigrostriatal pathway. *Brain Res.*, 229: 209–217.

Dunnett, S.B., Björklund, A., Stenevi, U. and Iversen, S.D. (1981c) Behavioral recovery following transplantation of substantia nigra in rats subjected to 6-ODHA lesions of the nigrostriatal pathway. II. Bilateral lesions. *Brain Res.*, 229: 457–470.

Freed, W.F., Perlow, M.J., Karoum, F., Seiger, A., Olson, L., Hoffer, B.J. and Wyatt, R.J. (1980) Restoration of dopaminergic function by grafting of fetal rat substantia nigra to the caudate nucleus: Long-term behavioural, biochemical and histochemical studies. *Ann. Neurol.*, 8: 510–519.

Gash, D.M. and Scott, D.E. (1980) Fetal hypothalamic transplantation in the third ventricle of the adult brain. *Cell Tiss. Res.*, 211: 191–206.

Gash, D.M. and Sladek, J.R., Jr. (1980) Vasopressin neurons grafted into Brattleboro rats: Viability and activity. *Peptides*, 1: 11–14.

Gash, D.M., Sladek, J.R., Jr. and Sladek, C.D. (1980a) Functional development of grafted vasopressin neurons. *Science*, 210: 1367–1369.

Gash, D.M., Sladek, C.D. and Sladek, J.R., Jr. (1980b) A model system for analyzing functional development of transplanted peptidergic neurons. *Peptides*, 1, Suppl. 1: 125–134.

Gash, D.M., Warren, P.H., Dick, L.B., Sladek, J.R., Jr. and Ison, J.R. (1982) Behavioral modification in Brattleboro rats due to vasopressin administration and neural transplantation. *Ann. N.Y. Acad. Sci.*, in press.

Jaeger, C.B. and Lund, R.D. (1980) Transplantation of embryonic occipital cortex to the tectal region of newborn rats: a light microscopic study of organization and connectivity of the transplants. *J. comp. Neurol.*, 194: 571–597.

Kovács, G.L., Bohus, B., Versteeg, D.H.G., De Kloet, E.R. and De Wied, D. (1979) Effect of oxytocin and vasopressin on memory consolidation: Sites of action and catecholaminergic correlates after local microinjection into limbic midbrain structures. *Brain Res.*, 175: 303–314.

Kovács, G.L., Buijs, R.M., Bohus, B. and Van Wimersma Greidanus, Tj.B. (1982) Microinjection of arginine 8-vasopressin antiserum into the dorsal hippocampus attenuates passive avoidance behavior in rats. *Physiol. Behav.*, 28: 45–48.

Krieger, D.T., Perlow, M.J., Gibson, M.J., Davies, T.F., Zimmerman, E.A., Ferin, M. and Charlton, H.M. (1982) Brain grafts reverse hypogonodism of gonodotropin releasing hormone deficiency. *Nature (Lond.)*, 298: 468–471.

LeMoal, M., Koob, G.F., Koda, L.Y., Bloom, F.E., Manning, M., Sawyer, W.H. and Rivier, J. (1981) Vasopressin receptor antagonist prevents behavioral effects of vasopressin. *Nature (Lond.)*, 291: 491–493.

Lewis, E.R., Mueller, J.C. and Cotman, C.W. (1979) Neonatal septal implants: Development of afferent lamination in the rat dentate gyrus. *Brain Res. Bull.*, 5: 217–221.

Lund, R.D. and Harvey, A.R. (1981) Transplantation of tectal tissue in rats. I. Organization of transplants and pattern of distribution of host afferents within them. *J. comp. Neurol.*, 202: 505–520.

Perlow, M.J., Freed, W.F., Hoffer, B.J., Seiger, A., Olson, L. and Wyatt, R.J. (1979) Brain grafts reduce motor abnormalities produced by destruction of nigrostriatal dopamine system. *Science*, 204: 643–647.

Perlow, M.J., Reppert, S.M., Artman, H.A., Fisher, D.A., Seif, S.M. and Robinson, A.G. (1982) Oxytocin, vasopressin, and estrogen-stimulated neurophysin: daily patterns of concentration in cerebrospinal fluid. *Science*, 216: 1416–1418.

Reppert, S.M., Artman, H.G., Swaminathan, S. and Fisher, D.A. (1981) Vasopressin exhibits a rhythmic daily pattern in cerebrospinal fluid but not in blood. *Science*, 213: 1256–1257.

Rigter, H. and Crabbe, J.C. (1979) Modulation of memory by pituitary hormones and related peptides. *Vitamins Hormones*, 37: 153–241.

Scheinberg, L.C., Edelman, F.L. and Levy, W.A. (1964) Is the brain "an immunologically priviledged site"? *Arch. Neurol.*, 11: 248–264.

Seiger, A. and Olson, L. (1977) Quantitation of fiber growth in transplanted central monoamine neurons. *Cell Tiss. Res.*, 179: 285–316.

Sokol, H.W., Zimmerman, E.A., Sawyer, W.H. and Robinson, A.G. (1976) The hypothalamic-neurohypophyseal system of the rat: localization and quantitation of neurophysin by light microscopic immunocytochemistry in normal rats and in Brattleboro rats deficient in vasopressin and a neurophysin. *Endocrinology*, 98: 1176–1188.

Stenevi, U., Björklund, A. and Svendgaard, N. (1976) Transplantation of central and peripheral monoamine neurons to the adult rat brain: techniques and conditions for survival. *Brain Res.*, 114: 1–20.

Stenevi, U., Björklund, A., Kromer, L.F., Paden, C.M., Gerlach, J.L., McEwen, B.S. and Silverman, A.J. (1980) Differentiation of embryonic hypothalamic transplants cultured on choroidal pia in brains of adult rats. *Cell Tiss. Res.*, 205: 217–228.

Swanson, L.W. and Sawchenko, P.E. (1983) Hypothalamic integration: Organization of the paraventricular and supraoptic nuclei. *Ann. Rev. Neurosci.*, in press.

Vandersande, F. and Dierickx, K. (1976) Immunocytochemical demonstration of the inability of the homozygous Brattleboro rat to synthesize vasopressin and vasopressin-associated neurophysin. *Cell Tiss. Res.*, 165: 307–316.

Van Wimersma Greidanus, Tj.B., Dogterom, J. and De Wied, D. (1975) Intraventricular administration of anti-vasopressin serum inhibits memory consolidation in rats. *Life Sci.*, 16: 637–644.

The Neurohypophysis: Structure, Function and Control, Progress in Brain Research, Vol. 60, edited by B.A. Cross and G. Leng

Possible Control by Oxytocin of Periodical and Synchronous Neurosecretory Bursts of Oxytocin Cells

M.J. FREUND-MERCIER, F. MOOS, Y. GUERNE and Ph. RICHARD

Laboratoire de Physiologie générale, LA 309 C.N.R.S., 21, rue René Descartes F 67084 Strasbourg Cedex
(France)

INTRODUCTION

In suckled rats, oxytocin is released periodically every 6–20 min (Wakerley and Lincoln, 1971). Each milk-ejection, shown by an increase in mammary pressure, appears 15–20 sec after a characteristic short high frequency burst of spikes from oxytocin cells (Lincoln et al., 1973; Lincoln and Wakerley, 1974; Wakerley and Lincoln, 1973). These neurosecretory bursts probably occur simultaneously in all oxytocin cells, inducing a pulsatile release of oxytocin. The frequency, amplitude and synchronization of these neurosecretory bursts are controlled by various neural factors. The neurotransmitter dopamine has the most clearly demonstrated effect (Moos and Richard, 1982) and is able to increase the frequency and amplitude of neurosecretory bursts and induce a milk-ejection reflex not established 1 h after the beginning of suckling. Similar effects have been noted after intraventricular injections of small doses of oxytocin (0.01, 0.1, 1 ng; Freund-Mercier and Richard, 1981).

The present paper gives some experimental data obtained in vivo and in vitro, to determine more precisely the central excitatory effect of oxytocin on its own release.

EFFECTS OF INTRAVENTRICULAR INJECTIONS OF AN OXYTOCIN ANTAGONIST ON NEUROSECRETORY BURSTS OF OXYTOCIN CELLS

Intraventricular injection of an oxytocin antagonist was used with or without previous similar administration of oxytocin, to verify the specificity of action of exogenous oxytocin, and to test the putative role of endogenous oxytocin on oxytocin cell activations during suckling (preliminary results may be found in Freund-Mercier and Richard, 1982).

The milk-ejection reflex was studied in urethane-anaesthetized rats according to a method derived from Wakerley and Lincoln (1973) and described in detail by Moos and Richard (1982). Eleven paraventricular oxytocin cells were identified according to both their antidromic response to electrical stimulation of the neurohypophysis and their short high frequency bursts of spikes 15–20 sec before each increase in mammary pressure. Oxytocin (Sandoz) and/or an oxytocin antagonist, $(1(\beta$-mercapto-β,β-cyclopentamethylene-propionic acid), 8 ornithine-)vasotocin, i.e. $d(CH_2)_5$ OVT (Bankowski et al., 1980), were injected in a constant volume of $1\,\mu l$ into the 3rd ventricle. Before and after peptide injections, the parameters studied were: the frequency of neurosecretory bursts or milk-ejections (mean number by 5 or 10 min periods) and the amplitude of bursts (total number of spikes) or milk-ejections (increase in mammary pressure).

198

Intraventricular injections of $d(CH_2)_5$ OVT ($1\mu l$, 10^{-4}M, i.e. $0.1\mu g$) after 3–4 regular milk-ejections resulted in an inhibition of the reflex 5–15 min later without modification of the mammary gland sensitivity. The frequency of bursts, the total number of spikes per burst and the amplitude of milk-ejections were decreased. These parameters reverted to normal 70–80 min later. Similarly, the oxytocin antagonist inhibited a milk-ejection reflex previously activated by the intraventricular injection of $1\mu l$ of 10^{-6}M oxytocin solution (i.e. 1 ng; Fig. 1B). The mean number of milk-ejections per 5 min period, which increased to as much as 2.0 after an oxytocin injection (vs 0.1–0.5 before), was decreased immediately and markedly to 0–0.3 by $d(CH_2)_5$ OVT. This inhibitory effect lasted 50 min.

Thus, in addition to its well-known peripheral effect, oxytocin plays a role at the central level, controlling both the frequency and amplitude of neurosecretory bursts of oxytocin cells.

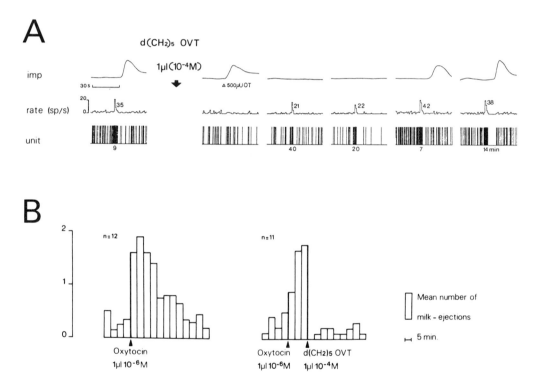

Fig. 1. The effects of an oxytocin antagonist on the milk-ejection reflex in anaesthetized rats. A: intramammary pressure (imp) was recorded simultaneously with the electrical activity of oxytocin cells (unit). Rate is the number of spikes per sec (sp/s). The total number of spikes per neurosecretory burst is given beside each burst and the time (minute) elapsing since the previous one underneath. Injection into the 3rd ventricle of an oxytocin antagonist $d(CH_2)_5$ OVT ($1\mu l$, 10^{-4}M, i.e. $0.1\mu g$) delays the next neurosecretory burst by 40 min, and burst frequency only returns to control values after injection. The oxytocin release induced by the two bursts following injection is not sufficient to increase intramammary pressure, although the sensitivity of mammary glands to the intravenous injection of 500μU oxytocin is not affected. B: mean numbers of milk-ejections over successive 5 min periods during suckling. Left, injection into the 3rd ventricle of oxytocin ($1\mu l$, 10^{-6}M, i.e. 1 ng) increases the milk-ejection frequency, n = 12; right, injection into the 3rd ventricle of an oxytocin antagonist, $d(CH_2)_5$ OVT ($1\mu l$, 10^{-4}M i.e. $0.1\mu g$) inhibited milk-ejection reflex enhanced 15 min before by intraventricular oxytocin injection ($1\mu l$, 10^{-6}M, i.e. 1 ng) n – 11.

OXYTOCIN RELEASE FROM ISOLATED PARAVENTRICULAR AND SUPRAOPTIC NUCLEI

In vitro studies were undertaken to investigate the mechanism and sites of action of oxytocin. The isolated paraventricular and supraoptic nuclei (PVN, SON) were used to assess the effects of exogenously applied oxytocin, isotocin, arginine-vasopressin, oxytocin with a Ca^{2+} channel blocker or an oxytocin antagonist, on oxytocin release measured by a radioimmunoassay (RIA) developed in our laboratory. The antibody anti-oxytocin developed by the method of Vance et al. (1969) was specific to oxytocin, no cross-reaction being observed with isotocin and arginine-vasopressin for the concentrations used in standard curves.

Isolated PVN or SON from male Wistar rats were incubated (two pairs in each vial) in a cerebrospinal fluid-like medium (Bridges et al., 1976) at 37°C and continuously oxygenated with carbogen (95% O_2, 5% CO_2). After an equilibration period of 20 min, the tissues were incubated in fresh medium for two 10-min periods, the drugs being tested during the 2nd period. Tissues were allowed to recover in normal medium before homogenization (in 0.5% acetic acid solution), heating (3 min in a water-bath at 95°C), centrifugation and freezing. Samples of the medium were acidified to pH 3.5 with acetic acid and frozen until RIA.

Hormone release per 10 min period was expressed as a percentage of the initial hormone content. On an average of 24 values, one pair of SON initially containing 5.06 ± 0.41 ng

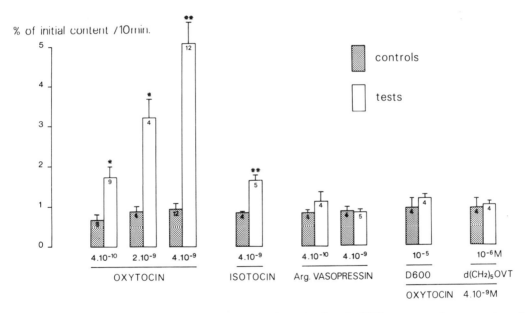

Fig. 2. Oxytocin release from isolated SON per 10 min. Oxytocin release by SON was expressed as a percentage of initial content. The tissues were incubated in the absence (controls) or presence (tests) of oxytocin, isotocin, arginine-vasopressin, oxytocin with D600 (a Ca^{2+} channel blocker) or d(CH₂)₅ OVT (an oxytocin antagonist). Each value was the mean ± S.E. of n determinations indicated in each column. * $P < 0.01$; ** $P < 0.001$ (Student's-t-test). Adding oxytocin ($4 \cdot 10^{-10}$, $2 \cdot 10^{-9}$, $4 \cdot 10^{-9}$M) to the incubation medium increased basal oxytocin release in a dose-dependent manner. A similar effect was obtained with $4 \cdot 10^{-9}$M isotocin, but arginine-vasopressin ($4 \cdot 10^{-10}$, $4 \cdot 10^{-9}$M) gave no result. The higher dose of oxytocin ($4 \cdot 10^{-9}$M) in the presence of 10^{-5}M D600, failed to induce an increase in oxytocin release. The oxytocin antagonist (10^{-6}M) also prevented the facilitatory effect of $4 \cdot 10^{-9}$M oxytocin, but this blockage was only observed when SON had been preincubated for 10 min with d(CH₂)₅ OVT alone just before the test period.

oxytocin, released 40 ± 3 pg of oxytocin per 10 min period, the percentage of oxytocin released corresponding to $0.83 \pm 0.075\,\%$ of initial SON content. For incubations in the presence of oxytocin, the amount of oxytocin released by SON was calculated by subtracting the amount of exogenous oxytocin from the total measured in the incubation medium. This correction was not necessary for isotocin and arginine-vasopressin since they do not cross-react with the anti-oxytocin.

Adding oxytocin increased basal hormone release significantly in a dose-dependent manner (Fig. 2): 2.3, 3.7 and 5.4 times increase respectively with $4 \cdot 10^{-10}$ M ($P < 0.01$), $2 \cdot 10^{-9}$ M ($P < 0.01$) and $4 \cdot 10^{-9}$ M ($P < 0.001$). Facilitation was also obtained with $4 \cdot 10^{-9}$ M isotocin ($P < 0.001$). Arginine-vasopressin ($4 \cdot 10^{-10}$ and $4 \cdot 10^{-9}$ M) did not affect basal oxytocin release from isolated SON (Fig. 2). These in vitro results tally with those obtained in vivo; both intraventricular injections of oxytocin and isotocin had an excitatory effect on the milk-ejection reflex (Freund-Mercier and Richard, in preparation) whereas arginine-vasopressin did not (Freund-Mercier and Richard, 1981).

D600 (10^{-5} M), a Ca^{2+} channel blocker, incubated with $4 \cdot 10^{-9}$ M oxytocin, prevented the facilitatory effect of the hormone. Thus, the release of oxytocin from isolated magnocellular nuclei was Ca^{2+}-dependent, as is that from the axonal endings in the neurohypophysis.

d(CH_2)$_5$ OVT (10^{-6} M), an oxytocin antagonist, also blocked the increase normally induced by $4 \cdot 10^{-9}$ M oxytocin, suggesting that the facilitatory effect of oxytocin was specific. However, the blockage by d(CH_2)$_5$ OVT was efficient only when a 10 min preincubation with the antagonist alone was realized, just before the test period (oxytocin with d(CH_2)$_5$ OVT). This would suggest a difference in the affinity of the receptors for oxytocin and its antagonist.

Similar results were obtained with isolated PVN.

CONCLUSIONS AND SUMMARY

These results provide evidence that oxytocin may be involved in the control of its own release. Injection into the 3rd ventricle of an oxytocin antagonist, d(CH_2)$_5$ OVT, inhibited the milk-ejection reflex in the rat, decreasing both the frequency and amplitude of neurosecretory bursts and milk-ejection. Moreover, this antagonist prevented the facilitatory effect of intraventricular injection of oxytocin on the milk-ejection reflex that we have previously described (Freund-Mercier and Richard, 1981). The level and mechanism of action of such a control remains to be discovered. Several data suggest a hypothalamic action. Oxytocin injections into the 4th ventricle were not sufficient to activate the milk-ejection reflex, and the effects observed after lateral ventricle injections were inferior to those obtained after 3rd ventricle injections (Freund-Mercier and Richard, in preparation). A direct effect on neurosecretory cells is possible, since microiontophoretic applications of oxytocin increases the firing of most neurosecretory cells in PVN (Moss et al., 1972). Such an effect is corroborated by our in vitro results, since oxytocin and isotocin increased oxytocin release, this effect being blocked by D600 (a Ca^{2+} channel blocker) and d(CH_2)$_5$ OVT (an oxytocin antagonist).

One could postulate that oxytocin is released by axon collaterals or dendrites into the extracellular spaces of the magnocellular nuclei, as is dopamine in the substantia nigra (see Cheramy et al., 1981). Such an increase of the endogenous oxytocin concentration during suckling could control the frequency and amplitude of the periodic activation of oxytocin cells. Finally, although we have no experimental data in favour of such an hypothesis, oxytocin could be a synchronizing factor of the bursting activation of oxytocin cells in the magnocellular nuclei.

ACKNOWLEDGEMENTS

This work was supported by grants from the CNRS (ATP 1780) and INSERM (CRL 79-1-234-4). Our grateful thanks are due to E. Waltisperger (CNRS) for technical assistance, Dr. M. Manning for generous supplies of the oxytocin antagonist, and Drs H. Friedli and H. Weidmann (Sandoz Laboratory) for oxytocin.

REFERENCES

Bankowski, K., Manning, M., Seto, J., Haldar, J. and Sawyer, W.H. (1980) Design and synthesis of potent in vivo antagonists of oxytocin. *Int. J. Peptide Protein Res.*, 16: 382–391.

Bridges, T.E., Hillhouse, E.W. and Jones, M.T. (1976) The effect of dopamine on neurohypophysial hormone release in vivo and from the rat neural lobe and hypothalamus in vitro. *J. Physiol. (Lond.)*, 260: 647–666.

Cheramy, A., Lievel, V. and Glowinski, J. (1981) Dendritic release of dopamine in the substantia nigra. *Nature (Lond.)*, 289: 537–542.

Freund-Mercier, M.J. and Richard, Ph. (1981) Excitatory effects of intraventricular injections of oxytocin on the milk ejection reflex in the rat. *Neurosci. Lett.*, 23: 193–198.

Freund-Mercier, M.J. and Richard, Ph. (1982) Oxytocin as a putative factor in control of periodic and synchronized neurosecretory bursts of oxytocinergic cells. *C.R. Acad. Sci, (Paris)*, 294: 497–500.

Lincoln, D.W., Hill, A. and Wakerley, J.B. (1973) The milk ejection reflex of the rat: an intermittent function not abolished by surgical levels of anaesthesia. *J. Endocr.*, 57: 459–476.

Lincoln, D.W. and Wakerley, J.B. (1974) Electrophysiological evidence for the activation of supraoptic neurones during the release of oxytocin. *J. Physiol. (Lond.)*, 242: 533–554.

Moos, F. and Richard, Ph. (1982) Excitatory effect of dopamine on oxytocin and vasopressin reflex releases in the rat. *Brain Res.*, 241: 249–260.

Moss, R.L., Dyball, R.E.J. and Cross, B.A. (1972) Excitation of antidromically identified neurosecretory cells of the paraventricular nucleus by oxytocin applied iontophoretically. *Exp. Neurol.*, 34: 95–102.

Vance, V.K., Schure, J.J. and Reichlin, M. (1969) Induction of antibodies to porcine ACTH in rabbits with non steroidogenic polymers of BSA and ACTH. In M. Margoulies (Ed.), *Protein and Polypeptide Hormones*, Excerpta Medica, New York, pp. 380–384.

Wakerley, J.B. and Lincoln, D.W. (1971) Milk-ejection in the rat: recordings of intramammary pressure during suckling. *J. Endoc.*, 51: 13–14.

Wakerley, J.B. and Lincoln, D.W. (1973) The milk ejection reflex of the rat: a 20 to 40 fold acceleration in the firing of paraventricular neurones during oxytocin release. *J. Endocr.*, 57: 477–493.

Biosynthesis of
the Neurohypophysial Hormones

The Neurohypophysis: Structure, Function and Control, Progress in Brain Research, Vol. 60, edited by B.A. Cross and G. Leng

Precursors of Vasopressin and Oxytocin

H. GAINER

Section on Functional Neurochemistry, Laboratory of Developmental Neurobiology, National Institute of Child Health and Human Development, National Institutes of Health, Bldg. 36, Rm. 2A21, Bethesda, MD 20205 (U.S.A.)

INTRODUCTION

The original proposal for the existence of a vasopressin precursor was put forth about 18 years ago (Sachs and Takabatake, 1964). Since that time a large number of peptide hormones have been shown to derive from the post-translational processing of larger precursor proteins. This mechanism accounts not only for the biosynthesis of peptide hormones, but also for the biosynthesis of a wide variety of secreted, membrane and viral proteins found in cells (see Freedman and Hawkins, 1980; Koch and Richter, 1980; Palade, 1975; Zimmerman et al., 1980). Considerable information is now available about the cell biological mechanisms which underly the biosynthesis and intracellular routing of secretory proteins, and it is now generally agreed that in addition to transcription and translation processes, various signal sequences and post-translational processing events are also involved in determining which peptides will be secreted by the cell.

As a consequence of the above developments, unequivocal criteria for the identification of precursors (e.g. prohormones) of peptides and proteins have been established. These criteria include: (1) demonstration in classical pulse-chase experiments in intact cellular systems (in vivo or in situ) that a larger form of the peptide is first synthesized and subsequently decreases in radioactivity as the radioactive peptide is formed. Chemical identity between putative precursor and products is usually established in such experiments by immunoprecipitation and peptide mapping procedures; (2) demonstration by in vitro (cell-free) translation experiments (i.e. mRNA is purified from the synthesizing tissue and incubated in the presence of heterologous cell-free translation systems — e.g. wheat germ and reticulocyte lysates), that a larger precursor form of the peptide is synthesized. These experiments can also provide information about the signal sequence of the prohormone, and when performed in the presence of microsomal membranes, it is possible to demonstrate several post-translational processes (e.g. signal sequence cleavage, glycosylation, etc.); (3) to utilize modern recombinant DNA techniques to clone cDNA obtained from a purified mRNA template using reverse transcriptase. The cloned cDNA can be rapidly sequenced, and from the nucleotide sequence the amino acid sequence of the precursor (i.e. pre-prohormone) can be deduced. All these criteria have been fulfilled in the case of the vasopressin precursor, and a brief description of some of these studies with regard to both vasopressin and oxytocin is presented below.

IDENTIFICATION OF VASOPRESSIN AND OXYTOCIN PRECURSORS

Historical aspects

Table I shows some of the landmark events which pertain to the search for vasopressin and oxytocin precursors. Without question the most important conceptual contribution was made by Howard Sachs and his colleagues who not only proposed the precursor hypothesis for vasopressin (Sachs and Takabatake, 1964), but also the "common precursor" hypothesis (Sachs et al., 1969) which argued that both vasopressin and neurophysin were synthesized via a single prohormone. It is not commonly known that these proposals preceded the discovery of proinsulin by 3 years, and the discovery of the "common precursor" of ACTH-endorphin by 8 years. Thus, the current state of prohormone research in general, stands as a tribute to the prescience of Sachs and his coworkers.

Although the efforts to test Sachs' hypothesis by identifying such precursors for vasopressin and neurophysin proceeded at a relatively slow pace (compared to other putative precursors), it is clear that the subsequent successes (see Table I) in this endeavour were more due to technological advances than conceptual ones. These advances included the utilization of the Brattleboro rat as an experimental model, the development of micropunch techniques for brain samples, the availability of antibodies adequate for immunoprecipitation procedures, and most recently the utilization of in vitro translation and recombinant DNA techniques.

Experimental evidence for precursors

The various early pulse-chase studies which attempted to identify these precursors (Sachs et al., 1969; Walter et al., 1977; Mendelson and Walter, 1978) were unsuccessful simply because methods to increase the "signal to noise" ratio in the biochemical analyses (e.g. punch techniques and immunoprecipitation procedures) were either not available or not utilized. Application of these techniques and approaches rapidly led to the identification of separate approximately 20,000 molecular weight precursors for vasopressin and oxytocin-associated neurophysins synthesized by the rat supraoptic nucleus in vivo (Gainer et al., 1977a, b; Brownstein and Gainer, 1977; Brownstein et al., 1977; Gainer and Brownstein, 1978). The use of the Brattleboro rat model system for in vivo biosynthesis and axonal transport studies, pioneered by Pickering and his colleagues (Burford and Pickering, 1973; Jones and Pickering, 1972; Pickering et al., 1975), was invaluable in establishing which of these precursors was related to vasopressin (Brownstein and Gainer, 1977; Gainer and Brownstein, 1978). Based on these data, and subsequent work on the neurophysin precursors synthesized in vivo (Russell et al., 1979, 1980, 1981), it was possible to provide evidence that these precursors (two forms for vasopressin with pI = 5.6 and 6.1, and two forms for oxytocin with pI = 5.1 and 5.4; see Fig. 1) were indeed common precursors as had been hypothesized by Sachs' group.

The properties of these precursors are summarized in Table IIA. From these data it could be concluded that the vasopressin precursor contained three peptide moieties: the vasopressin sequence, the vasopressin-associated neurophysin; and a < 10,000 molecular weight glycopeptide, in this order from amino to carboxyl terminus (Russell et al., 1981). Analyses of the various pI forms of these precursors, indicated that both forms of the vasopressin precursor (pI 5.6. and 6.1, in Fig. 1) were of comparable molecular weight (about 20,000 daltons) and contained all of the known peptide products. It is still unclear whether the pI 5.6. form is an intermediate formed from the pI 6.1. form (Fig. 1), or alternatively is a separate gene product differing in the glycopeptide moiety. In this regard, it is interesting that two distinct glycopep-

TABLE I

HISTORY OF OXYTOCIN AND VASOPRESSIN PRECURSORS

Year	Development	Reference
1963–1964	Vasopressin biosynthesis occurs in the hypothalamus and not in the pituitary. Synthesis is coupled to protein synthesis.	Sachs (1963); Sachs and Takabatake (1964); Takabatake and Sachs (1964)
1964	Hypothesis of a vasopressin precursor.	Sachs and Takabatake (1964)
1968–1969	Evidence for coordinate synthesis and secretion of vasopressin and neurophysin.	Fawcett et al. (1968); Sachs et al. (1969)
1969	Hypothesis of a common precursor for vasopressin and neurophysin. Supporting analogue (α-methylleucine, α-methylmethionine, histidinol) data.	Sachs et al. (1969)
1972–1973	Parallel synthesis and axonal transport of neurohypophysial hormones and neurophysin.	Jones and Pickering (1972); Burford and Pickering (1973)
1974–1975	Brattleboro rats deficient in synthesis, axonal transport, and storage of vasopressin and vasopressin-associated neurophysin.	Pickering et al. (1975); Valtin et al. (1974)
1977	Identification of separate precursors for oxytocin and vasopressin-associated neurophysins in in vivo experiments.	Gainer et al. (1977a,b); Brownstein and Gainer (1977); Brownstein et al. (1977)
1979	Identification of separate neurophysin precursors in in vitro translation experiments.	Guidice and Chaiken (1979); Lin et al. (1979); Schmale et al. (1979)
1979–1980	Peptide mapping data in favour of common precursor for vasopressin and its neurophysin. Evidence that vasopressin precursor is a glycoprotein but oxytocin precursor is not (in vivo, rat).	Russell et al. (1979, 1980)
1980–1981	Immunological evidence for common precursors of vasopressin and oxytocin and their respective neurophysins. Evidence that vasopressin precursor is a glycoprotein; oxytocin precursor is not (in vitro translation, bovine).	Richter et al. (1980); Ivell et al. (1981); Schmale et al. (1980, 1981a)
1981	Prediction of order of peptide components in vasopressin and oxytocin precursors derived from peptide mapping studies.	Russell et al. (1981); Schmale and Richter (1981c)
1982	Complete sequence of the bovine vasopressin-neurophysin II pre-prohormone elucidated by recombinant DNA techniques.	Land et al. (1982)

tides are transported to the pituitaries of normal rats, and that both are missing in Brattleboro rats (Russell et al., 1980). Similarly, the two forms of the oxytocin precursor (pI 5.1. and 5.4, in Fig. 1) are both about 15,000 daltons and both appear to contain oxytocin and its neurophysin (Table IIA).

An entirely separate approach to the identification of the precursors of oxytocin and vasopressin, i.e. using in vitro translation techniques, has led to similar conclusions (compare in vivo data in Table IIA to in vitro data in Table IIB). Several laboratories (Guidice and

208

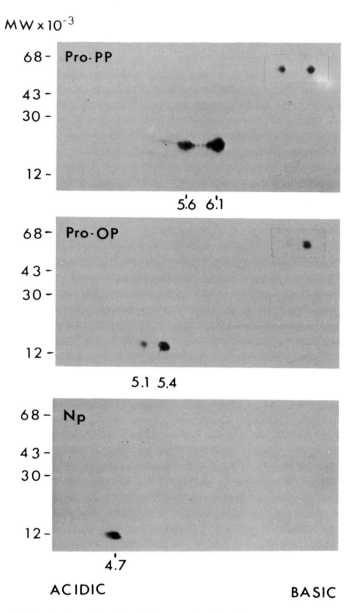

Fig. 1. Two-dimensional gel electrophoresis and fluorography of [^{35}S]cysteine-labelled Pro-PP (top), Pro-OP (middle) and neurophysin (Np, bottom) synthesized by rat supraoptic nuclei and isolated by Sephadex G-75 chromatography. Islets show two-dimensional gels containing labelled Pro-PP and Pro-OP immunoprecipitated by antibodies to rat neurophysin. (From Russell et al., 1981.) Pro-PP, propressophysin or rat vasopressin precursor; Pro-OP, prooxyphysin or rat oxytocin precursor.

Chaiken, 1979; Lin et al., 1979; Schmale et al., 1979) have shown that mRNA isolated from bovine, mouse, or rat hypothalami could serve as templates in cell-free translation systems to yield 20–25,000 molecular weight proteins which could be immunoprecipitated by antibodies raised against neurophysin. The most extensive series of cell-free translation experiments have

TABLE II

PROPERTIES OF OXYTOCIN AND VASOPRESSIN PRECURSORS

Precursor	Molecular weight (by SDS gel analysis)	Constituents		
		nonapeptide	neurophysin	carbohydrate [c]
(A) Rat: in vivo [a]				
Vasopressin prohormone	19,500	+	+	+
Oxytocin prohormone	15,000	+	+	−
(B) Bovine: in vitro [b]				
Vasopressin pre-prohormone	21,000	+	+	−
(+ membranes + tunicamycin)	19,000	+	+	−
(+ membranes − tunicamycin)	23,000	+	+	+
Oxytocin pre-prohormone	16,500	+	+	−
(+ membrane ± tunicamycin)	15,500	+	+	−

[a] From Russell et al., 1980, 1981.

[b] From Ivell et al., 1981; Richter et al., 1980; Schmale and Richter, 1980, 1981a–c; and Schmale et al., 1979.

[c] Refers only to carbohydrate moiety and not glycopeptide amino acid sequence.

been performed by Schmale and Richter and their colleagues (Schmale et al., 1979; Richter et al., 1980; Ivell et al., 1981; Schmale and Richter, 1980, 1981a–c).

By an elegant set of in vitro experiments the Schmale and Richter group have shown: (1) that bovine hypothalamic mRNA can be used to synthesize separate common precursors for vasopressin and bovine neurophysin II, as well as for oxytocin and bovine neurophysin I; (2) by including dog liver microsomes in the reticulocyte translation cocktail, both precursors can be shown to be converted from pre-prohormones to prohormones, but only the vasopressin prohormone is glycosylated; (3) the cell-free translated vasopressin pre-prohormone has a molecular weight (on SDS gels) of 21,000, is cleaved to a 19,000 molecular weight prohormone in the presence of tunicamycin (which prevents glycosylation) and microsomes, but is glycosylated to a molecular weight of 23,000 in the presence of microsomes without tunicamycin; (4) the oxytocin pre-prohormone is about 16,500 molecular weight, and is converted to a 15,500 molecular weight prohormone by liver microsomes (with no effect of tunicamycin); and (5) tryptic mapping of the vasopressin pre-prohormone and prohormone indicated that the vasopressin follows signal sequence and precedes the neurophysin II in the pre-prohormone. The conclusions from these in vitro translation studies in the cow are in complete agreement with those derived from the in vivo studies in the rat (see summary in Table II), thereby enhancing the credibility of these identifications of the oxytocin and vasopressin precursors.

Complete characterization of the vasopressin precursor

The entire nucleotide sequence of the cloned cDNA encoding the bovine vasopressin-neurophysin II pre-prohormone has recently been reported (Land et al., 1982). The corresponding amino acid sequence contains 166 amino acids, of which 19 appear to belong to the signal sequence. The order of the peptide components in the prohormone is the same as that which was predicted from the in vivo and in vitro experiments described above. Fig. 2 illustrates the essential features of the vasopressin pre-prohormone elucidated by this recombinant DNA analysis. The signal sequence (which begins with Met^{-19} at the N-terminus, has a central hydrophobic region, and terminates with an amino acid with a small neutral side chain, i.e.

Ala^{-1}) is immediately followed by the arginine-vasopressin sequence, which is separated from the neurophysin II sequence by Gly^{10}–Lys^{11}–Arg^{12}, which in turn is separated from the 39 amino acid C-terminal peptide by a single Arg^{108}. The latter 39 amino acid peptide is believed to be the glycopeptide moiety discussed earlier, since it contains a characteristic amino acid sequence, Asn^{114}–Ala^{115}–Thr^{116}, typical of N-asparagine-linked glycopeptides.

A number of new insights derive from this sequence. As mentioned earlier, the order of peptide components was predicted from previous in vivo and in vitro data. It was expected that the peptide components would be separated by basic amino acid residues as these are found in other prohormones, and due to the results of previous tryptic mapping studies. However, while the Gly^{10}–Lys^{11}–Arg^{12} sequence interposed between vasopressin and neurophysin II is typical of prohormone cleavage sites where amidation also occurs, the single basic residue, Arg^{108}, between neurophysin II and the glycopeptide is not characteristic of other prohormone cleavage sites. These usually contain pairs of basic amino acids. Curiously, the Arg–Arg site in positions 105–106, which would appear to be more appropriate as a cleavage site, appears not to be recognized by the converting enzyme. These residues are found intact in bovine neurophysin II in situ (Pickering and Jones, 1978).

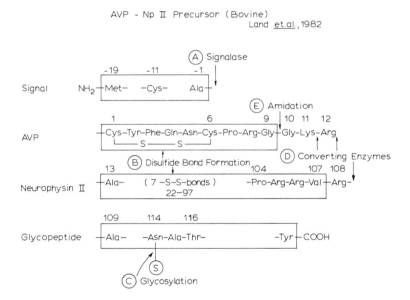

Fig. 2. Structure of the bovine arginine-vasopressin-neurophysin II precursor. (Modified from Land et al., 1982.) Arrows (A–E) denote post-translation events occurring at specific sites on the precursor. See text.

Perhaps the biggest surprise in this sequence was the identification of the 39 amino acid putative glycopeptide. The complete amino acid sequence of the glycopeptide is shown in Table III. A glycopeptide with the identical amino acid sequence had previously been extracted from bovine pituitary, isolated and sequenced by Smyth and Massey (1979). Similar glyco-peptides with remarkable conservation of sequences were also found by these authors in pig and sheep pituitaries. As these authors note in their paper, a similar 17 amino acid glycopeptide (corresponding exactly to the 1–17 amino acid sequence in Table III, except that position 2 is Ser in the pig) had been isolated earlier from pig posterior pituitary by Holwerda (1972). Although the amino acid sequence of this glycopeptide had been known for some time, it was not until the recombinant DNA studies that it was associated with vasopressin biosynthesis. In addition to the 1–17 and 1–39 glycopeptide sequences, several other fragments were found (corresponding to sequences 1–10, 1–19, 23–39 and 26–39). While these have been interpreted as "naturally occurring" peptides (Smyth and Massey, 1979), it remains to be determined whether they are formed by the biosynthetic process (during post-translational processing) in vivo, or are natural degradative products, or are formed as a result of proteolytic cleavages which occurred during the isolation procedures.

TABLE III

AMINO ACID SEQUENCE OF THE GLYCOPEPTIDE IN THE BOVINE VASOPRESSIN-NEUROPHYSIN II PRECURSOR

The amino acid order of the naturally found bovine glycopeptide (Smyth and Massey, 1979) is shown numbered from 1–39; the numbers in parentheses show the corresponding positions in the prohormone (Land et al., 1982).

<pre>
      1   3   10
NH2–Ala–Asn–Asp–Arg–Ser–Asn–Ala–Thr–Leu–Leu–
    (109)   (113)   (118)
     11   15   20
    –Asp–Gly–Pro–Ser–Gly–Ala–Leu–Leu–Leu–Arg–
    (119)   (123)   (128)
     21   25   30
    –Leu–Val–Gln–Leu–Ala–Gly–Ala–Pro–Glu–Pro–
    (129)   (133)   (138)
     31   35   39
    –Ala–Glu–Pro–Ala–Gln–Pro–Gly–Val–Tyr–COOH
    (139)   (143)   (147)
</pre>

Higher molecular weight vasopressin precursors

There have been several reports of much larger (i.e. about 80–140,000 daltons) vasopressin and neurophysin precursors (Camier et al., 1979; Lauber et al., 1979, 1981; Beguin et al., 1981). However, it is important to note that no in vivo and in vitro biosynthesis studies, nor recombinant DNA studies supporting these claims have been reported. Until such experiments are published, one should remain cautious about these larger putative precursors.

POST-TRANSLATIONAL PROCESSING OF PRECURSOR PROTEINS

The arrows in Fig. 2 denote the expected processing events for the vasopressin-neurophysin II precursor as deduced from its structure. The first three events, enzymatic cleavage of the signal peptide by a signalase, disulfide bond formation, and the initial stages of glycosylation, appear to occur during translation and are associated with the rough endoplasmic reticulum. A second stage of glycosylation occurs within the Golgi apparatus. The last two processes, enzymatic cleavage of the prohormone at the basic amino acid residues, and amidation of the C-terminal glycine of vasopressin, appear to occur after packaging, within the secretory vesicles.

Some insight as to the localization of the converting enzyme activity can be deduced from axonal transport studies. These studies show that most of the precursor is transported into the

212

axon, where it is converted to the final peptides during axonal transport (Gainer et al., 1977a, b; Gainer and Brownstein, 1978). Fig. 3 illustrates the presence of various labelled precursor forms in the posterior pituitary even as long as two hours after injection of [³⁵S]cysteine into the supraoptic nucleus. Since the neurosecretory vesicles are the principal vehicles for the axonal transport of neurophysin and vasopressin, it would follow logically that these organelles are the sites of prohormone conversion. A similar proposal, based on other data, had been suggested by the Sachs' group (Sachs et al., 1969), and localization of the conversion process in secretory vesicles has also been proposed in the biosynthesis of insulin, glucagon and somatostatin in islet cells of the pancreas (Fletcher et al., 1980, 1981).

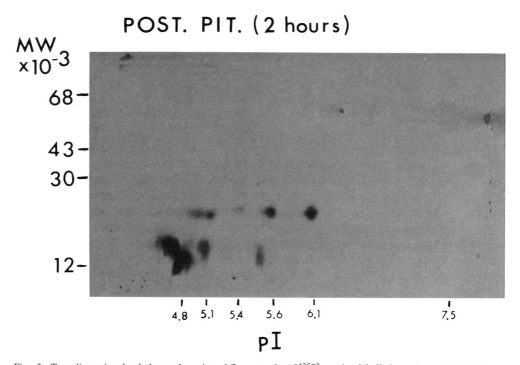

Fig. 3. Two-dimensional gel electrophoresis and fluorography of [³⁵S]cysteine-labelled proteins synthesized by rat supraoptic nuclei and transported to posterior pituitary (pituitary sample taken 2 h after injection). Note presence of labelled precursor forms as well as neurophysin. See text.

Given the above hypothesis that the secretory vesicle is the major site for enzymatic cleavage of the prohormone, then one would expect that appropriate converting enzymes should be present in the vesicles. Recent experiments indicate that this is the case for a variety of tissues. Converting enzyme activity has been detected and partially characterized in secretory vesicles isolated from anglerfish pancreas islet cells (Fletcher et al., 1980, 1981), neural and intermediate lobes of the rat pituitary (Loh and Gainer, 1982; Loh and Chang, 1982), and bovine posterior pituitary (Chang et al., 1982). Analysis of the converting enzyme activities found in all of these secretory vesicles indicates that they are acid, thiol proteases with specificities of cleavage at pairs of basic amino acids. Preliminary experiments in our laboratory indicate that the pro-opiocortin converting enzyme activity isolated from bovine neurosecretory vesicles (Chang et al., 1982) can release the vasopressin sequence from the rat vasopressin precursor (unpublished observations).

CONCLUSIONS

With the sequencing of the entire bovine vasopressin-neurophysin II precursor completed, the characterization of at least one form of this precursor can be considered finalized. It is expected that the oxytocin precursor will similarly be characterized by recombinant DNA methods soon. Many questions, however, remain to be answered. These include: (1) the nature of the post-translational processing enzymes and mechanisms which fashion the final peptide products; (2) the mechanisms underlying the transcriptional and translational regulation of the precursors during functional activity (e.g. dehydration, lactation, adrenalectomy); (3) the possible heterogeneity of these precursors in different cell groups in the hypothalamus; and (4) the function of the 39 amino acid glycopeptide derived from the vasopressin precursor. Thus, 18 years after the bold hypothesis by Sachs and Takabatake (1964), the vasopressin (and oxytocin) precursor concept has been brought to fruition by experimentation. Clearly, we are still only at the threshold of understanding about these precursors, and future studies will undoubtedly alter our views about their biological significance.

SUMMARY

A variety of biosynthesis studies conducted in vivo and in vitro have shown that the vasopressin precursor is a 19–23,000 molecular weight glycoprotein, which contains vasopressin at its N-terminus, neurophysin in the middle, and a 39 amino acid glycopeptide at the C-terminus. In contrast, the 15–16,000 molecular weight oxytocin precursor is not glycosylated. The vasopressin precursor has been completely sequenced by recombinant DNA methods, thereby providing insights into the nature of the glycopeptide as well as post-translational processing mechanisms.

REFERENCES

Beguin, P., Nicolas, P., Bousetta, H., Fahy, C. and Cohen, P. (1981) Characterization of the 80,000 molecular weight form of neurophysin isolated from bovine neurohypophysis. *J. biol. Chem.*, 256: 9289–9294.

Brownstein, M.J. and Gainer, H. (1977) Neurophysin biosynthesis in normal rats and in rats with hereditary diabetes insipidus. *Proc. nat. Acad. Sci. U.S.A.*, 74: 4046–4049.

Brownstein, M.J., Robinson, A.G. and Gainer, H. (1977) Immunological identification of rat neurophysin precursors. *Nature (Lond.)*, 269: 259–261.

Burford, G.D. and Pickering, B.T. (1973) Intracellular transport and turnover of neurophysins in the rat. *Biochem. J.*, 136: 1047–1052.

Camier, M., Lauber, M., Mohring, J. and Cohen, P. (1979) Evidence for higher molecular weight immunoreactive forms of vasopressin in the mouse hypothalamus. *FEBS Lett.*, 108: 369–373.

Chang, T.-L., Gainer, H., Russell, J.T. and Loh, Y.P. (1982) Proopiocortin converting enzyme activity in bovine neurosecretory granules. *Endocrinology*, 111: 1607–1614.

Fawcett, C.P., Powell, A.E. and Sachs, H. (1968) Biosynthesis and release of neurophysin. *Endocrinology*, 83: 1299–1310.

Fletcher, D.J., Noe, B.D., Bauer, G.E. and Quigley, J.P. (1980) Characterization of the conversion of a somatostatin precursor to somatostatin by islet secretory granules. *Diabetes*, 29: 593–599.

Fletcher, D.J., Quigley, J.P., Bauer, G.E. and Noe, B.D. (1981) Characterization of pro-insulin and pro-glucagon converting activities in isolated secretory granules. *J. Cell Biol.*, 90: 312–322.

Freedman, R.B. and Hawkins, H.C. (Eds.) (1980) *The Enzymology of Post-Translational Modification of Proteins*, Academic Press, New York.

Gainer, H. and Brownstein, M.J. (1978) Identification of the precursors of the rat neurophysins. In J.D. Vincent and C. Kordon (Eds.), *Cell Biology of Hypothalamic Neurosecretion*, CNRS, Paris.

Gainer, H., Sarne, Y. and Brownstein, J.J. (1977a) Neurophysin in biosynthesis: conversion of a putative precursor during axonal transport. *Science*, 195: 1354–1356.

Gainer, H., Sarne, Y. and Brownstein, M.J. (1977b) Biosynthesis and axonal transport of rat neurohypophysial proteins and peptides. *J. Cell Biol.*, 73: 366–381.

Guidice, L.M. and Chaiken, I.M. (1979) Cell-free biosynthesis of different high molecular forms of bovine neurophysin I and II coded by hypothalamic mRNA. *J. biol. Chem.*, 254: 11767–11770.

Holwerda, D.A. (1972) A glycopeptide from the posterior lobe of pig pituitaries. 2. Primary structure. *Europ. J. Biochem.*, 28: 340–346.

Ivell, R., Schmale, H. and Richter, D. (1981) Glycosylation of the arginine vasopressin/neurophysin II common precursor. *Biochem. Biophys. Res. Commun.*, 120: 1230–1236.

Jones, C.W. and Pickering, B.T. (1972) Intra-axonal transport and turnover of neurohypophysial hormones in the rat. *J. Physiol. (Lond)*, 227: 553–564.

Koch, G. and Richter, D. (Eds.) (1980) *Biosynthesis, Modification, and Processing of Cellular and Viral Polyproteins*, Academic Press, New York.

Land, H., Schütz, G., Schmale, H. and Richter, D. (1982) Nucleotide sequence of cloned cDNA encoding bovine arginine vasopressin-neurophysin II precursor. *Nature (Lond.)*, 295: 299–303.

Lauber, M., Camier, M. and Cohen, P. (1979) Immunological and biochemical characterization of distinct high molecular weight forms of neurophysin and somatostatin in mouse hypothalamus extracts. *FEBS Lett.*, 97: 343–347.

Lauber, M., Nicolas, P., Boussetta, H., Fahy, C., Beguin, P., Camier, M., Vaudry, H. and Cohen, P. (1981) The Mr 80,000 common forms of neurophysin and vasopressin from bovine neurohypophysis have corticotropin- and β-endorphin-like sequences and liberate by proteolysis biologically active corticotropin. *Proc. nat. Acad. Sci. U.S.A.*, 78: 6086–6090.

Lin, C., Joseph-Bravo, P., Sherman, T., Chen, L. and McKelvey, J.F. (1979) Cell-free synthesis of putative neurophysin precursors from rat and mouse hypothalamic poly(A)-RNA. *Biochem. Biophys. Res. Commun.*, 89: 943–950.

Loh, Y.P. and Chang, T.-L. (1982) Pro-opiocortin converting activity in rat intermediate and neural lobe secretory granules. *FEBS Lett.*, 127: 57–62.

Loh, Y.P. and Gainer, H. (1982) Characterization of pro-opiocortin converting activity in purified secretory granules from rat pituitary neurointermediate lobe. *Proc. nat. Acad. Sci. U.S.A.*, 79: 108–112.

Mendelson, I.S. and Walter, R. (1978) On the biosynthesis of putative neurophysin-vasopressin precursors in the hypothalamo-neurohypophysial gland of the guinea pig. In W. Voelter and D. Gupta (Eds.), *Hypothalamic Hormones*, Verlag Chemie, Weinheim.

Palade, G. (1975) Intracellular aspects of the process of protein synthesis. *Science*, 189: 347–358.

Pickering, B.T. and Jones, C.W. (1978) The neurophysins. *Hormone Proteins and Peptides*, 5: 103–158.

Pickering, B.T., Jones, C.W., Burford, G.D., McPherson, M., Swann, R.W., Heap, P.F. and Morris, J.F. (1975) The role of neurophysin proteins: suggestions from the study of their transport and turnover. *Ann. N.Y. Acad. Sci.*, 248: 15–35.

Richter, D., Schmale, H., Ivell, R. and Schmidt, C. (1980) hypothalamic mRNA-directed synthesis of neuropeptides: immunological identification of precursors to neurophysin II/arginine vasopressin and to neurophysin I/oxytocin. In G. Kock and D. Richter (Eds.), *Biosynthesis, Modification, and Processing of Cellular and Viral Polyproteins*, Academic Press, New York.

Russell, J.T., Brownstein, M.J. and Gainer, H. (1979) Trypsin liberates an arginine vasopressin-like peptide and neurophysin from a M_r 20,000 putative common precursor. *Proc. nat. Acad. Sci. U.S.A.*, 76: 6086–6090.

Russell, J.T., Brownstein, M.J. and Gainer, H. (1980) Biosynthesis of vasopressin, oxytocin, and neurophysins: Isolation and characterization of two common precursors (propressophysin and prooxyphysin). *Endocrinology*, 107: 1880–1891.

Russell, J.T., Brownstein, M.J. and Gainer, H. (1981) Biosynthesis of neurohypophyseal polypeptides: the order of peptide components in propressophysin and prooxyphysin. *Neuropeptides*, 2: 59–65.

Sachs, H. (1963) Studies on the intracellular distribution of vasopressin. *J. Neurochem.*, 10: 289–297.

Sachs, H. and Takabatake, Y. (1964) Evidence for a precursor in vasopressin biosynthesis. *Endocrinology*, 75: 943–948.

Sachs, H., Fawcett, P., Takabatake, Y. and Portanova, R. (1969) Biosynthesis and release of vasopressin and neurophysin. *Recent Progr. Horm. Res.*, 25: 447–491.

Schmale, H. and Richter, D. (1980) In vitro biosynthesis and processing of composite common precursors containing amino acid sequences identified immunologically as neurophysin I/oxytocin and as neurophysin II/vasopressin. *FEBS Lett.*, 121: 358–362.

Schmale, H. and Richter, D. (1981a) Immunological identification of a common precursor to arginine vasopressin and neurophysin II synthesized by in vitro translation of bovine hypothalamic mRNA. *Proc. nat. Acad. Sci. U.S.A.*, 78: 766–769.

Schmale, H. and Richter, D. (1981b) A direct comparison of the rat and bovine arginine vasopressin/neurophysin II common precursor. *Neuropeptides*, 2: 151–156.

Schmale, H. and Richter, D. (1981c) Tryptic release of authentic arginine vasopressin$_{1-8}$ from a composite arginine vasopressin/neurohysin II precursor. *Neuropeptides*, 2: 47–52.

Schmale, H., Leipold, B. and Richter, D. (1979) Cell-free translation of bovine hypothalamic mRNA: synthesis and processing of the preproneurophysins I and II. *FEBS Lett.*, 108: 311–316.

Smyth, D.G. and Massey, D.E. (1979) A new glycopeptide in pig, ox, and sheep pituitary. *Biochem. Biophys. Res. Commun.*, 87: 1006–1010.

Takabatake, Y. and Sachs, H. (1964) Vasopressin biosynthesis. III. In vitro studies. *Endocrinology*, 75: 934–942.

Valtin, H., Stewart, J. and Sokol, H.W. (1974) Genetic control of the production of posterior pituitary principles. In *Handbook of Physiology, Vol. 7*, pp. 131-171.

Walter, R., Audhya, T.K., Schlesinger, D.H., Shin, S., Saito, S. and Sachs, H. (1977) Biosynthesis of neurophysin proteins in the dog and their isolation. *Endocrinology*, 100: 162–174.

Zimmerman, M., Mumford, R.A. and Steiner, D.F. (Eds.) (1980) Precursor Processing in the Biosynthesis of Proteins. *Ann. N.Y. Acad. Sci.*, 343: 1–449.

Note added in proof

After this paper had gone to press, the complete amino acid sequence of the oxytocin precursor was published (Land, H., Grez, M., Ruppert, S., Schmale, H., Rehbein, M., Richter, D. and Schutz, G. (1983) Deduced amino acid sequence from the bovine oxytocin-neurophysin I precursor cDNA. *Nature (Lond.)*, 302: 342–344). The oxytocin precursor contains oxytocin at its N-terminus, separated from neurophysin I by a Gly Lys–Arg, and only an extra histidine at its C-terminus.

The Neurohypophysis: Structure, Function and Control, Progress in Brain Research, Vol. 60, edited by B.A. Cross and G. Leng

The Neurophysins: Production and Turnover

W.G. NORTH, H. VALTIN, S. CHENG and G.R. HARDY

Department of Physiology, Dartmouth Medical School, Hanover, NH 03756 (U.S.A.)

INTRODUCTION

The study of the biosynthesis of neurophysins has provided major insights on vasopressin and oxytocin production by hypothalamic neurones. The pulse-chase studies of Gainer and his colleagues (Gainer et al., 1977; Russell et al., 1979) resulted in the immunological identification of 20,000 and 15,000 dalton proteins that were possible precursors of neurophysins. Precursor forms were later demonstrated by cell-free translation using mRNA from bovine hypothalamus (Guidice and Chaiken, 1979; Schmale et al., 1979; Schmale and Richter, 1981) and from rat hypothalamus (Lin et al., 1979). The precursors generated by vasopressin neurones in these species are glycosylated (Russell et al., 1980; Schmale and Richter, 1981). Recently Land and co-workers (1982) deduced the amino acid sequence for a common precursor of vasopressin and its associated neurophysin from the nucleotide sequence of an mRNA of bovine hypothalamus. The primary structure of the precursor minus a proposed signal peptide of 19 amino acids is represented in Fig. 1. An N-terminal sequence representing vasopressin is joined to neurophysin through a tripeptide bridge, and the neurophysin is in turn joined to a C-terminal glycopeptide by an arginine bridge. It is likely that prohormones for oxytocin will have similar structures. Because neurophysins represent a major portion of the prohormone structure, we believe they can provide information about the evolution of the magnocellular system, the processing of prohormones, and the responsiveness of vasopressin and oxytocin neurones to different stimuli.

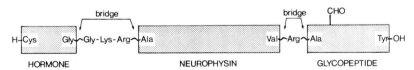

Fig. 1. Schematic representation of the structure of provasopressin from the data of Land et al. (1982). An N-terminal vasopressin is joined to neurophysin by the tripeptide bridge –Gly–Lys–Arg. Neurophysin is, in turn, joined to a glycopeptide by an arginine residue.

NOMENCLATURE AND PRIMARY STRUCTURE OF NEUROPHYSINS

In mammals, vasopressin neurones appear to produce one type of neurophysin together with vasopressin, and oxytocin neurones produce another type of neurophysin with oxytocin. At the last meeting of the neurohypophysis symposium (North et al., 1977a) we introduced a nomenclature for neurophysins which we now put forward for adoption: when a link has been established between a neurophysin and a particular hormone, the neurophysin should be given a name that denotes this association. The nomenclature would be VP-NP for vasopressin-associated neurophysins, OT-NP for oxytocin-associated neurophysins, MT-NP for mesotocin-associated neurophysins, and VT-NP for vasotocin-associated neurophysins. Metabolic derivatives of these proteins are assigned one or more primes, and species or family distinction is obtained by the insertion of a letter immediately before the NP, e.g., BNP for bovine neurophysins. This is the nomenclature used below.

All of the neurophysins so far sequenced have either 93 or 95 amino acid residues (Fig. 2). The N-terminal 9 residues make up a variable region, while the region represented by residues 10 through 74 is highly conserved. The C-terminal region from residue 75 through to 93 or 95, like the N-terminal regions, displays a high degree of variation. However, all of the neurophysins have an N-terminal alanine and a lipophilic residue (Gln, Val or Ala) at the C-terminus. From the evolutionary standpoint neurophysins can be viewed both as components of prohormones and as peptide-binding proteins.

```
                                Vasopressin-associated Neurophysins

                  5              10             15             20             25             30
VP-BNP  Ala-Met-Ser-Asp-Leu-Glu-Leu-Arg-Gln-Cys-Leu-Pro-Cys-Gly-Pro-Gly-Gly-Lys-Gly-Arg-Cys-Phe-Gly-Pro-Ser-Ile-Cys-Cys- Gly-Asp-Glu-Leu-Gly
VP-PNP  ________________________________________________________________________________________________________ _______________
VP-ENP  ________________________________________________________________________________________________________ _______________
VP-RNP  ___-Thr-______-Met-_____________________________________________________________________________________ Ala-___________
VP-HNP  ________________________________________________________________________________________________________ ______-Pro-_____

        35             40             45             50             55             60             65
VP-BNP  Cys-Phe-Val-Gly-Thr-Ala-Glu-Ala-Leu-Arg-Cys-Gln-Glu-Glu-Asn-Tyr-Leu-Pro-Ser-Pro-Cys-Gln-Ser-Gly-Gln-Lys-Pro-Cys- Gly-Ser-Gly-Gly-Arg
VP-PNP  ________________________________________________________________________________________________________ _______________
VP-ENP  ________________________________________________________________________________________________________ _______________
VP-RNP  _____-Leu-______-Leu-Val-_______________________________________________________________-Gly-___________ _______________
VP-HNP  _______________________________________________________________________________-Arg-______________ __________-Lys

            70             75             80             85             90             95
VP-BNP  Cys-Ala-Ala-Ala-Gly-Ile-Cys-Cys-Asn-Asp-Glu-Ser-Cys-Val-Thr-Glu-Pro-Glu-Cys-Arg-Glu-Gly-Val-Gly-Phe-Pro-Arg-Arg- Val
VP-PNP  ____________________________________________________________________________-Ala-Ser-___-Leu-_________ Ala
VP-ENP  ____________________________________________________________________________-Ala-___-Leu-_____________ Ala
VP-RNP  _ ______________________-Ser-_______________-Ala-_______________-Pro-___-Phe-Phe-Arg-Leu-Thr-___ ___
VP-HNP  _____________-Thr-__________-Ser-

                                Oxytocin-associated Neurophysins

                  5              10             15             20             25             30
OT-BNP  Ala-Val-Leu-Asp-Leu-Asp-Val-Arg-Thr-Cys-Leu-Pro-Cys-Gly-Pro-Gly-Gly-Lys-Gly-Arg-Cys-Phe-Gly-Pro-Ser-Ile-Cys-Cys- Gly-Asp-Glu-Leu-Gly
OT-PNP  ____________________________-Lys-___________________________________________________________________________________
OT-ENP  ___-Ala-____________________-Lys-___________________________________________________________________________________
OT-RNP  ___-Ala-___________-Met-___-Lys-____________________________________________________________________ Ala-____________
OT-HNP  ___-Ala-Pro-______-Glu-_____-Lys-___________________________________________________________________ Ala-Gly-___ ____

        35             40             45             50             55             60             65
OT-BNP  Cys-Phe-Val-Gly-Thr-Ala-Glu-Ala-Leu-Arg-Cys-Gln-Glu-Glu-Asn-Tyr-Leu-Pro-Ser-Pro-Cys-Gln-Ser-Gly-Gln-Lys-Pro-Cys- Gly-Ser-Gly-Gly-Arg
OT-PNP  _____________________________________________________________________________________________________________-Glu-_____
OT-ENP  ____________________________________________________________________________________________________________________
OT-RNP  _______________________________________________________-Ser-______________-Gly-____________________________________
OT-HNP  ________________________________________________________________________

            70             75             80             85             90
OT-BNP  Cys-Ala-Ala-Ala-Gly-Ile-Cys-Cys-Ser-Pro-Asp-Gly-Cys-His-Glu-Asp-Pro-Ala-Cys-Asp-Pro-Glu-Ala-Ala-Phe-Ser-Gln
OT-PNP  ____________________________-Asn-_____________-Arg-Phe-________________________-Thr-__________
OT-ENP  ___________________________________________-Leu-Ala-______-Ser-___-His-Asp-__________________
OT-RNP  _________-Thr-________________________________-Arg-Thr-_______________________-Ser__________
```

Fig. 2. Comparison of oxytocin-associated and vasopressin-associated neurophysins from ox (BNPs), pig (PNPs), horse (ENPs), rat (RNPs) and human (HNPs). The data are taken from Chauvet et al. (1981) and North and Mitchell (1981; and unpublished). In each instance identity of sequence with OT-BNP and VP-BNP is shown by solid lines for the other proteins. Residues about which there is lack of agreement are underlined. Only the partial sequences of the two human neurophysins are given.

Changes in genetic expression which have evolved provasopressins and pro-oxytocins from a possible ancestral provasotocin would *not* be expected to involve aspects of the amino acid sequence required to ensure the generation of active hormones. Such aspects could include the preservation of specific peptide bonds that are cleaved by intragranular enzymes and an arrangement of amino acids which gives rise to required topographic features. Conservation of topographic features certainly seems to be important for the ability to bind peptide hormones (Cohen et al., 1979). The highly conserved central region of neurophysins has been shown to be involved in this binding, particularly Tyr^{49} and Gln^{31} (Breslow, 1974; Cohen et al., 1979). Recently, Breslow and co-workers (1982) have obtained convincing evidence that the Arg^8 of neurophysins is also important for the formation of non-covalent complexes with vasopressin and oxytocin. C-terminally elongated forms of neurophysins do not appear to bind hormones (see below) and, as this binding seems to be important for the delivery of quantal pulses of hormone to sites for release, the bonds joining NPs to the C-terminal glycopeptides (or peptides) must be readily cleaved during processing. According to the data of Chauvet et al. (1981), Gln has been rigidly conserved at the C-terminus of OT-NPs, and either Val or Ala is the C-terminal residue of VP-NPs. Although C-terminally shortened NPs have been located in neural lobe and apparently result from proteolysis within neurosecretory granules (NSG) (North et al., 1977b, 1978), glycopeptides that have been isolated from ox, pig, sheep and human neural lobes, and which are probable fragments of provasopressins, all have an N-terminal alanine. Thus, generalizing from the ox structure, it seems likely that the single basic residue joining NPs to these glycopeptides is split out during processing.

Chauvet et al. (1975) have classified neurophysins into two groups: MSEL-neurophysins and LVDV-neurophysins, according to the nature of amino acid residues in positions 2, 3, 6 and 7, and these divisions seem to coincide with the division into VP-NPs and OT-NPs. However, these positions are not invariant within each group. Methionine is at position 5 in VP-RNP, and this would reduce their scheme for VP-NPs to SEL-neurophysins. Moreover, the known structures of OT-NPs reduce the VLDV-scheme completely, as none of the residues 2, 3, 6 and 7 are conserved (Fig. 2). In fact, if we consider residues that have been rigidly conserved in OT-NPs and VP-NPs through speciation in eutherian mammals, and therefore may reflect duplication of an original gene that gave rise to two hormones, only *five* such residues can be found. These are Pro^{76}, Asp^{77}, Gly^{78}, Asp^{82} and Gln^{88} for OT-NPs, and Asp^{76}, Glu^{77}, Ser^{78}, Glu^{82} and Gly^{88} for VP-NPs. Speciation in the eutherian mammals seems to have given rise to 12 changes within the sequence of OT-NPs and to 16 changes within the sequence of VP-NPs.

PROCESSING OF PRECURSORS IN NEUROSECRETORY GRANULES

Neurophysins are packaged into secretory granules in the Golgi apparatus almost certainly in the form of prohormones, and they are generated from these structures during migration of the granules from perikarya to axonal storage sites within the neural lobe. The pH within NSG appears to be between 4.5 and 5.5 from the studies of Morris and Cannata (1973) and Russell and Holz (1981). However, Scherman and Nordmann (1982) have proposed that it could be as high as pH 6.6. Proteolysis that liberates neurophysins (and hormones) presumably occurs somewhere in the pH range from 4.5 to 6.6.

The structure of bovine provasopressin determined by Land et al. (1982) would require that at least four peptide bonds be cleaved to liberate vasopressin, VP-BNP and glycopeptide. A transamidase (or endoaminoxidase, see below) is required to generate vasopressin, the cleavage of Arg–Ala and Val–Arg bonds is required to generate VP-BNP, and an Arg–Ala bond must be split to give free glycopeptide. However, other peptide bonds also seem to be susceptible to cleavage by intragranular enzymes: C-terminally shortened VP-NPs and OT-NPs located in NSG have resulted from the splitting of Phe–Leu, Leu–Arg and Phe–Ser bonds (North et al., 1977b, 1978). The same enzymatic action could account for the C-terminally shortened fragments of glycopeptides located in neural lobes (Smyth and Massey, 1979; Seidah et al., 1981). It is possible that combined actions of trypsin and carboxypeptidase B could yield neurophysin and intact glycopeptide as suggested by Russell and co-workers (1979). However, if this were so, it would be necessary to add to the regimen of enzymes within NSG an enzyme with α-chymotrypsin-like specificity, which would give rise to modified NPs and glycopeptides.

There is an alternative possibility for generating NPs and glycopeptides. Initially removal of hormone along with Gly^{10}, Lys^{11} and Arg^{12} could take place from the precursor described by Land et al. (Fig. 1), to form what might be called a proneurophysin. This glycoprotein would comprise residues 13 through 147 of the bovine provasopressin sequence. Proneurophysin could then be converted to NP by a proneurophysinase (proNPase) with α-chymotrypsin-like specificity splitting the bond between Val^{107} and Arg^{108}. It is even possible that Arg^{108} could be split out of the structure by such an enzyme to give glycopeptide because chymotrypsin appears to exhibit some capacity to split bonds on the carboxyl side of basic residues (Hirs, 1976). The action of this same enzyme would then account for the modified forms of NPs and glycopeptides. Such an enzyme has been described by us previously (North et al., 1977b, 1978; Valtin et al., 1978). It is an acid proteinase showing maximal activity between pH 4 and 5.5. Because this enzyme would seem to share properties with pepsin and renin, we would predict that its activity could be blocked by inhibitors such as pepstatin. We believe we have now succeeded in isolating the enzyme from bovine neural lobes. This was achieved by using an affinity resin, Nα-CBZ-D-phenylalanine triethylene tetramine Agarose, to bind enzymes in an extract at pH 5.0, and the bound material was then eluted at pH 8.0 (unpublished data). Following gel filtration on Sephadex G-75 a protein of 20,000 daltons was obtained as judged by its behaviour on SDS-electrophoresis. Amino acid composition reveals the protein to be rich in Asp, Thr, Gln, Gly, Ala, Leu, Lys, Arg and Cys, with Gln (24 residues) and Leu (20 residues) being the predominant amino acids present. Studies are now being initiated to examine the specific activity of this enzyme.

The evidence required to demonstrate that processing of provasopressin proceeds via intermediate formation of proneurophysin is the identification of a glycoprotein having VP-NP as its N-terminal structure. We have recently characterized such a protein of bovine neural lobes (North et al., 1983a). It represented about 90 % of the glycoprotein in the 12,000–20,000 dalton molecular weight range, and had a value of 16,000 daltons on SDS-electrophoresis. Automated sequencing of this glycoprotein through 25 cycles of Edman degradation showed it to have the N-terminal sequence of VP-BNP. C-terminal analysis revealed that about one-third of the protein had the C-terminal Tyr of intact glycopeptide (Tyr^{147}), while two-thirds appeared to represent a proneurophysin that had been cleaved in the region of Leu^{129} of the provasopressin sequence — a shortened or truncated proneurophysin through loss of a C-terminal fragment. Present as a 5–10 % contaminant of the proneurophysin(s) was a glycoprotein with the structure of vasopressin at the N-terminus, presumably provasopressin. The presence of these glycoproteins and their relative amounts in bovine neural lobes suggests the general scheme for processing shown in Fig. 3. This involves conversion of prohormone to proneurophysin and C-terminally truncated proneurophysins, and the generation from these of VP-NPs and glycopeptides by a proneurophysinase.

Bradbury et al. (1982) have isolated what appears to be an endoaminoxidase from porcine NSG. The enzyme, described by them as an amidase, can convert the synthetic substrate D-Tyr–Val–Gly to D-Tyr–Valamide at pH 7.4 and pH 7. The enzyme removes hydrogen from a C-terminal glycine when it is joined to an adjacent Gly, Val or Phe to form an imino bond which undergoes spontaneous hydrolysis to a C-terminal carboxamide group and glyoxylic acid. The enzyme has a molecular weight $\geq$ 60,000 daltons, and is probably responsible for forming active vasopressin from the provasopressin structure. The evidence to date indicates that Gly[10]-vasopressin must first be removed from the prohormone. It is not yet clear if the enzyme is active at the pHs thought to occur in NSG. If not, it could give rise to the possibility that the intragranular pH changes during the passage of NSG from perikarya to axonal storage sites. Hormone would be liberated from provasopressin at pH 7, and neurophysin from proneurophysin at pH 5.

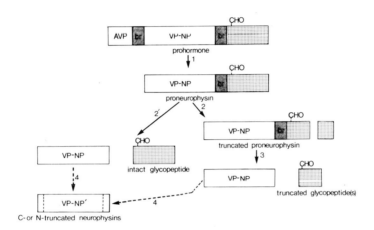

Fig. 3. A scheme for the manner in which prohormone (provasopressin) is processed to VP-NPs within the neurosecretory granules of vasopressin neurones. In this proposal, vasopressin and the bridging sequence (br) from the N-terminal structure of the prohormone are first liberated to form a proneurophysin. This proneurophysin is then either converted directly to neurophysin and an intact glycopeptide, or is first modified by loss of a peptide fragment(s) from the C-terminal end to form a truncated proneurophysin, which is then converted to neurophysin and a truncated glycopeptide(s). Both conversions are proposed. Generated VP-NP can be modified to VP-NP' by loss of N- or C-terminal peptide fragments. The scheme is based on the characterization of proneurophysins, truncated proneurophysins, truncated glycopeptides, and truncated VP-NPs as components of the neural lobe.

NEUROPHYSINS AS POSSIBLE MONITORS OF MAGNOCELLULAR ACTIVITY

In the rat neural lobe there are stored molar equivalents of vasopressin and VP-RNP (VP-RNP plus a metabolite, VP-RNP'), and of oxytocin and OT-RNP (OT-RNP plus a metabolite, OT-RNP') and these 1 : 1 molar ratios appear to hold not only for mature animals, but also for rats throughout postnatal development (North et al., 1978, 1983b). As the major products of proteolysis within NSG are released from the neural lobe into the circulation, the plasma or serum levels of these substances should provide some index of the activity within magnocellular neurones. Of course, this presupposes that the neural lobe is the chief or only source of oxytocin, vasopressin, OT-NPs and VP-NPs found in the general circulation. Wathes and Swann (1982) have demonstrated that oxytocin is present in corpora lutea, but it is still not clear that hormone(s) from this or other origins contribute significantly to the levels found in plasma or serum. On this supposition we have used serum values for OT-RNP and VP-RNP determined by radioimmunoassay, the half-lives of the NPs in the circulation, and their volumes of distribution, to arrive at estimates of rates of release by magnocellular neurones (North et al., 1983b). For conscious Long–Evans rats drinking ad libitum, this approach gave the following rates of production for VP-RNP: 32 pmol/day · 100 g body weight (males) and 41 pmol/day · 100 g body weight (females); and for OT-RNP, 55 pmol/day · 100 g body weight (males) and 81 pmol/day · 100 g body weight (females). These values are similar to those obtained by Pickering and co-workers (1975) for the rates of production of vasopressin and oxytocin in rats based on estimates from pulse-chase studies.

Trained, chronically catheterized rats (Gellai and Valtin, 1979) were recently used by us to evaluate the effects of an acutely administered salt-load on the release of neurophysins from the neural lobe. These animals were subjected to an i.v. infusion of 18 % saline while in the conscious state as well as under anaesthesia induced by ketamine hydrochloride (60 mg/kg body weight) plus sodium pentobarbital (21 mg/kg body weight). Conscious and anaesthetized conditions were compared because certain anaesthetics induce large changes in renal haemo-dynamics (Walker et al., 1983), and because it is possible that anaesthetics influence the release of neurohypophysial principles. Nine male Long–Evans rats (310–425 g) were used. They were each subjected initially to a baseline infusion of 0.45 % saline (20 μl/100 g body weight ·min) for 75 min, and then to 18 % saline (10 μl/100 g body weight ·min) for 60 min. Blood samples were taken at the following times: before infusion of 0.45 % saline; 15 min after initial administration of anaesthetic; at the end of the 0.45 % saline infusion; and at 10, 20, 40 and 60 min after the onset of hypertonic saline. On each occasion 0.7 ml of blood was withdrawn, the plasma taken for study, and the red cells (resuspended in 0.9 % saline) returned to the animal.

In conscious animals, the infusion of 0.45 % saline produced a small but significant decrease (3 mOsm/kg H_2O) in plasma osmolality as well as a fall in VP-RNP plasma levels from 287 to 213 pg/ml (Fig. 4). Values for VP-RNP rose during infusion of 18 % saline, while plasma osmolality increased from 292 to 336 mOsm/kg H_2O (plasma sodium concentration rose from 134 to 154 mEq/l). At plasma osmolalities above 300 mOsm/kg H_2O, the straight line relationship between P_{Osm} and VP-RNP (Fig. 4a) had a slope of 0.123, and a correlation coefficient of $+0.72$. The slope of this relationship is very similar to that obtained by Robertson (1977) between vasopressin and plasma osmolality in human subjects.

Anaesthesia alone produced a significant ($P < 0.001$) rise in plasma osmolality of 5 mOsm/kg H_2O but no change in VP-RNP. In response to the infusion of 18 % saline, anaesthetized animals displayed rates of change in plasma VP-RNP (Fig. 4b) and plasma osmolality that were similar to those seen in conscious animals, with a slight trend for larger rates of increase in both variables at later periods of infusion. Plasma osmolality rose from 295 to 362 mOsm/kg H_2O, while plasma sodium increased from 134 to 166 mEq/l. For the relationship of VP-RNP versus plasma osmolality, there was no significant difference between conscious and anaesthetized animals. These data suggest that, under anaesthesia, the responsiveness of magnocellular neurones to acute changes in plasma osmolality is no different from their responsiveness in the conscious state.

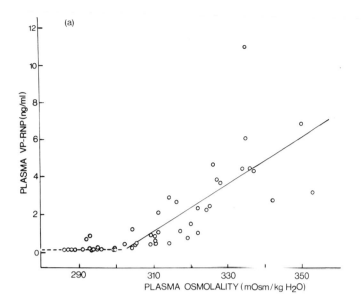

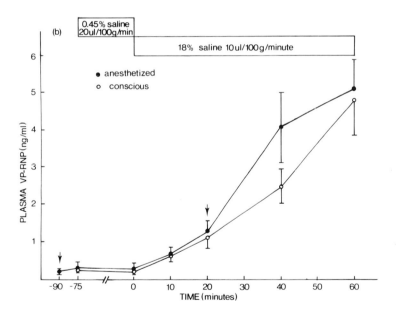

Fig. 4. a: relationship between plasma osmolality and plasma concentrations of VP-RNP for trained, conscious, chronically catheterized rats given an acute i.v. infusion of 18 % saline. The dotted lines represent the limit of detection for the radioimmunoassay used in the study. The solid line is a linear expression of best fit for plasma osmolalities exceeding 300 mOsm/kg H₂O; the line has a slope of 0.123 and the correlation coefficient is +0.72. b: plasma VP-RNP values recorded at different times of i.v. infusion of first 0.45 % saline, and then 18 % saline for chronically catheterized rats in the conscious state (o), and under ketamine and pentobarbital anaesthesia (●). The arrows designate the time when anaesthetic was given. Each point represents the mean ± 1 S.E.M. (n ⩾ 7).

CONCLUSIONS

The study of neurophysins is proving useful for elucidating pathways for the processing of secretory products within magnocellular neurones. Comparison between the primary structures of the neurophysins may provide clues to the manner in which oxytocin and vasopressin neurones have evolved from an ancestral neurone that produced a provasotocin. Processing of a common precursor for vasopressin and VP-NP within NSG may involve the intermediate formation of proneurophysin (after removal of the hormone), which is then converted to neurophysin by a proneurophysinase(s). On the assumption that plasma neurophysins provide an index of activity within magnocellular neurones, it would seem that pentobarbital anaesthesia does not significantly change the responsiveness of these neurones to acute changes in plasma osmolality.

ACKNOWLEDGEMENTS

We wish to thank Teresa Mitchell, Gary Allan and Geraldine North for technical assistance. Miklos Gellai provided helpful advice. This work was supported in part by USPHS Research Grants CA-19613, AM-08469, 5 T32 AM 07301, and Contract 1-CN-55199 from the National Cancer Institute. W.G.N. is recipient of USPHS Research Career Development award CA 00552, and S.C. is a fellow of the Albert J. Ryan Foundation.

REFERENCES

Bradbury, A.F., Finnie, M.D.A. and Smyth, D.G. (1982) Mechanism of C-terminal amide formation by pituitary enzymes. *Nature (Lond.)*, 298: 686–688.

Breslow, E. (1974) The neurophysins. *Advanc. Enzymol.*, 40: 271–333.

Breslow, E., Pagnozzi, M. and Tias-Telo (1982) Chemical modification or excision of neurophysin arginine-8 is associated with loss of peptide-binding ability. *Biochem. Biophys. Res. Commun.*, 106: 194–201.

Chauvet, M.-T., Chauvet, J. and Acher, R. (1975) Phylogeny of neurophysins: partial amino acid sequence of a sheep neurophysin. *FEBS Lett.*, 52: 212–215.

Chauvet, M.-T., Chauvet, J. and Acher, R. (1981) Identification of rat neurophysins: Complete amino acid sequences of MSEL- and VLDV-neurophysins. *Biochem. Biophys. Res. Commun.,* 103: 595–603.

Cohen, P., Nicolas, P. and Camier, M. (1979) Biochemical aspects of neurosecretion: neurophysin-neurohypophysial complexes. *Curr. Topics cell. Regulation*, 15: 263–318.

Gainer, H., Sarne, Y. and Brownstein, M.J. (1977) Biosynthesis and axonal transport of rat neurohypophysial proteins and peptides. *J. Cell Biol.*, 73: 366–381.

Gellai, M. and Valtin, H. (1979) Chronic vascular constrictions and measurements of renal function in conscious rats. *Kidney Int.*, 15: 419–426.

Guidice, L.C. and Chaiken, I.M. (1979) Immunological and chemical identification of a neurophysin-containing protein coded by messenger RNA from bovine hypothalamus. *Proc. nat. Acad. Sci. U.S.A.*, 76: 3800–3804.

Hirs, C.H.W. (1976) Specificity of chymotrypsin for hydrolysis of peptide bonds in proteins and polypeptides. In G.D. Fasman (Ed.), *Handbook of Biochemistry and Molecular Biology, Proteins, Vol. II*, 3rd edn., CRC Press, pp. 212–213.

Land, H., Schütz, G., Schmale, H. and Richter, D. (1982) Nucleotide sequence of cloned DNA encoding bovine arginine vasopressin-neurophysin II precursor. *Nature (Lond.)*, 295: 299–303.

Lin, C., Joseph-Bravo, P., Sherman, T. and McKelvy, J. (1979) Cell-free synthesis of putative neurophysin precursors from rat and mouse hypothalamic poly(A)-RNA. *Biochem. Biophys. Res. Commun.*, 89: 943–950.

Morris, J.F. and Cannata, M.A. (1973) Ultrastructural preservation of the dense core of posterior pituitary neurosecretory granules and its implications for hormone release. *J. Endocr.*, 57: 517–529.

North, W.G. and Mitchell, T.I. (1981) Evolution of neurophysin proteins: the partial sequence of rat neurophysins. *FEBS Lett.*, 126: 41–44.

North, W.G., Morris, J.F., LaRochelle, F.T., Jr. and Valtin, H. (1977a) Enzymatic interconversions of neurophysins. In A.M. Moses and L. Share (Eds.), *Neurohypophysis*, Karger, Basel, pp. 43–52.

North, W.G., Valtin, H., Morris, J.F. and LaRochelle, F.T., Jr. (1977b) Evidence for metabolic conversions of rat neurophysins within neurosecretory granules of the hypothalamo-neurohypophysial system. *Endocrinology*, 101: 110–118.

North, W.G., LaRochelle, F.T., Jr., Morris, J.F., Sokol, H.W. and Valtin, H. (1978) Biosynthetic specificity of neurons producing neurohypophysial principles. In K. Lederis and W.H. Veale (Eds.), *Current Studies of Hypothalamic Function*, Karger, Basel, pp. 62–76.

North, W.G., Mitchell, T.I. and North, G.M. (1983a) Characteristics of a precursor to vasopressin-associated bovine neurophysin. *FEBS Lett.*, 152: 29–34.

North, W.G., LaRochelle, F.T., Jr. and Hardy, G.R. (1983b) Development of radioimmunoassays to individual rat neurophysins. *J. Endocr.*, 96: 373–386.

Pickering, B.T., Jones, C.W., Burford, G.D., McPherson, M., Swann, R.W., Heap, P.F. and Morris, J.F. (1975) The role of neurophysin proteins: suggestions from the study of their transport and turnover. *Ann. N.Y. Acad. Sci.*, 248: 15–35.

Robertson, G.L. (1977) The regulation of vasopressin in health and disease. *Prog. Horm. Res.*, 33: 333–385.

Russell, J.T. and Holz, R.W. (1981) Measurement of pH and membrane potential in isolated neurosecretory vesicles from bovine neurohypophyses. *J. biol. Chem.*, 256: 5950–5953.

Russell, J.T., Brownstein, M.J. and Gainer, H. (1979) Trypsin liberates an arginine vasopressin-like peptide and neurophysin from a M_r 20,000 putative common precursor. *Proc. nat. Acad. Sci. U.S.A.*, 76: 6086–6090.

Russell, J.T., Brownstein, M.J. and Gainer, H. (1980) Biosynthesis of vasopressin, oxytocin and neurophysins: isolation and characterization of two common precursors (propressophysin and prooxyphysin). *Endocrinology*, 107: 1880–1891.

Schmale, H. and Richter, D. (1981) Immunological identification of a common precursor to arginine vasopressin and neurophysin II synthesized by in vitro translation of bovine hypothalamic mRNA. *Proc. nat. Acad. Sci. U.S.A.*, 78: 766–769.

Schmale, H., Leipold, B. and Richter, D. (1979) Cell-free translation of bovine hypothalamic mRNA. *FEBS Lett.*, 108: 311–316.

Schnerman, D. and Nordmann, J.J. (1982) Internal pH of isolated newly formed and aged neurohypophysial granules. *Proc. nat. Acad. Sci. U.S.A.*, 79: 476–479.

Seidah, N.G., Benjannet, S. and Chrétien, M. (1981) The complete sequence of a novel human pituitary glycopeptide homologous to pig posterior pituitary glycopeptide. *Biochem. Biophys. Res. Commun.*, 100: 901–907.

Smyth, D.G. and Massey, D. (1979) A new glycopeptide in pig, ox and sheep pituitary. *Biochem. Biophys. Res. Commun.*, 87: 1006–1010.

Valtin, H., North, W.G., LaRochelle, F.T., Jr., Sokol, H.W. and Morris, J.F. (1978) Biochemical and anatomical aspects of ADH production. In M. Bergeron (Ed.), *Proc. VIIth Int. Congr. Nephrol.*, Karger, Basel, pp. 313–320.

Walker, L.A., Buscemi-Bergin, M. and Gellai, M. (1982) Renal hemodynamics in conscious rats: effects of anesthesia, surgery, and recovery. *Amer. J. Physiol.*, in press.

Wathes, D.C. and Swann, R.W. (1982) Is oxytocin an ovarian hormone? *Nature (Lond.)*, 297: 225–227.

The Neurohypophysis: Structure, Function and Control, Progress in Brain Research, Vol. 60, edited by B.A. Cross and G. Leng

The Structure of the Precursor to Arginine-Vasopressin: A Model Preprohormone

D. RICHTER and H. SCHMALE

Institut für Physiologische Chemie der Universität Hamburg, Martinistrasse 52, 2000 Hamburg 20 (F.R.G.)

INTRODUCTION

The hypothalamic nonapeptide hormone arginine-vasopressin (AVP) is synthesized principally in the supraoptic and paraventricular nuclei of the hypothalamus, together with its corresponding "carrier" protein, neurophysin (NpII) (Brownstein et al., 1980). Within these nuclei AVP appears to be synthesized in magnocellular neurones, where it is packaged into neurosecretory vesicles and axonally transported into the neurohypophysis, to be either stored in the nerve endings or secreted into the blood stream.

Sachs et al. (1969) suggested that AVP and its corresponding neurophysin may be synthesized as a common precursor, to be cleaved by specific proteolytic enzymes into the functional end-products. The common precursor theory was strengthened when it was found that Brattleboro rats with hereditary diabetes insipidus are unable to synthesize AVP and one species of neurophysin (Valtin et al., 1974). Subsequently, this polyprotein model gained further support when precursors to neurophysins were immunologically identified from the hypothalami of rats (Brownstein and Gainer, 1977) and mice (Lauber et al., 1979) of approximately 20,000 and 17,000 dalton (20K and 17K), respectively. Pulse-chase experiments in vivo showed that these polypeptides were processed to smaller oligopeptides of about the size of neurophysin itself (ca. 10K). Moreover, trypsinization of the rat precursor gave rise to an AVP-like oligopeptide (Russell et al., 1979), though no cross-reactivity with anti-AVP antisera could be detected with the original longer precursor.

As in vitro translation systems became available, neurophysin precursors were detected in wheat germ, rabbit reticulocyte lysate (Schmale et al., 1979; Schmale and Richter, 1980; Guidice and Chaiken, 1979; Lin et al., 1979) and *Xenopus laevis* oocyte (Schmale and Richter, 1980) systems which had been supplemented with hypothalamic mRNA. Using specific antisera AVP- and bovine NpII-like amino acid sequences were identified within the precursor without recourse to trypsinization (Schmale and Richter, 1980, 1981a). Antisera and their use in identifying antigenic sequences in longer polypeptides are, however, notorious for the ambiguity that may arise due to problems of cross-reactivity with unrelated proteins. It was therefore essential to confirm the identification of the bovine AVP-NpII common precursor by a means independent of antisera and, if possible, to elaborate its primary structure. Here we outline the steps taken to achieve this aim using tryptic fingerprint analysis and recombinant DNA technology.

[227]

METHODS

The method for isolation of mRNA from bovine hypothalami, its translation in various cell-free systems and the immunological identification steps, have been published elsewhere (Richter et al., 1980). The tryptic fingerprint mapping as well as the cloning and sequencing of the cDNA encoding the AVP-NpII precursor have been reported in detail (Schmale and Richter, 1981b; Land et al., 1982).

RESULTS

In vitro biosynthesis of the AVP-NpII precursor

When bovine hypothalamic mRNA is translated in a wheat germ or a rabbit reticulocyte lysate system, a product with an M_r of 21K reacts specifically with both anti-NpII and anti-AVP antisera (Schmale and Richter, 1981a). The precursor can be labelled with N-for-myl-[^{35}S]methionine suggesting an intact N-terminus (Schmale and Richter, 1981b; Richter et al., 1982). The 21K polypeptide which can be considered as the preprohormone is converted into the glycosylated prohormone, when microsomal membranes from dog pancreas are added to the cell-free system (Schmale and Richter, 1981a). That this proform (M_r of 23K) is a glycoprotein has been shown by several criteria (Ivell et al., 1981): (i) it is quantitatively bound to concanavalin A-Sepharose and released from the lectin on subsequent washing with α-methylmannoside; (ii) when treated with jackbean α-mannosidase, the 23K proform is converted into a product migrating at approximately 19K, comparable to the unglycosylated proform obtained by translation with membranes inactive in the glycosylation reaction (Schmale and Richter, 1981a); (iii) microinjection experiments with the oocyte system shows incorporation of mannose, glucosamine and fucose into the 23K proform. Since neither the AVP nor NpII amino acid sequences contain a typical glycosylation site (Asn–X–Ser or Asn–X–Thr), it was suggested that the carbohydrate chain(s) is located in the cryptic region of the precursor (Ivell et al., 1981). This has been confirmed by the cDNA sequencing data which show that the glycosylation site is at the C-terminal part of the molecule (Land et al., 1982).

Synthesis and processing in Xenopus *oocytes*

Oocytes from *Xenopus laevis* microinjected with an appropriate mRNA are a useful tool for studying processing and modification events occurring during or after translation. When *Xenopus laevis* oocytes are microinjected with bovine hypothalamic mRNA, the synthesis of several polypeptides reacting with both anti-AVP and anti-NpII antisera have been found (Schmale and Richter, 1980). Dominant among these specific translation products is the 23K glycosylated proform. In addition, a smaller product of 14K is synthesized in the oocyte. Pulse-chase experiments indicate that the 14K protein is an intermediate product derived from the larger precursor. Because the 14K polypeptide shows antigenic reactivity towards both anti-AVP and anti-NpII, it was suggested that this molecule is a direct precursor to the products AVP and NpII, and that both are close neighbours in the primary sequence (Schmale and Richter, 1981c).

Besides being a useful "one-cell test tube", the oocyte is also a potent system for studying secretory events, such as the export of heterologous prohormones (Schmale and Richter,

1981b). The major products secreted into the incubation medium are a 25K precursor and the 14K intermediate. The 25K polypeptide cross-reacts with antisera against AVP and NpII and most likely contains a more complete carbohydrate chain(s) than the 23K proform. Co-secretion of the 14K intermediate suggests that cleavage between the AVP-NpII moiety and the cryptic region at the C-terminus occurs within the secretory vesicles of the oocyte. It also suggests that this cleavage site is readily accessible and recognizable by the proteolytic enzymes. Authentic NpII or AVP has been found neither in the oocyte nor in the incubation medium. Most likely this process — proteolysis and amidation — requires a tissue specific set of processing enzymes. It may well turn out that the trypsin- and carboxypeptidase B-like cleavage are directly coupled to amidation of the C-terminal glycine of the AVP. Whether the sequence of processing events observed are comparable to those taking place in the hypothalamo-neurohypophysial system remains to be established. Neither a 14K product nor other possible intermediate candidates, e.g. neurophysin-glycoprotein, have yet been isolated from brain tissues.

Tryptic peptide mapping

In order to obtain further information on the intramolecular organization of the AVP-NpII precursor, [^{35}S]cysteine- and/or [^{125}I]tyrosine-labelled precursors (21K, 23K and 14K) were treated with trypsin (Schmale and Richter, 1981c) and compared by two-dimensional chromatography.

Tryptic peptide mapping of bovine NpII yields nine tryptides, of which four contain cysteine and one of these four also tyrosine (Wuu and Crumm, 1976). Trypsinization of AVP yields glycinamide and the fragment AVP$_{1-8}$, containing two cysteine and one tyrosine residues. In all fingerprints of the 21K, 23K and 14K [^{35}S]cysteine-labelled products, four (spots 1–4) of the nine ninhydrin-stained NpII marker tryptides coincided with the radioactive spots (Schmale and Richter, 1981c). When labelling with [^{125}I]tyrosine alone, only one of the NpII tryptides (spot 4) was labelled, having a slightly altered mobility with respect to the authentic fragment probably due to the iodination (Richter and Schmale, 1983).

Another radioactive spot was evident in the fingerprints of the 21K, 23K and 14K [^{35}S]cysteine-labelled precursors. Whereas this spot was similar for the 23K and 14K precursors (spot 6), it migrated differently in the fingerprint of the 21K precursor (spot 5). Spot 6 was identified as the tryptide of AVP, since it co-migrated precisely with authentic AVP$_{1-8}$ in two different electrophoretic systems (Schmale and Richter, 1981c). Spot 5, only observed in the 21K fingerprint, clearly did not co-migrate with AVP$_{1-8}$; nonetheless, it apparently contained amino acid sequences immunologically identical to AVP, since it cross-reacted with anti-AVP antiserum.

These results pointed to a single unambiguous model for the structure of the AVP-NpII precursor. The key difference between the 21K and 23K or 14K precursor is that the 23K and 14K forms lack the pre-sequence; the AVP-like spot 5 appears to be substituted by AVP$_{1-8}$ (spot 6) when the pre-sequence is removed from the 21K preproform. Pre-sequences, in general, are not separated from their proforms by basic amino acids and consequently not accessible to trypsin. Spot 5 would therefore represent AVP$_{1-8}$ with an N-terminal extension comprising part or all of the pre-sequence. Since the 14K product implies a close neighbourhood of AVP and NpII within the molecule, NpII would be C-terminal to the AVP. Hence the cryptic region with the site of glycosylation should be at the C-terminus of the AVP/NpII precursor. This common precursor model was confirmed later by data obtained from sequencing of the cloned cDNA encoding the AVP-NpII precursor.

Nucleotide sequencing of cloned cDNA

To obtain conclusive structural evidence of the intramolecular organization of the AVP-NpII precursor, its complete primary amino acid sequence was deduced from the nucleotide sequence of cloned hypothalamic mRNA (Land et al., 1982). To this end double-stranded cDNA was prepared by standard procedures from total poly A$^+$ RNA isolated from bovine hypothalami and cloned in *Escherichia coli* 5K, using plasmid pBR322 as vector. Since the proportion of total poly A$^+$ RNA estimated to code for the AVP-NpII precursor is approximately 1% (Richter et al., 1982), the clones were preliminarily screened using AVP-NpII precursor mRNA enriched ten-fold by isokinetic sucrose gradient centrifugation and labelled with ^{32}P. Of the 550 initial colonies, 55 proved positive at this first screening. For further screening a strategy was adopted whereby restriction endonuclease cleavage sites in an unknown DNA sequence can be unambiguously predicted from the known sequence of amino acids. One of these restriction endonucleases is the enzyme *Sau* 96I, which cuts DNA at positions coding for the amino acid sequences Gly–Pro (GGNCCN). Such Gly–Pro dipeptides occur twice in the amino acid sequence of NpII, at positions 14–15 and 23–24. Consequently, DNA coding for neurophysin and digested with *Sau* 96I should yield a 27 base pair (bp) fragment. The analysis revealed that altogether seven positive clones could be identified, five of which carried sequences homologous to the bovine AVP-NpII precursor, and two specific for the oxytocin-neurophysin I precursor.

Plasmid pVNpII-1 was selected for further investigation because it contained the longest cDNA insert (ca. 750 bp) specific for the AVP-NpII precursor. The nucleotide sequence was determined by the method of Maxam and Gilbert (1977). Although a method was used to prepare the cDNA which preserved as much as possible of the 5′ end (Land et al., 1981), primer extension sequencing was additionally carried out to give a complete picture of the 5′ region of the mRNA.

Primary structure of the AVP-NpII common precursor

The amino acid sequence of the AVP/NpII precursor is schematically represented in Fig. 1; it substantiated fully our deductions based on the tryptic fingerprint analysis. There appears to be a pre-sequence of 19 amino acids, directly followed by the sequence of AVP, without an intervening basic amino acid. AVP is, in turn, followed by the triplet Gly–Lys–Arg, and the bovine NpII sequence. The latter is then separated by a single arginine from a polypeptide of 39 amino acids, which contains a glycosylation site Asn–X–Thr at residue 114–116. This glycoprotein, located at the C-terminus of the AVP common precursor, is completely homologous with a protein isolated and sequenced from the posterior pituitaries of several species (Holwerda, 1972; Smyth and Massey, 1979; Seidah et al., 1981). The function of this glycoprotein has not yet been established.

The Brattleboro rat as a model system for gene expression

A detailed knowledge of the mechanism of biosynthesis and structure of a precursor hormone is a prerequisite for any study of regulation. This aim has been established for the AVP-NpII precursor from the ox, an animal which for technical reasons proved well suited for this purpose. To extend these investigations of the expression of the vasopressin gene and its control we are now transferring our techniques to the rat. This animal not only offers a well characterized in vivo system, but also has the great advantage that in the Brattleboro rat, a

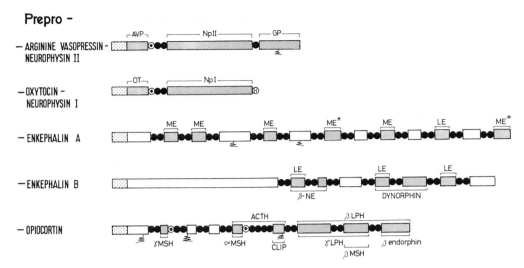

Fig. 1. Polyproteins as precursors to neuropeptides. AVP, arginine-vasopressin; NpII, bovine neurophysin II; GP, glycoprotein; OT, oxytocin; NpI, bovine neurophysin I; ME, methionine-enkephalin; LE, leucine-enkephalin; ME*, C-terminally extended Met-enkephalin; β-NE, β-neoendorphin; β- or γ-LPH; β- or γ-lipotropin; dotted regions, pre-sequence; striped regions, in vivo isolated peptides; open bars, "spacer" sequences; black circles, basic amino acids; open circle with dot, glycine residue; ⤸, glycosylation site; H, histidine residue. The precursors were deduced from the following publications: AVP-NpII, Land et al. (1982); OT-NpI, Land et al., in preparation; enkephalin A, Noda et al. (1982); enkephalin B, Kakidani et al. (1982); opiocortin, Herbert (1981).

mutant exists with hereditary hypothalamic diabetes insipidus (DI rat). Studies have shown that these animals lack biologically active vasopressin as well as its corresponding neurophysin carrier (Valtin et al., 1974). Characteristically, these rats show a high water uptake accompanied by excretion of an excessive amount of dilute urine. It is not known at which level of gene expression the defect occurs.

As cDNA probes encoding the bovine AVP-NpII precursor will hybridize to rat hypothalamic mRNA and to the rat AVP-NpII gene, tools are now available to approach the problem discussed above. Preliminary experiments analyzing supraoptic nuclei mRNA from DI rats either in cell-free translation experiments or by hybridization, indicate a significant reduced level of AVP-NpII mRNA. Exact confirmation, however will have to wait until DNA probes are available, encoding sequences uniquely present in the AVP-NpII precursor and not occurring in the partially homologous oxytocin-neurophysin precursor.

DISCUSSION

The AVP-NpII preprohormone can be considered as a typical representative of a polyprotein (Fig. 1). Like other polyproteins it is composed of several distinct biological entities. The processing of these polyproteins is generated by proteolytic enzymes, a reaction often directed by pairs of basic amino acids. The maturation process can be accompanied by modifications of the biologically active peptide, e.g. amidation of the AVP. This amidation reaction requires a glycine residue C-terminal to the hormone and is found in several precursors to amidated peptides.

The structure of the AVP-NpII precursor indicates, however, that this polyprotein has additional interesting features. Firstly, the hormone AVP is located immediately after the pre-sequence and consequently the latter is not separated from the hormone by basic amino acids. Secondly, NpII and the glycoprotein are separated only by one arginine residue (another example would be the human tumour somatostatin precursor, where somatostatin-28 is also separated from the cryptic region by one basic amino acid residue). Thirdly, it is probable that all three components of the vasopressin precursor are functional units, including the glycoprotein; although a physiological role for the latter moiety has not yet been identified, its high sequence conservation between species would imply some function. Thus, besides processing recognition signals, the vasopressin precursor does not include long "spacer" sequences separating functional units as found in the opiocortin and enkephalin precursors.

The primary sequence information reported here offers a framework for studying the regulation of the expression of the vasopressin gene at various levels. The DI rat model should be extremely helpful in answering how regulation of such composite preprohormones can be monitored at the level of transcription, translation and post-translation.

ACKNOWLEDGEMENTS

We thank Dr. Richard Ivell for stimulating discussions during preparation of the manuscript, and the Deutsche Forschungsgemeinschaft for financial support.

REFERENCES

Brownstein, M.J. Russell, J.T. and Gainer, H. (1980) Synthesis, transport, and release of posterior pituitary hormones. Science, 207: 373–378.

Guidice, L.C. and Chaiken, I.M. (1979) Immunological and chemical identification of a neurophysin-containing protein coded by messenger RNA from bovine hypothalamus. Proc. nat. Acad. Sci. U.S.A., 76: 3800–3804.

Herbert, E. (1981) Discovery of pro-opiomelanocortin — a cellular polyprotein. Trends Biochem., 6: 184–188.

Holwerda, D.A. (1972) A glycopeptide from the posterior lobe of pig pituitaries. Europ. J. Biochem., 28: 340–346.

Ivell, R., Schmale, H. and Richter, D. (1981) Glycosylation of the arginine vasopressin/neurophysin II common precursor. Biochem. Biophys. Res. Commun., 102: 1230–1236.

Kakidani, H., Furutani, Y., Takahashi, H., Noda, M., Morimoto, Y., Hirose, T., Asai, M., Inayama, S., Nakanishi, S. and Numa, S. (1982) Cloning and sequencing analysis of cDNA for porcine β-neo-endorphin/dynorphin precursor. Nature (Lond.), 298: 245–249.

Land, H., Grez, M., Hauser, M., Lindemaier, W. and Schütz, G. (1981) 5' Terminal sequences of eukaryotic mRNA can be cloned with high efficiency. Nucleic Acid Res., 9: 2251–2266.

Land, H., Schütz, G., Schmale, H. and Richter, D. (1982) Nucleotide sequence of cloned DNA encoding the bovine arginine vasopressin-neurophysin II precursor. Nature (Lond.), 295: 299–303.

Land, H., Grez, M., Rupert, S., Schmale, H., Rehbein, M., Richter, D. and Schütz, G. (1983) Deduced amino acid sequence from the bovine oxytocin-neurophysin I precursor cDNA. Nature (Lond.), 302: 342–344.

Lauber, M., Camier, M. and Cohen, P. (1979) Immunological and biochemical characterization of distinct high molecular weight forms of neurophysin and somatostatin in mouse hypothalamus extracts. FEBS Lett., 97: 343–347.

Lin, C., Joseph-Bravo, P., Sherman, T., Chan, L. and McKelvy, J.F. (1979) Cell-free synthesis of putative neurophysin precursors from rat and mouse hypothalamic poly (A)-RNA. Biochem. Biophys. Res. Commun., 89: 943–959.

Maxam, A. and Gilbert, W. (1977) A new method for sequencing DNA. Proc. nat. Acad. Sci. U.S.A., 74: 560–564.

Noda, M., Teranishi, Y., Takahashi, H., Toyosato, M., Notake, M., Nakanishi, S. and Numa, S. (1982) Isolation and structural organization of the human preproenkephalin gene. Nature (Lond.), 297: 431–434.

Richter, D. and Schmale, H. (1983) A cellular polyprotein from bovine hypothalamus: structural elucidation of the precursor to the nonapeptide hormone arginine vasopressin. In McKerns (Ed.), Regulation of Gene Expression by Hormones, Plenum Press, New York, pp. 235–252.

Richter, D., Ivell, R. and Schmale, H. (1980) Neuropolypeptides illustrate a new perspective in mammalian protein synthesis — the composite common precursor. In G. Koch and D. Richter (Eds.), *Biosynthesis, Modification, and Processing of Cellular and Viral Polyproteins*, Academic Press, New York, pp. 5–13.

Richter, D., Schmale, H., Ivell, R. and Kalthoff, H. (1982) Cellular polyproteins from pituitary and hypothalamus: composite precursors to oligopeptide hormones. In McKerns (Ed.), *Hormonally Active Brain Peptides: Structure and Function*, Plenum Press, New York, pp. 581–598.

Russell, J.T., Brownstein, M.J. and Gainer, H. (1979) Trypsin liberates an arginine vasopressin-like peptide and neurophysin from a M_r 20,000 putative common precursor. *Proc. nat. Acad. Sci. U.S.A.*, 76: 6086–60.

Sachs, H., Fawcett, P., Takabatake, Y. and Portanova, R. (1969) Biosynthesis and release of vasopressin and neurophysin. *Recent Progr. Horm. Res.*, 25: 447–491.

Schmale, H. and Richter, D. (1980) In vitro biosynthesis and processing of composite common precursors containing amino acid sequences identified immunologically as neurophysin I/oxytocin and neurophysin II/arginine vasopressin. *FEBS Lett.*, 121: 358–362.

Schmale, H. and Richter, D. (1981a) Immunological identification of a common precursor to arginine vasopressin and neurophysin II synthesized by in vitro translation of bovine hypothalamic mRNA. *Proc. nat. Acad. Sci. U.S.A.*, 78: 766–769.

Schmale, H. and Richter, D. (1981b) RNA-directed synthesis of a common precursor to the nonapeptide arginine vasopressin and neurophysin II: immunological identification and tryptic peptide mapping. *Hoppe Seyler's Z. Physiol. Chem.*, 362: 1551–1559.

Schmale, H. and Richter, D. (1981c) Tryptic release of authentic arginine vasopressin$_{1-8}$ from a composite arginine vasopressin/neurophysin II precursor. *Neuropeptides*, 2: 47–52.

Schmale, H., Leipold, B. and Richter, D. (1979) Cell-free translation of bovine hypothalamic mRNA. Synthesis and processing of the prepro-neurophysin I and II. *FEBS Lett.*, 108: 311–316.

Seidah, N.G., Rochemont, J., Hamelin, J., Banjannet, S. and Chretien, M. (1981) The missing fragment of the pro-sequence of human pro-opiomelanocortin sequence and evidence for C-terminal amidation. *Biochem. Biophys. Res. Commun.*, 102: 710–716.

Smyth, D.G. and Massey, D.E. (1979) A new glycopeptide in pig, ox, and sheep pituitary. *Biochem. Biophys. Res. Commun.*, 87: 1006–1010.

Wuu, T.C. and Crumm, S.E. (1976) Amino acid sequence of bovine neurophysin-II: a reinvestigation. *Biochem. Biophys. Res. Commun.*, 68: 634–639.

Valtin, H., Stewart, J. and Sokol, H.W. (1974) Genetic control of the production of posterior pituitary principles. *Handbook of Physiology, Vol. 7*, Hanover, NH, pp. 131–171.

The Neurohypophysis: Structure, Function and Control, Progress in Brain Research, Vol. 60, edited by B.A. Cross and G. Leng

Harbingers and Hormones: Inter-Relationships of Rat Neurohypophysial Hormone Precursors In Vivo

R.W. SWANN, C.B. GONZÁLEZ, S.D. BIRKETT and B.T. PICKERING

Department of Anatomy, The Medical School, University of Bristol (U.K.)

INTRODUCTION

To study the possible biosynthetic relationships between radiolabelled proteins and peptides isolated from the rat neural lobe we have developed a high-performance liquid chromatography (HPLC) system which, in a single chromatographic step, will separate all the known major neurohypophysial components of oxytocin and vasopressin biosynthesis. Using gel-permeation chromatography, immunoprecipitation and SDS-polyacrylamide gel electrophoresis, we have identified putative hypothalamic hormone precursors and characterized their behaviour on HPLC. With these techniques we have investigated the effects of colchicine, which blocks neurosecretory granule transport, on hormone biosynthesis and have extended our observations on the carbohydrate content of these biosynthetic components.

DEVELOPMENT OF AN HPLC SYSTEM

Although polyacrylamide gel electrophoresis has been used to advantage in the separation of the neurophysins and their precursors, it is not suited to the isolation of the hormones. In fact there has been no technique available whereby all the known components of hormone biosynthesis could be separated simply from one another and this has restricted the usefulness of data obtained from radioisotope incorporation studies. Furthermore, the precision in relating the amount of label in one component with that in another declines as the number of purification steps increases. We have overcome this problem to some extent by using a single HPLC step for the separation of all the known components of oxytocin and vasopressin biosynthesis found in the rat neural lobe (Swann et al., 1982). Using a 5 mm (i.d.) $\times$ 10 cm column packed with Hypersil ODS (5 μm) injected samples were eluted at 1 ml/min in 0.2 M NaH_2PO_4 (pH 2.1) with an increasing gradient of acetonitrile. The HPLC elution pattern of radioactivity obtained from acid extracts of rat neural lobes taken 24 h after bilateral supraoptic injection of a mixture of tritiated amino acids can be seen in Fig. 1(top). Five radioactive peaks can be detected which, in order of elution, correspond to vasopressin, oxytocin, oxytocin-neurophysin, vasopressin-neurophysin and vasopressin glycopeptide. Twenty-four hours after a similar injection of [^{35}S]cysteine all except the vasopressin-glycopeptide are labelled and the vasopressin-neurophysin/vasopressin ^{35}S ratio is about 7.0, suggesting an equimolar relationship between these molecules. The oxytocin-neurophysin/oxytocin ^{35}S ratio is generally higher, about 10.0, which may be due to the co-elution of labelled precursor molecules with

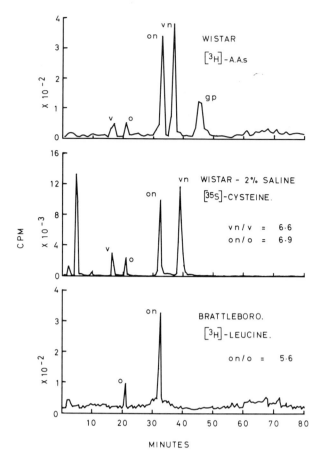

Fig. 1. HPLC of neurointermediate lobe extracts obtained from rats 24 h after an injection of isotope in the area of the supraoptic nucleus. Top: Wistar rats (n = 4) injected with tritiated amino acid mixture (minus methionine and cysteine). Middle: Wistar rats (n = 5) given 2% saline in place of drinking water for five days; [^{35}S]cysteine was injected at the end of the fourth day. Bottom: homozygous Brattleboro rats (n = 5) injected with [^{3}H]leucine. v, vasopressin; o, oxytocin; on, oxytocin-neurophysin; vn, vasopressin-neurophysin; gp, vasopressin glycopeptide.

oxytocin neurophysin (see below). In five-day saline-treated rats, 24 h after [^{35}S]cysteine injection, both of the neurophysin/hormone ^{35}S ratios are about 7.0 (Fig. 1, middle), which may reflect more completely processed material arriving in the neural lobe (Russell et al., 1981).

VASOPRESSIN GLYCOPEPTIDE

HPLC analysis of neural lobe extracts obtained from rats injected with various labelled amino acids has provided considerable information about the nature of the vasopressin glycopeptide which represents the C-terminus of provasopressin (Land et al., 1982). Twenty-four hours after [^{3}H]leucine injection, oxytocin, the neurophysins and the glycopeptide are the only tritiated components seen. The vasopressin-neurophysin/glycopeptide ratio of tritium counts is about 1.25, which is close to what would be expected if these molecules were present in equimolar amounts, vasopressin-neurophysin containing 7 moles leucine/mol while the vasopressin glycopeptides isolated so far (Smyth and Massey 1979; Seidah et al., 1981) have 6–7 moles leucine/mol.

Hypothalamic injections of [³H]fucose or [³H]glucosamine result in a single labelled-peak on HPLC which corresponds to the vasopressin glycopeptide. Similarly, only the hormones, the neurophysins and the vasopressin glycopeptide are labelled in the neural lobe by 24 h after an injection of a complete mixture of tritiated amino acids (containing all 19 commonly occurring amino acids minus methionine, cysteine, asparagine and glutamine). These data would suggest that the vasopressin glycopeptide is cleaved from the precursor molecule as the full 39 amino acid peptide and is only subsequently cleaved to the truncated forms which have also been found in mammalian pituitaries (Smyth and Massey, 1979). However, the possibility remains that these labelled fragments co-elute with the intact glycopeptide on HPLC.

THE CARBOXY-TERMINUS OF THE OXYTOCIN PRECURSOR

When Brattleboro rats are injected with [³H]leucine, a [³H]amino acid mixture or [³⁵S]cysteine and the neural lobes removed 24 h later, only two radioactive peaks are seen on HPLC of their acid extracts: these correpond to oxytocin and oxytocin-neurophysin (Fig. 1, bottom). Injections of [³H]fucose, [³H]glucosamine and [³H]mannose resulted in no apparent labelling of material chromatographing on the HPLC column. Not only have we been unable to detect a glycopeptide component of the oxytocin precursor, but we have also found no evidence for a comparable carboxy-terminal fragment of such a molecule. We are currently investigating the possibility that a small fragment might not be labelled sufficiently to be detected and/or co-elutes with another labelled component. Whatever the case, it is clear that the vasopressin and oxytocin precursors can be packaged and processed with very different structures at their carboxy-terminals.

IDENTIFICATION OF HORMONE PRECURSORS IN THE RAT SUPRAOPTIC NUCLEUS

Sephadex G-75 chromatography of supraoptic nucleus extracts, taken from rats injected directly into the area of the supraoptic nucleus with [³⁵S]cysteine, revealed three major peaks of radioactivity corresponding to 40K (peak B) and 20–30K proteins (peak C), and a third peak in the region of the 10K (peak D) neurophysins. Immunoprecipitation of these peaks with a rat neurophysin antiserum (which does not distinguish between the three rat neurophysins) followed by SDS-polyacrylamide gel electrophoresis, revealed labelled proteins of 21K and 19K in G-75 peaks B and C respectively, while peak D contained 15K labelled proteins. When run on HPLC the 19K and 15K proteins eluted in a similar position to rat oxytocin-neurophysin, but it is not clear where the 21K protein runs in this system. Using antisera raised to oxytocin and vasopressin to immunoprecipitate supraoptic nucleus extracts taken from rats 20 min after an injection of [³⁵S]cysteine, we have found that only the 21K and 19K proteins can be precipitated with anti-vasopressin serum, and only the 15K protein can be precipitated using the anti-oxytocin serum. Thus the 21K and 19K proteins are common precursors to vasopressin and vasopressin-neurophysin, while the 15K proteins are common precursors to oxytocin and oxytocin-neurophysin. Consistent with these observations is the finding that Brattleboro rats contain only the 15K labelled proteins in supraoptic nucleus extracts taken 20 min after isotope injection.

Both vasopressin precursors become labelled by 1 h after an injection of [^{3}H]fucose. As fucose is thought to be added during passage through the Golgi complex (see Munro et al., 1975), this would suggest that these precursors are both post-Golgi products. However, digestion of supraoptic nucleus extracts, taken 1 h after [^{35}S]cysteine injection, with the enzyme ENDO H (which removes only non-fucosylated (i.e. pre-Golgi) carbohydrate groups), gives rise to a new 17K anti-neurophysin immunoprecipitable protein, so that the extract must contain some labelled pre-Golgi material. Neither the 21K nor the 19K protein were substantially reduced by ENDO H, so it is not yet possible to determine if the pre-Golgi material arose from one or other of these components, or from both. Treatment with tunicamycin, an inhibitor of N-glycosylation, also results in the disappearance of the immunoprecipitable 21K and 19K bands and in the appearance of a 17K immunoprecipitable ^{35}S component. Whether the ENDO H- and tunicamycin-generated 17K molecules are the same and represent the common polypeptide chain of the vasopressin precursors is under investigation.

PROCESSING OF HORMONE PRECURSORS

Maturation of the precursor molecules to active hormones occurs, to a great extent, during their passage within the neurosecretory granules to the neural lobe (see Pickering, 1978). By injecting low doses of colchicine into the CSF of rats we have shown (Parish et al., 1981) that blockade of granule movement results in an increase of immunoreactive neurophysin in the supraoptic nucleus which is commensurate with the calculated biosynthetic output. Biosynthesis therefore seems to continue even when granule transport is halted: but is processing going on normally or is there an accumulation of hormone precursors in the supraoptic nucleus of colchicine-treated animals? To test this possibility rats were injected intracisternally with 7 μg colchicine and, after 24 h, were injected with [^{35}S]cysteine directly into the area of the supraoptic nucleus and the animals were killed and their supraoptic nuclei punched out either 20 min or 6 h afterwards. Animals injected with saline instead of colchicine were used as controls. The supraoptic nuclei were extracted in 0.1 M HCl (containing 10μg/ml phenyl-methanesulphonyl fluoride) and chromatographed on an upward-flow Sephadex G-75 column (Russell et al., 1980). Twenty minutes after isotope injection, more radioactivity was associated with the vasopressin precursor in peak C than with the oxytocin precursor and the neurophysins in peak D, irrespective of whether the animals had been given colchicine or not. However, by 6 h after isotope injection colchicine-treated animals had more radioactivity associated with 10K rather than 20–30K proteins when compared with saline controls. Furthermore, the increased 10K radioactivity is accompanied by an increase in immuno-reactive neurophysins which elute from HPLC in the position of authentic rat neurophysins. Processing of prohormones, then, appears to be initiated by the time the neurosecretory granule is formed and will proceed whether the granule is transported to the neural lobe or not. Maturation, in this instance, is a process involving time, not space.

PUTATIVE VASOPRESSIN PRECURSORS: SERIAL OR PARALLEL SYNTHESIS?

The presence of two major putative vasopressin precursors of different molecular sizes raises the question of whether they share a common biosynthetic origin. Six years ago Brownstein and Gainer (1977) were prompted to advance just such an idea to explain the presence in the rat supraoptic nucleus of 20K and 17K putative precursors to both neurohypophysial hormones, suggesting that the larger form gave rise to the smaller. Such a clear relationship does not appear to exist between the 21K and 19K putative vasopressin precursors described here. At no time after isotope injection has it been possible to show that one protein becomes labelled before the other, but rather, when isotope incorporation is followed from 5 min to 24 h, ^{35}S radioactivity appears in these proteins at the same time. It is clear that the 19K precursor is not an obligatory intermediate in the biosynthesis of vasopressin-neurophysin and vasopressin from the 21K precursor.

How, then, do these molecules differ? Immunoprecipitation data show that they both contain vasopressin and neurophysin sequences while the incorporation of [^{3}H]fucose and their binding to concanavalin A suggests the presence of glycopeptide. If this difference is due to the absence of part of the carboxy-terminal part of the molecule, then one should find corresponding glycopeptides in the neural lobe in the same proportion as the parent molecules. Our preliminary data do not support this. Alternatively, differences in glycosylation could be responsible for the apparent size difference. We are currently investigating the carbohydrate nature of both oxytocin and vasopressin precursors as the significance of this moiety is not certain, although an involvement in directing the intracellular fate of these molecules seems quite likely (González et al., 1981).

ACKNOWLEDGEMENTS

This work was supported by grants from the MRC and the Wellcome Trust, and benefitted from the able technical assistance of Peter Rees and Mandy Smith.

REFERENCES

Brownstein, M.H. and Gainer, M. (1977) Neurophysin biosynthesis in normal rats and in rats with hereditary diabetes insipidus, Proc. nat. Acad. Sci. U.S.A , 74: 4046–4049.

González, C.B., Swann, R.W. and Pickering, B.T. (1981) Effects of tunicamycin on the hypothalamo-neurohypophysial system of the rat. Cell Tiss. Res., 217: 199–210.

Land, M., Schütz, G., Schmale, H. and Richter, D. (1982). Nucleotide sequence of cloned cDNA encoding bovine arginine vasopressin-neurophysin II precursor. Nature (Lond.), 295: 299–303.

Munro, J.R., Narasimhan, S., Wetmore, S., Riordan, J.R. and Schachter, H. (1975) Intracellular Localization of GDP-1-Fucose: glycoprotein and CMP-sailic Acid: apolipoprotein glycosyltransferases in rat and pork livers. Arch. Biochem. Biophys., 169: 269–277.

Parish, D.C., Rodriguez, E.M., Birkett, S.D. and Pickering, B.T. (1981) Effects of small doses of colchicine on the components of the hypothalamo-neurohypophysial system of the rat. Cell Tiss. Res., 220: 809–827.

Pickering, B.T. (1978) The neurosecretory neurone: a model system for the study of secretion. Essays Biochem., 14: 45–81.

Russell, J.T., Brownstein, M.J. and Gainer, M. (1980) Biosynthesis of vasopressin, oxytocin and neurophysins: isolation and characterization of two common precursors (propressophysin and prooxyphysin). Endocrinology, 107: 1880–1891.

Russell, J.T., Brownstein, M.J. and Gainer, M. (1981) Time course of appearance and release of [^{35}S]cysteine labelled neurophysins and peptides in the neurohypophysis. Brain Res., 205: 299–311.

Seidah, N.G., Benjannet, S. and Chrétien, M. (1981) The complete sequence of a novel human pituitary glycopeptide homologous to pig posterior pituitary glycopeptide. Biochem. Biophys. Res. Commun., 100: 901–907.

Smyth, D.G. and Massey, D.E. (1979) A new glycopeptide in pig, ox and sheep pituitary. Biochem. Biophys. Res. Commun., 87: 1006–1010.

Swann, R.W., Gonzáles, C.B., Birkett, S.D. and Pickering, B.T. (1982) Precursors in the biosynthesis of vasopressin and oxytocin in the rat. Characteristics of all the components in high-performance liquid chromatography. Biochem. J., 208: 339–349.

The Neurohypophysis: Structure, Function and Control, Progress in Brain Research, Vol. 60, edited by B.A. Cross and G. Leng

The Neurophysin Domains in the Neurohypophysial Hormone Precursors

R. ACHER, J. CHAUVET, M.T. CHAUVET and D. HURPET

Laboratory of Biological Chemistry, University of Paris VI, 96 Bd Raspail, 75006 Paris (France)

INTRODUCTION

Since the discovery of stoichiometric and reversible complexes between oxytocin, vasopressin and neurophysins in mammals (Acher et al., 1955; Chauvet et al., 1960) the suggestion was made that they could be fragments of common precursors (Acher, 1968). The existence of such precursors was substantiated first by the work of Sachs and collaborators (1969) on pro-vasopressin, later by the results of Brownstein et al. (1982) for both hormone precursors, and finally by the identification of the cDNA sequences by Richter's team (Land et al., 1982). Because two neurohypophysial hormones are usually found in most vertebrates (Acher, 1980), two corresponding neurophysins should be identified in each species. In 1975, on the basis of preliminary structural data on mammalian neurophysins, we proposed a dual classification according to the N-terminal amino acid sequences (Chauvet et al., 1975). Using the one-letter symbols of amino acids, we distinguished the MSEL-neurophysins and the VLDV-neurophysins by the nature of residues in positions 2, 3, 6 and 7. The two neurophysins found in a given species differ by N-terminal and C-terminal sequences but have nearly identical central sequences. This distinction has so far been confirmed with seven mammalian species (Acher et al., 1981). It was assumed that in each precursor MSEL-neurophysin is bound with vasopressin and VLDV-neurophysin with oxytocin (Chauvet et al., 1979). This has been directly proved in bovine by cDNA studies (Land et al., 1982; Richter and Schmale, 1982).

Processing of the bovine vasopressin precursor gives three fragments: vasopressin (9 residues), MSEL-neurophysin (95 residues) and a glycopeptide (39 residues) (Land et al., 1982). Enzymatic cleavages occur usually in accessible regions of a native protein and may give separate domains that can conserve their initial conformations. Because the reassociation can easily be carried out between neurohypophysial hormones and neurophysins (Chauvet et al., 1960), it is clear that these fragments have largely conserved the conformation they had in the precursors. In contrast the third domain, that of the glycopeptide, is not found associated in the complex.

THE TWO TYPES OF NEUROPHYSINS

From the investigation of seven species of placental mammals, it can be deduced that in each species two types of neurophysins, MSEL-neurophysin and VLDV-neurophysin, exist in the neurohypophysis. They are very similar in size but differ by the amino acid sequence, essentially by the N- and C-terminal sequences.

Fig. 1 gives the complete amino acid sequences of six MSEL-neurophysins, namely those of sheep, ox, pig, horse, whale and rat. It is clear that there is virtually no substitution in N-terminal and central sequences. In contrast, between positions 89 and 95, many variations occur. The MSEL-neurophysins have usually 95 residues except those of rat (Chauvet et al., 1981) and man (Chauvet et al., 1982), which are slightly shorter (93 residues). A tandem of two arginine residues precedes the C-terminal residue except in rat protein.

Fig. 2 shows the complete amino acid sequences of four VLDV-neurophysins, namely those of pig, ox, horse and rat. These neurophysins have 93 residues. Again most of the substitutions are concentrated in the C-terminal part, between positions 80 and 93. There is no basic residues near the C-terminal residues.

The fourteen half-cystine residues are in the same locations in the two families of neurophysins so that it can be assumed that the seven disulfide bridges are identical.

When the two types of neurophysins are compared (Fig. 3), it appears that they differ essentially by the N-terminal (sequence 1–9) and C-terminal (sequence 75–95) parts but the central region (sequence 10–74) is virtually constant within the families and between the families. Because each type of neurophysin can bind either oxytocin or vasopressin, the hormone-binding site has often been located in this constant region (Breslow, 1974).

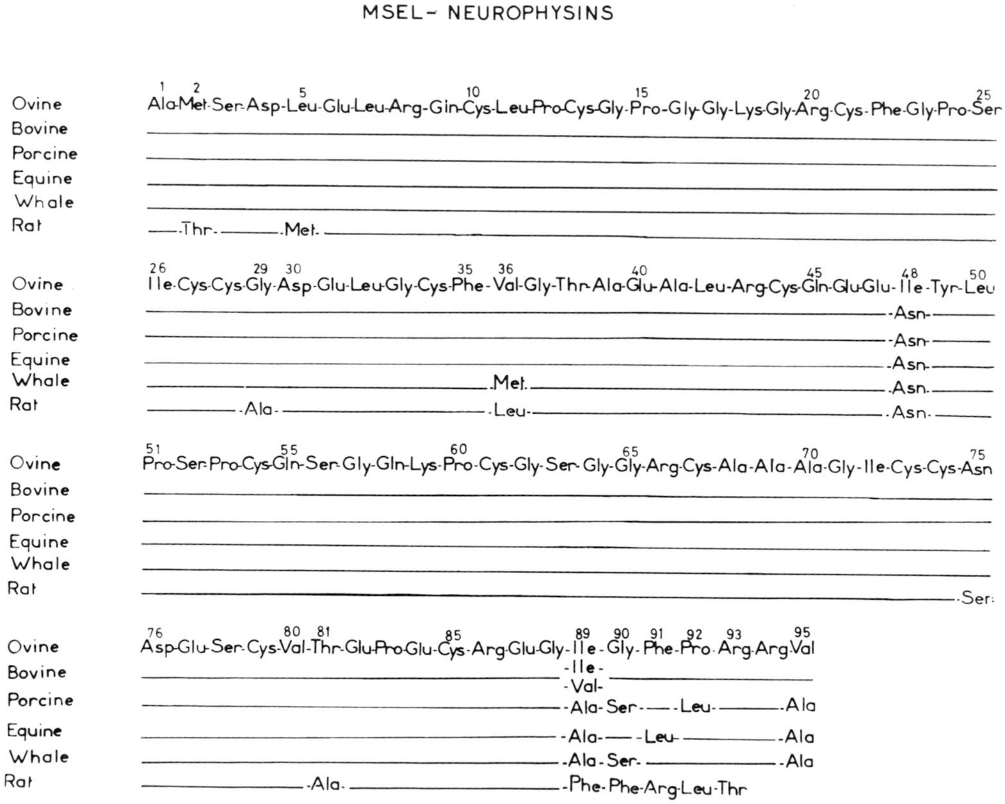

MSEL- NEUROPHYSINS

Fig. 1. The family of MSEL-neurophysins. Residues identical with those of ovine MSEL-neurophysins are indicated by solid lines.

VLDV-NEUROPHYSINS

```
          1 2         5     7     9 10           15                       20                   25
Porcine   Ala.Val.Leu.Asp.Leu.Asp.Val.Arg.Lys.Cys.Leu.Pro.Cys.Gly.Pro.Gly.Gly.Lys.Gly.Arg.Cys.Phe.Gly.Pro.Ser
Bovine    ---------------------------.Thr.------------------------------------------------------------------
Equine    ---.Ala.------------------------------------------------------------------------------------------
Rat       ---.Ala.---------------.Met.--------------------------------------------------------------------

          26      29  30                 35                 40                  45                     50
Porcine   Ile.Cys.Cys.Gly.Asp.Glu.Leu.Gly.Cys.Phe.Val.Gly.Thr.Ala.Glu.Ala.Leu.Arg.Cys.Gln.Glu.Glu.Asn.Tyr.Leu
Bovine    --------------------------------------------------------------------------------------------------
Equine    --------------------------------------------------------------------------------------------------
Rat       -----------.Ala.----------------------------------------------------------------------------------

          51              55                 60                  64  65              69  70              75
Porcine   Pro.Ser.Pro.Cys.Gln.Ser.Gly.Gln.Lys.Pro.Cys.Gly.Ser.Glu.Gly.Arg.Cys.Ala.Ala.Ala.Gly.Ile.Cys.Cys.Asn
Bovine    -------------------------------------------------.Gly.------------------------------------.Ser
Equine    -------------------------------------------------.Gly.------------------------------------.Ser
Rat       -------------------------------------------------.Gly.------------.Thr.-------------------.Ser

          76              80  81          84  85  86  87      89  90          93
Porcine   Pro.Asp.Gly.Cys.Arg.Phe.Asp.Pro.Ala.Cys.Asp.Pro.Glu.Ala.Thr.Phe.Ser.Gln
Bovine    ---------------.His.Glu.------------------------------.Ala.------------
Equine    ---------------.Leu.Ala.--------.Ser.---.His.Asp------.Ala.------------
Rat       -------------------.Thr.--------------------------.Ser.Ala.------------
```

Fig. 2. The family of VLDV-neurophysins. Residues identical with those of porcine VLDV-neurophysins are indicated by solid lines.

The last part of the sequence (residues 89–95) seems hypervariable. This part could be involved in the processing mechanism of the vasopressin precursor since only an arginine residue separates MSEL-neurophysin from the glycopeptide (Land et al., 1982). In contrast there is no additional peptide in the bovine oxytocin precursor (Richter and Schmale, 1982) and VLDV-neurophysins have very different C terminal sequences. There is about 80% homology between the two neurophysins of a given species.

CONFORMATION OF NEUROPHYSINS

The conformation of neurophysins seems unusual. It was first believed that the molecule is compact because of the presence of 7 disulfide bridges for 93–95 residues. However the accessibility to proteolytic enzymes on the one hand, and to reducing agents on the other, suggests an extended or extendable conformation. When native ovine MSEL-neurophysin was subjected to trypsin proteolysis in 0.1 M ammonium bicarbonate buffer, pH 8.0, virtually all the susceptible arginyl or lysyl bonds were split, as shown by peptide mapping (Chauvet et al., 1976), in the same way as for the protein unfolded by reduction or oxidation. This suggests that the susceptible bonds are exposed in the native state.

On the other hand, when ovine MSEL-neurophysin was submitted to reduction with dithiothreitol in the absence of urea and the resulting cysteine residues alkylated with iodoacetamide, it was observed, by mapping tryptic peptides, that the seven disulfide bridges were readily opened (Chauvet et al., 1976). Complete reduction of all the disulfide bridges is not observed in globular proteins in the absence of an unfolder such as urea and this suggests again that all the disulfide bridges are very exposed in neurophysins. These results could be

244

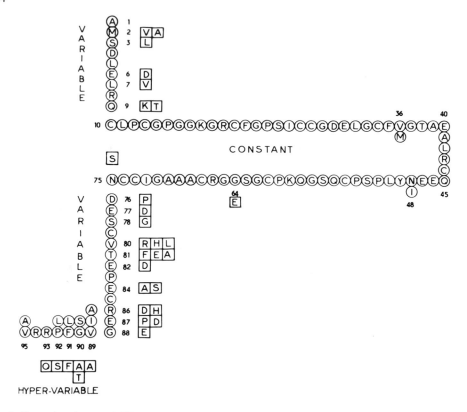

Fig. 3. Comparison between MSEL- and VLDV-neurophysins. Circles: residues of MSEL-neurophysins (substitutions in the family shown as adjacent circles). Squares: residues of VLDV-neurophysins *different* from those of MSEL-neurophysins (substitutions in the family shown as adjacent squares). The central sequence (residues 10–75) is nearly invariant within the families and between the families.

explained by an extended conformation or a flexible and easily extendable conformation. An analysis of the far-ultraviolet circular dichroism spectrum of bovine MSEL-neurophysin (neurophysin II) has shown that this protein has 40% β-structure and only about 5% α-helix (Breslow, 1974). A flat conformation built with β-sheet could explain the great accessibility of various bonds to enzymes and reagents and also a possible dimerization.

THE THREE DOMAINS OF THE VASOPRESSIN PRECURSOR

Because the oxytocin and vasopressin precursors isolated from hypothalamus by Brownstein et al. (1982) have a molecular weight of about 17,000–20,000 daltons, whereas the sum of the molecular weights of a neurohypophysial hormone and a neurophysin is about 11,000 daltons, additional peptides should also be components of the precursors. In the case of vasopressin precursor, which is glycosylated (Brownstein et al., 1982), a previously characterized glycopeptide isolated from pituitary glands (Seidah et al., 1981; Smyth and Massey, 1979) has been found to arise from the C-terminal part of the precursor (Land et al., 1982). Apparently the 20K vasopressin precursor is dissected by processing proteolytic enzymes, mainly into three fragments that must correspond to three distinct domains in the native protein

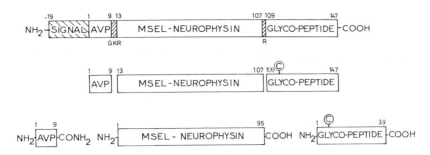

Fig. 4. The three domains of vasopressin precursor. (Redrawn from Land et al., 1982.) Negative numbering is used for the signal peptide removed from the pre-proprotein during the passage of the rough endoplasmic reticulum membrane. One-letter symbols (G, glycine; K, lysine; R, arginine) are employed for residues separating the arginine-vasopressin domain (AVP) from the MSEL-neurophysin domain and this latter from the glycopeptide domain. It is assumed that processing enzymes split after the arginine residues (R) and the connecting residues are removed by a carboxypeptidase B. For vasopressin, the amino group of the connecting glycine (G) gives the amide group (NH_2) possibly through dehydrogenation by a specific enzyme.

(Fig. 4) (Land et al., 1982; Russell et al., 1979). The conformation of the precursor, determined by the structural gene, must be built in such a way that processing enzymes can have access to the specific bonds. These processing enzymes seem to cleave either after a pair of basic amino acid residues (Peng Loh and Gainer, 1982) or after a single basic residue (trypsin-like proteinases). An enzyme of the first type is likely to be involved in the separation of the vasopressin domain from the MSEL-neurophysin domain by splitting after a Lys–Arg sequence (residues 10 and 11 of the precursor). This enzyme does not split after the Arg–Arg sequence found in positions 93 and 94 of the MSEL-neurophysin probably because of inaccessibility. On the other hand a trypsin-like enzyme splits after the arginine residue separating MSEL-neurophysin from the glycopeptide (residue 108 of the precursor) and apparently does not after the many other basic residues of the precursor, again probably for steric hindrance.

Study on the three-dimensional structures of neurohypophysial hormones and neurophysins through X-ray crystallography has not been successful up to now because of the instability of the crystals. However the complex between arginine vasopressin and MSEL-neurophysin, i.e. the association between the first two domains of the vasopressin precursor, could give better results by mutual stabilization. Recently crystals appropriate for X-ray investigation have been made by complexing porcine or bovine MSEL-neurophysin with Tyr–Phe amide (Pitts et al., 1980), or Phe Tyr amide (Yoo et al., 1979) respectively. The dipeptide Tyr–Phe corresponds to residues 2 and 3 of arginine- or lysine-vasopressins. Elucidation of the conformation of these binary complexes could give information not only on the mutual binding sites but also on the processing mechanism.

REFERENCES

Acher, R. (1968) Neurophysin and neurohypophysial hormones. *Proc. roy. Soc. B*, 170: 7–16.
Acher, R. (1980) Molecular evolution of biologically active polypeptides *Proc. roy. Soc. B*, 210: 21–43.
Acher, R., Manoussos, G. and Olivry, G. (1955) Sur les relations entre l'ocytocine et la vasopressine d'une part et la proteine de van Dyke d'autre part. *Biochim. biophys. Acta*, 16: 155–156.
Acher, R., Chauvet, J. and Chauvet, M.T. (1981) Neurohypophysial hormones and neurophysins: structures, precursors and evolution. In F. de Las Heras and S. Vega (Eds.), *Medicinal Chemistry Advances*, Pergamon Press, Oxford, pp. 473–485.

Breslow, E. (1974) The Neurophysins. In A. Meister (Ed.), *Advances in Enzymology, Vol. 40,* John Wiley, New York, pp. 271–333.

Brownstein, M., Russell, J. and Gainer, H. (1982) Biosynthesis of posterior pituitary hormones. In W.F. Gangong and L. Martini (Eds.), *Frontiers in Neuroendocrinology, Vol. 7,* Raven Press, New York, pp. 31-43.

Chauvet, J., Lenci, M.T. and Acher, R. (1960) L'ocytocine et la vasopressine du mouton: reconstitution d'un complexe hormonal actif. *Biochim. biophys. Acta,* 38: 266–272.

Chauvet, M.T., Chauvet, J. and Acher, R. (1975) Phylogeny of neurophysins: partial amino acid sequence of a sheep neurophysin. *FEBS Lett.,* 52: 212–215.

Chauvet, M.T., Chauvet, J. and Acher, R. (1976) Non-compact conformation of ovine MSEL-neurophysin. *FEBS. Lett.,* 71: 96–98.

Chauvet, M.T., Chauvet, J., Acher, R. and Robinson, A. (1979) Identification of MSEL and VLDV neurophysins in human pituitary gland. *FEBS. Lett.,* 101: 391–394.

Chauvet, M.T., Chauvet, J. and Acher, R. (1981) Identification of rat neurophysins; complete amino acid sequences of MSEL- and VLDV-neurophysins. *Biochem. Biophys. Res. Commun.,* 103: 595–603.

Chauvet, M.T., Hurpet, D., Chauvet, J. and Acher, R. (1982) The neurophysin domain of human vasopressin precursor. *FEBS. Lett.,* 143: 183–187.

Land, H., Schutz, G., Schmale, H. and Richter, D. (1982) Nucleotide sequence of cloned cDNA encoding bovine arginine vasopressin-neurophysin II precursor. *Nature (Lond.),* 295: 299–303.

Peng Loh, Y. and Gainer, H. (1982) Characterisation of pro-opiocortin-converting activity in purified secretory granules from rat pituitary neurointermediate lobe. *Proc. nat. Acad. Sci. U.S.A.,* 79: 108–112.

Pitts, J.E., Wood, S.P., Hearn, L., Tickle, I.J., Wu, C.W., Blundell, T.L. and Robinson, I.C.A.F. (1980) Crystallisation and preliminary crystallographic data of porcine neurophysin I–Tyr–Phe–NH_2 complex. *FEBS Lett.,* 121: 41–43.

Richter, D. and Schmale, H. (1982) A cellular polyprotein from bovine hypothalamus: the structure of the arginine vasopressin (AVP) neurophysins II (NPII) precursor. In *Abstracts, 12th International Congress of Biochemistry,* p. 150.

Russell, J.T., Brownstein, M. and Gainer, H. (1979) Trypsin liberates an arginine vasopressin-like peptide and neurophysin from a M_r 20,000 putative common precursor. *Proc. nat. Acad. Sci. U.S.A.,* 76: 6086–6090.

Sachs, H., Fawcett, P., Takabatake, Y. and Portanova, R. (1969) Biosynthesis and release of vasopressin and neurophysin. *Rec. Progr. Horm. Res.,* 25: 447–492.

Seidah, N.G., Benjannet, S. and Chrétien, M. (1981) The complete sequence of a novel human pituitary glycopeptide homologous to pig posterior pituitary glycopeptide. *Biochem. Biophys. Res. Commun.,* 100: 901–907.

Smyth, D.G. and Massey, D.E. (1979) A new glycopeptide in pig, ox and sheep pituitary. *Biochem. Biophys. Res. Commun.,* 87: 1006–1010.

Yoo, C.S., Wang, B.C., Sax, M. and Breslow, E. (1979) Crystals of a bovine neurophysin II–dipeptide amide complex. *J. molec. Biol.,* 127: 241–242.

The Neurohypophysis: Structure, Function and Control, Progress in Brain Research, Vol. 60, edited by B.A. Cross and G. Leng
© *1983 Elsevier Science Publishers B.V.*

Human Pituitary Neurophysin Precursors

J.G. VERBALIS and A.G. ROBINSON

University of Pittsburgh, Pittsburgh, PA 15261 (U.S.A.)

Based on the model of intragranular processing of precursor molecules to their respective neurophysins and neurohypophysial hormones during the axonal transport of granules from the hypothalamus to the pituitary (Sachs and Takabatake, 1964; Gainer et al., 1977), one would predict that some incompletely processed precursor forms might be stored within the neurosecretory granules of the neurohypophysis. Our initial finding that 4–12 % of the extracted neurophysin immunoreactivity from human pituitaries ran in the 17–20,000 dalton region by SDS-PAGE (Verbalis and Robinson, 1982) prompted further studies of the high molecular weight neurophysins found in human neurohypophyseal tissue.

Sephadex G-75 gel filtration of acid extracts of desiccated human posterior pituitaries in the presence of 6 M urea revealed four distinct peaks of neurophysin immunoreactivity (Fig. 1): Peak # 4 — the normal neurophysin peak which coeluted with [^{125}I]NSN — ran in the 10,000 dalton region by SDS-PAGE, and accounted for 80–90 % of the total neurophysin activity; Peak # 3 — directly preceding the normal neurophysin peak — ran predominantly (> 90 %) in the 19–20,000 dalton region by SDS-PAGE, and represented 10–16 % of the total neurophysin activity; Peak # 2 — a small peak which often appeared as a shoulder on the ascending limb of peak # 3 and was better separated using the sodium chloride-precipitated protein fraction from the initial acid extract — ran in the 26–30,000 dalton region by SDS-PAGE but with significant peaks in the 10,000 and 20,000 dalton regions as well, and represented < 1–2 % of the total neurophysin activity; Peak # 1 — the void volume (V_o) fraction which contained 2–3 % of the extracted neurophysin activity. In none of these peaks except # 1, the V_o fraction, was there any vasopressin (AVP) or oxytocin (OT) by radioimmunoassay, but a large peak of AVP and OT eluted after the 10,000 dalton neurophysin peak. When a crude extract of human neurohypophysial tissue was enriched with iodinated neurophysins, > 99 % of the γ radioactivity coeluted with the 10,000 dalton neurophysin peak, arguing against artifactual in vitro aggregation producing these higher molecular weight neurophysins.

Because numerous studies have shown a molecular weight of ≈ 20,000 daltons for neurophysin-AVP precursor molecules (Guidice and Chaiken, 1979; Lin et al., 1979; Russell et al., 1980; Land et al., 1982), the Peak # 3 neurophysins were isolated by affinity chromatography using anti-human neurophysin gamma globulin coupled to AH-Sepharose. This purified neurophysin fraction was stable to heating in the presence of SDS and reducing agents (100° C × 5 min in 1 % SDS, 40 mM dithiothreitol), but following short incubations with chymotrypsin the 20,000 dalton neurophysin immunoreactivity was partially converted to a 10,000 dalton form along with generation of increased AVP immunoreactivity. While this pattern is qualitatively similar to proteolysis of putative common precursor molecules from

248

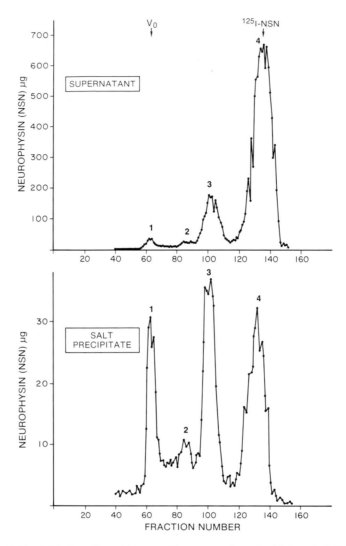

Fig. 1. Sephadex G-75 gel filtration of an acid extract of human neurohypophysial tissue in 0.1 M formic acid, 6 M urea. Top: the NSN elution pattern of the supernatant. Bottom: the NSN elution pattern of the NaCl-precipitated proteins. The four identified peaks of neurophysin activity are labelled sequentially on each panel.

other species, not all of the 20,000 dalton neurophysin activity was enzymatically converted to the 10,000 dalton form following short periods of proteolysis (quantification of longer enzymatic incubations is difficult since neurophysin immunoreactivity is progressively destroyed), and the AVP immunoreactivity generated was only $\approx 20\%$ of that expected on a molar ratio basis (although it is not known whether the cleaved AVP-like fragments possess normal AVP activity by our radioimmunoassay). Nonetheless, the data suggest that at least some fraction of the 20,000 dalton neurophysin immunoreactivity in human pituitaries represents incompletely processed precursor molecules, specifically propressophysin. However, unlike in the rat (Gainer et al., 1977) and in human lung cancer tissue (Yamaji et al., 1981), this pituitary neurophysin immunoreactivity showed no adsorption on concanavalin A affinity chromatography, suggesting the possibility that the propressophysin extracted from human pituitary tissue is deglycosylated. Proteolysis of the crude protein peak containing 26–30,000 dalton neurophysins yielded similar results, but its characterization as a precursor molecule remains uncertain at this time because of our inability to purify the 26–30,000 dalton form free from accompanying 10,000 and 20,000 dalton neurophysin activity.

To overcome some of the limitations inherent in the study of human post-mortem tissue, in vivo labelling studies were done in monkeys. Following L-[^{35}S]cysteine infusion into the lateral ventricles of dehydrated monkeys for 4–6 h, acid extracts of the posterior pituitary and hypothalamus were subjected to affinity chromatography using AH-Sepharose-coupled anti-human neurophysin gamma globulin and then analyzed by SDS-PAGE (Fig. 2). In both the hypothalamus and pituitary > 80 % of the affinity purified counts were found in the 10,000 dalton region, but 13–14 % of the counts ran in the 20,000 dalton and 4–6 % in the 25–26,000 dalton regions, consistent with the relative proportions of these forms in the extracts of human post-mortem neurohypophysial tissue.

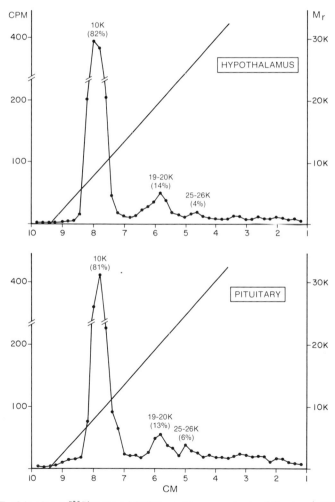

Fig. 2. SDS-PAGE of in vivo L-[^{35}S]cysteine-labelled monkey neurophysins following anti-human Np affinity purification. Top: the hypothalamus-median eminence extract. Bottom: the posterior pituitary extract.

250

Since an 80,000 dalton neurophysin-immunoreactive protein postulated to be a common precursor molecule for both ACTH-like and neurohypophysial peptides has been described in bovine neurohypophysial tissue (Beguin et al., 1981; Lauber et al., 1981), we also studied the human V_o neurophysin peak in collaboration with Dr. Anthony Liotta and Dr. Dorothy Krieger, Mount Sinai School of Medicine. This neurophysin activity remains in the V_o elution position despite treatment with a variety of denaturing agents which would be expected to dissociate simple aggregates (6 M and 10 M urea, 1 % Triton-X). However, heating this material to $100°C \times 5$ min in the presence of 1 % SDS causes conversion of most of the broad smear of $> 30,000$ dalton neurophysin immunoreactivity found on SDS-PAGE to discrete smaller 10,000 and 20,000 dalton peaks coincident with the de novo appearance of a large AVP-immunoreactive peak in the < 5000 dalton region (Fig. 3). Very similar results were found with hACTH and β-endorphin immunoreactivity. Further treatment of the V_o peak with reducing agents (5 % mercaptoethanol) prior to SDS-PAGE completely converted all measu-

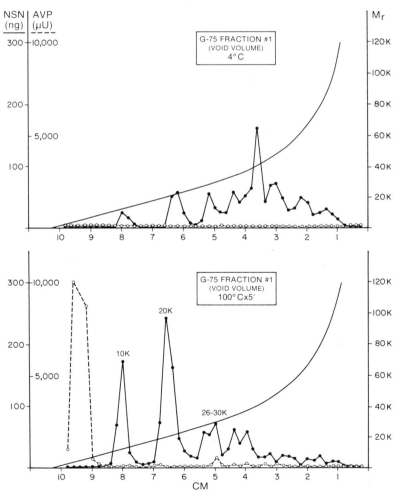

Fig. 3. SDS-PAGE of the human V_o neurophysin peak radioimmunoassayed for NSN and AVP. Top: electrophoretic profile of the unheated sample at 4°C. Bottom: electrophoretic profile of an aliquot of the same sample heated to 100°C for 5 min.

rable > 30,000 dalton ACTH and β-endorphin immunoreactivity to discrete peaks of the normal lower molecular weight forms (hACTH$_{1-39}$, β-endorphin and β-lipotropin), with the exception of a small residual peak in the area of proopiomelanocortin. However, since disulfide reduction destroys > 95 % of neurophysin immunoreactivity in our radioimmunoassays, this treatment could not be used for analysis of the V$_0$ neurophysin activity. These data suggest that in our human neurohypophysial tissue the G-75 V$_0$ fraction consisted largely of heat-dissociable aggregates of neurophysins, neurophysin precursors, AVP, OT, and other peptides including ACTH and opioids, rather than stable covalently bonded common neurophysin-ACTH precursor molecules of very high molecular weight. However, the relative stability of the V$_0$ neurophysin activity to denaturants, combined with our inability to demonstrate simple in vitro aggregation by extracting with iodinated neurophysins, raises the possibility that these aggregates are formed in vivo, possibly representing neurosecretory granule membrane proteins and lipids with non-covalently adherent or disulfide-linked peptides.

Finally, given the presence of incompletely processed neurophysin precursor molecules in the neurohypophysis, we would predict that following appropriate stimulation these forms are also released into the blood along with the normal neurophysins and neurohypophysial hormones. There is precedent for this in other cellular systems employing intragranular enzymatic processing of precursor molecules to final products, such as the pancreatic beta islet cells, where up to 5 % of the granular insulin content is incompletely processed proinsulin (Rubenstein and Steiner, 1971) which is released in measurable quantities into the blood. With the future development of methods to measure the levels of neurohypophysial precursor molecules and cleavage products in plasma, we may thereby gain new insights into the physiology and pathophysiology of neurohypophysial function in man.

REFERENCES

Beguin, P., Nicholas, P., Boussetta, H., Fahy, C. and Cohen, P. (1981) Characterization of the 80,000 molecular weight form of neurophysin isolated from bovine neurohypophysis. *J. biol. Chem.*, 256: 9289–9294.

Gainer, H., Sarne, Y. and Brownstein, M.J. (1977) Biosynthesis and axonal transport of rat neurohypophyseal proteins and peptides. *J. Cell Biol.*, 73: 366–381.

Guidice, L.C. and Chaiken, I.M. (1979) Immunological and chemical identification of a neurophysin-containing protein coded by messenger RNA from bovine hypothalamus. *Proc. nat. Acad. Sci. U.S.A.*, 76: 3800–3804.

Land, H., Schutz, G., Schmale, H. and Richter, D. (1982) Nucleotide sequence of cloned cDNA encoding bovine arginine vasopressin-neurophysin II precursor. *Nature (Lond.)*, 295: 299–303.

Lauber, M., Nicholas, P., Boussetta, H., Fahy, C., Beguin, P., Camier, M., Vaudry, H. and Cohen, P. (1981) The M$_r$ 80,000 common forms of neurophysin and vasopressin from bovine neurohypophysis have corticotropin- and endorphin-like sequences and liberate by proteolysis biologically active corticotropin. *Proc. nat. Acad. Sci. U.S.A.*, 78: 6086–6090.

Lin, C., Joseph-Bravo, P., Sherman, T., Chan, L. and McKelvy, J.F. (1979) Cell-free synthesis of putative neurophysin precursors from rat and mouse hypothalamic poly (A)-RNA. *Biochem. Biophys. Res. Commun.*, 89: 943–950.

Rubenstein, A.H. and Steiner, D.F. (1971) Proinsulin. *Ann. Rev. Med.*, 22: 1–24.

Russell, J.T., Brownstein, M.J. and Gainer, H. (1980) Biosynthesis of vasopressin, oxytocin, and neurophysins: isolation and characterization of two common precursors (propressophysin and prooxyphysin). *Endocrinology*, 107: 1880–1891.

Sachs, H. and Takabatake, Y. (1964) Evidence for a precursor in vasopressin biosynthesis. *Endocrinology*, 75: 943–948.

Verbalis, J.G. and Robinson, A.G. (1982) Identification of high molecular weight neurophysins in extracts of human neurohypophyseal tissue. *Brain Res.*, 237: 504–509.

Yamaji, T., Ishibashi, M. and Katayama, S. (1981) Nature of the immunoreactive neurophysins in ectopic vasopressin-producing oat cell carcinomas of the lung. *J. clin. Invest.*, 68: 388–398.

The Neurohypophysis: Structure, Function and Control, Progress in Brain Research, Vol. 60, edited by B.A. Cross and G. Leng
© *1983 Elsevier Science Publishers B.V.*

Characterization of the "Giant Precursors" (70–80K) of Vasopressin and Oxytocin in the Rat Hypothalamus

G.J. MOORE and J.C. ROSENIOR

Department of Medical Biochemistry, University of Calgary, Alberta T2N 1N4 (Canada)

Putative precursors of vasopressin and oxytocin with molecular weights of $\geq 70K$, $30–40K$, $17–19K$ and $9–15K$ have been detected in the supraoptic (SON) region of the rat hypothalamus (Rosenior et al., 1980, 1981). The possible occurrence of glycosylation of these "precursors"

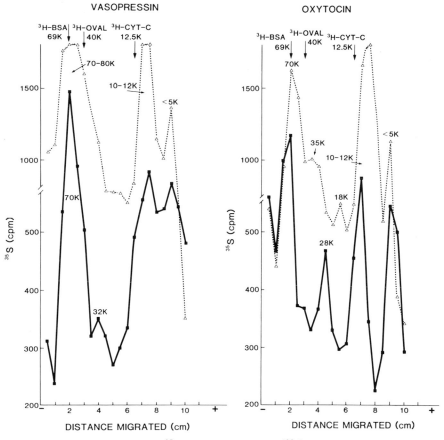

Fig. 1. SDS-PAGE showing migration of ^{35}S-labelled proteins from [^{35}S]-cysteine in vitro pulsed (60 min) rat hypothalamus (SON region) after immunoprecipitation with vasopressin or oxytocin antiserum and treatment with anhydrous HF at 0°C for 30 min ■, HF-treated; Δ, control.

254

has been investigated by treating ^{35}S-labelled immunoprecipitates with anhydrous hydrogen fluoride, and re-examining the molecular weights of the deglycosylated products (Fig. 1). The molecular weights of the largest detectable "precursors" (80K for vasopressin and 70K for oxytocin) demonstrated no significant change in migration on SDS-polyacrylamide gels (SDS-PAGE) after HF treatment, suggesting that these proteins may not be glycosylated or contain < 10% carbohydrate by weight. In contrast, the 30–40K species demonstrated decreases in molecular weight after HF treatment (vasopressin, 40K→32K; oxytocin, 35K→28K), indicating that these proteins contain ≈ 20% carbohydrate by weight. The 17–19K precursor of oxytocin may also be glycosylated, although the small amount of this species detected in this study renders this conclusion tentative. The 20–24K precursor of vasopressin is not detected by our vasopressin antiserum (Rosenior et al., 1981).

Evidence favouring the existence of separate "giant precursors" of vasopressin and oxytocin has been obtained from investigations of their susceptibilities to trypsin digestion. The 80K vasopressin/vasopressin-neurophysin "precursor" appears to be resistant to the action of trypsin, whereas the ≈ 40K species is not (Fig. 2A, B). In contrast, the 70K oxytocin/oxytocin-neurophysin "precursor" appears to be hydrolyzed by trypsin (Fig. 2C, D).

The finding that the 80K "precursor" of vasopressin from the bovine pituitary contains β-endorphin (Lauber et al., 1981) prompted us to examine our rat hypothalamic "precursors" for the presence of endorphin. Whereas immunoreactive proteins with molecular weights of 70–80K were observed for vasopressin, oxytocin and β-endorphin, no evidence was obtained to suggest that any of these species contained more than one of the three peptides (Fig. 3). However, it is possible that immunoprecipitation may cause irreversible changes in the antigenic properties of the "precursors".

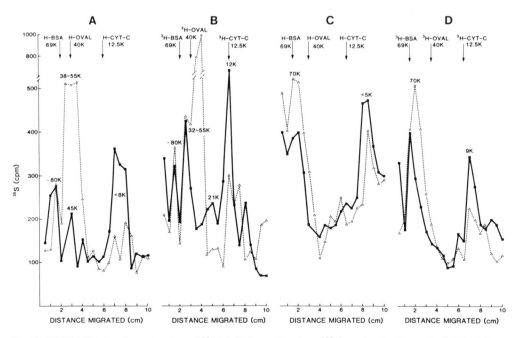

Fig. 2. SDS-PAGE showing migration of ^{35}S-labelled proteins from [^{35}S]cysteine in vitro pulsed (60 min) rat hypothalamus (SON region) after dialysis, trypsin treatment and immunoprecipitation with vasopressin (A), vasopressin-neurophysin (B), oxytocin (C) or oxytocin-neurophysin antiserum (D). ■, Trypsin-treated (0.01 mg/ml at 37°C for 30 min, pH 8.0); Δ, control.

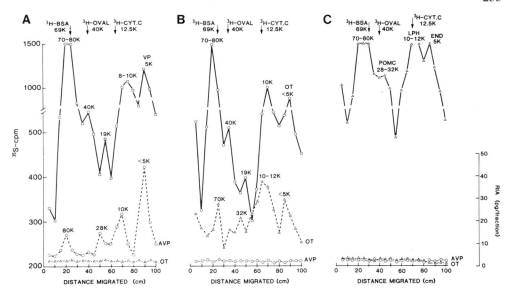

Fig. 3. SDS-PAGE showing migration of ^{35}S-labelled (solid lines) and RIA-immunoreactive (broken lines) proteins from [^{35}S]cysteine in vitro pulsed (60 min) rat hypothalamus (SON region) after immunoprecipitation with vasopressin (A), oxytocin (B) or β-endorphin antiserum (C).

Recent studies in our laboratory indicate that all of these "precursors" are acted on by proteases present in the hypothalamo-neurohypophysial system. Based on the terminology proposed by Russell et al. (1980) for the 19–20K precursors in this system, we suggest, until shown to be inappropriate or otherwise, the following extended nomenclature (Moore and Rosenior, 1983):

Vasopressin/Vasopressin-neurophysin
10–15K Pressophysin
17–24K Propressophysin
32–40K Macropressophysin
≈ 80K Gigantopressophysin

Oxytocin/Oxytocin-neurophysin
9–12K Oxyphysin
16–21K Prooxyphysin
28–35K Macrooxyphysin
≈ 70K Gigantooxyphysin

There is reasonable circumstantial evidence to suggest that the "pro" form is a precursor, whereas the "macro" and "giganto" (from the Greek for "long" and "giant" respectively) forms have not yet been shown to be precursors of the neurohypophysial hormones and neurophysins.

REFERENCES

Lauber, M., Nicolas, P., Bousetta, H., Fahy, C., Beguin, P., Camier, M., Vaudry, H. and Cohen, P. (1981) The M_r 80,000 common forms of neurophysin and vasopressin from bovine neurohypophysis have corticotropin- and endorphin-like sequences and liberate by proteolysis biologically active corticotrophin. *Proc. nat. Acad. Sci. U.S.A.*, 78: 6086–6090.

Moore, G.J. and Rosenior, J.C. (1983) Biosynthesis of neurohypophysial hormones: historical and current events. *Canad. J. Biochem.*, in press.

Rosenior, J.C., North, W.G., Lederis, K. and Moore, G.J. (1980) Studies on precursors of vasopressin and neurophysin in the rat hypothalamus. *J. Endocr.*, 87: 57P–58P.

Rosenior, J.C., North, W.G. and Moore, G.J. (1981) Putative precursors of vasopressin and neurophysin in the rat hypothalamus. *Endocrinology*, 109: 1067–1072.

Russell, J.T., Brownstein, M.J. and Gainer, H. (1980) Biosynthesis of vasopressin, oxytocin and neurophysins: isolation and characterization of two common precursors (propressophysin and prooxyphysin). *Endocrinology*, 107: 1880–1891.

SECTION V

Mechanisms of Release from the Neurohypophysis

The Neurohypophysis: Structure, Function and Control, Progress in Brain Research, Vol. 60, edited by B.A. Cross and G. Leng

Ultrastructural Manifestations of Increased Hormone Release in the Neurohypophysis

C. D. TWEEDLE

Department of Anatomy, Michigan State University, East Lansing, MI 48824 (U.S.A.)

INTRODUCTION

Electron microscopy (EM) of the mammalian neural lobe has been a valuable source of information in the understanding of neurosecretion. Light microscopic work indicated that hypothalamic magnocellular neurosecretory cells contained stainable neurosecretory material and send their axons to the neurohypophysis to terminate. This stainable material (now known to include oxytocin and vasopressin and their carrier proteins) could be released into the blood by appropriate stimuli (e.g., Bargmann, 1949; Bargmann and Scharrer, 1951). These studies were soon followed by ultrastructural investigations, including some of the earliest experimental EM work (Green and Van Breemen, 1955; Palay, 1955; Bargmann and Knoop, 1957; Hartmann, 1958). With improvements in tissue preservation and experience in interpretation, the fine structure of the neural lobe has gradually become fairly well described, though not completely understood. This article will focus on the ultrastructural changes which accompany altered hormone release, with current opinions and speculation about the role of the anatomical elements during hormone release. A more complete review of the ultrastructural aspects of neurosecretion has been given by Morris et al. (1978), which includes a discussion of the compartmentalization and involvement of dense core vesicles, microvesicles and vacuoles in hormone release. Unless indicated otherwise, the experimental results described in this article are from the rat.

AN OVERVIEW OF THE ELECTRON MICROSCOPY OF THE NORMAL NEURAL LOBE

The main components of the mammalian neural lobe are a variety of supportive cells, the most obvious being pituicytes (astrocytic glial cells closely associated with neurosecretory axons), and the varicose neurosecretory axons whose terminals end via "synaptoid" contacts onto pituicytes or onto a basement membrane which lines a ramifying perivascular space (Fig. 1). Some of the blood vessels in the space are fenestrated capillaries which allow released hormone to enter the general circulation. The neurosecretory axons contain the usual axonal organelles as well as 100–200 nm dense core vesicles. Packaging in these vesicles is thought to be the way in which neurosecretory material is transported to the neural lobe for release by exocytosis at nerve endings or for storage in the nerve swellings. Dense core vesicles are depleted from nerve endings abutting the perivascular space by acute stimulation and also from

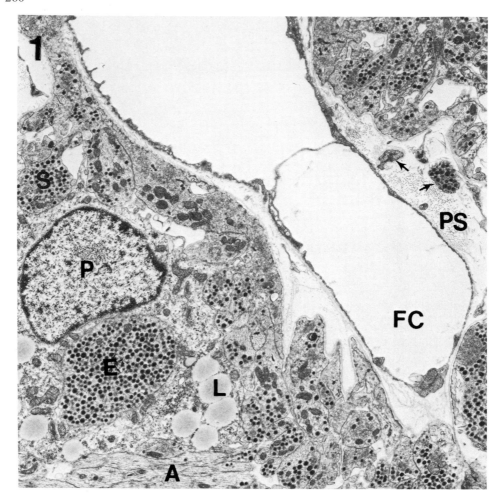

Fig. 1. Low-power electron micrograph of neural lobe. A pituicyte (P) with lipid droplets (L) can be seen to be surrounded by many neurosecretory axons (A) and swellings (S). One of the swellings (E) is enclosed by pituicyte cytoplasm. Hormone is released into the perivascular space (PS) around fenestrated capillaries (FC). A few axons (arrows) may be seen in the perivascular space. ×8100.

nerve swellings by more chronic stimulation. The amount of depletion seems to reflect closely the amount of hormone loss from the neural lobe (Morris et al., 1978). Some evidence suggests that non-vesicular neurosecretory material exists and may be transported down the axon via the smooth endoplasmic reticulum (Silverman and Zimmerman, 1975; Rougon-Rapuzzi et al., 1978; Alonso and Assenmacher, 1979; Dreyfuss et al., 1979; Castel and Dellmann, 1980). The existence of non-vesicular hormone remains controversial, however. The issue may eventually be resolved by better techniques for the EM immunocytochemistry of hormone localization. The large clumps of neurosecretory material (Herring bodies) previously visualized in the neural lobe and neurohypophysial tract at the light microscopic level turned out to be large swellings of individual axons which were full of dense core vesicles. Lysosomes are seen more in neurosecretory axons than in those of other neurones, and particularly in the Herring

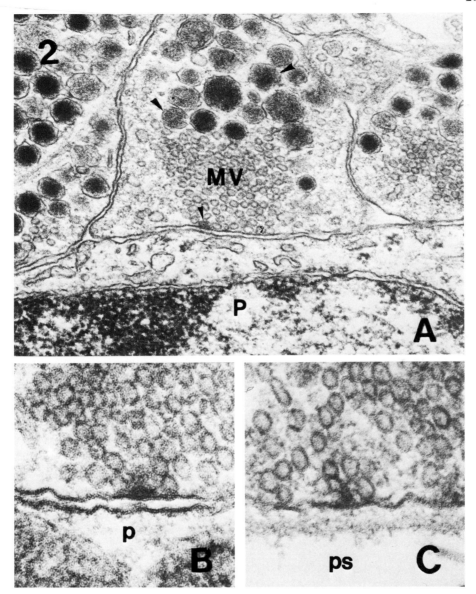

Fig. 2. A: medium-power electron micrograph of a synaptoid contact from a neurosecretory process onto a pituicyte. One can see dense core vesicles (larger arrowheads) and microvesicles (MV) as well as a pre-synaptic membrane specialization (small arrowhead). × 57,000. B: high-power electron micrograph of a synaptoid contact from an axonal ending onto a pituicyte (p). A membrane specialization and microvesicles are seen. C: electron micrograph at same magnification as B, showing the similarity of a synaptoid contact from a neurosecretory axon onto the basement membrane adjacent to the perivascular space (ps). × 145,000.

bodies and nerve endings. Herring bodies may mainly represent a store of neurosecretory material, as in normal rats they contain 60% of all dense core vesicles (Morris, 1976). Autoradiographic studies (Heap et al., 1975; Haddad et al., 1980) indicate that, with time, the labelled material accumulates in the Herring bodies. Stimulation of the neurosecretory system, on the other hand, brings about a preferential release of newly formed granules (e.g., Sachs and Haller, 1968). Thus, under normal circumstances older dense core vesicles tend to accumulate in the Herring bodies. The lysosomes found there may serve the purpose of autophagic degradation of old or unneeded vesicles (Dellmann and Rodriguez, 1970). The most conspicuous autophagic activity has been observed in terminal and preterminal parts of axons during rehydration after osmotic stimulation (Picard et al., 1977) or during recovery from lactation (Rufener, 1973), conditions when one might expect a previously activated synthetic and transport system to be piling up superfluous hormone in the neural lobe. Forty to 60 nm electron-lucent microvesicles are also found in neurosecretory axons, mainly in the axonal endings, and may be either dispersed or in clumps. At least some of these are involved in the calcium homeostasis of the nerve endings (Nordmann, this volume), while others may be a result of pinocytotic activity (Theodosis et al., 1977). The nerve endings have synaptoid specializations: these are membrane presynaptic specializations characterized by accumulations of electron-dense material often associated with aggregated microvesicles and contacting either the basement membrane or pituicytes (across a 10 nm cleft) (Monroe and Scott, 1966; Nakai, 1970; Fig. 2). Their role is unknown but their numbers change under certain functional conditions (see below). They are possibly involved in (bidirectional?) neuro/glial communication as well as hormone release.

Pituicytes lie in close association with the neurosecretory processes and make up 25–30% of the volume of the neural lobe (Reinhardt et al., 1969; Nordmann, 1977). In electron micrographs from normal rats these glial cells commonly have axonal processes indented into, or even apparently surrounded by, their cytoplasm (Figs. 1 and 3). They send long processes out among the neurosecretory axons or to the basement membrane of the perivascular zone where these processes cover that part not covered by neurosecretory terminals (Fig. 4). The cytoplasm of pituicytes contains abundant Golgi bodies, free ribosomes and (in the rat) characteristic lipid bodies. Immunocytochemical staining with antibodies to glial fibrillary acidic protein indicates that pituicytes are astrocytic (Suess and Pliška, 1981; Salm et al., 1982). Like other astrocytes, they are connected to one another by prominent gap junctions which indicate probable sites of electrotonic coupling. Several authors have classified pituicytes into two or more types (e.g., Romeis, 1940), and others into one morphologically variable type (Krsulovik and Brückner, 1969). In our studies we have not found any morphological alterations in pituicyte cytoplasm (including hypertrophy) following physiological conditions of hormone release such as 24 h dehydration, parturition or lactation (Tweedle and Hatton, 1980a, 1982). Wittkowski and Brinkmann (1974) reported the same even following a more profound stimulus (3 days of water deprivation). However, several days of water deprivation or NaCl imbibition can lead to pituicyte hypertrophy, mitosis and a large increase in the number of lipid bodies (Leveque and Small, 1959; Krsulovic and Brückner, 1969; Paterson and Leblond 1977). Such findings led to early (probably accurate) speculation about pituicytes having a role in neurosecretion. However, the particular changes observed may have been a reflection of the pathology created by unphysiological conditions of stimulation.

Quantitative measurements at the ultrastructural level have revealed that pituicyte changes also occur with physiological levels of hormone release. Short-term water deprivation (4–24 h), parturition or lactation significantly reduced the amount of glial enclosure of neurosecretory processes. Subsequent rehydration following the dehydration led to a re-establishment of the glial enclosure (Tweedle and Hatton, 1980a, 1982; see Table I and Fig. 3). The latter data indicate that a day-to-day role of pituicytes might consist of modifying the degree of exposure of the membranes of axonal processes (or endings) to glial membrane and/or the hormone release site at the basement membrane (see below). Following section of

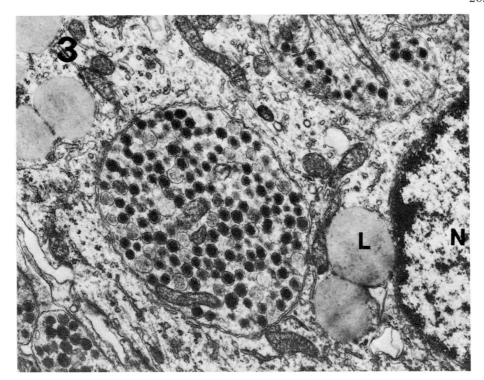

Fig. 3. A neurosecretory process enclosed within pituicyte cytoplasm. Extracellular space separates them. The incidence of these is less under conditions of greater hormone release. A part of the pituicyte nucleus (N) and lipid bodies (L) are present. × 22,600.

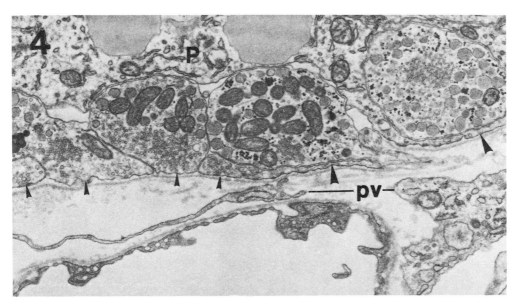

Fig. 4. Neurovascular contact zone showing apposition of both pituicyte processes (large arrowheads) and axon terminals (small arrowheads) to the basement membrane. Increased hormone release can lead to increased neural contact at this interface. Perivascular cell processes (pv) can be seen in the perivascular space. P, Pituicyte. × 18,200.

TABLE I

THE NUMBER OF NEUROSECRETORY AXONS ENCLOSED BY PITUICYTE CYTOPLASM DURING DIFFERENT TREATMENTS

Conditions of increased hormone release bring about a decreased enclosure. This can take place rapidly (e.g. at parturition), is reversible (e.g. with rehydration), and reflects the degree of hormone demand (e.g. 10-day saline treatment).

Animal treatment	Axons/100 μm^2 pituicyte cytoplasm (mean $\pm S.E.$)
Normal male rats[a]	2.1 ± 0.6
24-h water-deprived male rats[a]	0.7 ± 0.2*
Rehydrated male rats[a]	2.5 ± 0.6
Virgin female rats[b]	1.7 ± 0.5
Pre-partum female rats[b]	1.6 ± 0.4
Post-partum female rats[b]	0.6 ± 0.2*
Lactating rats[b]	0.5 ± 0.1*
Virgin female rats — 10 days of 2% saline treatment (n = 3)[c]	0.1 ± 0.04*

[a] Tweedle and Hatton (1980a); [b] based on data from Tweedle and Hatton (1982). Pituicyte area did not increase following birth or during lactation; [c] Tweedle and Hatton (unpublished).
* Significantly less than the appropriate control ($P < 0.02$ at least).

the pituitary stalk, the axons in the neural lobe degenerate and are phagocytosed by pituicytes (Dellmann, 1973). Phagocytosis may be a physiological role for pituicytes as there is evidence for degeneration (turnover?) of neurosecretory fibres (Dellmann and Rodriguez, 1970; Tweedle and Hatton, 1980a) and catecholamine fibres (Baumgarten et al., 1972) in the neural lobe of normal animals.

EVIDENCE FOR PITUICYTE INVOLVEMENT DURING HORMONE RELEASE

Morris (1976) and Nordmann (1977) classified the recognizable components of the rat neural lobe into the following categories: axonal *swellings* (non-terminal dilatations, containing neither microvesicles nor neurotubules); axonal *endings* (terminal dilatations, containing microvesicles but no neurotubules); *axons* (undilated, containing neurotubules but no or very few microvesicles); pituicytes; blood vessels; and extracellular space. The data of Bandaranayake (1971) for the number of neurones projecting to the neural lobe compared to the number of swellings and endings computed by Nordmann, led to the conclusion that there were around 400 swellings and 1800 endings per magnocellular neurosecretory neurone under normal conditions. This provides a large potential terminal area for hormone release per magnocellular neurone. However, there is evidence that hormone release following acute stimulation occurs only at those nerve endings that contact the basement membrane. Stimulation of hormone release did not deplete the dense core vesicles from those endings nor at the basement membrane or from axons per se or swellings (Nordmann and Morris, 1976). Work partially described above (Tweedle and Hatton, 1980a, b, 1982; Table I) has indicated that the number of neurosecretory axonal profiles surrounded by pituicyte cytoplasm can change apidly depending on conditions of hormone release. Increased hormone release induced by a variety of stimuli consistently brought about less glial wrapping of nerve processes. Serial thin section analysis showed that some of these neurosecretory axonal profiles terminated within pituicyte cytoplasm, i.e., they were axonal endings.

Tweedle and Hatton (1980a) suggested that enclosure by pituicytes either directly or indirectly inhibits hormone release from neurosecretory endings. This could occur in a number of ways.

(1) Preventing contact of axonal endings with the basement membrane. This implies that contact of the endings with the basement membrane per se is necessary for hormone release. Recent studies have indicated that the basement membrane at the neuromuscular junction has important roles in the accumulation of acetylcholine receptors (Bader, 1981) and in neuromuscular recognition (Sanes et al., 1978), and contains the inactivating enzyme acetylcholinesterase (McMahan et al., 1978). The basement membrane of the neural lobe could similarly be integral to release from neurosecretory endings.

(2) Glial degradation of released hormone (this would seem to be an inefficient and wasteful way to do things).

(3) Glial regulation of the extracellular ionic environment (especially K^+ or Ca^{2+}) around the neurosecretory axon or terminal which might influence stimulus–secretion coupling (see Dellmann et al., 1974).

(4) Release of GABA from pituicytes which could then inhibit the electrical activity of neurosecretory axons or terminals. GABA is taken up by pituicytes and can be released from isolated neural lobes either by electrical stimulation of the pituitary stalk or by elevated K^+ (56 mM) (Beart et al., 1974; Minchin and Nordmann, 1975). Thus, normal, spontaneous electrical activity may similarly release GABA into the extracellular space. In this model, the pituicyte release of axons during increased hormonal output would free the axons from constant inhibition of GABA. Zingg et al. (1979) have shown in isolated neural lobe preparations that increased GABA in the medium (10^{-3} M) reduced the amplitude and increased the latency of compound action potentials recorded from hypothalamo-neurohypophysial axons in response to electrical stimulation of the neural lobe. Although the concentration of GABA needed to elicit these effects was high, if small amounts of GABA were continually released into the narrow extracellular space around a neurosecretory ending completely surrounded by pituicyte cytoplasm, the effective concentration might be high enough to inhibit hormone release. However, GABA was found by Iversen et al. (1980) to have no effect on stimulation-evoked vasopressin release. Also, although GABA may be taken up and released from pituicytes, they do not seem to contain glutamate decarboxylase, the synthesizing enzyme. Any GABA they might release, therefore, must have previously been taken up and probably comes from the plexus of GABAergic fibres in the neural lobe (Vincent et al., 1982).

(5) Inhibition of hormone release by cyclic AMP activity at the axonal/pituicyte interface. Santolaya and Lederis (1980) found heavy deposits of adenylate cyclase reaction product on the external membrane surface of neurosecretory axons, especially where they contact pituicytes. Adenylate cyclase is the key enzyme in the synthesis of cyclic AMP. Exogenously added cyclic AMP has been reported to inhibit spontaneous release of vasopressin from the explanted neural lobe (Mathison and Lederis, 1980). Modulation of exocytosis at "enclosed" axonal endings via cyclic AMP is also a possibility due to the circumstantial evidence that the unstimulated neural lobe has more extracellular cyclic AMP than the stimulated lobe (Mathison and Lederis, 1980).

(6) Feedback inhibition of hormone release by enkephalin during glial enclosure of axonal endings. It has been reported in the rat (Martin and Voigt, 1981) and cat (Coulter et al., 1981) that enkephalin is found in the same terminals as the other peptide hormones. Enkephalin is

released from the neural lobe simultaneously with oxytocin and vasopressin during water deprivation (Rossier et al., 1979). Lincoln et al. (1981) and Coulter et al. (1981) have suggested that oxytocin and vasopressin release could be inhibited by the autoregulatory feedback of simultaneously-released enkephalin. Extracellular levels of enkephalin could be higher when the ending is sequestered by glia (as opposed to being "free" at the basement membrane) and thus have a more profound inhibitory effect. Recent evidence from Van Leeuwen and De Vries (this volume) contradicts the co-localization findings, however. They report that enkephalin-containing fibres in the neural lobe end only on pituicytes. The hypothesis this generates is that enkephalin modulation of hormone release might be carried out by an influence on the pituicytes.

Changes at the perivascular contact zone

Wittkowski and Brinkmann (1974) and Carithers et al. (1981) have reported that the proportion of the basement membrane of the perivascular space covered by nerve profiles (vs pituicyte processes) increased following 3 days of water deprivation. Recent work (Tweedle and Hatton, unpublished) has shown that there is also a significant and relatively rapid increase in the amount of contact by nerve endings at the basement membrane during parturition. The data indicate that this occurs because fewer pituicyte processes contact the basement membrane, and there is also an increase in the basement membrane contact length of the individual nerve profiles (Table II). The number of nerve endings per unit area did not increase. These phenomena could provide an increased terminal release area during hormone demand. Although our results corroborate those of Wittkowski and Brinkmann (1974), Morris and Nordmann (1980) did not find an increase in individual nerve ending contact lengths with the basement membrane following 15 min of in vitro stimulation in high potassium medium. The reasons for this discrepancy are not clear, although they may be temporal, since our animals were perfusion-fixed from 2 to 24 h after giving birth. This extra time following hormone release may have allowed further change in ending size and/or shape. In an interesting study by Carithers et al. (1981), lesions of the tissue surrounding the anterolateral third ventricle, which cause adipsia but no antidiuretic response (and thus elevated plasma osmotic pressure), produced an unusually large coverage of the perivascular surface of the rat neural lobe by glial cytoplasm. Dense core vesicles in neural lobe axonal swellings increased greatly but, accompanying the absence of release, much less basement membrane surface area was contacted by axonal endings. Incidentally, this study also suggests that the glial withdrawal from the perivascular zone seen during water deprivation is not primarily due to osmotic cues. Although the data in Table II do not support the notion that the *number* of functional axonal endings at the basement membrane might vary depending upon the demand for hormone release, more chronic stimuli might cause such changes. For example, when hormone release is not very great an increased number of nerve endings may be displaced from the basement membrane by being enwrapped or displaced by pituicyte processes. This would require that nerve endings make and break synaptoid contacts at the basement membrane, an idea that is perhaps not too alarming, considering other reports in the literature. For example, Scharrer and Kater (1969) reported an increase in synaptoid contacts (thought to be release sites) with the extracellular space in the corpus cardiacum of the cockroach following electrical stimulation of hormone release. The number of synaptoid contacts with pituicytes has also been reported to increase following 3 days of water deprivation in the rat (Wittkowski and Brinkmann, 1974) or following transfer from fresh to salt water in the eel (Knowles and Vollrath, 1966). We found (Tweedle and Hatton, 1982) that neither conditions leading up to parturition nor the prolonged

TABLE II

THE EFFECT OF HORMONAL RELEASE ON NEURAL vs GLIAL COVERAGE AT THE NEURAL LOBE PERIVASCULAR CONTACT ZONE

All conditions of increased hormone release shown brought about an increased amount of neural apposition at the basement membrane. This is through the presence of a decreased number of glial processes and more surface area covered per nerve ending. It is interesting that in the rats of Wittkowski and Brinkmann there is a higher glial coverage than in the other two studies. This is apparently mainly due to the larger number of glial processes present at the contact zone.

Animal treatment	Glial cytoplasm at perivascular surface (%)	Average length (μn) of individual perivascular neuronal contact (mean ± S.E.)	Number of pituicyte processes per 100 μn of contact zone	Number of neural processes per 100 μn of contact zone
Sham — with access to water[a]	25.9 ± 5.8 S.D.	—	—	—
Sham — 3-day water-deprived[a]	11.3 ± 2.3* S.D.	—	—	—
Pre-partum female rats (n = 4)[b]	32.6 ± 3.1 S.E.	0.94 ± 0.06	11.3 ± 0.8	43.0 ± 4.2
Post-partum female rats (n = 4)[b]	21.8 ± 2.0* S.E.	1.30 ± 0.17*	7.7 ± 1.6*	44.4 ± 2.5
Male rats with access to water[c]	48	1.1 ± 0.1	43.5	45.5
Male rats, 3-day water-deprived[c]	33*	1.6 ± 0.2*	31.2*	43.5

[a] Carithers et al. (1981). Sham refers to sham AV3V lesion; [b] Tweedle and Hatton (unpublished). Data collected from 12 micrographs per animal (× 7500). Pre-partum = day 21 of gestation; post-partum = 2–24 h after birth; [c] Wittkowski and Brinkmann (1974). Data recomputed for comparison.
* Stimulated significantly different from normal at least at P < 0.02.

stimulus of lactation brought about any detectable change in the number of synaptoid contacts onto pituicyte cell bodies, so the phenomenon may be stimulus-specific or may occur on portions of the glial cells not sampled by us. As the contents of dense core vesicles are released only at the basement membrane and therefore not necessarily at synaptoid contacts onto pituicytes (Morris and Nordmann, 1980), the chemical message (if any) that neurosecretory axons might use to communicate with pituicytes is unclear.

Similar findings in the median eminence

There have been several reports that the coverage of the basement membrane of the neurohaemal contact zone of the median eminence by tanycytes (specialized glia) changes under different physiological or experimental conditions (Hökfelt, 1973; Oota et al., 1974; Wittkowski and Scheurer, 1974; Lichtensteiger et al., 1978; Scheibler et al., 1978). These studies parallel the reports of changes in pituicyte contact with the neurohaemal zone, especially as the tanycytes also receive many synaptoid contacts (Kobayashi et al., 1970; Güldner and Wolff, 1973) from both neurosecretory (Scheibler et al., 1978) and dopamine fibres (Scott and Krobisch-Dudley, 1975). The cell bodies of the dopamine fibres are in the mediobasal hypothalamus (arcuate and periventricular nuclei) (Björklund et al., 1970). Acute electrical activation of these cells is followed by a decreased coverage of the neurohaemal contact zone by tanycyte foot processes (Stoeckart et al., 1975; Lichtensteiger et al., 1978). This was interpreted as evidence for a neural influence on the tanycytes. The changes could be seen at 30 and 60, but not 15 min after stimulation (Stoeckart et al., 1975). Apparently more than 15 min are required to elicit glial movement at the contact zone. With this in mind, it would be interesting to know if incubation of the neural lobe for more than 15 min in high potassium solution would alter the previously mentioned results of Morris and Nordmann (1980) in regard to the area of neural contact with the basement membrane. It is still unclear whether the site of the stimulus for an influence on tanycytes would be at the synaptoid contacts or through altered levels of release products at the contact zone. A similar doubt exists as to the stimulus that induces mobility of pituicytes in the neural lobe. For example, water deprivation can lead to increased release of oxytocin, vasopressin, neurophysin, cholecystokinin, enkephalin and dopamine from the neural lobe (Jones and Pickering, 1969; Mata et al., 1978; Rossier et al., 1979; Beinfeld et al., 1980; Holzbauer et al., 1978). Any (or a combination) of these or some other molecules could be an activating agent, perhaps taken up by endocytosis (Theodosis, 1979). The data indicate that any stimulus for hormone release from the neural lobe (dehydration, parturition, lactation) will cause pituicyte release (unwrapping) of neurosecretory processes, so pituicyte activation may be by something non-specific that accompanies enhanced neurosecretion, e.g. ionic changes along the axons or at the terminals. As glial cells, pituicytes may sequester K^+ released from axonal firing which could lead to changes in cell metabolism, shape and motility (Lipton and Heimbach, 1977; Narumi et al., 1978; Van Calker and Hamprecht, 1980). A considerable amount of evidence has accumulated that astrocytic processes between neurosecretory cell bodies in the supraoptic, paraventricular and circularis nuclei can withdraw during enhanced hormone release, bringing the cell bodies into greater direct contact (Tweedle and Hatton, 1977; Gregory et al., 1980; Theodosis et al., 1981; Hatton and Tweedle, 1982). The stimulus for this glial mobility may also be ionic.

The perivascular region and blood vessels

Moderate stimulation of hormone release is accompanied by increased blood flow and vasodilatation in the neural lobe (Sooriyamoorthy and Livingston, 1972, 1973; Livingston,

1975). Under conditions of more chronic hormone demand (2 weeks of 1.75% NaCl imbibition) in young rats there is also a significant increase in the proliferation of endothelial cells to generate increased vasculature in the hypertrophied neural lobe (Paterson and Leblond, 1977). Whether this also indicates the development of an increased total perivascular surface for hormone release is unknown. The same study also found increased proliferation of pituicytes and perivascular cells. The latter (Fig. 4) lie within the perivascular space and can sometimes be seen to have an intimate relationship with neurosecretory axons lying in this space. Although they do not receive axonal synaptoid contacts, the perivascular cells may completely enclose the axonal processes. Occasionally, axonal phagocytosis by perivascular cells may be seen (Olivieri-Sangiacomo, 1972). Perivascular cells could also be involved in production of collagen and basement membrane components found in the perivascular space.

SUMMARY

The anatomical elements of the neural lobe show a good deal of change during increased hormone release. The dense core vesicles of the axon terminals can be depleted and those in the axon swelling eventually recruited. Intra-axonal lysosomes increase, smooth endoplasmic reticulum proliferates, and microvesicles re-distribute. This article cites evidence that, at the levels of hormone release that produce the above changes, the area of overall and individual axonal ending contact with the basement membrane increases. The pituicyte processes withdraw from the basement membrane, possibly to provide a greater surface area for hormone release. Pituicytes also "unwrap" from around axonal processes, probably freeing axon terminals. Blood vessels dilate, filling up more of the perivascular space.

Indeed, all of the classifiable components of the neural lobe (Morris, 1976) show ultrastructural changes during increased hormone release. The meaning of certain of these (presumably functional) alterations is finally becoming clear, while the meaning of others can only be guessed at and provide the basis for continued investigation. Studies of the median eminence and magnocellular cell bodies of the hypothalamus suggest that the anatomical flexibility seen in the neural lobe may exist in these regions as well.

ACKNOWLEDGEMENTS

I am grateful to Drs. P. Cobbett, W. M. Falls, W. Gregory and G. Hatton and Ms. L. Perlmutter for comments on an earlier draft of the manuscript, and B. Rogers and B. Schmidt for technical and typing assistance. The author's research was supported by NIH Grant NS09140.

REFERENCES

Alonso, G. and Assenmacher, I. (1979) The smooth endoplasmic reticulum in neurohypophysial axons of the rat: possible involvement in transport, storage and release of neurosecretory material. *Cell Tiss. Res.*, 199: 415–429.

Bader, D. (1981) Density and distribution of α-bungarotoxin sites in postsynaptic structures of regenerated skeletal muscle. *J. Cell Biol.*, 83: 338–345.

Bandaranayake, R.C. (1971) The morphology of the accessory neurosecretory nuclei and the retrochiasmatic part of the supraoptic nucleus of the rat. *Acta anat.*, 80: 14–22.

Bargmann, W. (1949) Über die neurosekretorische Verknüpfung von Hypothalamus und Neurohypophyse. *Z. Zellforsch.*, 34: 610–634.

Bargmann, W. and Knoop, A. (1957) Elektronen mikroskopische Beobachtungen an der Neurohypophyse. *Z. Zell-forsch.*, 46: 242–251.

Bargmann, W. and Scharrer, E. (1951) The site of origin of the hormones of the posterior pituitary. *Amer. Sci.*, 39: 255–259.

Baumgarten, H. G., Björklund, A., Holstein, A. F. and Nobin, A. (1972) Organization and ultrastructural identification of the catecholamine nerve terminals in the neural lobe and pars intermedia of the rat pituitary. *Z. Zellforsch.*, 126: 483–517.

Beart, P. M., Kelly, J. S. and Schon, F. (1974) GABA in the rat peripheral nervous system, pineal and posterior pituitary. *Biochem. Soc. Trans.*, 2: 266–268.

Beinfeld, M. C., Meyer, D. K. and Brownstein, M. J. (1980) Cholecystokinin octapeptide in the rat hypothalamo-neurohypophysial system. *Nature (Lond.)*, 288: 376–377.

Björklund, A., Falck, A., Hromek, F., Owman, C. and West, K. (1970) Identification and terminal distribution of the tuberohypophysial monoamine fiber systems in the rat. *Brain Res.*, 17: 1–23.

Carithers, J., Dellmann, H. D., Bealer, S. L., Brody, M. J. and Johnson, A. K. (1981) Ultrastructural aspects of anterolateral third ventricle lesions on supraoptic nuclei and neural lobes of rats. *Brain Res.*, 220: 13–29.

Castel, M. and Dellmann, H. D. (1980) Thiamine pyrophosphatase activity in the axonal smooth endoplasmic reticulum of neurosecretory neurons. *Cell Tiss. Res.*, 210: 205–221.

Coulter, H. D., Elde, R. P. and Unverzagt, S. L. (1981) Co-localization of neurophysin- and enkephalin-like immunoreactivity in cat pituitary. *Peptides*, 2: 51–55.

Dellmann, H. D. (1973) Degeneration and regeneration of neurosecretory systems. *Int. Rev. Cytol.*, 36: 215–315.

Dellmann, H. D. and Rodriguez, E. M. (1970) Herring bodies: an electron microscopic study of local degeneration and regeneration of neurosecretory axons. *Z. Zellforsch.*, 111: 293–315.

Dellmann, H. D., Stoeckel, M. E., Porte, A. and Stutinsky, F. (1974) Ultrastructure of neurohypophysial glial cells following stalk transection in rat. *Experientia*, 30: 1220–1222.

Dreyfuss, F., Burlet, A., Chateau, M. and Czernichow, P. (1979) Localization ultrastructurale par immunocyto-chimie de la vasopressine dans la neurohypophyse du rat. *Biol. Cell.*, 35: 141–146.

Green, J. D. and Van Breemen, V. L. (1955) Electron microscopy of the pituitary and observations on neurosecretion. *Amer. J. Anat.*, 97: 177–228.

Gregory, W. A., Tweedle, C. D. and Hatton, G. I. (1980) Ultrastructure of neurons in the paraventricular nucleus of normal, dehydrated and rehydrated rats. *Brain Res. Bull.*, 5: 301–306.

Güldner, F.-H. and Woolff, J. R. (1973) Neurono-glial synaptoid contacts in the median eminence of the rat: ultrastructure, staining properties and distribution on tanycytes. *Brain Res.*, 61: 217–234.

Haddad, A., Guaraldo, S. P., Pelletier, G., Brasiliero, I.L.G. and Marchi, F. (1980) Glycoprotein secretion in the hypothalamo-neurohypophysial system of the rat. *Cell Tiss. Res.*, 209: 399–409.

Hartmann, J. F. (1958) Electron microscopy of the neurohypophysis in normal and histamine treated rats. *Z. Zellforsch.*, 48: 291–308.

Hatton, G. I. and Tweedle, C. D. (1982) Magnocellular neuropeptidergic neurons in hypothalamus: increases in membrane apposition and number of specialized synapses from pregnancy to lactation. *Brain Res. Bull.*, 8: 197–204.

Heap, P. F., Jones, C. W., Morris, J. F. and Pickering, B. T. (1975) Movement of neurosecretory product through the anatomical compartments of the rat neural lobe. *Cell Tiss. Res.*, 156: 483–492.

Hökfelt, T. (1973) Possible site of action of dopamine in the hypothalamic pituitary control. *Acta physiol. scand.*, 89: 606–608.

Holzbauer, M., Sharman, D. F. and Godden, U. (1978) Observations on the function of dopaminergic nerves innervating the pituitary gland. *Neuroscience*, 3: 1251–1260.

Iversen, L. L., Iversen, S. D. and Bloom, F. E. (1980) Opiate receptors influence vasopressin release from nerve terminals in rat neurohypophysis. *Nature (Lond.)*, 284: 350–351.

Jones, C. W. and Pickering, B. T. (1969) Comparison of the effects of water deprivation and sodium chloride imbibition on the hormone content of the neurohypophysis of the rat. *J. Physiol. (Lond.)*, 203: 449–458.

Knowles, F. and Vollrath, L. (1966) Neurosecretory innervation of the eels *Anguilla* and *Conger*. *Proc. roy. Soc. B*, 250: 311–327.

Kobayashi, H., Matsui, T. and Ishii, S. (1970) Functional electron microscopy of the hypothalamic median eminence. *Int. Rev. Cytol.*, 29: 281–315.

Krsulovik, J. and Brückner, G. (1969) Morphological characteristics of pituicytes. *Z. Zellforsch.*, 99: 210–220.

Leveque, F. and Small, M. (1959) The relationship of the pituicyte to the posterior lobe hormones. *Endocrinology*, 65: 909–915.

Lichtensteiger, W., Richards, J. G. and Kopp, H. G. (1978) Possible participation of non-neuronal elements of median eminence in neuroendocrine effects of dopaminergic and cholinergic systems. In: D. E. Scott, G. P.

Kozlowski and A. Weindl (Eds.), *Brain-Endocrine Interaction III. Neural Hormones and Reproduction*, Karger, Basel, pp. 251–262.

Lincoln, D. W., Clarke, G. and Merrick, L. (1981) An opiate-mediated inhibition of peptide release from neurosecretory terminals. In D. S. Farner and K. Lederis (Eds.), *Neurosecretion: Molecules, Cells, Systems*, Plenum Press, New York, pp. 269–280.

Lipton, P. and Heimbach, C. J. (1977) The effect of extracellular potassium on protein synthesis in guinea pig hippocampal slice. *J. Neurochem.*, 28: 1347–1354.

Livingston, A. (1975) Morphology of the perivascular regions of the rat neural lobe in relation to hormone release. *Cell Tiss. Res.*, 159: 551–561.

Martin, R. and Voigt, K. H. (1981) Enkephalins co-exist with oxytocin and vasopressin in nerve terminals of rat neurohypophysis. *Nature (Lond.)*, 289: 502–504.

Mata, M. M., Gainer, H. and Klee, W. A. (1978) Effect of dehydration on the endogeneous opiate content of the rat neuro-intermediate lobe. *Life Sci.*, 21: 1159–1162.

Mathison, R. and Lederis, K. (1980) A mechanism for adenosine 3'5'-monophosphate regulation of vasopressin secretion. *Endocrinology*, 106: 842–848.

McMahan, U. J., Sanes, J. R. and Marshall, L. M. (1978) Cholinesterase is associated with the basal lamina at the neuromuscular junction. *Nature (Lond.)*, 271: 172–174.

Minchin, M.C.W. and Nordmann, J. J. (1975) The release of [^{3}H]gamma-aminobutyric acid and neurophysin from the isolated rat pituitary. *Brain Res.*, 90: 75–84.

Monroe, B. and Scott, D. (1966) Ultrastructural changes in the neural lobe of the hypophysis during lactation and suckling. *J. Ultrastruct. Res.*, 14: 497–517.

Morris, J. F. (1976) Distribution of neurosecretory granules among the anatomical compartments of the neurosecretory processes of the pituitary gland: a quantitative ultrastructural approach to hormone storage in the neural lobe. *J. Endocr.*, 68: 225–234.

Morris, J. F. and Nordmann, J. J. (1980) Membrane recapture after hormone release from nerve endings in the neural lobe of the rat pituitary gland. *Neuroscience*, 5: 639–647.

Morris, J. F., Nordmann, J. J. and Dyball, R.E.J. (1978) Structure–function correlation in mammalian neurosecretion. *Int. Rev. exp. Path.*, 18: 1–95.

Nakai, Y. (1970) Electron microscopic observations on synapse-like contacts between pituicytes and different types of nerve fibers in the anuran pars nervosa. *Z. Zellforsch.*, 110: 27–39.

Narumi, S., Kimelburg, H. K. and Bourke, R. S. (1978) Effects of norepinephrine on the morphology and some enzyme activities of primary monolayer cultures from rat brain. *J. Neurochem.*, 31: 1479–1490.

Nordmann, J. J. (1977) Ultrastructural morphometry of the rat neurohypophysis. *J. Anat.*, 123: 213–218.

Nordmann, J. J. and Morris, J. F. (1976) Membrane retrieval at neurosecretory axon endings. *Nature (Lond.)*, 261: 723–724.

Olivieri-Sangiacomo, C. (1972) On the fine structure of the perivascular cells in the neural lobe of rats. *Z. Zellforsch.*, 132: 25–34.

Oota, N., Kobayashi, H., Nishioka, R. S. and Bern, H. (1974) Relationship between the neurosecretory axon and ependymal terminals on capillary walls in median eminence of several vertebrates. *Neuroendocrinology*, 16: 127–136.

Palay, S.L. (1955) An electron microscope study of the neurohypophysis in normal, hydrated and dehydrated rats. *Anat. Rec.*, 121: 348.

Paterson, J. A. and Leblond, C. P. (1977) Increased proliferation of neuroglia and endothelial cells in the supraoptic nucleus and hypophysial neural lobe in young rats drinking hypertonic sodium chloride solution. *J. comp. Neurol.*, 175: 373–390.

Picard, D., Boudier, J. A. and Tasso, F. (1977) Intracellular regulatory mechanisms of neurosecretory activity. In D. E. Scott, G. Kozlowski and A. Weindl (Eds.), *Brain–Endocrine Interaction III. Neural Hormones and Reproduction*, Karger, Basel, pp. 33–45.

Reinhardt, H. F., Henning, L. C. and Rohr, H. P. (1969) Morphometrische-ultrastrukturelle Untersuchungen am Nucleus supraopticus der Ratte nach Dehydration. *Z. Zellfosch.*, 102: 172–181.

Romeis, B. (1940) Hypophyse. In W. von Möllendorff (Ed.), *Handbuch der Mikroskopischen Anatomie des Menschen*, Vol. 6, part 3, Springer, Berlin, pp. 393–430.

Rossier, J., Battenburg, E., Pittman, Q., Bayon, A., Koda, L., Miller, R., Guillemin, R. and Bloom, F. (1979) Hypothalamic enkephalin neurones may regulate the neurohypophysis. *Nature (Lond.)*, 277: 653–655.

Rougon-Rapuzzi, G., Cau, P., Boudier, J. A. and Cupo, A. (1978) Evolution of vasopressin levels in the hypothalamo-posthypophysial system of the rat during rehydration following water deprivation. *Neuroendocrinology*, 27: 46–62.

Rufener, C. (1973) Autophology of secretory granules in rat neurohypophysis. *Neuroendocrinology*, 13: 314–320.

Sachs, H. and Haller, E. W. (1968) Further studies on the capacity of the neurohypophysis to release vasopressin. *Endocrinology*, 83: 251–262.

Salm, A. K., Hatton, G. I. and Nilaver, G. (1982) Immunoreactive glial fibrillary acidic protein in pituicytes of the rat neurohypophysis. *Brain Res.*, 236: 471–476.

Sanes, J. R., Marshall, L. M. and McMahan, U. J. (1978) Reinnervation of muscle fiber basal lamina after removal of myofibers. *J. Cell Biol.*, 78: 176–198.

Santolaya, R. and Lederis, K. (1980) Localization of adenylate cyclase in the neurointermediate lobe of the rat pituitary. *Cell Tiss. Res.*, 207: 387–394.

Scharrer, B. and Kater, S. (1969) Neurosecretion XV. An electron microscopic study of the corpora cardiaca of *P. americana* after experimentally-induced hormone release. *Z. Zellforsch.*, 95: 177–186.

Scheibler, T. H., Leranth, C., Zaborsky, L., Bitsch, P. and Rützel, H. (1978) On the glia of the median eminence. In D. E. Scott, G. Kozlowski and A. Weindl (Eds.), *Brain–Endocrine Interaction III. Neural Hormones and Reproduction*, Karger, Basel, pp. 46–56.

Scott, D. E. and Krobisch-Dudley, G. (1975) Ultrastructural analysis of the mammalian median eminence. In K. Knigge, H. Kobayashi, D. Scott and S. Ishii (Eds.), *Brain–Endocrine Interaction II. The Ventricular System*, Karger, Basel, pp. 29–39.

Silverman, A. and Zimmerman, E. (1975) Ultrastructural immunocytochemical localization of neurophysin and vasopressin in the median eminence and posterior pituitary of the guinea pig. *Cell Tiss. Res.*, 159: 291–301.

Sooriyamoorthy, T. and Livingston, A. (1972) Variations in the blood volume of the neural and anterior lobes of the pituitary of the rat associated with neurohypophysial hormone releasing stimuli. *J. Endocr.*, 54: 407–415.

Sooriyamoorthy, T. and Livingston, A. (1973) Blood flow changes in pituitary neural lobe of rabbit associated with neurohypophysial hormone releasing stimuli. *J. Endocr.*, 57: 75–85.

Stoeckart, R., Kreike, A. J. and Jansen, H. G. (1975) Effect of electrochemical preoptic stimulation on the ultrastructural distribution of nonneuronal processes in the rat median eminence. *J. Endocr.*, 64: 57P.

Suess, U. and Pliška, V. (1981) Identification of pituicytes as astroglial cells by indirect immunofluorescence staining for the glial fibrillary acidic protein. *Brain Res.*, 221: 27–33.

Theodosis, D. T. (1979) Endocytosis in glial cells (pituicytes) of the rat neurophypophysis demonstrated by incorporation of horseradish peroxidase. *Neuroscience*, 4: 417–426.

Theodosis, D. T., Dreifuss, J. J. and Orci, L. (1977) Two classes of microvesicles in the neurohypophysis. *Brain Res.*, 123: 159–163.

Theodosis, D. T., Poulain, D. A. and Vincent, J.-D. (1981) Possible morphological bases for synchronization of neuronal firing in the rat supraoptic nucleus during lactation. *Neuroscience*, 6: 919–929.

Tweedle, C. D. and Hatton, G. I. (1977) Ultrastructural changes in rat hypothalamic neurosecretory cells and their associated glia during minimal dehydration and rehydration. *Cell Tiss. Res.*, 181: 59–72.

Tweedle, C. D. and Hatton, G. I. (1980a) Evidence for dynamic interactions between pituicytes and neurosecretory endings in the neurohypophysis of the rat. *Neuroscience*, 5: 661–667.

Tweedle, C. D. and Hatton, G. I. (1980b) Glial cell enclosure of neurosecretory endings in the rat. *Brain Res.*, 192: 555–559.

Tweedle, C. D. and Hatton, G. I. (1982) Magnocellular neuropeptidergic terminals in neurohypophysis: rapid glial release of enclosed axons during parturition. *Brain Res. Bull.*, 8: 205–209.

Van Calker, D. and Hamprecht, B. (1980) Effects of neurohormones on glial cells. In S. Federoff and L. Hertz (Eds.), *Cellular Neurobiology, Vol. 1*, Academic Press, New York, pp. 31–67.

Vincent, S. R., Hökfelt, T. and Wu, J.-Y. (1982) GABA neuron systems in hypothalamus and pituitary gland. *Neuroendocrinology*, 34: 117–125.

Wittkowski, W. and Brinkmann, H. (1974) Changes of extent of neurovascular contacts and number of neuro-glial synaptoid contacts in the pituitary posterior lobe of dehydrated rats. *Anat. Embryol.*, 146: 157–165.

Wittkowski, W. and Scheuer, A. (1974) Functional changes of the neuronal and glial elements at the surface of the external layer of median eminence. *Z. Anat. Entwickl.-Gesch.*, 143: 255–262.

Zingg, H. H., Baertschi, A. J. and Dreifuss, J. J. (1979) Action of gamma-aminobutyric acid on hypothalamo-neurohypophysial axons. *Brain Res.*, 171: 453–459.

The Neurohypophysis: Structure, Function and Control, Progress in Brain Research, Vol. 60, edited by B.A. Cross and G. Leng
© *1983 Elsevier Science Publishers B.V.*

Intracellular Membrane Movements Associated With Hormone Release in Magnocellular Neurones

D.T. THEODOSIS

I.N.S.E.R.M., U.176, Unité de Recherches de Neurobiologie des Comportements, Domaine de Carreire, Rue Camille Saint Saëns, 33077 Bordeaux Cedex (France)

EXO-ENDOCYTOSIS IN NEUROSECRETORY TERMINALS

Once synthesized and packaged into membrane-bound granules, oxytocin and vasopressin, together with their carrier proteins, the neurophysins, are transported anterogradely from cell bodies in the supraoptic and paraventricular nuclei of the hypothalamus to axon terminals in the neural lobe of the pituitary. The secretory material is then released directly into the perivascular space by exocytosis. Exocytosis involves fusion of the secretory granule membrane with the plasmalemma, thereby creating an opening through which the secretory products can be discharged. In the process of exocytosis, a considerable amount of membrane is inserted into the cell surface. Subsequent endocytosis, or membrane internalization by pinocytotic budding from the plasma membrane, ensures the maintenance of the cell surface (Palade, 1975).

Conventional electron microscopy of thin-sectioned neurosecretory fibres reveals few exocytotic profiles, even in stimulated preparations (Nagasawa et al., 1970; Theodosis et al., 1978a, b). As membrane fusion induces changes in the structure of the interacting membranes, exocytotic profiles are more readily visualized in replicas of freeze-fractured neurohypophyses. The technique of freeze-fracture splits membranes in the middle of their lipid bilayers and thus produces extensive en face views of the two faces of the membrane interior: the inner P face, adjacent to the cytoplasm, and the outer E face, adjacent to the extracellular space (Branton, 1971). Both fracture faces show smooth regions, corresponding to the phospholipid domains of the membrane, interrupted by protruding intramembrane particles, representing, for the most part, integral membrane proteins (Yu and Branton, 1976).

In thin-sectioned neurosecretory terminals, the occasional exocytotic images are characterized by invaginations of the terminal membrane that contain the granule core exposed to the extracellular space (Fig. 1a). In replicas of freeze-fractured neurosecretory fibres, associated granule core substance also serves to identify exocytotic profiles. These profiles consist of circular depressions in the P leaflet of the axolemma that contain material interpreted as the exposed granule core (Fig. 1b–d). Fortuitous fractures that pass into the cytoplasm show that the depressions represent the granule membrane continuous with the plasmalemma (Fig. 1b). The membrane leaflet surrounding the exocytotic openings often has few or no intramembranous particles, in contrast to the rest of the membrane leaflet where particles are numerous and evenly distributed (Fig. 1c). These completed exocytotic openings more than double in replicas of stimulated neurohypophyses (Theodosis et al., 1978a, b). Earlier stages of exocytosis, i.e. prior to and during fusion, are not yet clearly characterized in neurosecretory endings. In en face views of the P face of the axolemma, bulges devoid of particles (Fig. 1e) increase in

274

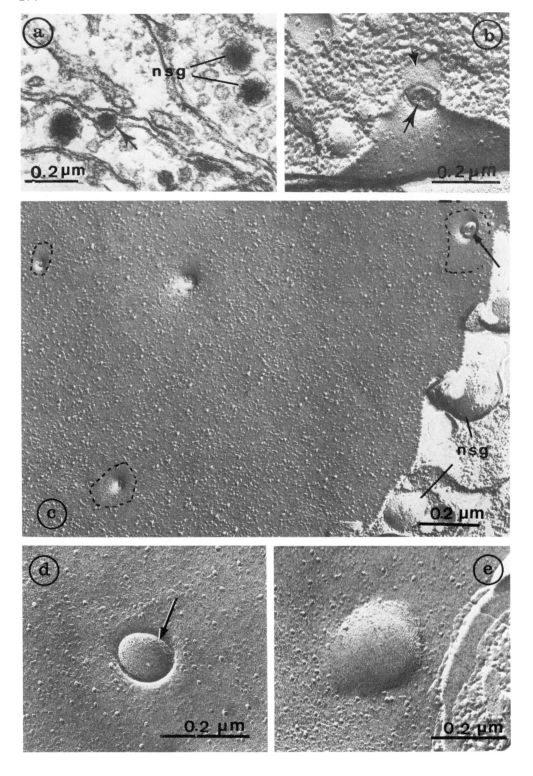

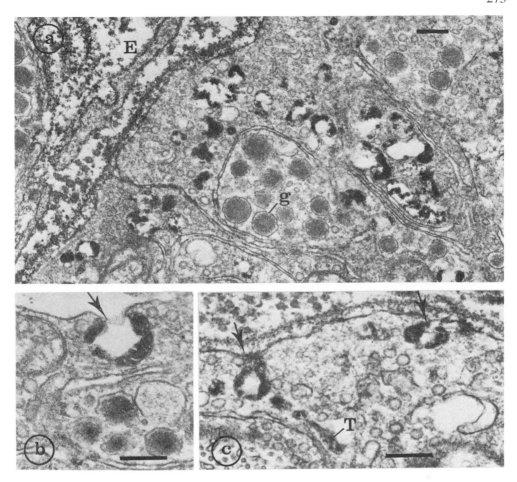

Fig. 2. Thin sections of neurohypophysial axons from rats injected with HRP (Sigma type VI) 5 min before stimulation of hormone release. a: terminals from a rat killed 5 min after the onset of haemorrhage. Peroxidase reaction product is seen intracellularly mainly in large vacuolar profiles. E, extracellular space; g, neurosecretory granules. ×40,000. b and c: terminals from a rat killed within 2 min after electrical stimulation of the pituitary stalk. Large, circular HRP-containing profiles appear to be invaginating at the cell surface (arrows). A tubular structure (T) also is labelled. ×53,000. All bars = 0.2 μm. (Adapted from Theodosis et al., 1976.)

Fig. 1. Electron micrographs of membrane changes indicative of exocytosis in neurohypophysial terminals. a: in this thin section, a round mass (arrow) of electron density similar to that of the cores of neurosecretory granules (nsg) in the axon cytoplasm fills an invagination in the cell membrane; the presence of core material identifies the invagination as resulting from the fusion of the granule and plasma membranes during exocytosis. ×70,000. b: in this replica of a freeze-fractured axon, the fracture passed along the P face of the plasmalemma and into the cytoplasm, thus revealing the fused granule and plasma membranes (arrowhead); a cross-fractured granule core fills the exocytotic opening (arrow). ×92,000. c: a large area of the axolemma P face shows several exocytotic openings, one of which contains granule core material (arrow). The dotted lines delineate areas poor in intramembranous particles. nsg, neurosecretory granules. ×66,000. d: a smooth-surfaced granule core (arrow) fills a circular depression in the membrane. ×130,000. e: axolemma P face showing a smooth circular bulge that could represent a neurosecretory granule closely applied to the inner leaflet of the plasma membrane. ×33,000. (Adapted from Theodosis et al., 1978b.)

276

frequency in stimulated glands, and they could represent granules closely applied to the cell surface and in the process of fusing with it (Dempsey et al., 1973; Theodosis, 1978b).

In neurohypophysial axons, membrane movements associated with endocytosis appear to be tightly coupled to those of exocytosis since no increase in the surface area of the neurosecretory endings is apparent even after strong stimulation (Nordmann and Morris, 1976). That retrieval of membrane associated with hormonal release is rapid is also apparent from studies tracing the uptake of the extracellular marker, horseradish peroxidase (HRP): after as little as 1 min of electrical stimulation of the pituitary stalk, the relative volume occupied by intracellular profiles labelled with the tracer is three times that of corresponding controls (Theodosis et al., 1976). Originally, secretion-related endocytosis in this system was thought to occur by micropinocytosis and to give rise to the numerous microvesicles found in the axons (Douglas, 1974). However, endocytotic vacuoles in neurosecretory fibres are as large as or larger than the neurosecretory granules (Fig. 2a), and they appear to arise directly from large invaginations of the cell surface (Fig. 2b, c). Morphometric analyses of neurohypophyses after stimulation of hormone release invariably show an increase in the frequency of large membranous profiles, whilst that of microvesicles remains the same (Nordmann and Morris, 1976; Theodosis et al., 1976, 1977). The role of the microvesicles may be to take up the excess Ca resulting from hormone release and so control intracellular Ca ion concentrations (Nordmann and Chevalier, 1980).

The identity of membrane internalized during endocytosis cannot be determined by tracing the uptake of tracers such as HRP, which, in fact, are labelling extracellular fluid passively taken up at the same time as the internalized membrane. Some clues to the problem may be

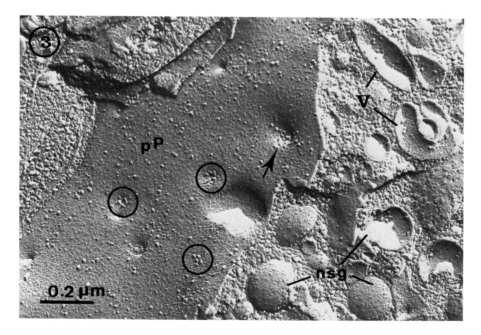

Fig. 3. Images of membrane modifications related to endocytosis as seen in replicas of freeze-fractured neurosecretory axons. Clusters of large particles (circles) in the axolemma P face (pP) are often associated with depressions in the membrane (arrow). In the cross-fractured cytoplasm are seen large ovoid or cup-shaped vacuoles (V) whose P-face contains particles of the same dimension as those in clusters and in the depressions in the plasma membrane leaflet. nsg, neurosecretory granules. × 67,000. (Adapted from Theodosis et al., 1978b.)

provided by freeze-fracture views of neurohypophysial terminals (Fig. 3). In addition to randomly distributed particles (mean diameter, 8 nm), the P leaflet contains clusters of 6–12 particles (mean diameter, 12 nm) that are often associated with depressions in the membrane. Such images are thought to represent incipient endocytosis: they increase significantly following stimulation (Theodosis et al., 1978b), and, in the cytoplasm of cross-fractured fibres, one finds large membrane profiles (similar to those marked with HRP in thin sections) whose P face also contains mainly large intramembranous particles (mean diameter, 11.5 nm). As the P face of neurosecretory granule membranes also contains mainly large particles, (mean diameter, 12 nm), the fragments of the axolemma that contain the clustered particles could represent granule membrane added to the plasmalemma by exocytosis. Compensatory endocytosis would then preferentially internalize the areas of surface membrane where granule membrane has been incorporated.

FATE OF THE MEMBRANE RESULTING FROM ENDOCYTOSIS

Most studies of endocytosis in magnocellular neurones have been concerned mainly with the immediate consequences of this event in the neurohypophysial axons (Castel, 1974; Morris and Nordmann, 1980; Nordmann et al., 1974; Nordmann and Morris, 1976; Theodosis et al., 1976, 1977) and very little has been known about the subsequent fate of the internalized membrane. From recent observations (Broadwell et al., 1980; Theodosis, 1982), it has become probable that such membrane does not remain in the neurosecretory axons but is removed by retrograde axonal transport to their hypothalamic perikarya where it gradually becomes sequestered in lysosomes.

In studies where systemically injected HRP is used to trace membrane uptake, morphometric analysis indicates that HRP-labelled profiles do not accumulate in the neurosecretory fibres (Theodosis, 1982). Neurosecretory cells are similar to other neurones in most respects, yet membrane internalized by endocytosis is not immediately reutilized to form new secretory granules at the terminals (Winkler, 1977). Thus, since endocytosis is presumably a continuous process, and as HRP, when injected, is available for labelling for several hours, the endocytotically derived material is either degraded in situ or transported elsewhere. The latter possibility is most likely: by 4 h after HRP injection, peroxidase-labelled structures, of various shape and size (Fig. 4), are seen in magnocellular perikarya in the hypothalamic nuclei, where the blood–brain barrier is effective (Broadwell and Brightman, 1976) and prevents direct passage of the tracer to the cell bodies. Comparative analysis of the intracellular distribution of HRP, both in neurohypophysial axons and their hypothalamic perikarya demonstrates that uptake of the tracer at the terminals is closely related to secretion, and also its accumulation in the perikarya: 8 h after HRP injection, the mean volume density of HRP-labelled organelles in supraoptic nucleus perikarya of dehydrated animals is more than three times greater than that in non-dehydrated controls (Theodosis, 1982).

One of the most common structures that contain HRP in the perikarya are multivesicular bodies (Fig. 4), organelles implicated in the sequestration of endocytotically derived membrane in numerous systems (for review see Holtzman et al., 1977). Peroxidase-labelled multivesicular bodies are also seen in neurohypophysial terminals, especially after long periods of exposure to the tracer, but it is in the perikarya that they increase in frequency with increasing time after HRP injection. It is probable, then, that one of the first steps in the sequestration of the endocytotic membrane occurs in these organelles, either in the terminals after transformation from the large vacuoles or within the perikarya. These organelles can

278

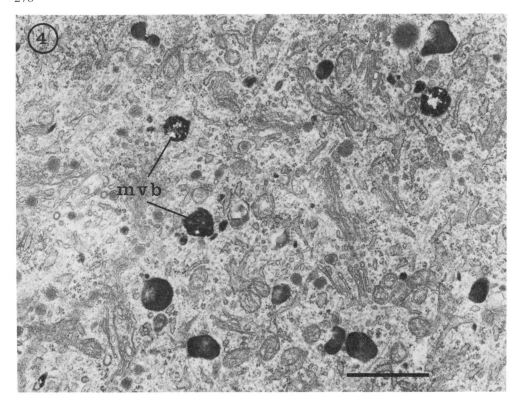

Fig. 4. Transmission electron micrograph of a thin-sectioned magnocellular perikaryon from the SO nucleus of a dehydrated rat that had been injected with HRP 8 h earlier. The section has not been stained with lead, and allows to see the dense reaction product within numerous vacuoles of various size, dense bodies and multivesicular bodies (mvb). Bar = 1 μm. × 21,000.

move retrogradely in axon cytoplasm (LaVail et al., 1980; Tsukita and Ishikawa, 1980) and they could thus also serve to transport the membrane to the perikarya. Multivesicular bodies occur in neurosecretory axons and cell bodies not exposed to any tracer and their volume density significantly increases in stimulated neurosecretory cells (Theodosis, 1982), suggesting that the membrane movements made visible by HRP normally occur in these cells and are not the result of exposure to a foreign protein.

By 24 h after HRP injection, very little tracer is seen in the terminals; in the perikarya, it is found mainly in lysosomal dense bodies, presumably to be degraded. Nevertheless, whether all the material internalized at neurosecretory terminals is ultimately degraded in the perikaryal lysosomes cannot be determined from such studies. Recent observations from other secretory systems (for reviews see Holtzman et al., 1977; Herzog and Miller, 1979) suggest that only partial degradation occurs and that the membrane or its constituents may be later reutilized.

REFERENCES

Branton, D. (1971) Freeze-etching studies of membrane structure. *Phil. Trans. roy. Soc. B*, 261: 133–138.
Broadwell, R.D. and Brightman, M.W. (1976) Entry of peroxidase into neurons of the central and peripheral nervous systems from extracerebral and cerebral blood, *J. comp. Neurol.*, 166: 257–284.

Broadwell, R.D., Oliver, C. and Brightman, M.W. (1980) Neuronal transport of acid hydrolases and peroxidase within the lysosomal system of organelles: involvement of agranular reticulum-like cisterns, *J. comp. Neurol.,* 190: 519–532.

Castel, M. (1974) In vivo uptake of tracers by neurosecretory axon terminals in normal and dehydrated mice, *Gen. comp. Endocr.,* 22: 336–337.

Dempsey, G.P., Bullivant, S. and Watkins, W.B. (1973) Ultrastructure of the rat posterior pituitary gland and evidence of hormone release by exocytosis as revealed by freeze-fracturing. *Z. Zellforsch.,* 143: 465–484.

Douglas, W.W. (1974) Mechanism of release of neurohypophysial hormones: stimulus secretion coupling. In E. Knobil and H.W. Sawyer (Eds.), *Handbook of Physiology, Vol. IV, Sect. 7, Part 1,* Amer. Physiol. Soc., Washington, pp. 191–220.

Herzog, V. and Miller, F. (1979) Membrane retrieval in secretory cells. In C.R. Hopkins and C.J. Duncan (Eds.), *Secretory Mechanisms,* Cambridge Univ. Press, pp. 101–116.

Holtzman, E., Schacher, S., Evans, J. and Teichberg, S. (1977) Origin and fate of the membranes of secretion granules and synaptic vesicles: membrane circulation in neurons, gland cells and retinal photoreceptors. In G. Poste and G.L. Nicolson (Eds.), *Cell Surface Reviews, Vol. 4,* Elsevier, Amsterdam, pp. 165–246.

LaVail, J.H., Rapisardi, S. and Sugino, I.K. (1980) Evidence against the smooth endoplasmic reticulum as a continuous channel for the retrograde transport of horseradish peroxidase, *Brain Res.,* 191: 3–20.

Morris, J.F. and Nordmann, J.J. (1980) Membrane recapture after hormone release from nerve endings in the neural lobe of the rat pituitary gland, *Neuroscience,* 5: 639–649.

Nagasawa, J., Douglas, W.W. and Schultz, R.A. (1970) Ultrastructural evidence of secretion by exocytosis and of "synaptic vesicle" formation in posterior pituitary glands. *Nature (Lond.),* 227: 407–409.

Nordmann, J.J. and Chevalier, J. (1980) The role of microvesicles in buffering $(Ca^{2+})_i$ in the neurohypophysis. *Nature (Lond.),* 287: 54–56.

Nordmann, J.J. and Morris, J.F. (1976) Membrane retrieval at neurosecretory axon endings. *Nature (Lond.),* 261: 723–725.

Nordmann, J.J., Dreifuss, J.J., Baker, P.F., Ravazzola, M., Malaise-Lagae, F. and Orci, L. (1974) Secretion-dependent uptake of extracellular fluid by the rat neurohypophysis. *Nature (Lond.),* 250: 155–157.

Palade, G. (1975) Intracellular aspects of the process of protein synthesis. *Science,* 189: 347–358.

Theodosis, D.T. (1982) Secretion-related accumulation of horseradish peroxidase in magnocellular cell bodies of the rat supraoptic nucleus. *Brain Res.,* 233: 3–16.

Theodosis, D.T., Dreifuss, J.J., Harris, M.C. and Orci, L. (1976) Secretion-related uptake of horseradish peroxidase in neurohypophysial axons. *J. Cell Biol.,* 70: 294–303.

Theodosis, D.T., Dreifuss, J.J. and Orci, L. (1977) Two classes of microvesicles in the neurohypophysis. *Brain Res.,* 123: 159–163.

Theodosis, D.T., Burlet, C., Boudier, J.L. and Dreifuss, J.J. (1978a) Morphology of membrane changes during neurohypophyseal hormone release in a hibernating rodent. *Brain Res.,* 154: 371–376.

Theodosis, D.T., Dreifuss, J.J. and Orci, L. (1978b) A freeze-fracture study of membrane events during neurohypophysial secretion. *J. Cell Biol.,* 78: 542–553.

Tsukita, S. and Ishikawa, H. (1980) The movement of membranous organelles in axons. Electron microscopic identification of anterogradely and retrogradely transported organelles. *J. Cell Biol.,* 84: 513–530.

Winkler, H. (1977) The biogenesis of adrenal chromaffin granules, *Neuroscience,* 2: 657–683.

Yu, J. and Branton, D. (1976) Reconstitution of intramembrane particles in recombinants of erythrocyte protein band 3 and lipid: effects of spectrin–actin association. *Proc. nat. Acad. Sci. U.S.A.,* 73: 3891–3895.

The Neurohypophysis: Structure, Function and Control, Progress in Brain Research, Vol. 60, edited by B.A. Cross and G. Leng

Stimulus–Secretion Coupling

J.J. NORDMANN

I.N.S.E.R.M., U. 176, Rue Camille Saint-Saëns, 33077 Bordeaux Cedex (France)

INTRODUCTION

The past decade of research on the mechanism by which oxytocin and vasopressin are released from neurosecretory nerve terminals leaves little doubt that hormone release occurs by exocytosis (Baker, 1974; Douglas, 1968, 1973, 1974a, b; Dreifuss, 1975; Morris et al., 1978; Nordmann, 1978; Normann, 1970). This conclusion is derived from three main experimental findings.

(1) The amount of a given intragranular molecule released upon stimulation is independent of the size of the molecule (Douglas, 1974a, b; Fawcett et al., 1968; Nordmann, 1978; Nordmann et al., 1971; Uttenthal et al., 1971). Stimulation of the neurohypophysis results in a parallel release of both neurohormones (oxytocin and vasopressin; molecular weight $\approx$ 1000) and their associated neurophysin (NpI and NpII; MW $\approx$ 10,000) (Fig. 1). The linear relationship between hormone and neurophysins implies that the magnitude of the stimulus does not influence the ratio of neurophysin: hormone released. In other words, there is no apparent diffusion barrier (except presumably the time during which the granule content is in direct contact with the extracellular space) between the interior of the granule and the extracellular space.

(2) The simultaneous release of different types of intragranular molecules does not seem to be due to a general increase in the cell membrane permeability, since there is no associated increase in the efflux of cytoplasmic marker proteins such as adenylate kinase (Edwards et al., 1973) or lactic dehydrogenase (Matthews et al., 1973).

(3) The time course of hormone release upon stimulation parallels that of the volumetric density of neurosecretory granules (NSG; Lescure and Nordmann, 1980). When neurohypophyses are stimulated with 50 mM K^+ or veratridine there is a marked increase in the amount of hormone released. When the volumetric density of NSG (which is directly related to the number of granules located in the nerve endings) is measured, there is an excellent correlation between the disappearance of granules and the amount of hormone released (Fig. 2). In other experiments, we calculated (Morris and Nordmann, 1980) that neural lobes stimulated with K^+ ions for 15 min release about 83 mU hormone (oxytocin + vasopressin), though this would be an underestimate in view of the hormone that is released but remains trapped within the gland (Müller et al., 1975; Ingram et al., 1982). Each granule has been calculated to contain 6×10^{-8} mU hormone (Morris, 1976; and this volume); the 83 mU hormone would therefore be contained in 1.4×10^9 NSG and stereological measurement of the granule population during such a stimulus gives a loss of 1.9×10^9 NSG. The reasonable agreement between hormone

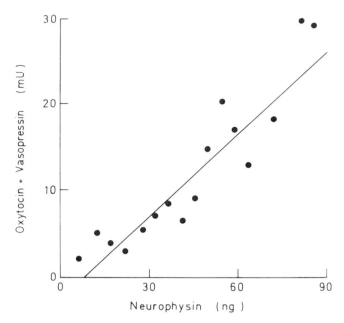

Fig. 1. Relationship between hormone release and neurophysin release following electrical stimulation of isolated neural lobes (Modified from Nordmann et al., 1971.)

assay and the stereological data strongly suggests that all the hormone released is derived from the neurosecretory granules which were lost from the terminals during acute stimulation.

With the exception of the work of Morris and Dyball (1974) and Reinhardt et al. (1969), most of the experiments involving hormone release and stereology have been done on isolated glands. I have recently analyzed hormone and granule depletion in neurohypophyses from rats subjected to dehydration. The results were similar to those observed in vitro, i.e. the time course of hormone (oxytocin + vasopressin) depletion during four days of dehydration was very similar to the decrease in the volumetric density of the NSG. In further experiments performed in collaboration with J.F. Morris (Oxford), Brattleboro rats were injected with

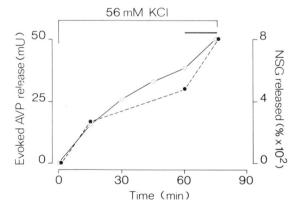

Fig. 2. Effects of prolonged depolarization on hormone release (●) and disappearance of neurosecretory granules (○). Veratridine was present during the time indicated by the heavy bar. (Modified from Lescure and Nordmann, 1980.)

exogenous vasopressin. These animals are unable to synthesize vasopressin, and exhibit a steady hypersecretion of oxytocin as a result of the osmotic imbalance caused by their diabetes insipidus. The number of NSG was reduced in both types of nerve endings in the hypersecreting Brattleboro rats, but increased as a result of vasopressin treatment. Thus, changes of the number of granules in the neural lobe are not only observed when hormone release is increased, but also when secretion is inhibited (Morris and Nordmann, 1982).

IS THERE A CYTOPLASMIC POOL?

Although these experiments demonstrate that neurohypophysial hormone is released by exocytosis, it remains to be discussed whether a proportion of the hormone is present within the cytoplasm.

Both hormone and neurophysin are found in the granule-free supernatant of homogenized neural lobes, and a greater proportion of free hormone can be found in supernatants derived from dehydrated, haemorrhaged and lactating rats (Barer et al., 1963; Daniel and Lederis, 1966; Norström, 1972). As newly synthesized hormone (Sachs and Haller, 1968) and newly formed granules (Nordmann and Labouesse, 1981) are preferentially released, it is to be expected that NSG remaining in stimulated animals are relatively older, and thus more liable to rupture during homogenization. We have already discussed (Morris et al., 1978) the description of cytoplasmic neurophysin but not vasopressin, and have commented that this might be due to an artefact. Recent experiments have demonstrated that neurosecretory granules are very fragile. This fragility might explain why neurophysin can be found either in the supernatant of homogenized glands or in the cytoplasm of fixed tissue. Older granules are particularly sensitive to osmotic damage during fixation (Cannata and Morris, 1973) and during homogenization (Nordmann, 1982). Whereas newly formed granules are insensitive to the surrounding osmotic pressure, older granules are permeable, as judged from the change in their diameter under different osmotic pressure (Nordmann et al., 1979). However, if glands are homogenized in a hyperosmotic medium, more than 95% of the total hormone is found within the granule fraction. Furthermore, after four days dehydration and two days rehydration, i.e. at a stage where most of the granules within the neural lobe can be considered as newly formed, up to 98% of the total hormone is found in a fraction corresponding to the NSG. These experiments suggest that all the hormone is located within the granules.

The experiment described above, showing that the amount of hormone released upon K^+ depolarization corresponds to the amount of hormone contained within the granules which have disappeared after stimulation, suffers the intrinsic disadvantage of its assumption of exclusive intragranular storage of hormone. To overcome this problem, we have recently designed an experiment (Morris and Nordmann, unpublished) in which NSG were mixed with a known number of Latex particles. Stereology and hormone and neurophysin assay were then used to calculate the number of NSG and thus measure their content. For osmotically stable granules (i.e. newly formed NSG) we found that each granule contains an average of 84,000 molecules of hormone and 95,000 molecules of neurophysin. This is consistent with the calculation of Morris (1976) and therefore validates the assumption that all hormone is in the granules.

Early descriptions suggested that, following exocytotic discharge of the content of NSG, the membrane is recaptured in the form of electron-lucent microvesicles (diameters of ca. 50 nm) (Douglas et al., 1971; Nagasawa et al., 1970). Such microvesicles were also shown to take up the extracellular marker horseradish peroxidase (Nagasawa et al., 1971). The idea that

284

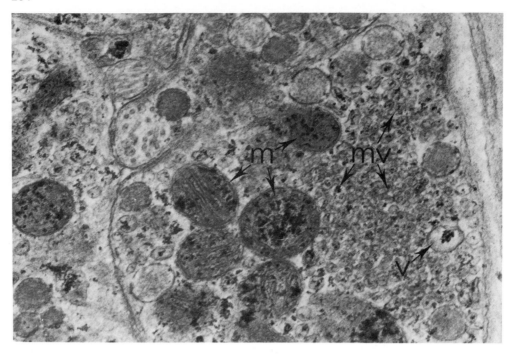

Fig. 3. Electron micrograph of the neural lobe. The neurohypophysis was fixed according to the method of Shaw and Morris (1981). Note the presence in the microvesicles (mv), in the mitochondria (m) and in a vacuole (v) of Ca deposit. Courtesy of Fraser Shaw and John Morris.

microvesicles are responsible for membrane reuptake came originally from the work of Bunt (1969) and Normann (1969, 1970). Working with invertebrate neurosecretory axon endings, they observed an increase in microvesicle *clusters* in the region of exocytosis. Some microvesicles were seen to be labelled with extracellular markers such as Thorotrast (Bunt, 1969) or ferritin (Smith, 1970). Douglas et al. (1971) calculated that in the neural lobe the membrane of a single granule would be sufficient to form 25 microvesicles. The volume occupied by these 25 microvesicles being less than that of a single granule, these authors concluded that microvesiculation would liberate space within the neurohypophysial terminals, and permit fresh NSG easier access to the neurosecretory terminal membrane.

A few years ago we were interested to determine how much extracellular Ca would be taken up by microvesicles during endocytosis. Using different isotope-labelled extracellular markers, we were surprised to find that the volume taken up by the terminals after exo-endocytosis was much larger than that expected if microvesiculation occurred, and was very close to the volume which would be taken into the nerve terminals by organelles of a similar size to the NSG (Nordmann et al., 1974). This prompted us to repeat the experiment with horseradish peroxidase as an extracellular marker. The striking observation was that most of the marker in the nerve ending was located in organelles of a size similar to that of NSG, which we named vacuoles (Fig. 3; see also Castel, 1974). Further experiments involving combined stereology and hormone assay confirmed these observations (Lescure and Nordmann, 1980; Morris and Nordmann, 1980, 1982; Nordmann and Morris, 1976; Theodosis et al., 1976). The vacuole hypothesis was supported by the experiments of Swann and Pickering (1976), who labelled NSG with radioactive lipids and followed the fate of the granule membrane. After stimulation of hormone release, they found that the label ([3H]choline) remained in the granular fraction, suggesting that the membrane is retrieved in the form of organelles of the same size as NSG and that the granules do not give rise to microvesicles after liberation of their content.

It could be argued that the acute experiments, and especially those conducted in vitro, have the defect that severe stimuli were used (potassium- or veratridine-induced depolarization, or haemorrhage) and that vacuoles are artefacts of this form of stimulation. However, in the experiment described above in which Brattleboro rats were given exogenous vasopressin, we observed concomitantly an *increase* of the volumetric density of the NSG and a *decrease* of that of vacuoles. Thus, for both acute and chronic hormone release, it is the vacuoles which are responsible for membrane reuptake.

One question which remains is: which membrane is retrieved? Is it the granule membrane itself, or is it part of the plasmalemma? In the neurohypophysis we favour the former because of the following.

(1) As mentioned above, Swann and Pickering (1976) found that after hormone release most of the labelled membrane of granules is found in the granule fraction.

(2) Brattleboro rats contain two types of NSG: one type is of a similar size to those found in normal rats, and presumably contain oxytocin; the second type has a mean diameter of about 100 nm. The content of these smaller granules is unknown. In both types of endings vacuoles can be found, and their diameter is very similar to that of the granules which are located in the same ending (Morris and Nordmann, 1982). Thus, in Brattleboro rats as in normal rats the size of the endocytotic vacuoles are directly related to the size of the NSG.

(3) Preliminary experiments in collaboration with Fraser Shaw (London) also suggest that the granule membrane itself is taken up into the nerve terminal after exocytosis. The outside surface of the membrane of neurosecretosomes (isolated nerve endings) was labelled with lectins coupled to ferritin or horseradish peroxidase. After washing out the unbound material, release was triggered with Ca containing liposomes or Ca ionophores in the presence of the extracellular marker. The interesting observation was that the vacuole membrane were not labelled with lectin, suggesting that no mixing between the granule membrane and the plasmalemma occurs during the exo-endocytotic process. Similar conclusions have been reached for mast cells with the use of rapid freezing (Chandler and Heuser, 1980). Because there is no mixing between the NSG and plasma membranes, the time during which the granule is in direct contact with the extracellular space is likely to be extremely short. The duration of the exocytotic event in the neural lobe has not yet been measured, but in mast cells, where release of granules can be observed at the light microscope level, the use of rapid photography at 5000 frames/sec suggests that exocytosis takes about 5 msec (Douglas, 1974b). Thus in the neural lobe the time for the membrane to fuse with the plasmalemma and to be retrieved should be of the same order of magnitude. This would explain why exocytotic figures are very rarely observed in the neural lobe (see Morris et al., 1978).

CALCIUM HOMEOSTASIS IN NEUROSECRETORY NERVE TERMINALS

To understand the role of intracellular Ca in the process of neurohormone release, it is necessary to look at the mechanisms of control of the ionized Ca in the neurosecretory nerve terminals. Unfortunately, in the neural lobe the absolute values of $[Ca]_i$ at rest or when hormone release, i.e. Ca uptake, is increased are very uncertain and we can only infer the concentration in the neurohypophysial nerve terminals from other systems. In the sinus gland of the crab, the inside of the neurosecretory nerve terminal membrane is about 70 mV negative with respect to the outside (Cooke, 1977). Because the external Ca concentration is in the millimolar range it follows that, if Ca is passively distributed across the nerve terminal plasmalemma, Ca should be highly concentrated inside the ending. This has never been observed in any system in which cytoplasmic Ca ion activities could be measured. There is general agreement in the literature for a cytoplasmic ionized Ca concentration of 10^{-7} M or below (for review see Requena and Mullins, 1979). However, recent work on both the neural lobe and another neurosecretory system, the adrenal medulla, allows an indirect estimation of the internal ionized Ca concentration.

Using NSG isolated from rat neurohypophyses, Gratzl et al. (1977) have shown by freeze-cleaving electron microscopy that external Ca concentrations above 10^{-6} M induce a small but significant increase in the number of fused granules. Because fused granules are extremely rarely observed in fixed tissue this suggests, but does not prove, that under resting conditions the internal ionized Ca concentration in the neurosecretory nerve endings is below 10^{-6} M. Furthermore, microvesicles located in the nerve terminals can accumulate Ca with an affinity constant ranging from 0.4 to 0.2 μM, and this uptake is maximal at $[Ca]_i$ of 10^{-6} M (Nordmann and Chevallier, 1981). Because there is an increase in Ca concentration in these organelles just after depolarization of the nerve terminals, one can estimate that in the neurohypophysial nerve endings $[Ca]_i$ is smaller than 10^{-6} M. Recent experiments on isolated chromaffin cells also suggest such a concentration. Cells were exposed to intense electrical fields for brief periods of time. Under these conditions, the plasmalemma undergoes a dielectric breakdown without obvious damage of the cell membrane. The cells are then freely accessible to low molecular weight solutes of the bathing medium, and do not show any significant loss of cytoplasmic molecules such as lactic dehydrogenase. In these so-called "leaky" cells secretion is half-maximally activated at $[Ca]_i$ of about 10^{-6} M and is arrested at a Ca concentration of about 10^{-7} M (Baker and Knight, 1981).

In summary, it is probable that, in the neurohypophysial nerve terminals, the ionized cytoplasmic concentration is about 10^{-7} M.

How is the cytoplasmic concentration maintained?

After Ca has entered the nerve ending during depolarization, its cytoplasmic concentration has to be reduced rapidly. If this were not the case secretion would proceed, possibly giving rise to physiological abnormalities. The ionized cytoplasmic Ca in excess of 10^{-7} M could: (1) be bound to cytoplasmic molecules; (2) be transferred into cellular organelles, or (3) be pumped out of the nerve terminal.

(1) Specific Ca-binding proteins have been identified in squid or *Myxicola* axoplasm (Baker and Schlaepfer, 1978). In the neural lobe, only the group of Thorn has tried to isolate Ca-binding proteins. Their main finding is that in the soluble fraction there is a protein of approximately 15,000 daltons (Russell and Thorn, 1977; Thorn et al., 1978). This protein is electrophoretically distinct from the neurophysins and the protein S-100 which has been shown to bind Ca ions (Calissano et al., 1969). Furthermore, it has an apparent dissociation constant for Ca of 1.1×10^{-5} M which is rather high if one considers the internal Ca concentration. However, because we do not know the exact concentration of Ca at the inner site of the membrane where fusion of the granule occurs (see Matthews, 1979), this protein might play a role in maintenance of a low Ca concentration.

(2) Electron microscopy reveals at least three types of subcellular organelles in the neuro-hypophysial nerve terminals: NSG, mitochondria, and microvesicles. The latter might be part of the endoplasmic reticulum as suggested by observations at high voltage of relatively thick section (Alonso and Assenmacher, 1979).

The NSG apparently contain a high concentration of Ca. Thorn et al. (1975) found that a fraction enriched in NSG contains a mean of 73 nEq/mg of proteins. Recent experiments with J.F. Morris (unpublished) show that each newly formed NSG contains about 2.2 fg of protein. Thus it can be calculated that the amount of Ca found in the NSG-containing fraction corresponds to an intragranular concentration of 0.14 mM. This is very similar to the

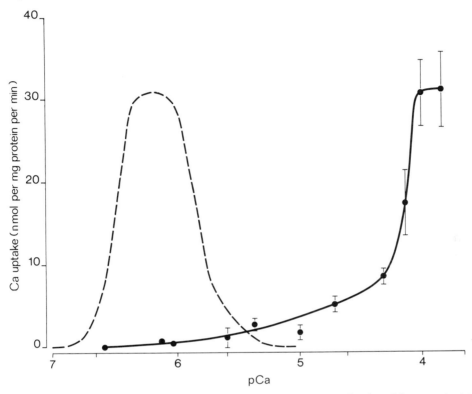

Fig. 4. Ca uptake into isolated microvesicles (dashed line) and mitochondria as a function of the external calcium concentration. The dashed line is drawn according to the data of Nordmann and Chevallier (1981).

concentration of Ca found in the chromaffin granules (0.1 mM) calculated on the basis that each granule contains 660 Ca ions (review by Winkler and Westhead, 1980) and has a mean volume of 1.1×10^7 nm^3. Flux studies of ^{45}Ca ions show that the Ca within the granules is only very slowly exchangeable (Russell and Thorn, 1975). However, recent experiments demonstrated that the pH gradient of the NSG, which in the neural lobe is governed by Donnan equilibrium, is much reduced in the presence of external Ca, suggesting some permeability of the NSG membrane for Ca ions (Scherman and Nordmann, 1982). Similar findings to those reported by Russell and Thorn have been described for the insulin storage granules (Howell et al., 1975; Borowitz and Matthews, 1980).

In a variety of tissues mitochondria have been suggested to be responsible for Ca homeostasis. Neural lobes fixed in the presence of oxalate and post-fixed with OsO_4 solution contaaaaining potassium antimonate show heavily stained mitochondria (Shaw and Morris, 1981). The mitochondria retained their precipitates after the tissue had been washed in phosphate buffer, but no deposit could be observed when the neural lobes were incubated in EGTA-containing medium before post-fixation.

The first biochemical evidence for Ca uptake by mitochondria in the neural lobe was published by Russell and Thorn (1975). The uptake depends on the presence of ATP and is considerably reduced in the presence of azide, an uncoupler of oxidative phosphorylation. Furthermore, in a recent study I have found that this uptake has an affinity constant for Ca of about 9×10^{-5} M and that the uptake is maximal around 10^{-4} M $[Ca]_o$ (Fig. 4). Although the capacity of mitochondria to accumulate Ca is relatively high (30 nmol/mg/min), the affinity constant of the sequestering mechanism renders it unlikely that the mitochondria are the sole organelles for controlling the ionized cytoplasmic concentration.

Microvesicles in the neural lobe have the advantage, when compared with studies on the neuromuscular junction or brain isolated synaptosomes, that they are very different in size and electron density from the storage organelles, i.e. the NSG. I have already argued that microvesicles are probably not responsible for membrane reuptake after exocytosis. This is not to say that these organelles are not involved in stimulus–secretion coupling. Normann (1970), in his study on the corpus cardiaca of the blowfly, observed an *increase* of the microvesicle *clusters* near the exocytotic sites. In our studies we observed no increase in the number of microvesicles in nerve endings after stimulation of hormone release, but rather a redistribution of the microvesicles towards the plasmalemma abutting the basement membrane (Morris and Nordmann, 1980). This is where exocytosis and possibly Ca uptake should occur because stimulation of hormone release indicates that it is a 600 nm wide zone of the endings immediately adjacent to the contact zone with the basement membrane that becomes most significantly depleted of granules. The observation of Stoekel et al. (1975) which demonstrated that microvesicles contain Ca precipitate prompted us to analyze in detail the uptake of Ca into a fraction containing microvesicles. Previous experiments had shown that a microsomal fraction isolated from the neurohypophysis (i.e. pituicytes and neuronal elements) accumulates Ca (Russell and Thorn, 1975). The amount of Ca taken up by this fraction (ca. 8 nmol/mg protein), however, is small in comparison with the quantity accumulated by the mitochondria. To avoid contamination by organelles derived from pituicytes, we isolated a fraction of neurosecretosomes, and from this prepared a microsomal fraction containing microvesicles (Nordmann and Chevallier, 1981). This fraction accumulates large amounts of Ca (ca. 240 nmol/mg protein). The accumulation is ATP-dependent and has an apparent K_m^{Ca} of about 0.5μM. This is in the range of the cytosolic $[Ca]$, and is much lower than the affinity constant of the Ca uptake mechanism in mitochondria. Neither the time course nor the amount of Ca uptake is affected by addition of mitochondrial inhibitors such as ruthenium red, antimycin or FFCP (carbonyl cyanide trifluomethoxyphenylhydrazone). These results show that fragments of mitochondria are not responsible for the ATP-dependent accumulation in the microvesicle-containing fraction. These data are confirmed by the experiments of Shaw and Morris (1981) who observed electron-dense deposits in microvesicles after fixation of the tissue in the presence of oxalate and post-fixation in the presence of potassium antimonate (Fig. 3). Precipitates remained localized in microvesicles and in the mitochondria after washing of the tissue in phosphate buffer.

The above mentioned data and those published by Torp-Pedersen et al. (1981) show that NSG are unlikely to participate to a large extent in Ca homeostasis, whereas microvesicles and mitochondria can accumulate Ca ions, the microvesicles having a much higher affinity for this divalent cation than mitochondria.

Ca extrusion at the plasmalemma of neurosecretory nerve terminals

Thus there is much evidence that, after depolarization of the nerve terminals, there is an increased Ca uptake. The resulting increase in $[Ca]_i$ may be buffered either by the microvesicles and/or by the mitochondria. Clearly the cell cannot accumulate Ca for long, and the nerve endings must eventually extrude the accumulated Ca. This is illustrated by the experiments of Russell and Thorn (1974a), where electrical stimulation of isolated pituitaries increases hormone release but failed to show a significant augmentation of Ca content when the glands have been stimulated for long periods of time.

How the Ca accumulated in microvesicles is released is not known. Electron micrographs often show fusion of these organelles with the plasmalemma, and so Ca could be released by exocytosis. Alternatively, Ca could be released slowly into the cytoplasm and long-term Ca homeostasis controlled by transporting systems located at the plasma membrane. That microvesicles can release their Ca by exocytosis or possibly into the cytoplasm comes from the observation that accumulation of Ca by microvesicles is maximal after 10 min of Ca challenge but then decreases with time (Nordmann and Chevallier, 1981). Also if, after K^+ depolarization or electrical depolarization in the presence of radioactive Ca, microvesicles are rapidly isolated, a significant increase in their radioactive Ca content is observed. However, 15–20 min after termination of the depolarization much less Ca is found in the microvesicles, which suggests that these organelles accumulate Ca only transiently (Fig. 5).

What are the mechanisms involved in the extrusion of Ca at the surface of neurosecretory nerve terminals? This extrusion is against an electrochemical gradient as the ionized Ca concentration in the cytoplasm is about 10^4 times less than in the extracellular space. Three different mechanisms have been described so far. The first is activated by external Na ions (Na_o), the second by external Ca (Ca_o) and the third is probably activated by a Ca-dependent ATPase (Nordmann and Zyzek, 1982).

The effect of Na_o on Ca efflux

When the external Na ions are replaced by choline, which presumably does not penetrate the nerve terminals, there is a significant (ca. 32%) decrease in the Ca efflux. The decrease is proportional to the magnitude of $[Na]_o$ reduction (Fig. 6). The data, according to the Hill representation, suggest that at normal (2.2 mM) Ca_o the extrusion of one Ca ion involves probably three Na ions (Hill coefficient = 2.8). According to the observed kinetics, $Ca_i/Ca_o = Na_i/Na_o$. Assuming that the ratio Na_i/Na_o in the neural lobe is similar to that found in other systems (ca. 1/10), the Na gradient would maintain in the nerve endings an ionized Ca concentration of ca. 2 μM, which is higher than the expected concentration (see p. 286).

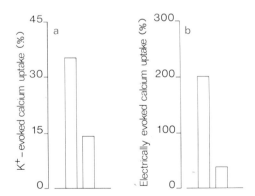

Fig. 5. Ca accumulation in microvesicles after K-depolarization (a) and electrical stimulation (b). On each panel the column on the left represents the Ca uptake measured 6 min after stopping the stimulation whereas the righthand columns are the values measured about 23 min after termination of the stimulation.

290

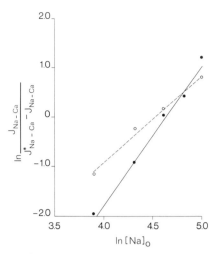

Fig. 6. Hill plot of the Na_o-dependent ^{45}Ca efflux. The calculated (least squares) slopes for the neural lobes incubated in the presence ($\bullet$) or the absence ($\circ$) of Ca_o are 2.8 and 1.7, respectively.

However, the Hill coefficient gives a minimum figure, and it is possible that four Na ions are involved in the extrusion of one Ca ion. This would maintain the ionized cytosolic Ca concentration at about 10^{-7} M. Under normal conditions half-activation of the Ca efflux occurs at 100 mM Na_o whereas removal of external Ca increases the affinity of the transporting system for Na_o. Under these conditions the affinity constant for Na_o is about 88 mM, with a Hill coefficient of 1.7 (Fig. 6). Assuming that in so-called Ca-free media (without chelating agent) the external Ca concentration is 10^{-5} M at the most, one can calculate that, under these conditions, $[Ca]_i$ would be around 10^{-7} M.

The role of Ca_o on Ca efflux

The Ca efflux from the neurohypophysis is decreased by more than 30% after removal of external Ca. Furthermore this Ca-dependent Ca efflux is inhibited by Na ions. Whereas in Na-free media the Ca-activated Ca efflux has a K_m of ca. 20 μM, at normal $[Na]_o$ this is increased to 0.8 mM. Although at present we have no evidence concerning the mechanism by which external Ca can modulate the extrusion of internal Ca, it seems likely that Ca activates the efflux of the ionized cellular Ca at the external surface of the cell membrane. The low affinity of Ca_o for the transporting system would render a counter mechanism inefficient.

ATP-dependent Ca efflux

Part of the Na_o- and Ca_o-independent or uncoupled Ca efflux from isolated neural lobes is inhibited by vanadate, which is a powerful inhibitor of the Ca-stimulated ATPase. Although in the neural lobe the uncoupled Ca efflux represents about only one-third of the Ca efflux, it is possible that in vivo a larger part of the total efflux is dependent on the cellular ATP level. Indeed, in squid axons at very low $[Ca]_i$ (ca. 0.04 μM), ATP requirement for the Ca efflux is critical (Dipolo, 1977). The large effect of internal ATP on Ca efflux can be understood by assuming that ATP changes the affinity for Na at the internal and possibly the external sites of the plasma membrane. Moreover, it is not necessary to postulate hydrolysis of the ATP. Unfortunately we have no means of controlling the ATP concentration in the neural lobe.

THE RELATIONSHIP BETWEEN Ca AND HORMONE RELEASE

At the beginning of this section I would like to "rendre hommage" to W.W. Douglas who, in the early 1960s, had already demonstrated with his colleagues Mikiten, Poisner and Rubin, that external Ca ions were essential for hormone release. Their experiments allowed them to formulate the by now well-known concept of stimulus–secretion coupling. Their main results were as follows.

(1) Incubation of isolated neurohypophyses in a high K solution or electrical stimulation of the gland in vitro, gives rise to an increase in vasopressin release.

(2) The K-induced increase in hormone release can occur (and even be potentiated) in low Na-containing medium.

(3) Whereas external Ca ions are essential for hormone release, the presence of Cl ions in the bathing medium is not. Furthermore, high Mg concentrations (10–20 mM) block the K-induced hormone release.

(4) Associated with the K-induced vasopressin release there is an increase in Ca uptake. Inhibition of release by Mg ions is accompanied by a decrease in Ca uptake.

Recently, the use of a voltage-sensitive dye (the fluorescence of which is a function of the potential of the membrane to which it is bound) has confirmed directly that K_o depolarizes neurosecretory nerve terminals of the neural lobe (Nordmann et al., 1982). However, whereas depolarization is a linear function of $[K]_o$ (between 10 and 100 mM), hormone release is not (Fig. 7). Assuming a resting membrane potential of -70 mV (see Nordmann et al., 1982), the maximum rate of change in hormone release occurs at a membrane potential of ca -30 to -20 mV. This is very close to the membrane potential of the squid giant synapse at which maximal release occurs. Although changes of external $[K]_o$ might give rise to profound and unphysiological changes in the ionic composition of the nerve endings, there is little doubt that in the presence of external Ca ions an increase in neurohormone release is induced by the depolarizing effect of $[K]_o$. This conclusion is strengthened by the increased hormone release induced by veratridine (Nordmann and Dyball, 1978), an alkaloid known to maintain Na channels in an open state.

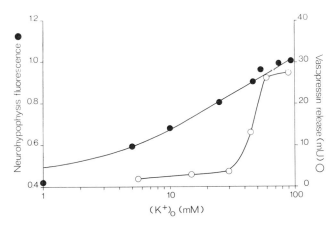

Fig. 7. Effects of external K concentration on the relationship between fluorescence of the dye diS-C$_3$-(5) and the amount of hormone release. The fluorescence fits the equation $F = A \log (K_o + 0.06 \, Na_o) + B$, where $A = 0.41$ and $B = 0.19$. (From Nordmann et al., 1982.)

Evidence for a depolarization-induced entry of Ca into the nerve terminals

Douglas and Poisner (1964a, b) found that in the neural lobe there is an increased Ca uptake associated with hormone release. However, until recently we did not know whether this uptake reflects a net entry of Ca or an exchange between internal and external ions. Recent experiments favour the first hypothesis. Firstly, removal of external Na increases Ca uptake but considerably reduces Ca efflux from the neural lobe. Secondly, K-depolarization increases hormone release and Ca uptake for prolonged periods (although both decline with time, see p. 294) but has only a very transient effect on Ca efflux. Finally, when veratridine is added to the bathing medium it induces a large increase in Ca uptake, but there is no change of the Ca efflux. Taken together with the more compelling evidence from the squid giant synapse in which a small depolarization of the presynaptic nerve terminal induces transmitter release but large depolarizations are ineffective (i.e. the potential at which transmitter release is blocked corresponds approximately to the Ca equilibrium potential), the data obtained on the neural lobe suggest strongly that depolarization of the terminals induces an increase in Ca entry.

Membrane permeability for Ca

How does Ca penetrate into the nerve terminals? The neural lobe contains glial as well as neuronal elements, and washout curves of ions from a tissue are difficult to extrapolate to the quantity of an ion crossing a unit surface area of membrane. Therefore, only a general impression of Ca fluxes in the neural lobe can be achieved.

At rest Ca entry is not a linear function of the external Ca concentration and can be described by the section of a rectangular hyperbola with a K_m^{Ca} of about 0.25 mM (Nordmann and Zyzek, 1982). In an attempt to calculate the amount of Ca which enters the neurohypophysis at rest I recently used a "rapid" washing technique which involves loading the gland with ^{45}Ca and then a short incubation in a Na-, Ca-free medium containing the chelating agent EGTA. Although the results are very approximate, at physiological external Ca concentration (2.2 mM) the uptake of Ca is about 40 pmol/mg protein/20 min. During K-depolarization this uptake increased significantly, as shown by Douglas and Poisner (1964b). We have no direct evidence that the Ca uptake induced by high-K is voltage-sensitive. However, experiments on ^{45}Ca uptake during short exposure to high-K solutions (Nordmann, 1976; unpublished) suggest that this is the case. The rate of hormone release increases steeply in the range of the presumed membrane potentials which correspond, in the squid giant synapse, to the maximum Ca current. Taking into account the time for the hormone to diffuse out of the tissue (Ingram et al., 1982), it is clear that hormone release stops immediately after return to 5 mM K solution. The neurohormone release can therefore be used as a sort of "Ca electrode" for the nerve terminal (see below). From its characteristics it is likely that, in the neurohypophysis as in other excitable systems, the major entry of Ca during depolarization is by a voltage-sensitive mechanism.

What is the route for this Ca entry? Some experiments have shown that tetrodotoxin (TTX), which blocks Na channels specifically, also blocks hormone release (Ishida, 1967). Although this could indicate a common route for Na and Ca ions, other experiments have shown that this is not the case (Nordmann and Dreifuss, 1972). Firstly, K-induced Ca uptake and hormone release are not blocked by TTX. Secondly, TTX in the medium does not always block electrically stimulated hormone release in vitro; this is due to different methods used for current delivery (suction electrode, "shishkebab" etc...; unpublished). This can be explained in the following way. Either the electrically induced depolarization is large enough to increase

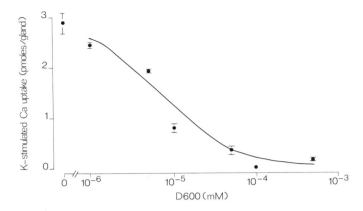

Fig. 8. Effects of D600 on K-induced Ca uptake in the neurohypophysis. The curve has been drawn according to J_{Ca} = $\bar{J}_{Ca}/1 + (D600/K)$, where $\bar{J}_{Ca}$ represent the uptake observed in the absence of D600 and K is the inhibitory constant with a value of 7 μM.

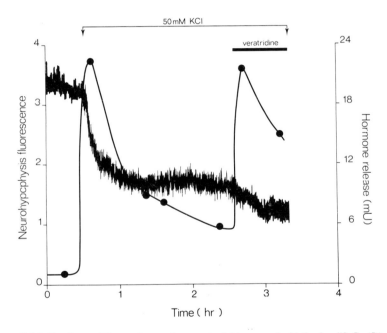

Fig. 9. Effects of high-K and veratridine on the membrane potential (measured with the dye diS-C_3-(5)) and hormone release. Note that the increased hormone release induced by K and veratridine is correlated with depolarization of the neural lobe. (From Dyball and Nordmann, 1977 and Nordman et al., 1982.)

Ca permeability directly or, if smaller, it can do so via activation of Na channels. Although we cannot exclude the possibility that some Ca ions enter the nerve terminals through the TTX-sensitive Na channels, the results so far suggest that during depolarization the Ca uptake occurs through the so-called "late" Ca channel. The term "late" comes from the observation that in the squid giant axon Ca entry occurs in two phases: an early phase which is parallel to the increase in Na permeability and a *late* phase which *turns on* later (Baker et al., 1973a). Ca

294

entry into the neural lobe is blocked by Mg, Mn and Co ions and the drug D600 (Dreifuss et al., 1973; Russell and Thorn, 1974b; Fig. 8). These agents similarly block the late Ca channel in the squid giant axon and the Ca inward current at the squid giant synapse. Endocytosis cannot contribute to a large extent to the observed Ca uptake, because the Ca taken up by the vacuoles would represent 5% at the most of the evoked Ca entry.

Does the late Ca channel in the neurohypophysis inactivate? This is a difficult question because only indirect methods can be used to analyze Ca entry into the neurosecretory nerve terminals. One observation can be interpreted as showing inactivation of the late Ca channel. During prolonged K-depolarization Ca uptake is not maintained but declines with time. Furthermore, the time course of Ca uptake is very similar to that of hormone release (Nordmann, 1976). This is not due to the repolarization of the membrane potential because depolarization measured with the fluorescent probe diS-C$_3$-(5) is maintained (Fig. 9) and,

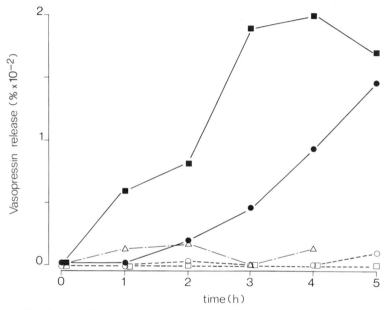

Fig. 10. Effects of incubation of isolated neurosecretosomes with liposomes on hormone release. The closed symbols represent the increase in hormone release induced by liposomes containing 5 mM CaCl$_2$. The open symbols represent the release observed in the absence of liposomes (○, □) and in the presence of liposomes loaded with 5mM MgCl$_2$ (Δ). The results are expressed as the percent of increase compared with that at time zero.

moreover, addition of veratridine further depolarizes the membrane and increases hormone release (Dyball and Nordmann, 1977; Nordmann et al., 1982). Also, addition of Ca after maintained K-depolarization in Ca-free medium always results in a smaller Ca uptake (and hormone release) than that observed at the onset of depolarization in a Ca-containing medium. These data suggest that channels are voltage-sensitive and inactivate slowly during membrane depolarization. Further depolarization by veratridine activates either new or inactivated channels. Recovery from inactivation is very slow, and seems to depend upon the time during which the preparation has been depolarized (Shaw, Dyball and Nordmann, in preparation). Similar observations have been made for the squid giant axon (Baker et al., 1973b). After exposure to high K for 2–3 min, the response to a second exposure to the same K concentration is much reduced and recovery is half-complete in about 3–4 min.

Evidence that neurohormone release is triggered by a rise in [Ca]$_i$

The next question is whether exocytosis results from the transport of Ca across the plasmalemma, or the rise in cytosolic Ca. Interesting data have been obtained in this respect from studies on the effect of Ca ionophores on Ca fluxes and hormone release (Nordmann and Currell, 1975; Nordmann and Dyball, 1975; Nakazato and Douglas, 1974; Russell et al., 1974). These lipophilic compounds transport Ca across biological membranes. These are not entirely specific for Ca, e.g. the ionophore X-537A transports Na and other cations. However, this problem can be overcome by incubating the gland in Na-free media, and this does not modify the response to the ionophore. Neural lobes incubated in presence of these ionophores release large amounts of hormone, and this effect is unlikely to result from any depolarization induced by these compounds (Nordmann and Desmazes, unpublished). Hormone release occurs in the absence of external Ca and, moreover, Ca flux studies show that the ionophore gives rise to a large increase of the Ca efflux which presumably arises from an increased cytosolic Ca concentration. Mitochondria and microvesicles are, as discussed on p. 287, good candidates for releasing Ca into the cytoplasm. Other experiments also suggest that an increase of [Ca]$_i$ is sufficient to promote vasopressin and oxytocin release. Neurosecretosomes (isolated nerve endings) were isolated as early as 1965 by La Bella and Sanwal. However, it seems that depolarization does not release hormone from neurosecretosomes. They do respond to cold stimulation, but the mechanism by which hormone is released is not known (Baker and Hope, 1976; Baker et al., 1975). The lack of release upon K-depolarization might arise from the haemorrhage of the animal (ox) which precedes removal of the gland. This might release the 20–30% of gland hormone content which can be released by acute stimuli (Nordmann and Dyball, 1975). Recently I have tried to increase the cytoplasmic Ca by adding liposomes containing 5 mM Ca to the neurosecretosome preparation. Fusion of the liposomes with the nerve endings gives rise to a large increase in vasopressin output (Fig. 10). This release is Ca-specific (although I have not yet tried to induce release with Sr- or Ba-containing liposomes) because Mg loaded liposomes do not significantly increase the basal release. The neurosecretosomes also respond to the ionophore X-537A, and a preliminary study in collaboration with Fraser Shaw (London) shows that Ca-containing liposomes or X-537A both induce exo-endocytotic coupling observed in the neural lobe. Thus, although the membrane potential of isolated nerve endings probably respond to change of [K]$_o$, one step (Ca entry?) seems to be lacking in the stimulus–secretion coupling mechanism.

In conclusion, these data suggest that a rise in cytoplasmic Ca is sufficient to promote hormone release, and that depolarization is not a prerequisite for secretion. This is supported by the findings of Douglas and Sorimachi (see Douglas, 1974a) who found that removal of external Na gives rise to a slow but significant increase in vasopressin output. This can be explained by an increase of [Ca]$_i$ resulting from blockage of the Na–Ca exchange (see p. 289). All the experiments published so far show quite clearly that neurohormone release and Ca uptake are closely linked. Mg, Co and Mn ions and D600 block both K-induced Ca entry and oxytocin and vasopressin release (Dreifuss, 1975; Dreifuss et al., 1973; Nordmann, 1976; Russell and Thorn, 1974b). Removal of external Na potentiates both mechanisms either under resting conditions (unpublished) or during K-depolarization. Whereas the relationship between [Na]$_o$ and hormone release suggest that two Na compete for one Ca ion (Dreifuss et al., 1971a), the interpretation of ^{45}Ca flux studies is unclear. Plots of Ca uptake and vasopressin release as a function of [Ca]$_o$ fit the section of a rectangular hyperbola with K_m values of 0.25 mM and 0.60 mM, respectively. Hill plots of the data give a slope of one for both phenomena. From these data I have tried (Fig. 11) to correlate the hormone release at different Ca concentrations with the basal uptake of Ca. The relationship is linear in the range of 0.11 to 2.2 Ca_o, and has a slope smaller than one. This suggests that one Ca ion can promote the release of one hormone unit or quantum (possibly the content of a single granule). This is not surprising

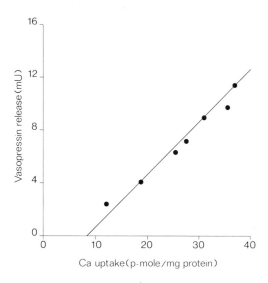

Fig. 11. The effect of external Ca concentration on vasopressin release. The hormone data are those published by Douglas and Poisner (1964a).

because Gage and Quastel (1966) and Crawford (1973) also observed that, at the neuromuscular junction, low external Ca concentration gives rise to a linear relationship between Ca and release. Furthermore, from the data of Ingram et al. (1982) one can calculate that electrical stimulation of isolated neural lobes produces a ten-fold increase in hormone output during the first minute of stimulation. This would correspond to a Ca concentration of 10^{-6} M during this period. If more than one Ca ion were involved in the release of such a quantum one would expect, with an identical rise in free Ca_i, to have much more hormone released. For example, if the ten-fold increase in hormone release observed by Ingram et al., (1982) involves a square relationship between Ca uptake and secretion, one would expect the ionized Ca concentration to rise by only a tenth of the resting $[Ca]_i$. This is extremely unlikely, because under such circumstances very small fluctuations of $[Ca]_i$ would give rise to a large amount of hormone release. Clearly, the above-mentioned calculations are somewhat speculative and only a new methodology for measuring the free Ca concentration will help to clarify the situation.

THE SIGNIFICANCE OF NEURONAL FIRING PATTERNS FOR HORMONE RELEASE

Magnocellular neurones of the hypothalamus show specific patterns of electrical discharge during activities such as suckling, haemorrhage and dehydration (for review see Poulain and Wakerley, 1982). What is the relevance of these patterns as far as hormone release is concerned? In isolated neural lobes stimulated electrically in a medium in which action potentials can propagate, the release of hormone is maximal at a frequency of ca. 35 Hz

(Dreifuss et al., 1971b). Less release is observed at higher frequencies. Similarly, electrical stimulation of isolated neural lobes in Na-free media (i.e. without propagated action potentials) gives rise to hormone release, but this increases up to a frequency of 100 Hz (Nordmann and Dreifuss, 1972; Fig. 12). The most likely explanation for this discrepancy is that the axons of the pituitary stalk fail to conduct action potentials at high frequencies. In collaboration with

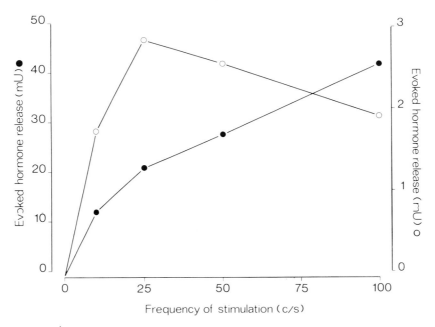

Fig. 12. The effect of frequency of stimulation on hormone release from neural lobe incubated in vitro. Glands were incubated in Na-containing (o) or Na-free media (●). (Modified from Dreifuss et al., 1971b and Nordmann and Dreifuss, 1972.)

Ian Cooke (Honolulu) we have used an in vitro preparation to check this possibility. The pituitary stalk was stimulated by a suction electrode and unit(s) in the neural lobe were recorded extracellularly (Fig. 13). The data show that the units (probably nerve endings) respond to frequencies up to 20 Hz through 30 sec of stimulation, but at 50 Hz no response could be observed after 30 sec of stimulation. Moreover, other recordings have shown that, at 50 Hz, the response of the units was abolished by the end of a 10 sec stimulation period. Similar results have also been obtained by recording in the neural lobe the compound action potentials evoked by stimulation of the stalk (Dreifuss et al., 1971b). This is of some importance when one tries to correlate hormone release with the rate of firing of the neurone. For example, an "oxytocin" cell can have a frequency discharge above 60 Hz at the onset of the burst (Poulain and Wakerley, 1982) but the depolarization effect on the nerve terminals would be of short duration due of the failure of the axons to conduct high frequency action potential trains for long periods of time.

Recent experiments by Dutton and Dyball (1979) have given some clue to the firing pattern observed in the hypothalamo-neurohypophysial tract. They used isolated neural lobes and compared the amount of hormone released by pulses given at a constant frequency with the output of hormone induced by a phasic pattern of stimuli identical to that of a "vasopressin" neurone. Although the mean frequencies were identical, the phasic pattern was more powerful

298

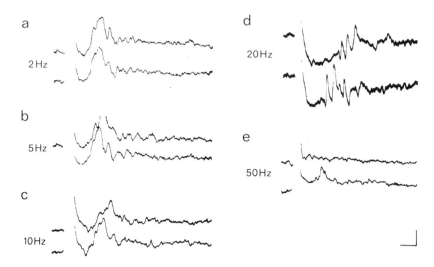

Fig. 13. The effect of frequency of stimulation on the extracellular recordings of units in the neurohypophysis. The frequency is indicated at the left of each recording. Bottom trace, onset of stimulation; top trace, 30 sec after the beginning of stimulation. Abscissa, 2 msec; ordinate, 0.2 mV except for d, where it is 0.1 mV. (I.M. Cooke and J.J. Nordmann, unpublished.)

in releasing vasopressin (Fig. 14). In other words, not only the frequency but also the pattern of firing is important for inducing hormone release.

To determine the mechanism by which phasic pattern enchances the release of hormone, I studied the Ca uptake into electrically stimulated neural lobes. The neurohypophyses were stimulated via the stalk by a stimulator triggered by a train of spikes previously recorded in vivo by Dominique Poulain (Fig. 15). One burst of stimuli (mean firing rate, 13.3 Hz) gives rise to an evoked Ca uptake of 272 pmol/gland. Moreover, whereas four bursts with intervals of 21.1 sec between each increase the evoked Ca uptake to a value of 751 pmol, the same number of bursts, but without silent periods, enhances Ca uptake to a value of 278 pmol. This is very similar to that observed after stimulation with a single burst. Also, four bursts of stimuli given at a *constant* frequency of 13.3 Hz with 21.1 sec intervals increased the Ca uptake by only 306 pmol. Similar results were observed with stimuli which mimic the pattern of discharge of an "oxytocin" neurone (not illustrated).

These data show that the discharge pattern of the magnocellular neurones has some facilitatory effect on Ca entry and hence on hormone release. We do not know exactly at which step of the stimulus–secretion coupling mechanism facilitation occurs, but the data above suggests that the phasic pattern of discharge has some effects on the late Ca channel. Plausible explanations are that it increases either (1) the number of channels activated at a given time or (2) the time for a channel to inactivate.

In experiments involving electrical stimulation of the gland with a stimulation triggered by trains of spikes previously recorded in vivo, one only looks at the effect of the frequency of pulses of the *same* duration. This might not be the case in vivo. In invertebrate neurones there is a considerable increase in the duration of action potentials during a burst of activity. If this is also the case at the neurohypophysial terminals, one would expect an even greater effect of the pattern of discharge on Ca entry and hence on hormone release.

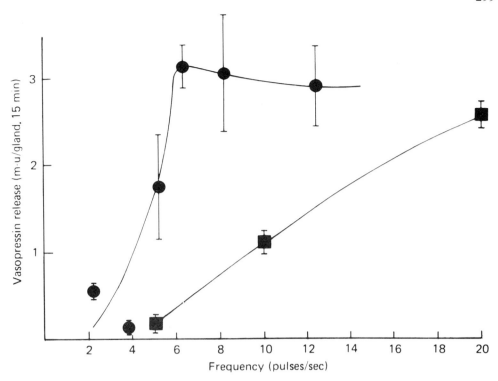

Fig. 14. The effect of the frequency of pulses applied on vasopressin release. The closed circles represent the amount of hormone release when glands were stimulated with trains of spikes previously recorded in vivo from identified vasopressin cells firing at 2.2, 3.8, 5.2, 6.3 and 8.2 spikes/sec. The squares represent the values obtained with a regular pattern given at 5, 10 and 20 Hz. (From Dutton and Dyball, 1979.)

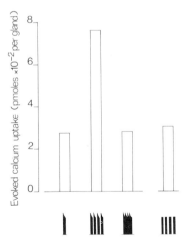

Fig. 15. Evoked Ca uptake induced by electrical stimulation of isolated neural lobes. The stimulator was triggered by train of spikes previously recorded in vivo by D. Poulain from an identified vasopressin cell. The bottom part indicates (from left to right) that Ca uptake was triggered by: one burst (348 spikes, 26.7 sec duration, 13 Hz mean frequency); four bursts with intervals of 21.2 sec; four bursts without intervals, and four bursts of regular pulses given at a constant frequency of 13 Hz (21.2 sec interval duration).

CONCLUSIONS

In this review I have tried to outline the main findings concerning Ca release and buffering in neurohypophysial nerve terminals and the process of exo-endocytosis. Although there has been some progress in this field during the last 20 years, there is a second, largely unknown, step of the stimulus–secretion coupling mechanism, i.e. the step during which Ca promotes hormone release. This is true not only for the neural lobe, but also for other secretory systems. Other second messengers (cAMP and cGMP) have been investigated by different groups, but their roles, if any, in the release process remain unknown (Mathison and Lederis, 1977; O'Dea et al., 1978; Torp-Pedersen et al., 1979; Thorn et al., 1978, 1979; Vale and Hope, 1982). This applies also to the fashionable molecule calmodulin (Dartt et al., 1981). Clearly, most of the experiments which will clarify the role of Ca in promoting hormone release remain to be done.

ACKNOWLEDGEMENTS

Supported by Grants DGRST 79.7.1057. and ERA 493. I thank Isabelle Lefranc for typing the manuscript and John Morris and Fraser Shaw for helpful comments.

REFERENCES

Alonso, G. and Assenmacher, I. (1979) The smooth endoplasmic reticulum in neurohypophysial axons of the rat: possible involvement in transport, storage and release of neurosecretory material. *Cell Tiss. Res.*, 199: 415–429.

Baker, P.F. (1974) Excitation–secretion coupling. In *Recent Advances in Physiology, Vol. 9,* Churchill-Livingstone, London, pp. 51–86.

Baker, P.F. and Knight, D.E. (1981) Calcium control of exocytosis and endocytosis in bovine adrenal medullary cells. *Phil. Trans. roy. Soc. B,* 296: 83–103.

Baker, P.F. and Schlaepfer, W.W. (1978) Uptake and binding of calcium by axoplasm isolated from giant axons of *Loligo* and *Myxicola*. *J. Physiol. (Lond.),* 276: 103–125.

Baker, P.F., Meves. H. and Ridgway, E.B. (1973a) Effects of manganese and other agents on the calcium uptake that follows depolarization of squid axons. *J. Physiol. (Lond.),* 231: 511–526.

Baker, P.F., Meves, H. and Ridgway, E.B. (1973b) Calcium entry in response to maintained depolarization of squid axons. *J. Physiol. (Lond.),* 231: 527–548.

Baker, R.V. and Hope, D.B. (1976) The effect of gradual changes in temperature on the release of hormones from nerve endings isolated from bovine neural lobes. *J. Neurochem.,* 27: 197–202.

Baker, R.V., Vilhardt, H. and Hope, D.B. (1975) Cold-induced release of hormones and proteins from nerve endings isolated from bovine neural lobes. *J. Neurochem.,* 24: 1091–1093.

Barer, R., Heller, H. and Lederis, K. (1963) The isolation, identification and properties of the hormonal granules of the neurohypophysis. *Proc. roy. Soc. B,* 158: 388–416.

Bicknell, R.J., Flint, A.P.F., Leng, G. and Sheldrick, E.L. (1982) Phasic pattern of electrical stimulation enhances oxytocin secretion from the isolated neurohypophysis. *Neurosci. Lett.,* 30: 47–50.

Borowitz, J.J. and Matthews, E.K. (1980) Calcium exchangeability in subcellular fractions of pancreatic islets cells. *J. Cell Sci.,* 41: 233–243.

Bunt, A.H. (1969) Formation of coated and "synaptic" vesicles within neurosecretory axon terminals of the crustacean sinus gland. *J. Ultrastruct. Res.,* 28: 411–421.

Calissano, P., Nevore, B.W. and Friesen, A. (1969) Effect of calcium ion on S-100, a protein of the nervous system. *Biochemistry,* 8: 4318–4326.

Cannata, M.A. and Morris, J.F. (1973) Changes in the appearance of hypothalamo-neurohypophysial neurosecretory granules associated with their maturation, *J. Endocr.,* 57: 531–538.

Castel, M. (1974) In vivo uptake of tracers by neurosecretory axon terminals in normal and dehydrated mice. *Gen. comp. Endocr.,* 22: 336–337.

Chandler, D.E. and Heuser, J.E. (1980) Arrest of membrane fusion events in mast cells by quick-freezing. *J. Cell Biol.*, 86: 666–674.

Conigrave, A.D., Treiman, M., Saermark, T. and Thorn, N.A. (1981) Stimulation by calmodulin of Ca^{2+} uptake and $(Ca^{2+}-Mg^{2+})$ ATPase activity in membrane fractions from ox neurohypophyses. *Cell Calcium*, 2: 125–136.

Cooke, I.M. (1977) Electrical activity of neurosecretory terminals and control of peptide hormone release. In H. Gainer (Ed.), *Peptides in Neurobiology*, Plenum Press, New York, pp. 345–374.

Crawford, A.C. (1973) Evoked transmitter release at the frog neuromuscular junction in very low calcium solutions. *J. Physiol. (Lond.)*, 231: 47–48 P.

Daniel, A.R. and Lederis, K. (1966) Effects of ether anaesthesia and haemorrhage on hormone storage and ultrastructure of the rat neurohypophysis. *J. Endocr.*, 34: 91–104.

Dartt, D.A., Torp-Pedersen, C. and Thorn, N.A. (1981) Effects of Ca^{2+} and calmodulin on cyclic nucleotide metabolism in neurosecretosomes isolated from ox neurohypophyses. *Brain Res.*, 204: 121–128.

Dipolo, R. (1977) Characterization of the ATP-dependent calcium efflux in dialyzed squid giant axons. *J. gen. Physiol.*, 69: 795–813.

Douglas, W.W. (1963) A possible mechanism of neurosecretion: release of vasopressin by depolarization and its dependence on calcium. *Nature (Lond.)*, 197: 81–82.

Douglas, W.W. (1968) Stimulus–secretion coupling: the concept and clues from chromaffin and other cells. *Brit J. Pharmacal.*, 34: 451–474.

Douglas, W.W. (1973) How do neurones secrete peptides? Exocytosis and its consequences, including "synaptic vesicle" formation in the hypothalamo-neurohypophysial system. In E. Zimmerman, W.H., Gispen, B.H., Marks and D. de Wied (Eds.), *Drug Effects or Neuroendocrine Regulation, Progress in Brain Res., Vol. 39*, Elsevier, Amsterdam, pp. 21–39.

Douglas, W.W. (1974a) Mechanism of release of neurohypophysial hormones: stimulus–secretion coupling. In R.O. Greep and E.B. Astwood (Eds.), *Handbook of Physiology. Section VII Endocrinology, Vol. IV. The Pituitary Gland and its Neuroendocrine Control, Part I*, American Physiological Society, Washington, DC, pp. 191–224.

Douglas, W.W. (1974b) Exocytosis and the exocytosis-vesiculation sequence: with special reference to neurohypophysis, chromaffin and mast cells, calcium and calcium ionophores. In N.A. Thorn and O.H. Petersen (Eds.), *Secretory Mechanism of Exocrine Glands*, Munksgaard, Copenhagen, pp. 116–129.

Douglas, W.W. and Poisner, A.M. (1964a) Stimulus–secretion coupling in a neurosecretory organ: the role of calcium in the release of vasopressin from the neurohypophysis. *J. Physiol. (Lond.)*, 172: 1–18.

Douglas, W.W. and Poisner, A.M. (1964b) Calcium movements in the neurohypophysis of the rat and its relation to the release of vasopressin. *J. Physiol. (Lond.)*, 172: 19–30.

Douglas, W.W., Nagasawa, J. and Schulz R. (1971) Electron microscopic studies on the mechanism secretion of the posterior pituitary hormones and significance of microvesicles ("synaptic vesicles"): evidence of secretion by exocytosis and formation of microvesicles as a byproduct of this process. *Mem. Soc. Endocr.*, 19; 353–378.

Dreifuss, J.J. (1975) A review on neurosecretory granules: their contents and mechanisms of release. *Ann. N.Y. Acad. Sci.*, 248: 184–201.

Dreifuss, J.J., Grau, J.D. and Bianchi, R.E. (1971a) Antagonism between Ca and Na ions at neurohypophyseal nerve terminals. *Experientia*, 27: 1295–1296.

Dreifuss, J.J., Kalnins, I., Kelly, J.S. and Ruf, K.B. (1971b) Action potentials and release of neurohypophysial hormones in vitro. *J. Physiol., (Lond.)*, 215: 805–817.

Dreifuss, J.J., Grau, J.D. and Nordmann, J.J. (1973) Effects of isolated neurohypophysis of agents which affect the membrane permeability to calcium. *J. Physiol. (Lond.)*, 231: 96–98 P.

Dutton, A. and Dyball, R.E.J. (1979) Phasic firing enhances vasopressin release from the rat neurohypophysis. *J. Physiol. (Lond.)*, 290: 433–440.

Dyball, R.E.J. and Nordmann, J.J. (1977) Reactivation by veratridine of hormone release from K^+-depolarized rat neurohypophysis. *J. Physiol. (Lond.)*, 269: 65–66 P.

Edwards, B.A., Edwards, M.E. and Thorn, N.A. (1973) The release in vitro of vasopressin unaccompanied by the axoplasmic enzymes: lactic dehydrogenase and adenylate kinase. *Acta Endocr.*, 72: 417–424.

Fawcett, C.P., Powell, A.E. and Sachs, H. (1968) Biosynthesis and release of neurophysin. *Endocrinology*, 83: 1299–1310.

Gage, P.W. and Quastel, D.M.J. (1966) Competition between sodium and calcium ions in transmitter release at a mammalian neuromuscular junction, *J. Physiol. (Lond.)*, 185: 95–123.

Gratzl, M., Dahl, G., Russell, J.T. and Thorn, N.A. (1977) Fusion of neurohypophyseal membranes in vitro. *Biochim. biophys. Acta*, 470: 45–57.

Howell, S.R., Montague, W. and Tyhurst, M. (1975) Calcium distribution in islets of Langerhans: a study of calcium concentrations and of calcium accumulation in B cell organelles. *J. Cell Sci.*, 19: 395–409.

302

Ingram, C.D., Bicknell, R.J., Brown, D. and Leng, G. (1982) Rapid fatigue of neuropeptide secretion during continual electrical stimulation. *Neuroendocrinology,* 35: 424–428.

Ishida, A. (1967) The effect of tetrodotoxin on calcium-dependent link in stimulus-secretion coupling in neurohypophysis. *Jap. J. Physiol.,* 17: 308–320.

La Bella, F.S. and Sanwal, M. (1965) Isolation of nerve endings from the posterior pituitary gland. *J. Cell Biol.,* 25: 179–191.

Lescure, H. and Nordmann, J.J. (1980) Neurosecretory granule release and endocytosis during prolonged stimulation of the rat neurohypophysis in vitro. *Neuroscience,* 5: 651–659.

Mathison, R. and Lederis, K. (1977) Cyclic nucleotides in the hypothalamo neurohypophyseal system and the release of vasopressin. In A.M. Moses. and L. Share (Eds.), *Neurohypophysis,* Karger, Basel, pp. 58–66.

Matthews, E.K. (1979) Calcium translocation and control mechanisms for endocrine secretion. In C.R. Hopkins and C.J. Duncan (Eds.), *Secretory Mechanisms,* Cambridge Univ. Press., Cambridge, pp. 225–249.

Matthews, E.K., Legros, J.J., Grau, J.D., Nordmann, J.J. and Dreifuss, J.J. (1973) Release of neurohypophysial hormones by exocytosis. *Nature (Lond.),* 241: 86–88.

Mikiten, T.M. and Douglas, W.W. (1965) Effect of calcium and other ions on vasopressin release from rat neurohypophyses stimulated electrically in vitro. *Nature (Lond.),* 207: 302.

Morris, J.F. (1976) Hormone storage in individual neurosecretory granules of the pituitary gland: a quantitative ultrastructural approach to hormone storage in the neural lobe. *J. Endocr.,* 68: 209–224.

Morris, J.F. and Cannata, M.A. (1973) Ultrastructural preservation of the dense core of posterior pituitary neurosecretory granules and its implications for hormone release. *J. Endocr.,* 57: 517–529.

Morris, J.F. and Dyball, R.E.J. (1974) A quantitative study of the ultrastructural changes in the hypothalamo-neurohypophysial system during and after experimentally induced hypersecretion. *Cell. Tiss. Res.,* 149: 525–535.

Morris, J.F. and Nordmann, J.J. (1980) Membrane recapture after hormone release from nerve endings in the neural lobe of the rat pituitary gland. *Neuroscience,* 5: 639–649.

Morris, J.F. and Nordmann, J.J. (1982) Membrane retrieval by vacuoles after exocytosis in the neural lobe of Brattleboro rats. *Neuroscience,* 7: 1631–1639.

Morris, J.F., Nordmann, J.J. and Dyball, R.E.J. (1978) Structure–function correlation in mammalian neurosecretion. *Int. Rev. exp. Path.,* 18: 1–95.

Müller, J.R., Thorn, N.A. and Pedersen, C. (1975) Effects of calcium and sodium on vasopressin release in vitro induced by a prolonged potassium stimulation. *Acta endocr.,* 79: 51–59.

Nagasawa, J., Douglas, W.W. and Schulz, R.A. (1970) Ultrastructural evidence of secretion by exocytosis and of "synaptic vesicle" formation in posterior pituitary glands. *Nature (Lond.),* 227: 407–409.

Nagasawa, J., Douglas, W.W. and Schulz R.A. (1971) Micropinocytotic origin of coated and smooth microvesicles ("synaptic vesicles") in neurosecretory terminals of posterior pituitary glands demonstrated by incorporation of horseradish peroxidase. *Nature (Lond.),* 332: 341–342.

Nagazato, J. and Douglas, W.W. (1974) Vasopressin release from the isolated neurohypophysis induced by a calcium ionophore, X-537A. *Nature (Lond.),* 249: 479–481.

Nordmann, J.J. (1976) Evidence for calcium inactivation during hormone release in the rat neurohypophysis. *J. exp. Biol.,* 65: 669–683.

Nordmann, J.J. (1978) Hormone release and membrane retrieval in neurosecretion. In J.D. Vincent and C. Kordon (Eds.), *Biologie Cellulaire des Processus Neurosécrétoires Hypothalamiques,* CNRS, Paris, pp. 619–636.

Nordmann, J.J. (1982) Evidence for an aging process within neurosecretory granules. In A.J. Baertschi and J.J. Dreifuss (Eds.), *Vasopressin, Corticoliberin and ACTH-Related Peptides,* Academic Press, London, pp. 11–20.

Nordmann, J.J. and Chevallier, J. (1981) The role of microvesicles in buffering $[Ca]_i$ in the neurohypophysis. *Nature (Lond.),* 287: 54–56.

Nordmann, J.J. and Currell, G.A. (1975) The mechanism of calcium ionophore-induced secretion from the rat neurohypophysis. *Nature (Lond.),* 253: 646–647.

Nordmann, J.J. and Dreifuss, J.J. (1972) Hormone release evoked by electrical stimulation of rat neurohypophyses in the absence of action potentials. *Brain Res.,* 45: 604–607.

Nordmann, J.J. and Dyball, R.E.J. (1975) New calcium mobilising agent. *Nature (Lond.),* 255: 414–415.

Nordmann, J.J. and Dyball, R.E.J. (1978) Effects of veratridine on Ca fluxes and the release of oxytocin and vasopressin from the isolated rat neurohypophysis. *J. gen. Physiol.,* 72: 297–304.

Nordmann, J.J. and Labouesse, J. (1981) Neurosecretory granules: evidence for an aging process within the neurohypophysis. *Science,* 211: 595–597.

Nordmann, J.J. and Morris, J.F. (1976) Membrane retrieval at neurosecretory axon endings. *Nature (Lond.),* 261: 723–725.

Nordmann, J.J. and Zyzek, E. (1982) Calcium efflux from the rat neurohypophysis *J. Physiol. (Lond.),* 325: 281–299.

Nordmann, J.J. Dreifuss, J.J. and Legros, J.J. (1971) A correlation of release of polypeptide hormones and of immunoreactive neurophysin from isolated rat neurohypophyses. *Experientia,* 27: 1344–1345.

Nordmann, J.J., Dreifuss, J.J., Baker, P.F., Ravazzola, M., Malaisse-Lagae, F. and Orci, L. (1974) Secretion dependent uptake of extracellular fluid by the rat neurohypophysis. *Nature (Lond.),* 250: 155–157.

Nordmann, J.J., Louis, F. and Morris, S.J. (1979) Purification of two structurally and morphologically distinct populations of rat neurohypophysial secretory granules. *Neuroscience,* 4: 1367–1379.

Nordmann, J.J., Desmazes, J.P. and Georgescault, D. (1982) The relationship between the membrane potential of neurosecretory nerve endings, as measured by a voltage-sensitive dye, and the release of nerohypophysial hormones, *Neuroscience,* 7: 731–737.

Normann, T.C. (1969) Experimentally induced exocytosis of neurosecretory granules. *Exp. Cell Res.,* 55: 285–287.

Normann, T.C. (1970) The mechanism of hormone release from neurosesecretory axon endings in the insect *Calliphora erythraocephala.* In W. Haromann and B. Scharrer (Eds.), *Aspects of Neuroendocrinology. V International Symposium on Neurosecretion,* Springer, Berlin, pp. 30–42.

Norström, A. (1972) Release in vitro of neurohypophysial proteins from neural lobe tissue slices and from isolated neurosecretory granules of the rat. *Z. Zellforsch.,* 129: 114–139.

O'Dea, R.F., Gagnon, C. and Zatz, M. (1978) Regulation of guanosine, 3′, 5′-cyclic monophosphate in rat pineal and posterior pituitary glands, *J. Neurochem.,* 31: 733–738.

Poulain, D.A. and Wakerley, J.B. (1982) Electrophysiology of hypothalamic magnocellular neurones secreting oxytocin and vasopressin. *Neuroscience,* 7: 773–808.

Reinhardt, H.E., Henning, L.C. and Rohr, H.P. (1969) Morphometrischultrastrukturelle Untersuchungen am Hypophysenhinterlappen der Ratte nach Dehydration. *Z. Zelforsch.,* 102: 182–192.

Requena, J. and Mullins, L.J. (1979) Calcium movement in nerve fibres. *Quart. Rev. Biophys.,* 12: 371–460.

Russell, J.T. and Thorn, N.A. (1974a) Calcium and stimulus–secretion coupling in the neurohypophysis slices from ox neurohypophyses stimulated electrically or by a high potassium concentration. *Acta endocr.,* 76; 449–470.

Russell, J.T. and Thorn, N.A. (1974b) Calcium and stimulus–secretion coupling in the neurohypophysis. II, Effects of lanthanum, a verapamil analogue (D600) and prenylamine on 45-calcium transport and vasopressin release in isolated rat neurohypophyses. *Acta endocr.,* 76: 471–487.

Russell, J.T. and Thorn, N.A. (1975) Adenosine triphosphate dependent calcium uptake by subcellular fractions from bovine neurohypophyses. *Acta physiol. scand.,* 93: 364–377.

Russell, J.T. and Thorn, N.A. (1977) Isolation and purification of calcium-binding proteins from bovine neurohypophyses. *Biochem. biophys. Acta,* 491: 398–408.

Russell, J.T. Hansen, E.L. and Thorn, N.A. (1974) Calcium and stimulus-secretion coupling in the neurohypophysis. III, Ca^{2+}-ionophore (A-23187)-induced release of vasopressin from isolated rat neurohypophyses. *Acta endocr.,* 77: 443–450.

Sachs, H. and Haller, E.W. (1968) Further studies on the capacity of the neurohypophysis to release vasopressin. *Endocrinology,* 83: 251–262.

Scherman, D. and Nordmann, J.J. (1982) Internal pH of isolated newly formed and aged neurohypophysial granules. *Proc. nat. Acad. Sci. U.S.A.,* 79: 476–479.

Shaw, F.D. and Morris, J.F. (1981) Ca localization in the rat neurohypophysis. *Nature (Lond.),* 287: 56–58.

Smith, U. (1970) The origin of small vesicles in neurosecretory axons. *Tissue and Cell,* 2: 427–433.

Stoeckel, M.E., Hindelang-Gertner, C., Dellman, H.D., Porte, A. and Stutinsky, F. (1975) Subcellular localization of calcium in the mouse hypophysis. I. Calcium distribution in the adeno- and neurohypophysis under normal conditions. *Cell Tiss. Res.,* 157: 307–322.

Swann, R.W. and Pickering, B.T. (1976) Incorporation of radioactive percursors into the membrane and contents of the neurosecretory granules of the rat neurohypophysis as a method of studying their fate. *J. Endocr.,* 68: 95–108.

Theodosis, D.T., Dreifuss, J.J., Harris, M.C. and Orci, L. (1976) Secretion related uptake of horseradish peroxidase in neurohypophysial axons. *J. Cell Biol.,* 70: 294–303.

Thorn, N.A., Russell, J.T. and Vilhardt, H. (1975) Hexosamine, calcium and neurophysin in secretory granules and the role of calcium in hormone release. *Ann. N.Y. Acad. Sci.,* 248: 202–217.

Thorn, N.A., Russell, J.T., Torp-Pedersen, C. and Treiman, M. (1978) Calcium and neurosecretion. *Ann. N.Y. Acad. Sci.,* 307: 618–638.

Thorn, N.A., Torp-Pedersen, C., Treiman, M., Dartt, D.A. and Worm-Petersen, S. (1979) In W. Wuttke, A. Weindl, K.H. Voigt and R.R. Dries (Eds.), *Brain and Pituitary Peptides,* Karger, Basel, pp. 118–124.

Torp-Pedersen, C., Treiman, M. and Thorn, N.A. (1979) Subcellular distribution of cyclic AMP phosphodiesterase in the ox neurohypophysis. *J. Neurochem.,* 32: 1085–1091.

Torp-Pedersen, C., Saemark, T., Bundgaard, M. and Thorn, N.A. (1981) ATP-dependent Ca^{2+} accumulation by microvesicles isolated from bovine neurohypophyses. *J. Neurochem.,* 35: 552–557.

304

Uttenthal, L.O., Livett, B.G. and Hope, D.B. (1971) Release of neurophysin together with vasopressin by a Ca^{++} dependent mechanism. *Phil. Trans. roy Soc. B,* 261: 379–380.

Vale, M.R. and Hope, D.B. (1982) Cyclic nucleotides and the release of vasopressin from the rat posterior pituitary. *J. Neurochem.,* 39: 569–573.

Winkler, H. and Westhead, E. (1980) The molecular organization of adrenal chromaffin granules. *Neuroscience,* 5: 1803–1823.

The Neurohypophysis: Structure, Function and Control, Progress in Brain Research, Vol. 60, edited by B.A. Cross and G. Leng
© 1983 Elsevier Science Publishers B.V.

Mechanisms of Inactivation of Neurohypophysial Hormone Release

F.D. SHAW, R.E.J. DYBALL* and J.J. NORDMANN[1]

Department of Anatomy, King's College London, Strand, London WC2R 2LS (U.K.) and [1]Institut National de la Recherche Medicale, Rue Camille Saint-Saens, 33077 Bordeaux Cedex (France)

INTRODUCTION

Inactivation of hormone release: the problem

The biosynthesis of the neurohypophysial hormones, followed by packaging into granules and transport to neurosecretory swellings and terminals (see Morris et al., 1978), provides a large pool of stored product from which hormone secreted into the blood is derived. The mechanisms which regulate the release of available hormone are fundamental to the physiology of the magnocellular neurosecretory system, and are probably of relevance to peptidergic neurones in general.

The application in vivo of appropriate stimuli to release hormone is associated with an increase in the firing rates of magnocellular neurones (see Poulain and Wakerley, 1982). A direct relationship between supply and demand for neurohypophysial hormones might reasonably be inferred, but this is demonstrably not the case. As long ago as 1960, Sachs and his colleagues discovered that, in dogs subjected to haemorrhage, an increased blood concentration of vasopressin is not maintained beyond the first few minutes of the stimulus (Weinstein et al., 1960). Later experiments showed that a much reduced secretory response is elicited by a haemorrhagic stimulus applied 1 h after an initial stimulus of only 10 min duration (Sachs et al., 1967). Hormone release from isolated neurohypophyses subjected to a prolonged depolarizing stimulus in vitro has also been shown to decline at a rate greater than can be accounted for by depletion of the total hormone store (Sachs et al., 1967; Sachs and Haller, 1968; Thorn, 1966).

These results were originally interpreted as evidence for the existence of two separate hormone pools, one of which was "readily releasable" and constituted 5–20% of the total store. It was postulated that this pool was constituted by the free cytoplasmic hormone then thought to exist (Ginsburg, 1968; Thorn, 1966), or alternatively by those granules situated close to the release site (Sachs et al., 1967; Sachs and Haller, 1968). However, it has since been demonstrated that stimulation in vitro can release 30% or more of the stored hormone (Müller et al., 1975; Nordmann, 1976). It was accordingly suggested that the "readily releasable pool" might represent those granules present in the secretory terminals, which account for some 30% of the total granule population in the unstimulated neurohypophysis

---

* Author for correspondence at present address: Department of Anatomy, Downing Street, Cambridge, CB2 3DY, U.K.

(Nordmann, 1976, 1977). The decrease (inactivation) of hormone release during prolonged stimulation in vitro was attributed to a decline in membrane calcium conductance, similar to that first described in the squid giant axon (Baker et al., 1973b). The existence of such a mechanism has been demonstrated in a number of cell types (e.g. D'Amore and Shepro, 1977; Foreman and Garland, 1974; Maddrell and Gee, 1974), and is thought, for instance, to limit catecholamine release by adrenal medullary cells (Baker and Rink, 1975).

However, many questions remain. Is the calcium channel inactivation hypothesis a sufficient explanation for all the observed features of the inactivation of hormone release? Is the mechanism exclusively depolarization-dependent, as suggested by the earlier work? Does an exactly similar mechanism operate when hormone release is elicited by the transient depolarization which follows the arrival of action potentials at the secretory terminals, rather than by the maintained depolarization employed in previous experiments? What is the physiological significance of inactivation of release, and can the same mechanisms be demonstrated in vivo? The present experiments were thus undertaken to re-examine the calcium entry hypothesis, and to extend the observations to electrical stimulation in vitro and to the intact system in vivo. The characteristics of hormone release inactivation will be shown to be rather more complex than previously supposed.

EXPERIMENTAL APPROACHES

Most of the experiments described employed an isolated neural lobe preparation maintained in vitro, which permits manipulation of the ionic environment and the precise determination of the time course of secretory response. Hormone release was evoked either by raising extracellular potassium, which is known to cause maintained depolarization (Nordmann et al., 1982), or by application of electrical stimulus pulses. The pulses were delivered at 10 Hz, a frequency similar to those recorded from the cell bodies of magnocellular neurones in rats subjected to haemorrhage or dehydration (see Poulain and Wakerley, 1982). Hormone release was stimulated in vivo by the administration of a 2% solution of NaCl in place of drinking water (Jones and Pickering, 1969) and the neurohypophyses were subsequently removed and incubated in vitro.

The bicarbonate-buffered incubation medium was maintained at 37° C, constantly bubbled with 95% O_2 and 5% CO_2, and had the following basic composition: NaCl 150 mM; $KHCO_3$ 5.6 mM; $MgCl_2$ 1.0 mM; $CaCl_2$ 2.2 mM, and glucose 10 mM. During potassium stimulation, KCl was increased to 56 mM and NaCl reduced to 100 mM; in other experiments using a reduced sodium concentration, choline chloride was added for osmotic compensation. Tissue to be electrically stimulated was impaled upon one of a pair of platinum electrodes immersed in the incubation medium (Dutton and Dyball, 1979). The medium was changed every 15 min, and the collected samples assayed by the rat milk-ejection method (Bisset et al., 1967). Experimental decay constants for hormone release inactivation were calculated together with their correlation coefficients, as described by Nordmann (1976). Significance levels quoted in the text all refer to Student's t-test.

RESULTS

Inactivation and reactivation in vitro: potassium stimulation

Stimulation for 2 h with 56 mM potassium in the presence of 100 mM sodium resulted in progressive inactivation of hormone release from isolated neurohypophyses (Fig. 1a), similar to the observations of Müller et al. (1975) and Nordmann (1975, 1976). The inactivation could be described by a single exponential with a decay constant (k) of 0.012 min^{-1} $(r = 0.96)$. If calcium was omitted from the incubation medium or if 0.1 mM D600 was present, hormone release failed to increase over basal levels during stimulation, again in accordance with previous results (Dreifuss et al., 1973). Inactivation cannot be attributed to a non-specific decline in viability of the tissue, as it is shown below that neurohypophyses first stimulated after as long as 5 h in vitro exhibit normal responsiveness.

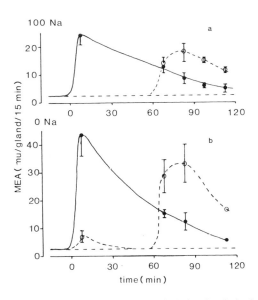

Fig. 1.a: hormone released from the isolated rat neurohypophysis during depolarization with a raised (56 mM) K$^+$ concentration added at time 0 and a sodium concentration of 100 mM. In each case hormone release is shown as milk-ejection activity (MEA) expressed in terms of mU of synthetic oxytocin. In this and the following figures, the horizontal dotted line indicates basal release (control, •——• ; experiments in which calcium was omitted for the first 60 min, o——o). b: similar experiments carried out in the absence of sodium. Both experiments show that, in the absence of calcium, inactivation was less severe and imply that calcium is important for inactivation.

To investigate the calcium-dependence of inactivation, a second group of neurohypophyses, incubated in parallel with the above experiment, were stimulated for 1 h in the absence of calcium, after which time calcium was reintroduced and the subsequent hormone release determined over a further 1 h (Fig. 1a). The release during the first sample period after calcium addition was similar to the corresponding value when calcium was present throughout, suggesting that inactivation had occurred by a calcium-independent mechanism (Nordmann, 1976). However, the following samples all contained significantly more hormone $(P < 0.01)$ than the relevant controls. It would thus appear that prolonged depolarization in the absence of calcium provokes only a limited degree of inactivation, and that a major component is calcium-dependent. The delayed increase in secretion may represent the time required for calcium to infiltrate the extracellular space, and also to reach the appropriate concentration since extracellular binding sites would also demand reoccupation.

A similar pair of experiments was performed in the absence of extracellular sodium (Fig. 1b). When calcium was present throughout the period of stimulation, initial hormone release was much greater than in 100 mM sodium, in accord with previous accounts of

308

antagonism between extracellular sodium and calcium in secretory systems (Kelly, 1965; Dreifuss et al., 1971). The subsequent inactivation proceeded more rapidly than in 100 mM sodium, with $k = 0.021$ min^{-1} ($r = 0.98$) rather than at a rate similar to that previously reported and cited as evidence for calcium channel inactivation (Nordmann, 1976). When calcium was introduced after 1 h of stimulation, release was higher than the corresponding controls throughout the following 1 h period (Fig. 1b). This occurred despite the small increase in secretion during the initial 1 h stimulation without added calcium, due presumably to the remaining extracellular calcium, as chelaters were not employed. Hormone release inactivation therefore showed a major dependence on extracellular calcium, both in the presence and absence of sodium, and a relatively minor dependence upon depolarization.

These results led to the consideration of recovery from inactivation, referred to here as "reactivation". Different groups of neurohypophyses were potassium-stimulated for 1 h (in the presence of sodium), returned to a normal medium for different time intervals, and then exposed once again to the stimulus. The results are expressed in Fig. 2a, in terms of the percentage of the initial release achieved by each neurohypophysis. Hormone release had significantly inactivated ($P < 0.01$) by the final 15 min period of the initial stimulation, and fell

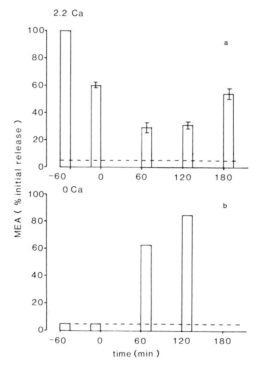

Fig. 2.a: hormone released (expressed as % initial MEA release) at different intervals after a 1 h potassium stimulus in the presence of 2.2 mM calcium, which ended at time 0. Reactivation occurs only slowly and is not complete after 3 h. b: similar experiments in which the initial stimulation was carried out in the absence of calcium. Inactivation was less severe and had recovered to values not significantly below control within 2 h. This implies the existence of at least two mechanisms of inactivation: a potential-dependent one which reactivates quickly and a calcium-dependent one which does not. (Error bars are added in a since the values were derived by comparing initial and subsequent release. They were not added in b since there was no initial release, and the release which followed the second stimulus was compared with that from a separate control series of neurohypophyses.)

to the basal levels by 30 min after its termination. Restimulation after intervals of 1 and 2 h evoked an increase in hormone output, but only to levels significantly lower ($P < 0.01$) than that from the same neurohypophyses at the end of the initial stimulation period. After a 3 h interval some recovery of secretory capacity was observed, but secretion nevertheless achieved only 54 % of its initial rate. It is unlikely that any damage was caused by the initial 1 h stimulus as the rate of loss of the cytoplasmic enzyme lactate dehydrogenase was unaltered throughout the incubation period, and as electron microscopy failed to reveal any structural alterations. A potassium stimulus therefore exerts chronic effects on subsequent hormone release.

The calcium-dependence of reactivation was investigated by stimulating for 1 h in the absence of calcium, followed by an interval and restimulation in its presence (Fig. 2b). The releases evoked by restimulation were compared with those for control neurohypophyses, treated identically except that they were not depolarized during the initial 1 h. As can be appreciated by comparison of Fig. 2a and b, recovery following stimulation was much more rapid in the absence of calcium. After a 1 h interval, release was 63 % of the control, but was nevertheless significantly less ($P < 0.01$), while after a 2 h interval release was not significantly different from the control. These results presumably represent the characteristics of the depolarization-dependent, calcium-independent process, and it would thus appear that the calcium-dependent process is responsible for long-term inactivation.

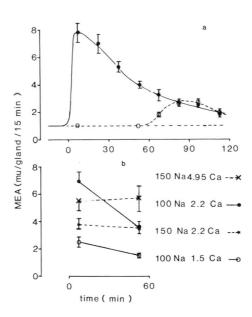

Fig. 3.a: hormone released (expressed as in Fig. 1) during a 2 h period of electrical stimulation at 10 Hz with a sodium concentration of 100 mM, begun at time 0 (control, ●———● ; experiments in which calcium was omitted for the first 60 min, o———o). With electrical stimulation, omission of calcium did not appear to impair the degree of inactivation (but lowered external sodium may have enhanced it). b: the effects of manipulation of calcium and sodium concentration on inactivation. Significant inactivation occurred only in those experiments with lowered external sodium concentration.

Inactivation and reactivation: in vitro electrical stimulation

Hormone release during 2 h of electrical stimulation is shown in Fig. 3a. It should be noted that the neurohypophyses were incubated in a medium containing 100 mM sodium (see below). Stimulated release could be abolished by the omission of calcium, and by the presence of 0.1 mM D600 or 10^{-7} g/ml tetrodotoxin, this last suggesting that propagation of sodium-dependent action potentials to the neurosecretory terminals was involved. The rate of secretion was initially about one-third of that obtained with potassium stimulation in the presence of 100 mM sodium, but inactivation actually proceeded more rapidly, with $k = 0.020$ min^{-1} ($r = 0.99$).

This result prompted investigation of the effects of external sodium and calcium on electrically stimulated release (Fig. 3b). The rapid inactivation during electrical stimulation in 100 mM sodium was initially interpreted as arising from activation of a calcium-mediated potassium permeability, as identified in both invertebrate and vertebrate neurones (see Meech, 1976), due to the increased calcium influx during stimulation. Such an increase in potassium permeability would reduce the duration of the action potential, and hence the rate of calcium entry and of hormone release. However, this explanation was rendered unlikely by the finding that significant inactivation occurs after 1 h of stimulation in a medium containing 100 mM sodium and only 1.5 mM calcium, despite the much reduced initial release (Fig. 3b). Further, prolonged stimulation in media containing 150 mM sodium did not result in inactivation after 1 h, whether a normal or a raised (4.95 mM) calcium concentration was employed, despite the large initial calcium influx which must have occurred in the latter case (Fig. 3b). These results suggest that inactivation caused by electrical stimulation at this frequency is a quite specific effect of lowering the sodium concentration of the medium, regardless of the calcium concentration or the ratio between the two ions. The effect of adding calcium after 1 h of stimulation in its absence (Fig. 3a) is consistent with the hypothesis of a sodium-dependent, calcium-independent effect. Addition of calcium resulted in an increased rate of secretion, but only to values almost identical with the corresponding controls.

Reactivation following electrical stimulation in 100 mM sodium is shown in Fig. 4. After an initial stimulus of only 30 min, and an interval of 30 min, restimulated release was significantly reduced ($P < 0.01$), amounting to only 52 % of the initial rate. More surprisingly, release of only about 30 % of the initial rate was observed after intervals of 1 and 4 h (Fig. 4a). Hormone release from control neurohypophyses which were stimulated after incubation in vitro for an equivalent time to the experimental group subjected to a 4 h interval, was not significantly below the initial release rate and was significantly higher ($P < 0.01$) that the restimulated release at that time (Fig. 4a). Further, there was no increase in lactate dehydrogenase release, and no ultrastructural changes were observed at that time, so it may be presumed that the tissue was fully functional. Long-term effects were also seen after only 15 min initial electrical stimulation, although the results were more variable and the inactivation not so profound (Fig. 4b).

By contrast, neurohypophyses stimulated for 30 min in the absence of calcium, followed by an interval of 30 min and restimulation in its presence, released hormone equivalent to 81 % of the control level, and not significantly different from it. Reactivation after a relatively short initial electrical stimulus thus apparently displays a calcium-dependence similar to that of potassium stimulation. However, it remains possible that the sodium-dependent effect also contributes to long-term inactivation; more experiments are required to determine whether further inactivation occurs after intervals of 1–4 h, as was observed following an initial 30 min stimulus in the presence of calcium (Fig. 4a).

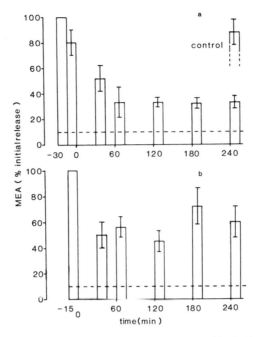

Fig. 4.a: hormone release (expressed as in Fig. 2) at different intervals after 30 min electrical stimulation at 10 Hz, which ended at time 0. Restimulation after an interval of 1 h released less hormone than after an interval of 30 min and there was no recovery within the 4 h incubation period; control release at this time confirmed the viability of the tissue. b: similar experiments after only 15 min initial stimulation.

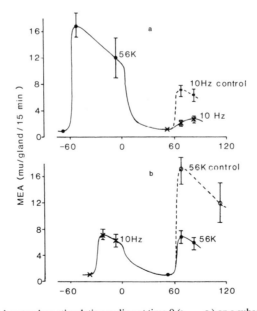

Fig. 5.a: the influence of 1 h potassium stimulation ending at time 0 (●——●) on a subsequent electrical stimulation (×——×) after an interval of 1 h; also shown are the equivalent values for control electrical stimulation (∗---∗). b: the influence of 30 min electrical stimulation (×——×), ending at time 0 on a subsequent potassium stimulation (●——●). Also shown are the equivalent values for a control potassium stimulation (o---o). Both initial stimuli impaired the effectiveness of the second stimulus, so that potassium and electrical stimulation clearly interact.

Interaction between potassium and electrical stimulation

The results outlined above suggest that there are three apparently separate processes governing inactivation, dependent upon depolarization, extracellular calcium and extracellular sodium. As the characteristics of inactivation and reactivation associated with either potassium or electrical stimulation were generally similar, the effect of one upon the other was investigated. Neurohypophyses were stimulated with raised potassium for 1 h or electrically for 30 min, followed by an interval of 1 h and application of the alternative stimulus (Fig. 5a, b). Initial potassium stimulation significantly ($P < 0.05$) reduced the hormone release evoked by a subsequent electrical stimulus, to 30 % of the control values (Fig. 5a). Tissue initially stimulated with electrical pulses also released significantly less ($P < 0.05$) in response to a subsequent potassium stimulus than the appropriate controls, amounting to 33 % of the latter (Fig. 5b). Potassium and electrical stimulation thus interact, 1 h of the former being approximately equivalent to 30 min of the latter in terms of their subsequent effects on reactivation (see also Figs. 2a and 4a). It should nevertheless be noted that hormone release evoked by 30 min electrical stimulation is only about 20 % that evoked by 1 h potassium stimulation.

The results encourage the view that similar processes are responsible for the inactivation which follows both stimuli. Further, electrical stimulation followed after an interval by potassium constitutes an in vitro equivalent of the experiments of Sachs et al. (1967), who found that neurohypophyses taken from dogs subjected to a haemorrhagic stimulus released much less hormone when stimulated with high potassium than did controls. This in turn suggests that the process occurring in vivo is similar to that observed in vitro.

Inactivation in vivo and reactivation in vitro

The possibility of inactivation in vivo was here investigated using the chronic stimulus of substituting 2 % NaCl for drinking water, which is known to release both oxytocin and vasopressin (Jones and Pickering, 1969). After only 24 h of such treatment, neurohypophyses incubated in vitro and electrically stimulated released substantially less than controls, the

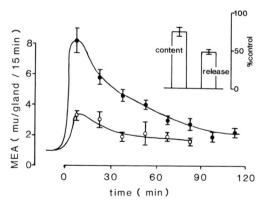

Fig. 6. Hormone release during 2 h electrical stimulation (beginning at time 0) from control glands (●——●) and neurohypophyses from rats that had been given 2 % NaCl to drink instead of water for 24 h (o——o). Inset are the values for the relative reduction in gland content and hormone release after 24 h of such treatment. Clearly drinking 2 % NaCl (in vivo) reduced the subsequent release from isolated glands in vitro and the relative reduction of release was significantly greater ($P < 0.01$) than that of gland content. This implies that inactivation of release also occurs in vivo.

initial release reaching only 48 % of the control level (Fig. 6). It is unlikely that the decrease was due entirely to depletion, as the treated neurohypophyses contained 76 % of the hormone content of controls, so the proportional decrease in release was significantly greater ($P < 0.01$) than that of neurohypophysial content.

It is thus likely that prolonged stimulation in vivo causes inactivation by mechanisms similar to those described above, although a far higher proportion of the gland content can ultimately be released in vivo than in vitro. This might be because the rate of hormone release in vivo, which in the present experiments amounted to approximately 2 mU/h for the 24 h (ignoring the effects of resynthesis), is sufficiently low to minimize inactivation. In addition, the characteristic discharge patterns of magnocellular neurones (Dutton and Dyball, 1979; Bicknell et al., 1981) might be adapted to optimize release relative to the extent of inactivation caused.

DISCUSSION

Is there a readily releasable pool?

The results presented here offer no support for the hypothesis of a readily releasable pool, at least in its original forms (see above). In the case of potassium stimulation, inactivation is demonstrable both in the presence of 100 mM sodium and in its absence, although far less hormone was released in the former case. Further, previous authors have shown that a second increase in secretion may be evoked by application of an appropriate stimulus, such as exposure to barium or lanthanum (Nordmann, 1976), or sodium withdrawal (when inactivation has proceeded in its presence: Müller et al., 1975; Nordmann, 1976). The alkaloid veratridine, which opens sodium channels permanently (Ohta et al., 1973), can also stimulate a second release (Dyball and Nordmann, 1977). Inactivation of release has also been demonstrated here with electrical stimulation, although 2 h of such stimulation in 100 mM sodium releases only about 25 % of that released by potassium stimulation in the absence of sodium. Further, inactivation associated with electrical stimulation depends not on the magnitude of hormone release, but on the sodium concentration of the incubation medium. It must be concluded that electrically evoked hormone release is normally not limited by availability of secretory product, although depletion may partially account for the declining release seen during potassium stimulation in the absence of sodium.

The actual "readily releasable pool", that is the granules available for release by sufficiently powerful stimuli, is therefore likely to represent at least the 30 % contained in the neurosecretory terminals. During prolonged stimulation, more hormone may also become available by migration of granules into the terminals from the axonal swellings. It should nevertheless be emphasized that a proportion of the granules within the terminals may only be accessible to more potent stimuli: for instance, the associated large calcium influx might penetrate deeper into the terminals, and recruit granules unavailable to weaker stimuli. Viewed in this way, the size of the release pool depends upon the particular stimulus employed. Evidence that exhaustion of this pool cannot account for release inactivation is provided by the findings for electrical stimulation in different sodium and calcium concentrations mentioned above. In addition, electrical stimulation causes inactivation of release in response to a subsequent potassium stimulation, which is proportionately greater than can be accounted for by the hormone released by the electrical stimulus itself. This in turn suggests that the mechanism of hormone release inactivation resides in a stage prior to the recruitment and exocytosis of the neurosecretory granules.

314

Since the original work of Douglas and Poisner (1964a, b), evidence has accumulated that an increase of the intracellular ionized calcium concentration is responsible for initiation of secretion (see Nordmann, this volume). It is extremely unlikely that inactivation is due to failure of the secretory mechanism, in view of evidence already discussed, such as the reactivation of potassium-stimulated hormone release by veratridine. Inactivation of hormone release might therefore occur because of limitation of the availability of calcium at exocytotic sites; this availability is influenced by the rate of calcium influx across the neurosecretory terminal membrane and release inactivation may thus reflect the properties of the membrane calcium permeability.

It remains to incorporate the depolarization-dependent, calcium-dependent and sodium-dependent elements of hormone release inactivation into a model of the mechanism involved. If the properties of inactivation described here are all attributable to the "late" calcium channel (Baker et al., 1973a, b; Nordmann, 1976), several modifications to these previous concepts of its operation are necessary. Baker et al. (1973b) demonstrated a potential-dependent inactivation of calcium conductance in the squid axon, and showed that recovery from previous stimulation was extremely slow by the standards of other membrane ion channels, being half-complete 3–4 min after 2–3 min of potassium depolarization. This bears some resemblance to the depolarization-dependent component of hormone release inactivation demonstrated here with potassium stimulation. However, an additional component of release inactivation was calcium-dependent, and it is of considerable interest that inactivation of calcium channels dependent upon the entry of calcium has been demonstrated in a number of cell types (e.g. Tillotson, 1979; Brehm et al., 1980). Further, Brown et al. (1981) have reported both calcium- and potential-dependent inactivation of calcium currents in *Helix* neurones.

The sodium-dependent component of hormone release inactivation is more difficult to incorporate into this model. One possibility is suggested by the work of Birks and Cohen (1968a, b), who showed that transmitter release at the neuromuscular junction is enhanced by an increase in intracellular sodium. It was postulated that sodium might displace calcium from an intracellular binding site, and thus exert the opposite effect on calcium entry to the extracellular antagonism observed in the same preparation (Kelly, 1965). Thus in the neurohypophysis, lowered extracellular sodium would allow increased access of calcium to its channels and hence increased hormone secretion, whereas lowered intracellular sodium would inhibit intracellular liberation of calcium, and hence decrease secretion. As no sodium-dependent effects were observed with potassium stimulation, it must be postulated that potassium stimulation did not alter intracellular sodium. Certainly, the potential-dependent sodium conductance would probably inactivate almost immediately. In the case of electrical stimulation, potential-dependent gating of sodium, potassium and calcium would occur with every pulse, causing activation of the sodium pump (Ritchie and Straub, 1957). It must be assumed that the activity of the pump would reduce intracellular sodium, and that this would occur more readily in a medium containing only 100 mM sodium, thus accounting for the sodium-dependent component of inactivation seen with electrical stimulation.

However, the extremely long time course of calcium-dependent release inactivation is difficult to reconcile with the rapid recovery of calcium conductance seen in systems investigated electrophysiologically (e.g. Brown et al., 1981). An alternative scheme, involving the sodium-calcium exchange mechanism known to be present in neurohypophysial membranes (Nordmann and Zyzek, 1982) is therefore presented as a further working hypothesis. If three or more sodium ions are exchanged for a single calcium ion without accompanying cations, the direction of exchange would vary with membrane potential, such that calcium flux would be directed predominantly outward at negative (resting) potentials, but would become predominantly inward at more positive (depolarized) potentials. A similar mechanism is thought to be responsible for tonic contraction in heart muscle (Horackova and Vassort, 1979). In this scheme, hormone release during potassium stimulation would be maintained by calcium influx in exchange for intracellular sodium, the release declining as the electrochemical gradient for outward movement of sodium decreases. This would also account for the enhanced release and increased rate of inactivation seen when extracellular sodium is reduced from 100 mM to zero.

In the case of electrical stimulation, depletion of intracellular sodium would proceed as described for the first model. It can be shown that relatively small changes in the intracellular sodium concentration would lead to a large decrease in intracellular calcium at a membrane potential around the resting level. Thus, inactivation induced by electrical stimulation could be due to failure of stimulus-induced calcium entry to increase the intracellular concentration by an increment great enough to cause hormone release. It is certainly feasible that alterations in the intracellular sodium concentration could persist following stimulation, as a facilitation of transmission in crayfish and crab motoneurones, attributable to sodium accumulation, remains undiminished after 2 h (Atwood et al., 1975). Both the above schemes explain the apparently disproportionate effect of electrical stimulation upon inactivation relative to the amount of hormone it releases, as intracellular sodium may thereby be altered independently of calcium influx.

The involvement of three processes in the mechanism of hormone release inactivation has thus been demonstrated, and their interaction provides evidence that all act upon the membrane calcium permeability. Similar processes, the nature of which could not have been envisaged by Sachs and his colleagues when the pioneering work on this subject was performed, are likely to operate during both acute and chronic stimulation of the magnocellular neurosecretory system in vivo. The precise mechanism by which the effects of calcium are exerted, together with the nature of the influence of the sodium concentration on inactivation, remain matters of conjecture.

SUMMARY

During prolonged stimulation, the rate of secretion from neurohypophyses stimulated in vivo or in vitro is not maintained at its original level, but declines at a rate higher than can be accounted for by depletion of the total hormone store. It has previously been suggested that this inactivation of hormone release is due either to depletion of a "readily releasable pool" of hormone, or to a potential-dependent reduction of membrane calcium permeability.

In the present experiments, the mechanism of inactivation was further investigated using both potassium and electrical stimulation in vitro, and the stimulus of 2 % saline drinking in vivo. It has been found that inactivation of release elicited by potassium stimulation is dependent not only on membrane potential, but also on calcium entry. Recovery from the potential-dependent component is much faster than from the calcium-dependent one. Calcium-dependent inactivation of hormone release can also be demonstrated with electrical stimulation, which additionally reveals a third component of inactivation dependent on external sodium. "Ex vivo" experiments, involving incubation of neurohypophyses from animals previously given 2 % NaCl rather than drinking water, suggest that similar mechanisms serve to limit hormone release in vivo.

It is proposed that all three components of inactivation exert their effects upon membrane calcium permeability, and that it is the magnitude of intracellular calcium entry during stimulation, rather than decreased availability of hormone or fatigue of the exocytotic mechanism, which is responsible for inactivation of release.

ACKNOWLEDGEMENTS

F.D. Shaw was in receipt of an MRC Studentship while much of this work was performed. We gratefully acknowledge the participation of P.G. Roe in the experiments shown in Fig. 6.

REFERENCES

Atwood, H.L., Swenarchuk, L.E. and Gruenwald, C.R. (1975) Long-term synaptic facilitation during sodium accumulation in nerve terminals. *Brain Res.*, 100: 198–204.

Baker, P.F. and Rink, T.J. (1975) Catecholamine release from bovine adrenal medulla in response to maintained depolarisation. *J. Physiol. (Lond.)*, 253: 593–620.

Baker, P.F., Meves, H. and Ridgway, E.B. (1973a) Effects of manganese and other agents on the calcium uptake that follows depolarisation of squid axons. *J. Physiol. (Lond.)*, 231: 511–526.

Baker, P.F., Meves, H. and Ridgway, E.B. (1973b) Calcium entry in response to maintained depolarisation of squid axons. *J. Physiol. (Lond.)*, 231: 527–548.

Bicknell, R.J., Dyball, R.E.J. and Shaw, F.D. (1981) Burst duration: a major determinant of electrically stimulated vasopressin release from the isolated rat neural lobe. *J. Physiol. (Lond.)*, 317: 39P.

Birks, R.I. and Cohen, M.W. (1968a) The action of sodium pump inhibitors on neuromuscular transmission. *Proc. roy. Soc. B*, 170: 381–399.

Birks, R.I. and Cohen, A.W. (1968b) The influence of internal sodium on the behaviour of motor nerve endings. *Proc. roy. Soc. B*, 170: 401–421.

Bisset, G.W., Clark, B.J., Holder, M.J., Harris, M.C., Lewis, G.P. and Rocha e Silva, M. (1967) The assay of milk-ejecting activity in the lactating rat. *Brit. J. Pharmacol.*, 31: 537–549.

Brehm, P., Eckert, R. and Tillotson, D. (1980) Calcium-mediated inactivation of calcium current in *Paramecium. J. Physiol. (Lond.)*, 306: 193–204.

Brown, A.M., Morimotok, T., Suda, Y. and Wilson, D.L. (1981) Calcium current-dependent and voltage dependent inactivation of calcium channels in *Helix aspersa. J. Physiol. (Lond.)*, 320: 193–218.

D'Amore, R. and Shepro, D. (1977) Stimulation of growth and calcium influx in cultured bovine aortic endothelial cells by platelets and vasoactive substances. *J. Cell Physiol.*, 92: 177–184.

Douglas, W.W. and Poisner, A.M. (1964a) Stimulus-secretion coupling in a neurosecretory organ: the role of calcium in the release of vasopressin from the neurohypophysis. *J. Physiol. (Lond.)*, 172: 1–18.

Douglas, W.W. and Poisner, A.M. (1964b) Calcium movement in the neurohypophysis of the rat and its relation to the release of vasopressin. *J. Physiol. (Lond.)*, 172: 19–30.

Dreifuss, J.J., Grau, J.D. and Bianchi, R.E. (1971) Antagonism between Ca and Na ions at neurohypophyseal nerve terminals. *Experientia*, 27: 1295–1296.

Dreifuss, J.J., Grau, J.D. and Nordmann, J.J. (1973) Effects on the isolated neurohypophysis of agents which affect the membrane permeability to calcium. *J. Physiol. (Lond.)*, 231: 96–98P.

Dutton, A. and Dyball, R.E.J. (1979) Phasic firing enhances vasopressin release from the rat neurohypophysis. *J. Physiol. (Lond.)*, 290: 433–440.

Dyball, R.E.J. and Nordmann, J.J. (1977) Reactivation by veratridine of hormone release from the K^+-depolarised rat neurohypophysis. *J. Physiol. (Lond.)*, 269: 65–66P.

Foreman, J.C. and Garland, L.G. (1974) Desensitisation in the process of histamine secretion induced by antigen and dextran. *J. Physiol. (Lond.)*, 239: 381–391.

Ginsburg, M. (1968) Molecular aspects of neurohypophyseal hormone release. *Proc. roy. Soc. B*, 170: 27–36.

Horackova, M. and Vassort, G. (1979) Sodium-calcium exchange in regulation of cardiac contractility. *J. gen. Physiol.*, 73: 403–424.

Jones, C.W. and Pickering, R.T. (1969) Comparison of the effects of water deprivation and sodium chloride imbibation on the hormone content of the neurohypophysis of the rat. *J. Physiol. (Lond.)*, 203: 449–458.

Kelly, J.S. (1965) Antagonism between Na^+ and Ca^{++} ions at the neuromuscular junction. *Nature (Lond.)*, 205: 296–297.

Maddrell, S.H.P. and Gee, J.D. (1974) Potassium-induced release of the diuretic hormones of *Rhodnius prolixus* and *Glossina austenii*: Ca dependence, time course and localisation of neurohaemal areas. *J. exp. Biol.*, 61: 155–171.

Meech, R.W. (1976) Intracellular calcium and the control of membrane permeability. *Soc. exp. Biol. Symp.*, 30: 161–191.

Morris, J.F., Nordmann, J.J. and Dyball, R.E.J. (1978) Structure–function correlation in mammalian neurosecretion. *Int. Rev. exp. Path.*, 18: 1–95.

Müller, J.R., Thorn, N.A. and Torp-Pedersen, C. (1975) Effects of calcium and sodium on vasopressin release in vitro induced by a prolonged potassium depolarisation. *Acta endocr.*, 79: 51–59.

Nordmann, J.J. (1975) Hormone release and calcium-entry inactivation in the rat neurohypophysis. *J. Physiol. (Lond.)*, 249: 38–39P.

Nordmann, J.J. (1976) Evidence for calcium inactivation during hormone release in the rat neurohypophysis. *J. exp. Biol.*, 65: 669–683.

Nordmann, J.J. (1977) Ultrastructural morphometry of the rat neurohypophysis. *J. Anat.*, 123: 213–218.

Nordmann, J.J. and Zyzek, E. (1982) Calcium efflux from the rat neurohypophysis. *J. Physiol. (Lond.)*, 325: 281–299.

Nordmann, J.J., Desmazes, J.F. and Georgescault, D. (1982) The relationship between the membrane potential of neurosecretory nerve endings, as measured by a voltage-sensitive dye, and the release of neurohypophysial hormones. *Neuroscience*, 7: 731–737.

Ohta, M., Narahashi, T. and Keeler, R.F. (1973) Effects of veratrum alkaloids on membrane potential and conductance of squid and crayfish giant axons. *J. Pharmacol. exp. Ther.*, 184: 143–154.

Poulain, D.A. and Wakerley, J.B. (1982) Electrophysiology of hypothalamic magnocellular neurones secreting oxytocin and vasopressin. *Neuroscience*, 7: 773–808.

Ritchie, J.M. and Straub, R.W. (1957) The hyperpolarisation which follows activity in mammalian non-medullated fibres. *J. Physiol. (Lond.)*, 136: 80–97.

Sachs, H. and Haller, E.W. (1968) Further studies on the capacity of the neurohypophysis to release vasopressin. *Endocrinology*, 83: 251–262.

Sachs, H., Share, L., Osinchak, J. and Carpi, A. (1967) Capacity of the neurohypophysis to release vasopressin. *Endocrinology*, 81: 755–770.

Thorn, N.A. (1966) In vitro studies of the release mechanism for vasopressin in rats. *Acta endocr.*, 53: 644–654.

Tillotson, D. (1979) Inactivation of calcium conductance dependent on entry of Ca ions in molluscan neurons. *Proc. nat. Acad. Sci. U.S.A.*, 76: 1497–1500.

Weinstein, M., Berne, R.M. and Sachs, H. (1960) Vasopressin in blood: effect of haemorrhage. *Endocrinology*, 66: 712–718.

The Neurohypophysis: Structure, Function and Control, Progress in Brain Research, Vol. 60, edited by B.A. Cross and G. Leng

Presynaptic Interactions in the Neurohypophysis: Endogenous Modulators of Release

Q.J. PITTMAN, D. LAWRENCE and K. LEDERIS

Department of Pharmacology and Therapeutics, Faculty of Medicine, University of Calgary, 3330 Hospital Dr. N.W., Calgary, Alb. T2N 4N1 (Canada)

INTRODUCTION

The modulation of neurohypophysial secretion by putative neurotransmitter substances and other pharmacological agents has been the subject of extensive study. As there are no neuronal cell bodies within the posterior pituitary, much of the study has been directed at interactions in the hypothalamus where the cell bodies of neurohypophysial neurones are located. Nevertheless, the observations that the innervation of the posterior pituitary extends beyond the fibres containing arginine-vasopressin (AVP) and oxytocin have prompted examination of potential presynaptic influences on neurohypophysial secretion. This review will survey some of the evidence for such presynaptic influences. Consideration will be given to: (1) the existence, within the neural lobe, or access to the neural lobe of endogenous substances; (2) evidence of release upon appropriate stimulation; (3) the presence of receptors; (4) pharmacological studies demonstrating influences on release of AVP or oxytocin, and (5) studies demonstrating altered release during physiological or experimental stimulation.

IONS

Almost 20 years ago Douglas (1963) reported on the utility of the neural lobe as a means of studying peptide release in vitro. Subsequent observations (Douglas and Poisner, 1964) established the requirement for calcium ions in the release of hormone and thereby demonstrated the similarity of these terminals in their ionic requirements to the squid giant axon. Neurophysiological studies in the latter preparation had demonstrated the effect of high frequency activity in facilitating transmitter release, probably through increased calcium availability (Katz, 1969); a similar effect has been demonstrated for the release of AVP from the neural lobe (Dutton and Dyball, 1979). The latter authors discovered that phasic stimulation of the neural lobe (an activity pattern characteristic of the putative AVP secreting cells) released more AVP than did an equal number of regularly spaced shocks. Dutton and Dyball concluded that short inter-spike intervals facilitated hormone release and suggested that this could be due to the action of residual calcium in the presynaptic terminal. Subsequent studies by Bicknell and Leng (1981) and Bicknell et al. (1982) demonstrated the increased effectiveness of phasic stimulation on both AVP and oxytocin release, but suggested that phasic stimulation obviates a rapid fatigue in transmitter release accompanying continuous, high frequency stimulation.

Our recent electrophysiological findings (Pittman, 1980) support the idea that high frequency stimulation of neurohypophysial axons may not be conducive to efficient transmitter release. Following electrical stimulation of neurohypophysial axons at frequencies as low as 20 Hz, the antidromic potential recorded extracellularly from paraventricular or supraoptic neurones increased in latency and often failed (Fig. 1). This phenomenon could be mimicked in hypothalamic slices by increasing the extracellular potassium concentration during 1 Hz stimulation; it is possible that the high frequency of action potentials in the neurohypophysial axons elevated extracellular potassium to levels sufficient to depolarize the axon and result in transmission failure. There may, of course, be other undetermined factors which could affect the fidelity of transmission in this system.

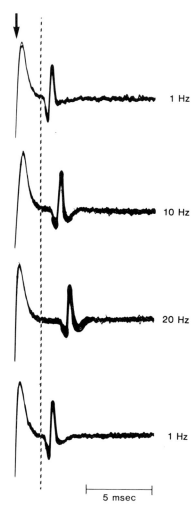

Fig. 1. Oscilloscope traces recording the electrical activity of a supraoptic neurone, in vivo, demonstrating antidromic invasion following stimulation in the pituitary stalk (arrow). Each trace represents 1–2 superimposed traces following 1 min stimulation at the indicated frequency.

These studies indicate that release of peptide from the neurohypophysis can be modulated by previous activity of the neurohypophysial neurones; these activity-related alterations in hormone release appear to be a consequence of altered ionic concentrations in the vicinity of the axons.

BIOGENIC AMINES

Noradrenaline, dopamine and 5-hydroxytryptamine have all been visualized by fluorescence histochemistry in both the intermediate and the neural lobes (Björklund et al., 1970; Baumgarten et al., 1972). Enzymes necessary for the synthesis and metabolism of these amines have also been found in the neurohypophysis (Saavedra et al., 1975). Dopamine is the most abundant amine in the neurohypophysis (Björklund et al., 1967) and dopaminergic processes have been reported to make close contact with neurosecretory axons and pituicyte processes (Baumgarten et al., 1972). This evidence, along with the demonstration of dopamine binding sites in the neural lobe (Creese et al., 1977; Cronin and Weiner, 1979), makes dopamine an attractive candidate for the regulation of hormone release from the neurohypophysis. Despite a number of studies carried out either in vivo or in vitro to determine the influence of dopamine on pituitary secretion, there is considerable confusion as to its role in the neurohypophysis (Mathison, 1981). An in vivo study reported that electrical stimulation of the dopamine cell bodies in the arcuate nucleus suppressed multi-unit activity from the neurohypophysis; since pimozide (a dopamine antagonist) prevented the suppression and dopamine superfusion of the neurohypophysis reduced it, this inhibition was considered to be mediated by dopamine release onto axons of the magnocellular neurones. Studies in isolated neurohypophyses have generally supported the idea of the inhibitory action of dopamine on AVP and oxytocin release, although increases or even no effects on the release of the hormones have been reported (Bridges et al., 1976; Hisada et al., 1977; Vizi and Volbekas, 1980; Lightman et al., 1982a). These variations have been attributed to the use of different dopamine concentrations or to the presence of possible presynaptic dopamine autoreceptors inhibiting endogenous dopamine release (Passo et al., 1981). Thus it is possible that high concentrations of dopamine inhibit AVP release through a direct action on neurosecretory terminals, whereas lower concentrations activate only dopamine autoreceptors on the dopaminergic nerve terminals, thereby reducing the endogenous dopamine inhibition of neurosecretion. This theory has not yet been tested experimentally. Racké et al. (1982a, b) used specific D-1 and D-2 receptor antagonists to obtain evidence implicating a D-1 receptor in the facilitation of AVP release and a D-2 receptor in the inhibition process.

Investigations into the functions of the dopamine innervation of the pituitary have been carried out by measuring turnover and content of dopamine under various conditions known to stimulate release of neurohypophysial hormones. Holzbauer et al. (1978) reported a decrease in pituitary dopamine content and an increase in its turnover during lactation in rats. The same authors reported an increase in the pituitary dopamine content in rats undergoing water deprivation and sodium chloride ingestion, but unfortunately the turnover was not reported; Alper et al. (1982) reported that the latter conditions were accompanied by increased dopamine synthesis (as determined by the rate of DOPA accumulation). Neither of these studies established whether the alterations in dopamine synthesis and content are reflected in altered secretion of this amine. Nevertheless, they provide some evidence for an involvement of the dopamine innervation in neurohypophysial secretion.

There is less noradrenaline than dopamine in the neurohypophysis and much of the noradrenaline is restricted to sympathetic nerve endings on the vasculature (Baumgarten et al., 1972). However, at high concentrations noradrenaline increases release of AVP from the isolated neurohypophysis (Bridges et al., 1976; Hisada et al., 1977); this effect may occur through an interaction at α-adrenergic receptors or through partial agonism at a dopamine receptor site. Racké et al. (1982b) also reported evidence indicating the presence within the neurohypophysis of a β adrenoceptor facilitating AVP secretion, and suggested that this stimulation is through an adenylate cyclase system. However, the evidence for an involvement of cyclic nucleotides in neurohypophysial secretion remains controversial (Mathison and Lederis, 1976).

Histamine and 5-hydroxytryptamine have also been found in the neurohypophysis, although these may be associated with mast cells (Saavedra et al., 1975). There is little evidence implicating these amines in modulation of neurohypophysial secretion (Mathison, 1981).

ACETYLCHOLINE

There is good evidence for a cholinergic innervation of the neurohypophysis as indicated by the presence of acetylcholine in nerve terminal vesicles (Lederis and Livingston, 1970) and of both synthesizing (choline acetyltransferase) and metabolizing (acetylcholinesterase) enzymes (Lederis and Livingston, 1969) in the neurohypophysis. There are also muscarinic receptor binding sites in the neurohypophysis (Tolliver et al., 1981). Although acetylcholine appears to be relatively ineffective in altering AVP or oxytocin release from the isolated neural lobe (Daniel and Lederis, 1967), it appears to stimulate release from hypothalamo-neurohypophysial explants (Nordmann et al., 1971) and following injection directly into the posterior pituitary in vivo (Gosbee and Lederis, 1972). These findings raise the possibility that, rather than regulating the release of neurohypophysial hormones, acetylcholine may influence the availability or distribution of secreted hormones. In keeping with this idea, Sooriyamoorthy and Livingston (1973) have shown that the local increase in blood flow in the posterior pituitary, which is associated with hormone-releasing stimuli, is cholinergically mediated.

AMINO ACIDS

The inhibitory neurotransmitter γ-aminobutyric acid (GABA) and its synthesizing and metabolizing enzymes have been found in the posterior pituitary (Beart et al., 1974). Although the location of the GABA was thought to be exclusively in pituicytes, recent immunohistochemical studies have demonstrated the GABA synthesizing enzyme, glutamic acid decarboxylase, in nerve fibres in the posterior pituitary (Oertel et al., 1982; Vincent et al., 1982). The release of tritiated GABA from the neurohypophysis has been reported (Minchin and Nordmann, 1975) but a role for GABA has yet to be demonstrated. Iversen et al. (1980) were unable to demonstrate an effect of GABA on spontaneous or evoked release of AVP from isolated neural lobes. Nevertheless, superfusion with GABA reduces the amplitude of antidromically conducted compound action potentials in neurohypophysial axons together with a receptor-specific increase in chloride conductance, which suggests that GABA may modulate the secretion of neurohypophysial hormones by presynaptic action (Zingg et al., 1979; Mathison and Dreifuss, 1981). Further studies are required to determine the physiological significance of these receptors.

OPIOID PEPTIDES

Cox et al. (1975) first reported opiate-like activity in the pituitary and subsequent studies detected substantial quantities of enkephalin immunoactivity in the neural lobe of rats (Rossier et al., 1977; Duka et al., 1978). Using immunohistochemical and lesion techniques, we were able to demonstrate an enkephalinergic neurohypophysial pathway arising in the paraventricular and supraoptic nuclei (Rossier et al., 1979, Fig. 2). Several laboratories have confirmed the existence of this pathway in rats (Sar et al., 1978; Martin and Voigt, 1981; Watson et al., 1982; Van Leeuwen, 1982) and have also demonstrated it in cat (Micevych and Elde, 1980), monkey (Haber and Elde, 1982) and fish (Reaves and Hayward, 1979; Follenius and Dubois, 1981). Recent reports indicate that the opioid peptides dynorphin (Watson et al., 1982) and α-neoendorphin (Weber et al., 1982) exhibit a similar neurohypophysial distribution. With the discovery of the various opioid peptides in the hypothalamo-neurohypophysial pathways, the coexistence of enkephalins and dynorphin in AVP- or oxytocin-producing neurones has been suggested (Coulter et al., 1981; Martin and Voigt, 1981; Watson et al., 1982). In view of the potential for cross-reactivity among a number of the antibodies used to

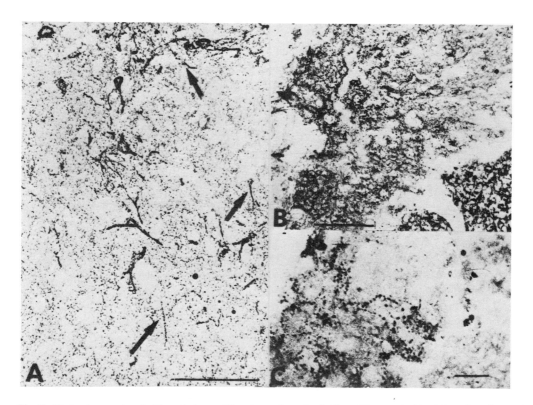

Fig. 2. Photomicrographs of rat hypothalamus (A) and neurohypophysis (B and C) reacted with rabbit anti-Leu^5-enkephalin and a horseradish peroxidase-tagged goat-anti-rabbit IgG. A: after intracerebroventricular colchicine, neurones in the lateral pole of the paraventricular nucleus exhibit positive immunoreactivity in their perikarya, dendrites, and in some finer varicose fibres. B: neurohypophysis and intermediate lobe (lower right) of normal rat. C: higher magnification view of immunoreactive fibres at the perimeter of the neurohypophysis. (From Rossier et al., 1979, with permission from Nature (Lond.), Macmillan Journals Ltd.)

324

date, and the uncertainty as to the biosynthetic relationship of the enkephalin–dynorphin family (cf. Cox et al., 1982; Watson and Akil, 1982), the fundamental questions of what peptide coexists with what require confirmation. Nevertheless, whether the presence of opioid peptides in the neural lobe is restricted to AVP or oxytocin fibres, or whether they orginate in independent neuronal systems, the opioid peptides are likely candidates as modulators of neurohypophysial secretion. That some such interaction may occur was suggested by observations that conditions favouring AVP or oxytocin release also altered pituitary levels of opioid peptides (Mata et al., 1977; Rossier et al., 1979, 1980; Hollt et al., 1981; Cox et al., 1982). Furthermore, it has been reported that opiate receptors are present in the neurohypophysis (Simantov and Snyder, 1977) and that opiates could influence vasopressin secretion (De Bodo, 1944).

A direct inhibitory effect of opioid peptides on vasopressin release from the neural lobe in vitro has been demonstrated (Lutz-Bucher and Koch, 1980; Iversen et al., 1980; Fig. 3).

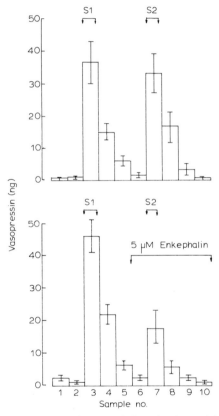

Fig. 3. Release of immunoreactive vasopressin from rat pituitary in vitro and inhibition by a stable enkephalin analogue. Rat pituitary pars nervosa/pars intermedia fragments were attached by the pituitary stalk to suction electrodes and incubated in Krebs–bicarbonate medium for 60 min before starting to collect sequential 15-min samples. During the experiment each gland was subjected to two periods of electrical stimulation (S1 and S2) through the pituitary stalk (30 V, 0.2 msec duration, 30 Hz in 10 sec trains with 10 sec intervals between trains for a total of 10 min). In 14 control experiments (top) the release of the vasopressin evoked during S2 was similar to that observed during S1. A stable enkephalin analogue (D-Ala^2,D-Leu^5-enkephalin = 5 μM Enkephalin) was added 15 min before S2 (bottom, eight experiments) and vasopressin was measured by radioimmunoassay. Results are expressed as ng Arg^8-vasopressin equivalents; each value is the mean ± S.E.M. for the number of experiments indicated. (From Iversen et al., 1980; with permission from Nature (Lond.), Macmillan Journals Ltd.)

Similarly, Clarke et al. (1979) demonstrated an opiate-mediated inhibition of oxytocin release from the pituitary of the lactating rat in the absence of any apparent effects on the electrical activity recorded from the hypothalamic cell body (Fig. 4). These studies raised the possibility that AVP and oxytocin nerve fibres were under a tonic opiate-mediated inhibition. Bicknell and Leng (1982) presented evidence to support such an inhibitory action of opiates on oxytocin secretion in vitro. In their experiments, the presence of naloxone in the perifusing fluid augmented the electrically stimulated release of oxytocin. However, in confirmation of previous observations of Iversen et al. (1980), they could not demonstrate a potentiation by naloxone of AVP release. Consequently, Bicknell and Leng (1982; see also this volume) suggested that an endogenous opiate does not appear to regulate release from the vasopressin-secreting terminals. This conclusion must be taken with caution however, as it implies specific distribution and access of endogenous opioids to *oxytocin* terminals to the exclusion of *AVP* terminals. Another possibility is that opiate receptors on vasopressin terminals are less susceptible to naloxone antagonism than receptors on the oxytocin terminals. For example, the evidence indicates that the receptors for dynorphin are of the κ variety (Chavkin et al., 1982) which differ from the μ and δ opioid receptors in their sensitivity to naloxone antagonism (Chang and Cuatrecasas, 1979).

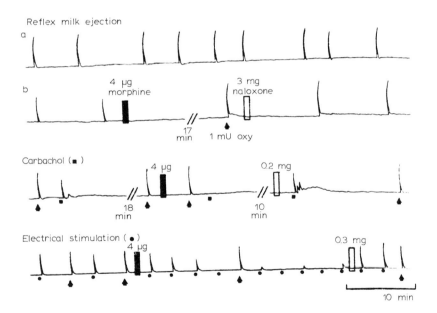

Fig. 4. Intramammary pressure recordings from four lactating rats anaesthetized with urethane to illustrate the effect of morphine on the suckling-induced and experimentally evoked release of oxytocin. Reflex milk ejection was induced by continuous sucking of the uncannulated nipples by a litter of 10 pups. a: normal pattern of milk ejection, characterized by uniform rises in intramammary pressure at intervals of 5–10 min. b: this intermittent pattern of oxytocin release has been abolished by intracerebroventricular injection of morphine (4 μg). Carbachol (■), 0.2 μg injected into the cerebral ventricles, evoked a mammary contraction of several minutes' duration; no evidence of oxytocin release was observed in response to this pharmacological treatment after administration of morphine. Similarly, the amount of oxytocin released by electrical stimulation of the neurohypophysis (●) (5 sec at 50 Hz) was reduced progressively and finally eliminated by i.v.t. injection of morphine. Naloxone totally reversed all three examples of morphine-induced inhibition of oxytocin release. Neither morphine nor naloxone changed the sensitivity of the mammary glands to exogenous oxytocin; the arrows each indicate a bolus injection of 1 mU oxytocin into a saphenous vein. (From Clarke et al., 1979; with permission from Nature (Lond.), Macmillan Journals, Ltd.)

326

The mechanism by which endogenous opiates inhibit the release of neurohypophysial hormone is not established. Evidence obtained in dorsal root ganglion cells in vitro indicates that enkephalin can reduce the calcium component of the action potential (Mudge et al., 1979). If such a phenomenon exists at the level of the terminal, the reduced calcium current would release less transmitter. In support of this idea, Lightman et al. (1982a) found that a high concentration of calcium in the perfusate antagonized the inhibitory effects of D-Ala^2,D-Leu^5-enkephalin on AVP release from the neural lobe in vitro. However, recent observations suggest that opiate effects may be mediated by a novel mechanism involving the pituicytes of the neural lobe. Van Leeuwen (1982; see also Van Leeuwen and De Vries, this volume) reported that enkephalin-immunoreactive fibres contacted pituicytes "in a synaptoid fashion". After pituitary stalk section in rats, which leads to degeneration of the nerve fibres in the neural lobe, opiate receptors increased rather than decreased in number (Lightman et al., this volume). These findings suggest that these receptors are located on the pituicytes. How such a receptor distribution might alter release from the neural lobe remains unknown. It should be borne in mind that an involvement of pituicytes in neurohypophysial hormone release has been suggested repeatedly (for reviews see Lederis, 1964; Tweedle, this volume).

OTHER PEPTIDES

Thyrotropin-releasing hormone (TRH), angiotensin II (AII), somatostatin (SRIF), cholecystokinin (CCK), corticotropin-releasing factor (CRF), glucagon and neurotensin have all been demonstrated by radioimmunoassay or immunohistochemistry in the neurohypophysis (Hökfelt et al., 1975; Johansson and Hökfelt, 1980; Kahn et al., 1980; Tager et al., 1980; Kilcoyne et al., 1980; Beinfeld et al., 1981; Vanderhaegen et al., 1981; Bloom et al., 1982). For most of these peptides, there is little evidence as to their function in the neural lobe. It will be important to resolve whether these peptides innervate the neural lobe, or whether their reported presence is due to their location in the median eminence which often extends into the proximal parts of the neural lobe (Van Leeuwen et al., 1979). Nevertheless, TRH (Lackoff and Jackson, 1981) and SRIF (Patel et al., 1977) can be released from the neural lobe in a calcium-dependent manner.

The presence of AII, which may be produced in the same neurones as AVP (Kilcoyne et al., 1980), and the occurrence of AII receptors and angiotensin converting enzyme (ACE) in the neurohypophysis, point towards AII as a likely candidate for modulation of AVP release (Saavedra et al., 1982). Homozygous Brattleboro rats, which have a genetic deficiency in AVP production, have high ACE activity (Chevillard and Saavedra, 1982) but greatly reduced numbers of AII receptors in the neurohypophysis (Van Houten et al., 1981). However, whereas central stimulation of vasopressin release by AII has been demonstrated (Keil et al., 1975), local stimulation of release from the neural lobe has been questioned (Ruoff et al., 1974; Gagnon et al., 1975; Sladek and Joynt, 1979).

Immunoreactive CCK-8 cell bodies have been found in the supraoptic and paraventricular nuclei and it has been suggested that CCK-8 coexists in oxytocin cell bodies (Vanderhaegen et al., 1981). This evidence for coexistence is supported by reports of reduced levels of CCK-8 in the neurohypophysis after hypertonic NaCl treatment or lactation in rats (Beinfeld et al., 1980). We have not found an effect of CCK-8 on AVP release from isolated neurointermediate lobes (Fig. 5).

Although AVP has long been known to have corticotropin-releasing activity (reviewed in Saffran and Schally, 1977) a 41-amino acid hypothalamic peptide discovered by Vale et al.

(1981) has been shown to have considerably higher potency in releasing corticotropin in vitro and in vivo. This corticotropin releasing factor (CRF) has been localized immunocytochemically in paraventricular cell bodies and pituitary fibres (Bloom et al., 1982). The precise interaction between the hypothalamic CRF and AVP in regulating corticotropin secretion remains to be elucidated.

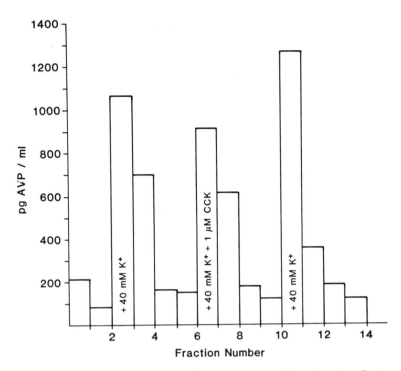

Fig. 5. Release of immunoreactive vasopressin (AVP) from rat neurointermediate lobe in vitro. Each sample consists of a 10 min serial perfusion of eight pooled lobes with a gassed Krebs–bicarbonate solution. AVP release was induced by addition of 40 mM KCl to the perfusate for 10 min during the three times indicated. During the second stimulation period 1 μM of CCK octapeptide was added to the medium. This caused little alteration in the amount of AVP appearing in the perfusate.

SUMMARY

The neurohypophysis contains many substances in addition to AVP and oxytocin. These may be present in the same cells as the neurohypophysial peptides or in independent neural systems. For some of these substances, evidence is accumulating that they may be released under physiological or experimental conditions and may modulate the release of AVP or oxytocin. Whether this interaction occurs via a presynaptic receptor on the neurohypophysial axon or involves the intervention of non-neural elements in the neurohypophysis, is not known. Electrical activity in neurohypophysial axons and the release of peptide may also be influenced by the ionic milieu resulting from previous activity or by circulating substances which pass through the fenestrated capillaries into the neural lobe.

328

Some of the potential interactions leading to presynaptic modulation of release are illustrated in Fig. 6. Considerable experimentation will be required before these interactions can be considered as much more than speculation. For example, to the best of our knowledge there are no reports of classical axo-axonic synapses in the neurohypophysis; whether the "osmiophilic membrane textures" or synaptoid features alluded to in previous studies (Baumgarten et al., 1972) represent the correlate of an axo-axonic synapse in the neurohypophysis remains to be determined.

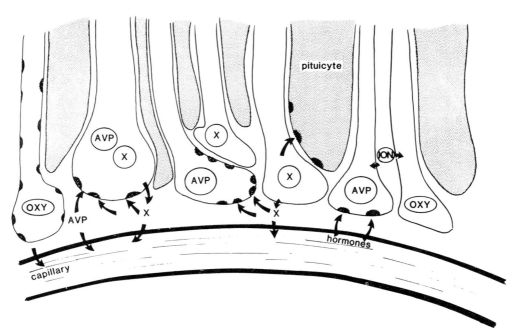

Fig. 6. Schematic of the neurohypophysis indicating possible interactions among cellular elements in the lobe. Among possible interactions are those resulting from an unidentified endogenous molecule (X) released either in association with neurohypophysial peptides or from independent fibres. Presynaptic receptors on AVP or oxytocin fibres may be accessible in the perivascular space to the released substance. Other possibilities include axo-axonic synapses onto AVP or oxytocin fibres or onto pituicytes in the neural lobe. Presynaptic receptors on neurohypophysial fibres may also be accessible to circulating substances in the blood. Finally, interactions between neurohypophysial fibres may result when high levels of activity alter ionic constituents in the vicinity and thereby affect membrane properties of adjacent fibres (right).

Finally, we are left to question why the brain has developed a mechanism for presynaptic regulation of transmitter release which requires generation and transmission of action potentials which will not release hormones. We can only speculate that this provides a fine control of neurosecretion additional to that which is known to occur at the level of the cell body (cf. Renaud et al., 1979).

ACKNOWLEDGEMENTS

Valuable discussions, ideas, and provision of data by Drs. F. Bloom, H. Gainer, L. Iversen, A. Baertschi, G. Leng and G. Clarke are gratefully acknowledged. Supported by MRC (Canada).

REFERENCES

Alper, R.H., Demarest, T. and Moore, K.E. (1982) Changes in the rate of dopamine synthesis in the posterior pituitary during dehydration and rehydration: relationship to plasma sodium concentrations. *Neuroendocrinology*, 34: 252–257.

Baumgarten, H.G., Björklund, A., Holstein, A.F. and Nobin, A. (1972) Organization and ultrastructural identification of the catecholamine nerve terminals in the neural lobe and pars intermedia of the rat pituitary. *Z. Zellforsch.*, 126: 483–517.

Beart, P.M., Kelly, J.S. and Schon, F. (1974) γ-Aminobutyric acid in the rat peripheral nervous system, pineal and posterior pituitary. *Biochem. Soc. Trans.*, 2: 266–268.

Beinfeld, M.C., Meyer, D.K. and Brownstein, M.J. (1980) Cholecystokinin octapeptide in the rat hypothalamo-neurohypophysial system. *Nature (Lond.)*, 288: 376–378.

Beinfeld, M.C., Meyer, D.K., Eskay, R.L., Jensen, R.T. and Brownstein, M.J. (1981) The distribution of cholecystokinin immunoreactivity in the central nervous system of the rat as determined by radioimmunoassay. *Brain Res.*, 212: 51–57.

Bicknell, R.J. and Leng, G. (1981) Relative efficiency of neural firing patterns for vasopressin release in vitro. *Neuroendocrinology*, 33: 295–299.

Bicknell, R.J. and Leng, G. (1982) Endogenous opiates regulate oxytocin but not vasopressin secretion from the neurohypophysis. *Nature (Lond.)*, 298: 161–162.

Bicknell, R.J. Flint, A.P.R., Leng, G. and Sheldrick, E.L. (1982) Phasic pattern of electrical stimulation enhances oxytocin secretion from the isolated neurohypophysis. *Neurosci. Lett.*, 30: 47–50.

Björklund, A., Falck, B. and Rosengren, E. (1967) Monoamines in the pituitary gland of the pig. *Life Sci.*, 6: 2103–2110.

Björklund, A., Falck, B., Hromek, F., Owman, C. and West, K.A. (1970) Identification and terminal distribution of the tubero-hypophyseal monoamine fibre systems in the rat by means of stereotaxic and microspectrofluorimetric techniques. *Brain Res.*, 17: 1–23.

Bloom, F.E., Battenberg, E.L.F., Rivier, J. and Vale, W. (1982) Corticotropin releasing factor (CRF): immunoreactive neurones and fibers in rat hypothalamus. *Regulat. Peptides*, 4: 43–48.

Bridges, T.E., Hilhouse, E.W. and Jones, M.T. (1976) The effect of dopamine on neurohypophysial hormone release in vivo and from the rat neural lobe and hypothalamus in vitro. *J. Physiol. (Lond.)*, 260: 647–666.

Chang, K.-J. and Cuatrecasas, P. (1979) Multiple opiate receptors. *J. biol. Chem.*, 254: 2610–2618.

Chavkin, C., James, I.F. and Goldstein, A. (1982) Dynorphin is a specific endogenous ligand of the κ pioid receptor. *Sience*, 215: 413–415.

Chevillard, C. and Saavedra, J.M. (1982) High angiotensin-converting enzyme activity in the neurohypophysis of Brattleboro rats. *Science*, 216: 646–647.

Clarke, G., Wood, P., Merrick, L. and Lincoln, D.W. (1979) Opiate inhibition of peptide release from the neurohumoral terminals of hypothalamic neurones. *Nature (Lond.)*, 282: 746–748.

Coulter, H.D., Elde, R.P. and Unverzagt, S.L. (1981) Co-localization of neurophysin- and enkephalin-like immunoreactivity in cat pituitary. *Peptides*, Suppl. 2: 51–55.

Cox, B.M., Opheim, K.E., Teschemacher, H. and Goldstein, A. (1975) A peptide-like substance from pituitary that acts like morphine. *Life Sci.*, 16: 1777–1782.

Cox, B.M., Baer, E.R. and Goldstein, A. (1982) Dynorphin immunoreactivity in pituitary. In E. Costa and M. Trabucchi (Eds.), *Regulatory Peptides: From Molecular Biology to Function*, Raven Press, New York, pp. 43–50.

Creese, I., Schneider, R. and Snyder, S.H. (1977) [³H]Spiroperidol labels dopamine receptors in pituitary and brain. *Europ. J. Pharmacol.*, 46: 377–381.

Cronin, M.J. and Weiner, R.I. (1979) [³H]Spiroperidol (spiperone) binding to a putative dopamine receptor in sheep and steer pituitary and stalk median eminence. *Endocrinology*, 104: 307–311.

Daniel, A. and Lederis, K. (1967) Release of neurohypophysial hormones in vitro. *J. Physiol. (Lond.)*, 190: 171–187.

De Bodo, R.C. (1944) The antidiuretic action of morphine and its mechanism. *J. Pharmacol. exp. Ther.*, 82: 74–85.

Douglas. W.W. (1963) A possible mechanism of neurosecretion: release of vasopressin by depolarization and its dependence on calcium. *Nature (Lond.)*, 197: 81–82.

Douglas, W.W. and Poisner, A.M. (1964) Stimulus–secretion coupling in a neurosecretory organ: the role of calcium in the release of vasopressin from the neurohypophysis. *J. Physiol. (Lond.)*, 172: 1–18.

Duka, T., Hollt, V., Przewlocki, R. and Wesche, D. (1978) Distribution of methionine and leucine enkephalin within the rat pituitary gland measured by highly specific radioimmunoassays. *Biochem. Biophys. Res. Commun.*, 85: 1119–1127.

Dutton, A. and Dyball, R.E.J. (1979) Phasic firing enhances vasopressin release from the rat neurohypophysis. *J. Physiol. (Lond.)*, 290: 433–440.

Follenius, E. and Dubois, M.P. (1981) Contribution of endorphinergic and enkephalinergic pathways to brain–pituitary relationships. In D.S. Farner and K. Lederis (Eds.), *Neurosecretion: Molecules, Cells, Systems*, Plenum, New York, pp. 79–92.

Gagnon, D.J., Sirois, P. and Boucher, P.J. (1975) Stimulation by angiotensin II of the release of vasopressin from incubated rat neurohypophyses — possible involvement of cyclic AMP. *Clin. exp. Pharmacol. Physiol.*, 2: 305–313.

Gosbee, J.L. and Lederis, K. (1972) In vivo release of antidiuretic hormone by direct application of acetylcholine or carbachol to the rat neurohypophysis. *Canad. J. Physiol. Pharmacol.*, 50: 618–620.

Haber, S. and Elde, R. (1982) The distribution of enkephalin immunoreactive fibers and terminals in the monkey central nervous system: an immunohistochemical study. *Neuroscience*, 7: 1049–1095.

Hisada, S., Fujimoto, S. and Kamiya, T. (1977) Antidiuresis of centrally administered amines and peptides and release of antidiuretic hormone from isolated rat neurohypophysis. *Jap. J. Pharmacol.*, 27: 153–161.

Hökfelt, T., Efendic, S., Hellerstrom, C., Johansson, O., Luft, R. and Arimura, A. (1975) Cellular localization of somastatin in endocrine-like cells and neurons of the rat with special references to the A_1-cells of the pancreatic islets and to the hypothalamus. *Acta endoc.*, Suppl. 200: 5–41.

Hollt, V., Haarmann, I., Seizinger, B.R. and Herz, A. (1981) Levels of dynorphin$_{1-13}$ immunoreactivity in rat neurointermediate pituitaries are concomitantly altered with those of leucine enkephalin and vasopressin in response to various endocrine manipulations. *Neuroendocrinology*, 33: 333–339.

Holzbauer, M., Sharman, D.F. and Godden, U. (1978) Observations on the function of the dopaminergic nerves innervating the pituitary gland. *Neuroscience*, 3: 1251–1262.

Iversen, L.L., Iversen, S.D. and Bloom, F.E. (1980) Opiate receptors influence vasopressin release from nerve terminals in rat neurohypophysis. *Nature (Lond.)*, 284: 350–351.

Johanssen, O. and Hökfelt, T. (1980) Thyrotropin releasing hormone, somatostatin and enkephalin: distribution studies using immunohistochemical techniques. *J. Histochem. Cytochem.*, 28: 364–366.

Kahn, D., Abrams, G.M., Zimmerman, E.A., Carraway, R. and Leeman, S.E. (1980) Neurotensin neurons in the rat hypothalamus: an immunocytochemical study. *Endocrinology*, 107: 47–53.

Katz, B. (1969) *The Release of Neural Transmitter Substances*. Thomas Springfield, IL.

Keil, L.C., Summy-Long, J. and Severs, W.B. (1975) Release of vasopressin by angiotensin II. *Endocrinology*, 96: 1063–1065.

Kilcoyne, M.M., Hoffman, D.L. and Zimmerman, E.A. (1980) Immunocytochemical localization of angiotensin II and vasopressin in rat hypothalamus: evidence for production in the same neuron. *Clin. Sci.*, 59: 57s-60s.

Lackoff, A. and Jackson, I.M.D. (1981) Calcium dependency of potassium-stimulated thyrotropin-releasing hormone secretion from rat neurohypophysis in vitro. *Neurosci. Lett.*, 27: 177–181.

Lederis, K. (1964) Neurosecretion and the functional structure of the neurohypophysis. In *Handbook of Physiology, Endocrinology IV, Part 1*, American Physiological Society, Washington, DC, pp. 81–102.

Lederis, K. and Livingston, A. (1969) Acetylcholine and related enzymes in the neural lobe and anterior hypothalamus of rabbit. *J. Physiol. (Lond.)*, 201: 695–709.

Lederis, K. and Livingston, A. (1970) Neuronal and subcellular localization of acetylcholine in the posterior pituitary of the rabbit. *J. Physiol. (Lond.)*, 210: 187–204.

Lightman, S.L., Iversen, L.L. and Forsling, M.L. (1982a) Dopamine and [D-Ala^2, D-Leu^5] enkephalin inhibit the electrically stimulated neurohypophyseal release of vasopressin in vitro: evidence for calcium-dependent opiate action. *J. Neurosci.*, 2: 78–81.

Lightman, S.L., Ninkovic, M. and Hunt, S.P. (1982b) Neurohypophysial opiate receptors: are they on pituicytes? In *Proc. 3rd International Conference on the Neurohypophysis*, p. 16.

Lutz-Bucher, B. and Koch, B. (1980) Evidence for a direct inhibitory effect of morphine on the secretion of posterior pituitary hormones. *Europ. J. Pharmacol.*, 66: 375–378.

Martin, R. and Voigt, K.H. (1981) Enkephalins co-exist with oxytocin and vasopressin in nerve terminals of rat neurohypophysis. *Nature (Lond.)*, 289: 502–504.

Mata, M.M., Gainer, H. and Klee, W.A. (1977) Effect of dehydration on the endogenous opiate content of rat neurointermediate lobe. *Life Sci.*, 21: 1159–1162.

Mathison, R. (1981) Regulation of secretion from the neurohypophysis: role of locally acting agents. In D.S. Favner and K. Lederis (Eds.), *Neurosecretion: Molecules, Cells, Systems*, Plenum Press, New York, pp. 167–175.

Mathison, R. and Dreifuss, J.J. (1981) Chloride-dependent action of gaba on the infundibular-neurohypophysial compound action potential. *Neurosci. Lett.*, 22: 309–312.

Mathison, R. and Lederis, K. (1976) Cyclic nucleotides in the hypothalamo-neurohypophysial system and the release of vasopressin. In *Proc. Neurohypophysis, Int. Conf.*, Key Biscayne, Fla., pp. 110–117.

Micevych, P. and Elde, R. (1980) Relationship between enkephalinergic neurons and the vasopressin-oxytocin neuroendocrine system of the cat: an immunohistochemical study. *J. comp. Neurol.*, 190: 135–146.

Minchin, M.C.W. and Nordmann, J.J. (1975) The release of [³H] gamma-aminobutyric acid and neurophysin from the isolated rat posterior pituitary. *Brain Res.*, 90: 75–84.

Mudge, A.W., Leeman, S.E. and Fischbach, G.D. (1979) Enkephalin inhibits release of substance P from sensory neurons in culture and decreases action potential duration. *Proc. nat. Acad. Sci. U.S.A.*, 76: 526–530.

Nordmann, J.J., Bianchi, R.E., Dreifuss, J.-J. and Ruf, K.B. (1971) Release of posterior pituitary hormones from the entire hypothalamo-neurohypophysial system in vitro. *Brain Res.*, 25: 669–671.

Oertel, W.H., Mugnaini, E., Tappaz, M.L., Weise, V.K., Dahl, A.D., Schmechel, D.E. and Kopin, I.J. (1982) Central GABAergic innervation of neurointermediate pituitary lobe: biochemical and immunocytochemical study of the rat. *Proc. nat. Acad. Sci. U.S.A.*, 79: 675–679.

Passo, S.S., Thornborough, J.R. and Ferris, C.F. (1981) A functional analysis of dopaminergic innervation of the neurohypophysis. *Amer. J. Physiol.*, 241: E186–E190.

Patel, Y.C., Zingg, H.H. and Dreifuss, J.J. (1977) Calcium-dependent somatostatin secretion from rat neurohypophysis in vitro. *Nature (Lond.)*, 267: 852–853.

Pittman, Q.J. (1980) Increases in antidromic latency of neuro-hypophysial neurons during sustained activation. *Proc. Canad. Physiol. Soc.*, 11: 111.

Racké, K., Ritzel, H., Trapp, B. and Muscholl, E. (1982a) Dopaminergic modulation of evoked vasopressin release from the isolated neurohypophysis of the rat: possible involvement of endogenous opioids. *Arch. Pharmacol.*, 319: 56–65.

Racké, K., Rothlander, M. and Muscholl, E. (1982b) Isoprenaline and forskolin increase evoked vasopressin release from rat pituitary. *Europ. J. Pharmacol.*, 82: 97–100.

Reaves, T.A. and Hayward, J.N. (1979) Immunocytochemical identification of enkephalinergic neurons in the hypothalamic magnocellular preoptic nucleus of the goldfish *Carassius auratus*. *Cell Tiss. Res.*, 200: 147.

Renaud, L.P., Pittman, Q.J. and Blume, H.W. (1979) Neurophysiology of hypothalamic peptidergic neurons. In K. Fuxe, T. Hökfelt and R. Luft (Eds.), *Central Regulation of the Endocrine System*, Plenum, New York, P., pp. 119–136.

Rossier, J., Vargo, T.M., Minick, S., Ling, N., Bloom, F.E. and Guillemin, R. (1977) Regional dissociation of β-endorphin and enkephalin contents in brain pituitary. *Proc. nat. Acad. Sci. U.S.A.*, 74: 5162–5165.

Rossier, J., Battenberg, E., Pittman, Q., Bayon, A., Koda, L., Miller, R., Guillemin, R. and Bloom, R. (1979) Hypothalamic enkephalin neurons may regulate the neurohypophysis. *Nature (Lond.)*, 277: 653–655.

Rossier, J., Pittman, Q., Bloom, F. and Guillemin, R. (1980) Distribution of opioid peptides in the pituitary: a new hypothalamic-pars nervosa enkephalinergic pathway. *Fed. Proc.*, 39: 2555–2560.

Ruoff, H.J., Gosbee, J.L. and Lederis, K. (1974) Substances affecting the release of neurohypophysial hormones. In K. Lederis and K.E. Cooper (Eds.), *Recent Studies of Hypothalamic Function*, Karger, Basel, pp. 62–79.

Saavedra, J.M., Palkovits, M., Kizer, J.S., Brownstein, M. and Zivin, J.A. (1975) Distribution of biogenic amines and related enzymes in the rat pituitary gland. *J. Neurochem.*, 25: 257–260.

Saavedra, J.M., Fernandez-Pardal, J. and Chevillard, C. (1982) Angiotensin-converting enzyme in discrete areas of the rat forebrain and pituitary gland. *Brain Res.*, 245: 317–325.

Saffran, M. and Schally, A.V. (1977) The status of corticotropin releasing factor (CRF). *Neuroendocrinology*, 24: 359–375.

Sar, M., Stumpf, W.E., Miller, R.J., Chang, K.J. and Cuatrecasas, P. (1978) Immunohistochemical localization of enkephalin in rat brain and spinal cord. *J. comp. Neurol.*, 182: 17–38.

Simantov, R. and Snyder, S.H. (1977) Opiate receptor binding in the pituitary gland. *Brain Res.*, 124: 178–184.

Sladek, C.D. and Joynt, R.J. (1979) Angiotensin stimulation of vasopressin release from the rat hypothalamo-neurohypophysial system in organ culture. *Endocrinology*, 104: 148–153.

Sooriyamoorthy, T. and Livingston, A. (1973) Blood flow changes in the pituitary neural lobe of the rabbit associated with neurohypophysial hormone-releasing stimuli. *J. Endocr.*, 57: 75–85.

Tager, H., Hohenboken, M., Markese, J. and Dinerstein, R.J. (1980) Identification and localization of glucagon-related peptides in rat brain. *Proc. nat. Acad. Sci. U.S.A.*, 77: 6229–6233.

Tolliver, J.M., Taylor, R.L. and Burt, D.R. (1981) Muscarinic receptors in the posterior pituitary gland. *Neuroendocrinology*, 32: 33–37.

Vale, W., Spiess, J., Rivier, C. and Rivier, J. (1981) Characterization of a 41-residue ovine hypothalamic peptide that stimulates secretion of corticotropin and β-endorphin. *Science*, 213: 1394–1397.

Vanderhaeghen, J.J., Lotstra, F., Vierendells, G., Gilles, C., Deschepper, C. and Verbanck, P. (1981) Cholecystokinins in the central nervous system and neurohypophysis. *Peptides*, Suppl. 2: 81–88.

Van Houten, M., Schiffrin, E.L. and Posner, B.I. (1981) Subnormal concentrations of brain circumventricular angiotensin II receptors in hereditary diabetes insipidus. *Soc. Neurosci. Abstr.*, 6: 508.

Van Leeuwen, F.W. (1982) Enkephalin immunoreactivity in fibres terminating in a synaptoid fashion on pituicytes in the rat neural lobe. In E. Costa and M. Trabucchi (Eds.), *Regulatory Peptides: From Molecular Biology to Function*, Raven Press, New York, pp. 203–208.

332

Van Leeuwen, F.W., De Raay, C., Swaab, D.F. and Fisser, B. (1979) The localization of oxytocin, vasopressin, somatostatin and luteinizing hormone releasing hormone in the rat neurohypophysis. *Cell Tiss. Res.*, 202: 189–201.

Vincent, S.R., Hökfelt, T. and Wu, J.-Y. (1982) GABA neuron systems in hypothalamus and the pituitary gland: immunohistochemical demonstration using antibodies against glutamate decarboxylase. *Neuroendocrinology*, 34: 117–125.

Vizi, E.S. and Volbekas, V. (1980) Inhibition by dopamine of oxytocin release from isolated posterior lobe of the hypophysis of the rat; disinhibitory effect of β-endorphin/enkephalin. *Neuroendocrinology*, 31: 46–52.

Watson, S.J. and Akil, H. (1982) Recent studies on dynorphin and enkephalin precursor fragments in central nervous system. In E. Costa and M. Trabucchi (Eds.), *Regulatory Peptides: From Molecular Biology to Function*, Raven Press, New York, pp. 35–42.

Watson, S.J., Akil, H., Fischli, W., Goldstein, A., Zimmerman, E. and Nilaver, G. (1982) Dynorphin and vasopressin: common localization in magnocellular neurons. *Science*, 216: 85–87.

Weber, E., Evans, C.J. and Barchas, J.D. (1982) Mapping of hypothalamic opioid peptide neurons by a novel immunohistochemical technique: relation to α-neo-endorphin and vasopressin systems. In E. Costa and M. Trabucchi (Eds.), *Regulatory Peptides: From Molecular Biology to Function*, Raven Press, New York, pp. 519–526.

Zingg, H.H., Baetschi, A.J. and Dreifuss, J.J. (1979) Action of γ-aminobutyric acid on hypothalamo-neurohypophysial axons. *Brain Res.*, 171: 453–459.

The Neurohypophysis: Structure, Function and Control, Progress in Brain Research, Vol. 60, edited by B.A. Cross and G. Leng
© 1983 Elsevier Science Publishers B.V.

Differential Regulation of Oxytocin- and Vasopressin-Secreting Nerve Terminals

R.J. BICKNELL and G. LENG

A.R.C. Institute of Animal Physiology, Babraham, Cambridge CB2 4AT (U.K.)

INTRODUCTION

Until recently it could be presumed that differences in the secretion of oxytocin and vasopressin from the neurohypophysis were solely a consequence of differences in the neural regulation of the cell bodies of the secretory neurones in the hypothalamus. However, recent experiments have demonstrated that differential control also occurs at the level of the neurohypophysis. First, some aspects of stimulus–secretion coupling at the secretory terminals are different for the two hormones, which may partly explain the differences between the "neural codes" of action potential discharge which control oxytocin and vasopressin release respectively. Second, the endogenous opiate innervation of the neurohypophysis may be confined in its action to the oxytocin terminals.

THE NEURAL CODE FOR HORMONE RELEASE

A series of now classic electrophysiological experiments (see Poulain and Wakerley, 1982) established that the oxytocin- and vasopressin-secreting neurones in the rat hypothalamus may be discriminated by the characteristics of their electrical activity. The vasopressin cells fire phasically under conditions of active hormone secretion, with periods of discharge at 8–15 Hz for 20–60 sec separated by silent periods of 15–40 sec duration. In contrast, the oxytocin cells discharge continuously, typically at 2–6 Hz but in a lactating rat this continuous activity is occasionally interrupted by a brief and massive discharge, at 30–80 Hz for 2–4 sec, when the suckling of a litter of pups evokes a reflex milk ejection.

Dutton and Dyball (1979) advanced an elegant hypothesis to explain the significance of the phasic discharge of the vasopressin cells. For a given mean frequency of action potential discharge, "clustering" in a phasic pattern will reduce the mode inter-spike interval. They suggested that facilitation of secretion occurs when spikes are grouped closely, possibly because intracellular calcium levels remain elevated for some time and will potentiate the effectiveness of any subsequent action potential that arrives within a sufficiently short time. Dutton and Dyball were able to demonstrate that electrical stimulation of the isolated rat neural lobe in vitro evoked more vasopressin release when stimuli were presented in a phasic pattern than when the same number of stimuli were presented at a regular frequency.

However, few cells in the hypothalamus fire regularly. While phasic firing as seen among the vasopressin cells is rare, many neurones, including the "continuous" oxytocin cells, fire

334

irregularly enough to have as many or more short interspike intervals as the vasopressin cells. Thus while phasic discharge may lead to more vasopressin secretion than the equivalent number of regularly spaced stimuli, does this mean that phasic discharge is any more efficient than the many other neural firing patterns seen in the hypothalamus?

We confirmed the conclusion that phasic firing is indeed highly efficient for the release of vasopressin (Bicknell and Leng, 1981). In these experiments the vasopressin released by phasically patterned stimuli was compared with that released by continuously patterned stimuli, using recordings of the electrical activity of a vasopressin neurone and an oxytocin neurone, respectively.

The results suggest, however, that the explanation for the superior efficiency of phasic firing does not lie in an increased preponderance of short inter-spike intervals. The firing patterns used in our experiments were matched both for the same overall mean rate, and for a similar distribution of inter-spike intervals, and yet the phasic pattern was still more effective. Therefore, another facet of the firing pattern seems to be responsible for the superior efficiency.

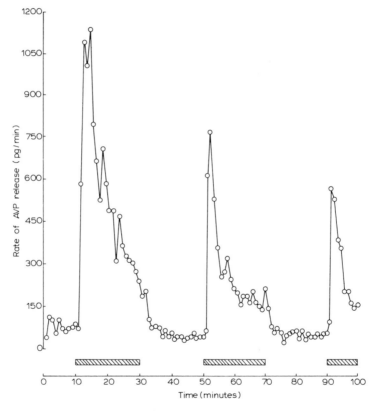

Fig. 1. Vasopressin (AVP) secretion from a rat neural lobe in vitro. The gland, with the pars intermedia attached, was impaled on a platinum stimulating electrode, and continuously perifused with warm, oxygenated medium (see Bicknell et al., 1982b). Fractions of the perifusate were collected at 1 min intervals, and the vasopressin content of each fraction was measured by specific radioimmunoassay. The hatched bars mark periods of 13 Hz electrical stimulation of the neural lobe (matched biphasic pulses, 2 msec pulse width, 5 mA peak–peak). Electrically stimulated vasopressin secretion is subject to a reversible fatigue: the stimulation evokes a high initial release of vasopressin which is not maintained, but declines within a few minutes to a "plateau" level. After a recovery period, subsequent stimulation again evokes a transient peak of secretion.

A study of the temporal profile of hormone secretion during maintained stimulation has provided a possible explanation of what this other facet might be. During sustained regular electrical stimulation, the secretion of vasopressin from the isolated rat neural lobe is not maintained at a constant level, but is subject to a quite dramatic fatigue (Fig. 1). A peak rate of secretion is attained within a minute of the onset of stimulation, but within a few minutes the rate of secretion drops to about 10–20 % of the peak rate. However, a second stimulation — after an intervening recovery period without stimulation — will again elicit a high but transient peak rate of secretion (Ingram et al., 1982).

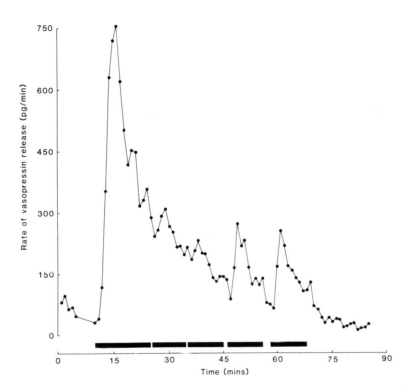

Fig. 2. Vasopressin secretion from a single rat neural lobe in vitro as described in the legend to Fig. 1. The onset of stimulation evokes a high initial release rate which is not maintained, but declines markedly due to a reversible fatigue of the release mechanism. However, silent periods of 30 sec, 30 sec, 1 min and 2 min each produce some recovery from this fatigue: transiently higher rates are attained on the resumption of stimulation after each gap.

Subsequent experiments have demonstrated that peak rates of secretion begin to decline after as little as 20–40 sec of 13 Hz stimulation, and that 30–60 sec of silence is sufficient to enable recovery from this fatigue to be demonstrated (Fig. 2). A comparison of these times with the typical discharge characteristics of phasic vasopressin cells given earlier invites the conclusion that the vasopressin neurone generates a phasic discharge pattern in order to be able to maintain a high tonic secretion of vasopressin with the least number of action potentials by avoiding the fatigue that accompanies continuous stimulation of the secretory terminals.

336

The mechanism of this fatigue is not determined. One possibility suggested by studies of other secretory systems is that inactivation of membrane calcium channels may occur (Nordmann, 1976). If the cause of fatigue is not peculiar to the vasopressin terminals, but perhaps is a common feature of peptide-secreting terminals, then why are phasic firing patterns found only infrequently in other areas of the hypothalamus (Leng, 1982)? In particular, why do the oxytocin neurones not also fire phasically?

One possible answer is that oxytocin neurones never need to maintain a high tonic level of secretion. Neurohypophysial oxytocin, insofar as we know its role, is required in spurts for reflex milk ejection and in labour, and it may be that the neural organization of the hypothalamus is designed to facilitate the synchronous, explosive discharge of oxytocin neurones rather than to sustain with efficiency a high tonic rate of secretion. This view is supported by the finding that phasic discharge is also highly efficient for releasing oxytocin from the isolated rat neural lobe (Bicknell et al., 1982a). However, although the continued stimulation of vasopressin endings leads to a relatively trivial release of vasopressin — at only about 10–20 % of the peak release rate at the onset of a period of stimulation — the fatigue is not so dramatic for the oxytocin endings (Fig. 3). Thus although the continuous background activity of an oxytocin neurone may not be optimally efficient for hormone release, neither does it appear to be quite as irrelevant as a similar discharge pattern might be for a vasopressin neurone. Indeed previous experiments have already shown (Brimble et al., 1978) that the background activity of oxytocin neurones produces a measurably elevated oxytocin concentration in plasma.

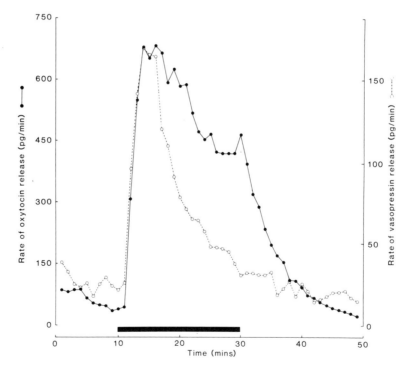

Fig. 3. Oxytocin and vasopressin secretion from a rat neural lobe in vitro. The gland was electrically stimulated at 13 Hz during the periods indicated by the shaded bars. The stimulated release of both hormones is subject to a reversible fatigue (see Figs. 1 and 2). However, the fatigue is much more dramatic for the vasopressin secreting terminals than for the oxytocin secreting terminals. Thus by the end of a 20 min period of stimulation, oxytocin is released at about 63 % of the measured peak rate while oxytocin release is only at about 17 % of the peak rate.

THE OPIATE INNERVATION OF THE NEUROHYPOPHYSIS

Although much interest has focussed over the years on the influences of opiates on vasopressin release (see Pittman et al. and Wakerley et al., this volume), less attention has been paid to their influence on oxytocin release. Recently it has been shown that the neurohypophysis itself receives an opiate peptide innervation from cell bodies in the hypothalamus (Rossier et al., 1979). The precise nature and origin of these projections remain to be established. Various groups have reported evidence for the presence in the neurohypophysis of leucine-enkephalin (Rossier et al., 1977), methionine-enkephalin (Martin and Voigt, 1981), dynorphin$_{1-17}$ (Goldstein et al., 1981), dynorphin$_{1-8}$ and α-neoendorphin (Weber et al., 1982). β-Endorphin is almost absent from the neurohypophysis, although present in large amounts in the intermediate lobe (Rossier et al., 1979).

Exogenous morphine and opiate peptides have been reported to inhibit both vasopressin (Iversen et al., 1980) and oxytocin release (Clarke et al., 1979) at the level of the neurohypophysis. However, we have recently reported evidence that the endogenous opiate innervation of the neurohypophysis inhibits the release of oxytocin, but not of vasopressin, and that the inhibition is quite dramatic in its extent (Bicknell and Leng, 1982). Thus although there are relatively few opiate fibres, if their action is inhibited by the opiate antagonist naloxone, the amount of oxytocin that is released by electrical stimulation of the neural lobe in vitro is about doubled. Electrically evoked vasopressin secretion is unaffected by naloxone, in agreement with previous reports (Iversen et al., 1980).

Such a differential regulation of oxytocin and vasopressin secretion by opiates suggests that the opiate innervation of the neural lobe may be restricted to the oxytocin terminals, which in the rat are concentrated in the periphery of the gland (Van Leeuwen et al., 1979). Rossier et al. (1979) reported that the leucine-enkephalin fibres were indeed concentrated on the perimeter of the rat neural lobe and more or less absent from the centre of the tissue. However, Van Leeuwen et al. (1981) found leucine-enkephalin fibres in the centre of the gland as well as on the perimeter.

The intermediate lobe of the pituitary contains large quantities of opiate peptides, but, as we have found recently (unpublished results), naloxone will still potentiate oxytocin secretion from the isolated neural lobe after removal of the intermediate lobe. However, while we may thus be reasonably sure that the specific opiate inhibition of oxytocin secretion is indeed mediated by hypothalamo-neurohypophysial opiate peptide fibres, the mechanism of this inhibition is unknown.

There is no ultrastructural evidence to support a mechanism in the neurohypophysis that would be analogous to classical presynaptic inhibition: the opiate terminals do not appear to make direct synaptic contact with neurosecretory terminals. However, there is evidence for a novel type of control involving the pituicytes: astrocytic glial cells that occur in close association with the neurosecretory processes in the neural lobe. Immunocytochemical studies at the electron microscopic level have shown that some opiate peptide-containing fibres appear to make synaptic contact with the pituicytes (Van Leeuwen and De Vries, this volume), and recently it has been found that opiate receptors persist in the deafferented neurohypophysis after degeneration of the neural elements (Lightman et al., this volume).

Each pituicyte encapsulates a number of neurosecretory processes, which may help to explain how a limited opiate innervation can exert such a considerable influence upon oxytocin release. However, the manner in which pituicytes might influence secretion is open to speculation. The pituicytes are linked by gap junctions, but there is no ultrastructural evidence that they are electrically linked to the secretory terminals.

338

Recent work (see Tweedle, this volume) has shown that the degree to which pituicytes encapsulate the secretory terminals alters under conditions of prolonged hypersecretion of oxytocin and vasopressin. If this structural reorganization has a functional significance for stimulus–secretion coupling, then it is a possible target of an opiate control system. However, the effect of naloxone upon oxytocin secretion is very rapid (Fig. 4): the stimulated release of oxytocin from the isolated neural lobe is potentiated within 1.8 min of exposure to naloxone, which suggests that any structural change would have to be accomplished rapidly.

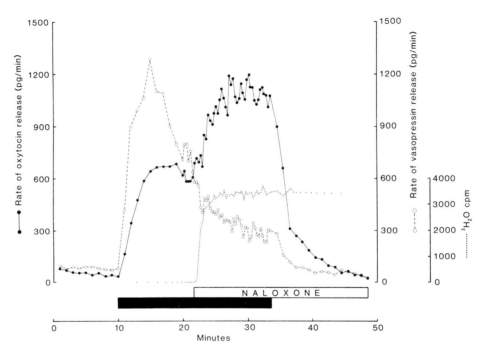

Fig. 4. Oxytocin and vasopressin secretion from a rat neural lobe in vitro. The solid bar marks a period of 13 Hz stimulation of the gland. Naloxone (5×10^{-6} M) was introduced into the perifusate after 10 min of stimulation along with a tritiated water "marker". The presence of naloxone in the fractions of perifusate may be inferred from the given measure of the presence of tritiated water. The vasopressin release in response to electrical stimulation follows a pattern of decline following an initial peak that has been described in detail, and this pattern is unaffected by the presence of naloxone. However, the arrival of naloxone causes an increase in the rate of oxytocin secretion. Within 1.8 min the measured oxytocin level exceeds the highest level previously obtained, and continuous to rise still higher. Electrical stimulation of the neural lobe releases oxytocin and vasopressin, and also endogenous opiates. The opiates inhibit the release of oxytocin but not that of vasopressin. The opiate antagonist naloxone removes the opiate influence on oxytocin release.

Alternatively, pituicytes may influence the neurosecretory terminals either via a secretory product, or by an influence upon the extracellular ionic environment (see Tweedle, this volume, for a discussion of these possibilities).

Various workers have suggested that GABA may be released by pituicytes (see Tweedle, and Pittman et al., this volume, for full discussions). However, as we have failed to find any marked effect of the GABA agonist muscimol or the GABA antagonist picrotoxin upon oxytocin release from the isolated neural lobe (Fig. 5), it seems unlikely that GABA mediates the opiate inhibition.

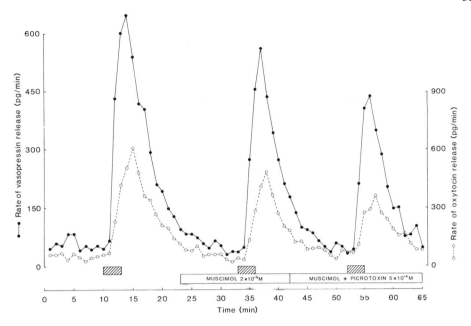

Fig. 5. Oxytocin and vasopressin secretion from a rat neural lobe in vitro. The hatched bars mark 3 min periods of 13 Hz electrical stimulation. During the periods indicated, the GABA agonist muscimol and/or the GABA antagonist picrotoxin were included in the perifusate. Neither compound markedly affected electrically stimulated hormone secretion: the decline in the amounts of hormone released in response to identical stimulations is similar to that seen in control experiments. Using a similar protocol we have shown that the opiate antagonist naloxone approximately doubles the amount of oxytocin released during such stimulation (Bicknell and Leng, 1982).

Finally, there is some evidence (Martin and Voigt, 1981; Watson et al., 1982) that opiates co-exist with oxytocin or vasopressin in the secretory terminals, and thus they may influence secretion by "auto-feedback". No explanation has been suggested of how the secretion of co-existing peptides could be under differential control, and thus the utility of such an organization seems limited, if the primary function of the neurohypophysial opiate peptides is indeed to modulate hormone secretion.

Thus, evidence is accumulating that the pituicytes influence hormone secretion from the neurohypophysis. If this influence proves to be under opiate control, then a reconsideration of the function of glia elsewhere in the CNS may follow. Even if the opiate–pituicyte hypothesis is false, it seems likely that the opiate inhibition of oxytocin secretion from the neurohypophysis involves a novel mechanism.

SUMMARY

Oxytocin and vasopressin nerve terminals do not respond in an identical way to electrical stimulation. During sustained electrical stimulation, vasopressin release from the rat neural lobe in vitro shows a dramatic but reversible "fatigue". The phasic firing patterns observed in vasopressin neurones may serve to avoid this fatigue, and enable a high tonic level of secretion to be maintained. Oxytocin release, on the other hand, shows a much less dramatic fatigue, and appreciable release will accompany continuous stimulation. The oxytocin neurones do not fire phasically, and although phasic stimulation is still a more efficient way of releasing hormone from the oxytocin terminals, it may be that the neural control of the oxytocin neurones puts a higher priority on organizing the synchronized burst discharge associated with reflex milk ejection, than on optimizing the efficiency of background release.

A further difference in the regulation of oxytocin and vasopressin nerve terminals is that opiate peptides released from the neural lobe by electrical stimulation exert a profound inhibitory influence upon oxytocin release, but do not appear to affect vasopressin release. It is likely that a novel mechanism of inhibition is involved, possibly mediated by an opiate control of the pituicytes.

ACKNOWLEDGEMENTS

Various major contributions have been made by D. Brown, C. Chapman and C. Ingram to the experiments and the ideas described in this article.

REFERENCES

Bicknell, R.J. and Leng, G. (1981) Relative efficiency of neural firing patterns for vasopressin release in vitro. *Neuroendocrinology*, 33: 295–299.

Bicknell, R.J. and Leng, G. (1982) Endogenous opiates regulate oxytocin but not vasopressin secretion from the neurohypophysis. *Nature (Lond.)*, 298: 161–162.

Bicknell, R.J., Flint, A.P.F., Leng, G. and Sheldrick, E.L. (1982a) Phasic pattern of electrical stimulation enhances oxytocin secretion from the isolated neurohypophysis. *Neurosci. Lett.*, 30: 47–50.

Bicknell, R.J., Chapman, C. and Leng, G. (1982b) A perifusion system for studying neurosecretion from the isolated rat neurohypophysis in vitro. *J. Neurosci. Meth.*, 5: 95–101.

Brimble, M.J., Dyball, R.E.J. and Forsling, M.L. (1978) Oxytocin release following osmotic activation of oxytocin neurones in the paraventricular and supraoptic nuclei. *J. Physiol. (Lond.)*, 278: 69–78.

Clarke, G., Wood, P., Merrick, L. and Lincoln, D.W. (1979) Opiate inhibition of peptide release from the neurohumoral terminals of hypothalamic neurones. *Nature (Lond.)*, 282: 746–748.

Dutton, A. and Dyball, R.E.J. (1979) Phasic firing enhances vasopressin release from the rat neurohypophysis. *J. Physiol. (Lond.)*, 290: 433–440.

Goldstein, A., Fischli, W., Lowrey, L.I., Hunkapiller, M. and Hood, L. (1981) Porcine pituitary dynorphin: complete amino acid sequence of the biologically active heptadecapeptide. *Proc. nat. Acad. Sci. U.S.A.*, 78: 7219–7223.

Ingram, C.D., Bicknell, R.J., Brown, D. and Leng, G. (1982) Rapid fatigue of neuropeptide secretion during continual electrical stimulation. *Neuroendocrinology*, 35: 424–428.

Iversen, L.L., Iversen, S.D. and Bloom, F.E. (1980) Opiate receptors influence vasopressin release from nerve terminals in rat neurohypophysis. *Nature (Lond.)*, 284: 350–351.

Leng, G. (1982) Phasic neurones in the lateral hypothalamus of anaesthetised rats. *Brain Research*, 230: 390–393.

Martin, R. and Voigt, K.H. (1981) Enkephalins co-exist with oxytocin and vasopressin in nerve terminals of rat neurohypophysis. *Nature (Lond.)*, 289: 503–504.

Nordmann, J.J. (1976) Evidence for calcium inactivation during hormone release in the rat neurohypophysis. *J. exp. Biol.*, 65: 669–683.

Poulain, D.A. and Wakerley, J.B. (1982) Electrophysiology of hypothalamic magnocellular neurones secreting oxytocin and vasopressin. *Neuroscience*, 7: 773–808.

Rossier, J., Vargo, T.M., Minick, S., Ling, N., Bloom, F.E. and Guillemin, R. (1977) Regional dissociation of beta-endorphin and enkephalin contents in the rat brain and pituitary. *Proc. nat. Acad. Sci. U.S.A.*, 74: 5162–5165.

Rossier, J., Battenberg, E., Pittman, Q.J., Bayon, A., Koda, L., Miller, R. and Bloom, F.E. (1979) Hypothalamic enkephalin neurones may regulate the neurohypophysis. *Nature (Lond.)*, 277: 653–655.

Van Leeuwen, F.W., De Raay, C., Swaab, D.F. and Fisser, B. (1979) The localisation of oxytocin, vasopressin, somatostatin and luteinizing hormone releasing hormone in the rat neurohypophysis. *Cell Tiss. Res.*, 202: 189–201.

Van Leeuwen, F.W., Pool, C. and Sluiter, A. (1983) Enkephalin immunoreactivity in synaptoid elements on glial cells in the rat neural lobe. *Neuroscience,* 8: 229–241.

Watson, S.J., Akil, H., Fischli, W., Goldstein, A., Zimmerman, E.A., Nilaver, G. and Van Wimersma Greidanus, Tj.B. (1982) Dynorphin and vasopressin: common localization in magnocellular neurons. *Science*, 216: 85–87.

Weber, E., Evans, C.J. and Barchas, J.D. (1982) Predominance of the amino-terminal octapeptide fragment of dynorphin in rat brain regions. *Nature (Lond.)*, 299: 77–79.

The Neurohypophysis: Structure, Function and Control, Progress in Brain Research, Vol. 60, edited by B.A. Cross and G. Leng
© *1983 Elsevier Science Publishers B.V.*

Enkephalin–Glial Interaction and Its Consequence for Vasopressin and Oxytocin Release from the Rat Neural Lobe

F.W. VAN LEEUWEN and G.J. DE VRIES

*Netherlands Institute for Brain Research,
IJdijk 28, 1095 KJ Amsterdam (The Netherlands)*

INTRODUCTION

Although the neural lobe does not contain neuronal perikarya, it is a highly organized protusion of the brain, composed of nerve fibres and glial cells. The nerve fibres contain not only vasopressin, oxytocin and their associated neurophysins but also various other peptides, amines and amino acids (for review see Van Leeuwen, 1982b; Pittman et al., this volume). The glial cells that were named pituicytes on the basis of a different morphology and peculiar staining properties and therefore considered as a special class of glia, later proved to be astrocytes (Hild, 1954; Christ, 1966; Salm et al., 1982); they occupy 25–30% of the neural lobe volume (Nordmann, 1977).

Under conditions of enhanced release of vasopressin and oxytocin into the bloodstream, the pituicytes show increased mitotic activity, a large hypertrophy of the nucleus and cell body, an increase in the number of cytoplasmic lipid droplets, an increased RNA-synthesizing capacity and reduced enclosure of nerve fibres by their processes (cf. Tweedle and Hatton, 1980a, b). Moreover, the number of synaptoid contacts between nerve fibres and pituicytes increases during dehydration (Wittkowski and Brinkman, 1974). On the basis of this parallelism in activity, many speculations have been raised about the role of pituicytes in the release of hormones from the neurohypophysis (cf. Boer, 1976; Wittkowski, 1980).

NERVE INPUT BY OPIOID PEPTIDES IN THE NEURAL LOBE

Simantov and Snyder (1977) and Wamsley et al. (1982) reported the presence of stereospecific opiate binding sites in the bovine and monkey neural lobe, respectively, and Rossier et al. (1977, 1979) found high levels of Met- and Leu-enkephalin by radioimmunoassay. These pharmacological and biochemical data were followed by immunocytochemical data (Rossier et al., 1979). Numerous enkephalin fibres were reported, especially in the peripheral parts of the neural lobe.

Subsequently a number of studies reported co-existence of Leu-enkephalin with vasopressin and Met-enkephalin with oxytocin (Lotstra et al., 1981; Martin and Voigt, 1981; Martin et al., 1982). A number of related opiate peptides (e.g. dynorphin$_{1-8}$, dynorphin$_{1-17}$ and α-neoendorphin) have also been found in the neural lobe (cf. Rossier, 1982; Weber et al., 1981, 1982). The presence of dynorphin had already been described in pig neural lobes (Cox et al., 1975)

344

and this peptide was later sequenced by Goldstein et al. (1980, 1981). Recently co-existence of α-neoendorphin with dynorphin was reported in the rat supraoptic nucleus (Weber et al., 1981). Watson et al. (1982) suggest that the aforementioned results of Martin and Voigt (1981) may be due to cross-reactivity of anti-Leu-enkephalin with dynorphin or a related compound. However, the distribution of dynorphin-immunoreactive fibres as shown by Watson et al. (1981) in the perimeter of the neural lobe points to a co-localization with oxytocin rather than with vasopressin (cf. Van Leeuwen et al., 1979, Fig. 1a, b). These differences might partly be due to the use of inappropriate specificity controls: these usually consist of blocking tests of the antiserum with the antigen to which it was raised. However, such controls do not exclude reaction with compounds possessing related antigenic determinants (cf. Swaab et al., 1977; Van Leeuwen et al., 1979; Van Leeuwen, 1982c). Unfortunately, sensitive peptide antigen identification techniques, which are required for the accurate interpretation of immunocytochemical results, are not available at present (Pool et al., 1983).

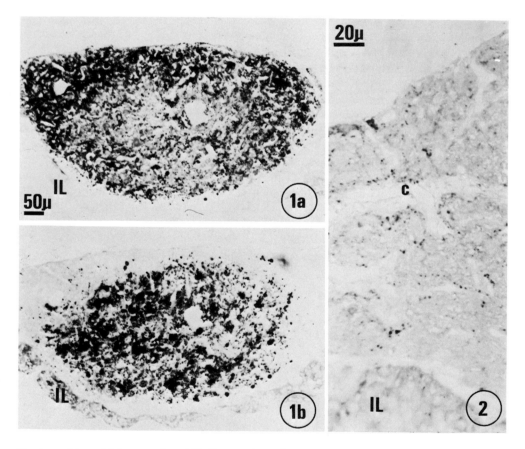

Fig. 1.a and b: serial transversal semithin Epon sections of rat neurointermediate lobe, immunocytochemically stained with purified anti-oxytocin (a) and anti-vasopressin (b). Note peripheral oxytocin fibres in neural lobe and vasopressin immunoreactivity in intermediate lobe (IL). (For details see Van Leeuwen et al., 1979.)

Fig. 2. Semithin sagittal Epon section of a part of the rat neurointermediate lobe immunocytochemically stained with anti-Leu-enkephalin serum showing immunoreactive fibres all over the neural lobe. IL, intermediate lobe.

In our studies we found no evidence for co-existence of Leu-enkephalin with vasopressin (Van Leeuwen, 1982b; Van Leeuwen et al., 1983). In fact, Rossier's results were confirmed and extended as we observed numerous Leu-enkephalin immunoreactive fibres not only in the perimeter of the neural lobe but also in the centre (Fig. 2). From these light microscopical data no conclusion could be drawn as to whether enkephalin fibres terminate upon vasopressin and oxytocin fibres, pituicytes and/or upon capillaries. A pre-embedding immunoelectron microscopical study was therefore performed in which synaptoid contacts of Leu-enkephalin terminals upon pituicytes were found (Figs. 3 and 4). Synaptoid contacts between enkephalin

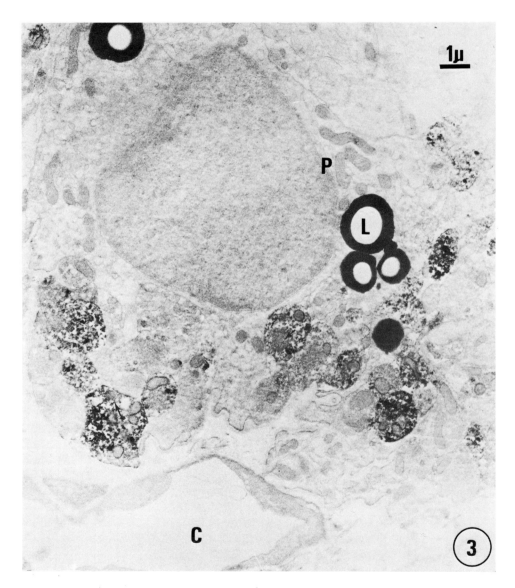

Fig. 3. Ultrathin section of a vibratome slice of the rat neurointermediate lobe showing Leu-enkephalin immunoreactive fibres surrounding a pituicyte (P). L, lipid droplet; ↑, clear vesicles, C, capillary.

346

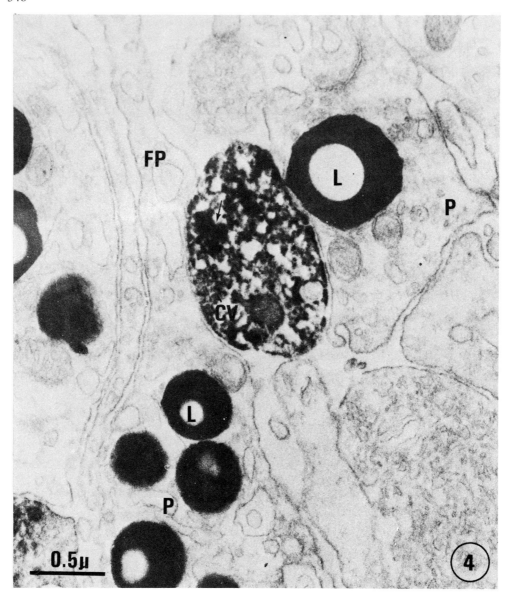

Fig. 4. Ultrathin section of a vibratome slice of the rat neurointermediate lobe showing a Leu-enkephalin immuno-reactive fibre making a synaptoid contact on a finger-like process (FP) of a pituicyte (P) recognized by the presence of lipid droplets (L). CV, clear vesicles, ↑, dense core vesicles.

fibres and glia may also occur in the guinea pig median eminence, as Beauvillain et al. (1980) reported "close proximity between enkephalin immunostained fibres and ependymocytes". Synaptoid contacts between nerve fibres and pituicytes have been reported in numerous electron microscopical studies in vertebrates (cf. Wittkowski, 1980). The presynaptoid elements contain dense core vesicles with a diameter of either 100 nm (infrequently) or 150 nm (frequently). From our immunoelectron microscopical studies and those of Beauvillain et al.

(1980, 1982), the infrequent 100 nm type dense core vesicles may contain enkephalin or a related opiate peptide (cf. Fig. 4). This would be another argument against co-localization of vasopressin and oxytocin with opiate peptides, as the former are present mainly in 150 nm vesicles (Van Leeuwen and Swaab, 1977; Martin et al., 1982).

NEURONAL–GLIAL INTERACTION IN THE NEURAL LOBE

Although there are about nine times more glial than nerve cells in the central nervous system (Kandel, 1981), knowledge of their role in brain function is still in its infancy (cf. Varon and Somjen, 1979; Abbott, 1981). The main reason may be that glial cells do not clearly advertise their function. An exception may be the neuronal–glial interaction in the neural lobe (see Introduction). Opiate peptides inhibit the release of vasopressin and oxytocin from the neural lobe (see Iversen et al., 1980; Aziz et al., 1981). As enkephalin immunoreactive synaptoid contacts are present on pituicytes, the opiate inhibitory action may be mediated via these cells rather than via a synaptic action upon neurosecretory terminals (cf. Clarke et al., 1979; Micevych and Elde, 1980). The presence of enkephalin synaptoid contacts on pituicytes, however, does not exclude the possibility that opiate receptors are also present on nerve terminals. Opiate receptors have been found in the neural lobe (Simantov and Snyder, 1977; Wamsley et al., 1982), however the autoradiographic technique used in the latter study usually displays a low resolution and a poor morphology. To overcome this difficulty Lightman et al. (this volume) decided to section the neurohypophysial stalk; a situation in which only pituicytes remain and nerve fibres disappear (Dellmann et al., 1974). After stalk-section opiate binding sites were indeed still found in the neural lobe. However, even with this approach there is still uncertainty about the presence of opiate binding sites on vasopressin and oxytocin nerve terminals. This problem may be solved by the use of antibodies directed against the opiate receptor protein(s) (Bidlack et al., 1981).

THE ROLE OF PITUICYTES IN VASOPRESSIN AND OXYTOCIN RELEASE

It is not clear how the pituicytes may influence the release of vasopressin and oxytocin. They may regulate the immediate environment of enclosed nerve terminals by uptake of potassium as in the mammalian spinal cord (Somjen, 1981; Sykova, 1981). The processes of pituicytes are connected via gap junctions (Dreifuss et al., 1975; Hatton and Ellisman, 1981) and so may form a syncytium and thereby act as a "spatial" buffer for potassium ions, as in the mammalian cortex (cf. Gardner-Medwin, 1981). Such a spatial buffer may be more effective if we consider the mechanism proposed by Tweedle and Hatton (1980a, b; Tweedle, this volume). During enhanced release of vasopressin and oxytocin they showed that there was less enclosure of neurosecretory endings by glial processes than under normal conditions: this might result in a diminished uptake of potassium ions. Thus enclosure of nerve endings may form the morphological framework for pituicyte involvement in inhibition and facilitation of hormone release. If opiate peptides inhibit the release of vasopressin and oxytocin this would mean that the pituicytes are stimulated to enclose the neurosecretory terminals via synaptoid contacts.

Calcium ions may also play a role in the regulation of hormone release by enkephalin. The release of vasopressin and oxytocin is accompanied by an influx of calcium into nerve terminals from the extracellular space. Recently Wright and Lincoln (1982) suggested that opiate inhibition of oxytocin release may be the result of a modulation of calcium influx.

348

Stoeckel et al. (1975) demonstrated calcium pyroantimonate deposits in both nerve fibres and pituicytes, while Karcsú et al. (1982) showed an increase of Ca^{2+} in mitochondria of nerve fibres after an i.v. injection of hypertonic saline. The role of pituicytes in calcium movements remains to be determined, however (cf. Orkand, 1982).

A way in which opiate peptides, vasopressin, oxytocin and pituicytes might interact is represented in Fig. 5. The release of hormone into the bloodstream would be influenced by pituicytes, the activity of which would be modulated by opiate peptides, and also by vasopressin and oxytocin. The effects of opiate peptides and vasopressin or oxytocin (which may be accomplished via synaptoid contacts) would be opposite. Morris (1976) reported that axon swellings especially exhibit such contacts. As these swellings are supposed to be storage sites for neurosecretory granules, the "message" of an overload of granules may be transmitted via

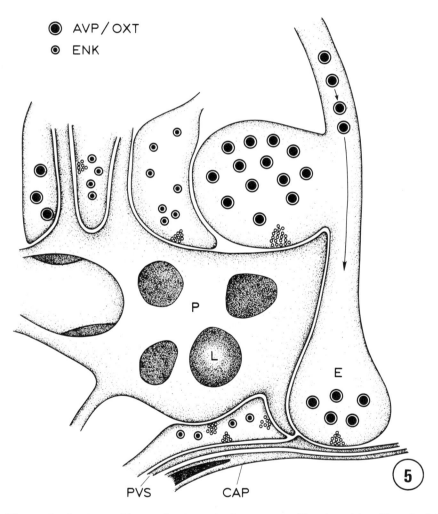

Fig. 5. Diagram showing the possible way of an interaction between nerve fibres (containing either enkephalin and vasopressin (AVP) or oxytocin (OXT) and a pituicyte, resulting in a modulation of vasopressin and oxytocin release into the perivascular space (PVS). CAP, capillary; E, ending; L, lipid droplet; P, pituicyte; PVS, perivascular space; S, swelling. (Reproduced with permission from the publisher of Neuroscience.)

these synaptoid contacts to the numerous pituicyte processes resulting in enhanced hormone release (e.g. by reduced enclosure of vasopressin or oxytocin terminals resulting in a less effective uptake of potassium ions).

Synaptoid contacts between nerve fibres and glial cells are not restricted to the neural lobe but have been described in various periventricular organs (for reference see Wolff et al., 1979; Wittkowski, 1980). In addition, although restricted to certain developmental stages, axo-glial synaptoid contacts have been found in other brain areas (cf. Wolff et al., 1979). It is clear that pituicytes may serve as an attractive model system for neuronal–glial interaction (see also Tweedle, and Bicknell and Leng, this volume).

SUMMARY

In the past few years it has become clear that the nervous input of the neural lobe not only consists of vasopressin and oxytocin, but is more complex, e.g. somatostatin, neurotensin and the enkephalins have been reported to occur. Recently it was proposed that opiate peptides would inhibit the release of vasopressin and oxytocin at the level of the neural lobe. Moreover, stereospecific opiate receptor binding was found in the bovine neural lobe. At the light microscope level we have observed Leu-enkephalin immunoreactive fibres all over the neural lobe. Contrary to recent literature, no co-existence in the same terminal of immunoreactivity for the enkephalins and vasopressin or oxytocin was found at the electron microscope level. Immunoreactive Leu-enkephalin fibres surround the pituicytes and make synaptoid contacts upon their soma and processes. The reaction product is localized both in dense core vesicles of 100 nm and diffusely spread over the cytoplasm. A working hypothesis is submitted in which pituicytes play an intermediary role in the regulation of vasopressin and oxytocin release by opiate peptides. The activity of pituicytes would be modulated by opiate peptides and vasopressin or oxytocin.

REFERENCES

Abbott, N.J. (1981) Glial–neurone interactions. *Trends Neurosci.*, 4: 14–16.

Aziz, L.A., Forsling, M.L. and Woolf, C.J. (1981) The effect of intracerebroventricular injections of morphine on vasopressin release in the rat. *J. Physiol. (Lond.)*, 311: 401–409.

Beauvillain, J.C., Tramu, G. and Croix, D. (1980) Electron microscopic localization of enkephalin in the median eminence and the adenohypophysis of the guinea-pig. *Neuroscience*, 5: 1705–1716.

Beauvillain, J.C., Tramu, G. and Poulain, P. (1982) Enkephalin-immunoreactive neurons in the guinea pig hypothalamus. *Cell Tiss. Res.*, 224: 1–13.

Bidlack, J.M., Abood, L.G., Osei-Gyimah, P. and Archer, S. (1981) Purification of the opiate receptor from rat brain. *Proc. nat. Acad. Sci. U.S.A.*, 78: 636–639.

Boer, G.J. (1976) *The Role of Pituicytes in the Rat Neurohypophysis : an Exploratory Investigation Using Histo- and Microchemistry*, Ph. D. Thesis, University of Amsterdam.

Bucy, P. (1930) The pars nervosa of the bovine hypophysis. *J. comp. Neurol.*, 50: 505–511.

Christ, J.F. (1966) Nerve supply, blood supply and cytology of the neurohypophysis. In G.W. Harris and B.T. Donovan (Eds.), *The Pituitary Gland*, Butterworths, London, pp. 62–130.

Clarke, G., Wood, P., Merrick, L. and Lincoln, D.W. (1979) Opiate inhibition of peptide release from the neurohumoral terminals of hypothalamic neurones. *Nature (Lond.)*, 282: 746–748.

Cox, B.M., Opheim, K.E., Teschemacher, H. and Goldstein, A. (1975) A peptide-like substance from pituitary that acts like morphine. *Life Sci.*, 16: 1777–1782.

Dellmann, H.D., Stoeckel, M.E., Porte, A. and Stutinsky, F. (1974) Ultrastructure of the neurohypophyseal glial cells following stalk transection in the rat. *Experientia*, 30: 1220–1222.

Dreifuss, J.J., Sandri, C., Akert, K. and Moor, H. (1975) Ultrastructural evidence for sinusoid spaces and coupling between pituicytes in the rat. *Cell Tiss. Res.,* 161: 33–45.

Gardner-Medwin, A.R. (1981) Possible roles of vertebrate neuroglia in potassium dynamics, spreading depression and migraine. *J. exp. Biol.,* 195: 111–127.

Goldstein, A. and Ghazarossian, V.E. (1980) Immunoreactive dynorphin in pituitary and brain. *Proc. nat. Acad. Sci. (U.S.A.)* 77: 6207–6210.

Goldstein, A., Fischli, W., Lowney, L.I., Hunkapiller, M. and Hood, L. (1981) Porcine pituitary dynorphin: complete amino acid sequence of the biologically active heptapeptide. *Proc. nat. Acad. Sci. U.S.A.,* 78: 7219–7223.

Hatton, J.D. and Ellisman, M.H. (1981) Distribution of orthogonal arrays and their relationship to intercellular junctions in neuroglia of the freeze-fractured hypothalamo-neurohypophyseal system. *Cell Tiss. Res.,* 215: 308–323.

Hild, W. (1954) Das morphologische, kinetische und endokrinologische Verhalten von hypothalamischen und neurohypophysären Gewebe in vitro. *Z. Zellforsch.,* 40: 257–312.

Iversen, L.I., Iversen, S.D. and Bloom, F.E. (1980) Opiate receptors influence vasopressin release from nerve terminals in rat neurohypophysis. *Nature (Lond.),* 284: 350–351.

Kandel, E.R. (1981) Nerve cells and behaviour. In E.R. Kandel and J.H. Schwartz (Eds.), *Principles of Neural Science,* Edward Arnold, London, p. 17.

Karcsú, S., Lászloó, F.A., Jancsó, G., Tóth, L. and Bácoy, E. (1982) Morphological evidence for the involvement of calcium in neurohypophyseal hormone release. *Brain Res.,* 238: 278–281.

Lotstra, F., Vierendeels, G. and Vanderhaeghen, J.J. (1981) Cholecystokinin, Met- and Leu-enkephalin in the hypothalamo-hypophyseal magnocellular system. *Neurosci. Lett.,* Suppl. 7: S248.

Martin, R. and Voigt, K.H. (1981) Enkephalin co-exists with oxytocin and vasopressin in nerve terminals of rat neurohypophysis. *Nature (Lond.),* 289: 502–504.

Martin, R., Schäfer, M. and Voigt, K.H. (1982) Enzymatic cleavage prior to antibody incubation as a method for neuropeptide immunocytochemistry. *Histochemistry,* 74: 457–467.

Micevych, P. and Elde, R. (1980) Relationship between enkephalinergic neurons and the vasopressin-oxytocin neuroendocrine system of the cat: an immunohistochemical study. *J. comp. Neurol.,* 190: 135–146.

Morris, J.F. (1976) Distribution of neurosecretory granules among the anatomical compartments of the neurosecretory processes of the pituitary gland: a quantitative ultrastructural approach to hormone storage in the neural lobe. *J. Endocr.,* 68: 225–234.

Morris, J.F., Nordmann, J.J. and Dyball, R.E.J. (1978) Structure–function correlation in mammalian neurosecretion. *Int. Rev. exp. Path.,* 18: 1–95.

Nordmann, J.J. (1977) Ultrastructural morphometry of the rat neurohypophysis. *J. Anat. (Lond.),* 123: 213–218.

Orkand, R.K. (1982) Signalling between neuronal and glial cells. In *Neuronal–Glial Cell Interrelationships, Life Sci. Res. Rep. 20,* Springer Verlag, Berlin, pp. 147–158.

Pool, C.W., Buijs, R.M., Swaab, D.F. Boer, G.J. and Van Leeuwen, F.W. (1983) On the way to a specific immunocytochemical localization. In A.C. Cuello (Ed.), *IBRO Handbook series: Methods in Neurosciences, Vol. 3,* John Wiley, New York, pp. 1–46.

Rossier, J. (1982) Opioid peptides have found their roots. *Nature (Lond.),* 298: 221–222.

Rossier, J., Vargo, T.M., Minick, S., Ling, N., Bloom, F.E. and Guillemin, R. (1977) Regional dissociation of beta-endorphin and enkephalin contents in rat brain and pituitary. *Proc. nat. Acad. Sci. U.S.A.,* 74: 5162–5165.

Rossier, J., Battenberg, E., Pittman, Q., Bayon, A., Koda, L., Miller, R., Guillemin, R. and Bloom, F. (1979) Hypothalamic enkephalin neurones may regulate the neurohypophysis. *Nature (Lond.),* 277: 653–655.

Salm, A.K., Hatton, G.I. and Nilaver, G. (1982) Immunoreactive glial fibrillary acidic protein in pituicytes of the rat neurohypophysis. *Brain Res.,* 236: 471–476.

Simantov, R. and Snyder, S.H. (1977) Opiate receptor binding in the bovine pituitary gland. *Brain Res.,* 124: 178–184.

Somjen, G.G. (1981) Neuroglia and spinal fluids. *J. exp. Biol.,* 95: 129–133.

Stoeckel, M.E., Hindelang-Gertner, C., Dellmann, H.D., Porte, A. and Stutinsky, F. (1975) Subcellular localisation of calcium in the mouse hypophysis. I. Calcium distribution in the adeno- and neurohypophysis under normal conditions. *Cell Tiss. Res.* 157: 307–322.

Swaab, D.F., Pool, C.W. and Van Leeuwen, F.W. (1977) Can specificity ever be proved in immunocytochemical staining? *J. Histochem. Cytochem.,* 25: 388–391.

Sykova, E. (1981) K$^+$ changes in the extracellular space of the spinal cord and their physiological role. *J. exp. Biol.* 95: 93–104.

Tweedle, C.D. and Hatton, G.I. (1980a) Glial cell enclosure of neurosecretory endings in the neurohypophysis of the rat. *Brain Res.,* 192: 555–559.

Tweedle, C.D. and Hatton, G.I. (1980b) Evidence for dynamic interactions between pituicytes and neurosecretory axons in the rat. *Neuroscience,* 5: 661–667.

Van Leeuwen, F.W. (1982a) Enkephalin immunoreactivity in fibres terminating in a synaptoid fashion on pituicytes in the rat neural lobe. In E. Costa and M. Trabacchi (Eds.), *Regulatory Peptides: From Molecular Biology to Function,* Raven Press, New York, pp. 203–208.

Van Leeuwen, F.W. (1982b) Enkephalin in the rat neural lobe. Immunocytochemical evidence for its presence within synaptic elements on pituicytes. In R.M. Buijs, D.F. Swaab and P. Pévet (Eds.), *Chemical Transmission in the Brain, Progress in Brain Research, Vol. 55,* Elsevier/North-Holland, Amsterdam, pp. 253–264.

Van Leeuwen, F.W. (1982c) Specific immunocytochemical localization of neuropeptides: a utopian goal? In G.R. Bullock and P. Petrusz (Eds.), *Techniques in Immunocytochemistry, Vol. 1,* Academic Press, New York, pp. 283–299.

Van Leeuwen, F.W. and Swaab, D.F. (1977) Specific immunoelectron microscopic localization of vasopressin and oxytocin in the neurohypophysis of the rat. *Cell Tiss. Res.,* 177: 493–501.

Van Leeuwen, F.W., De Raay, C., Swaab, D.F. and Fisser, B. (1979) The localization of oxytocin, vasopressin, somatostatin and luteinizing hormone releasing hormone in the rat neurohypophysis. *Cell Tiss. Res.,* 202: 189–201.

Van Leeuwen, F.W., Pool, C.W. and Sluiter, A. (1983) Enkephalin immunoreactivity in synaptoid elements in glial cells in the rat neural lobe. *Neuroscience,* 8: 229–241.

Varon, S S. and Somjen, G.G. (1979) Neuron–glia interactions. *Neurosci. Res. Progr. Bull.,* 17: 1–239.

Wamsley, J.K., Zarbin, M.A., Young, W.S., III and Kuhar, M.J. (1982) Distribution of opiate receptors in the monkey brain: an autoradiographic study. *Neuroscience,* 7: 595–613.

Watson, S.J., Akil, H., Ghazarossian, V.E. and Goldstein, A. (1981) Dynorphin immunocytochemical localization in brain and peripheral nervous system: Preliminary studies. *Proc. nat. Acad. Sci. U.S.A.,* 78: 1260–1263.

Watson, S.J., Akil, H., Fishli, W., Goldstein, A., Zimmerman, E., Nilaver, G. and Van Wimersma Greidanus, Tj. B. (1982) Dynorphin and vasopressin: common localization in magnocellular neurons. *Science,* 216: 85–87.

Weber, E., Roth, K.A. and Barchas, J.D. (1981) Colocalization of α-neo-endorphin and dynorphin immunoreactivity in hypothalamic neurons. *Biochem. Biophys. Res. Commun.,* 103: 951–958.

Weber, E., Evans, C.J. and Barchas, J.D. (1982) Predominance of the amino-terminal octapeptide fragment of dynorphin in rat brain regions. *Nature (Lond.),* 299: 77–79.

Wittkowski, W. (1980) Glia der Neurohypophyse. In A. Oksche (Ed.), *Handbuch der Mikroskopischen Anatomie des Menschen,* Springer Verlag, Berlin, pp. 667–756.

Wittkowski, W. and Brinkmann, H. (1974) Changes of extent of neurovascular contacts and number of neuro-glial synaptoid contacts in the pituitary posterior lobe of dehydrated rats. *Anat. Embryol.,* 146: 157–165.

Wolff, J.R., Rickmann, M. and Chronwall, B.M. (1979) Axo-glial synapses and GABA-accumulating glial cells in the embryonic neocortex of the rat. *Cell Tiss. Res.,* 201: 239–248.

Wright, D.M. and Lincoln, D.W. (1982) Do opiates interact with calcium mechanisms to inhibit neurosecretion? *Neurosci. Lett.,* Suppl. 10: S526.

The Neurohypophysis: Structure, Function and Control, Progress in Brain Research, Vol. 60, edited by B.A. Cross and G. Leng

Neurohypophysial Opiate Receptors:
Are They On Pituicytes?

S.L. LIGHTMAN*, M. NINKOVIC, and S.P. HUNT

MRC Neurochemical Pharmacology Unit, Medical Research Council Centre, Hills Road, Cambridge CB2 2QH
(U.K.)

INTRODUCTION

The administration of low doses of morphine and β-endorphin into the cerebral ventricles results in a fall in plasma vasopressin concentration (Van Wimersma Greidanus et al., 1979; Aziz et al., 1981). In vitro studies have shown that opioid peptides inhibit the release of vasopressin (Iversen et al., 1980; Lightman et al., 1982) and oxytocin (Bicknell and Leng 1982) at the level of neural lobe itself. The location of the opiate receptors responsible for this effect have been presumed to be on pre-terminal sites on the neurosecretory fibres themselves. However, recent light and electron microscopic immunohistochemical studies by Van Leeuwen (1981) suggested intimate contact between leucine-enkephalin fibres and pituicytes. This led to the suggestion that enkephalinergic fibres in the neural lobe acted on the pituicytes rather than directly on neurosecretory fibres.

We tested this hypothesis by measuring the opiate receptor population of the neural lobe in control rats and in rats in which the neurohypophysial neurosecretory fibres had degenerated following pituitary stalk transection two weeks previously. Studies by Dellman and his colleagues (1973) have previously confirmed that, in the rat, neurosecretory axons completely disappear from the pars nervosa within 10 days of pituitary stalk transection, leaving only glial cells and connective tissue. If opiate receptors were on glial cells we would therefore expect preservation of a sizeable proportion of binding sites even allowing for any loss of pituicytes that might arise due to postoperative blood flow changes and ischaemia. If the receptors were on neurosecretory axons, however, a massive loss of opiate binding sites should occur.

METHODS

Pituitary stalk sections were performed by stereotaxic manipulation of a blade through the pituitary stalk. The transection was not always total as assessed by measurement of the vasopressin content in the neural lobe. Successful stalk transections could however be separated from partial transections by measurement of the water intake of the rats. A water intake of over 200 ml/kg/day was always associated with a reduction of neural lobe vasopressin

---

* Present address: Medical Unit, Westminster Medical School, Page Street, London, SW1P 2AP, U.K.

[353]

354

to less than 5 % of the mean level found in control rats. Only rats with an intake of above 200 ml/kg/day over four successive days from day 10 to 13 postoperatively were assumed to have had total transections and were used in our studies.

On the experimental day, the rats were killed by cervical dislocation and their whole pituitary glands were rapidly dissected out, frozen, and mounted on a cryostat microtome. Sections of 13 μm were cut in a coronal plane, thaw-mounted onto cooled subbed slides and incubated in 2 nM [^{3}H]etorphine at 25° C for 20 min, with parallel incubations being performed with 1 μM levorphanol to assess non-specific binding. Emulsion-coated coverslips were then placed over the slides and they were allowed to remain for 6 weeks in the dark, before developing.

RESULTS AND DISCUSSION

The distribution of autoradiographic silver grains, representing the sites of specific [^{3}H]etorphine binding sites is seen in Fig. 1. The highest concentration of binding sites is in the neural lobe, with lower concentrations in the intermediate and anterior lobes. Pituitary stalk transection has no significant affect on the opiate receptor concentration in the intermediate or anterior lobe, but is associated with a significant ($P < 0.01$) increase in specific binding over the neural lobe, from 10.6 ± 0.29 to 17.8 ± 1.61 grains per 400 μm^2 (mean $\pm$ S.E.M., n = 6).

It can be seen in Fig. 1 that there has been apparent shrinkage of the neural lobe following stalk transection. This was formally quantitated in a separate study where whole pituitaries from control rats and rats with successful stalk transections were dissected out and cut on a cryostat microtome. After staining and mounting, the sections were viewed under bright-light illumination and the perimeter of the neural lobe drawn using a drawing tube. The areas were then obtained using a digitalizing pad attached to a computer. This confirmed that there had been a decrease in the volume of the neural lobe from 0.69 ± 0.06 to 0.25 ± 0.11 mm^3 (mean $\pm$ S.D.).

We have therefore been able to show that at two weeks after transection of the pituitary stalk there is a shrinkage of the neural lobe and an increase in the concentration of opiate receptor sites. Although the shrinkage of the neural lobe means that there has been an overall diminution of the opiate receptor population found in the intact gland, we have shown a very significant preservation of receptors, and indeed an increased concentration of opiate receptor sites, at a time when there is reported to be complete loss of neurosecretory axons (Dellman et al., 1973). This is in marked contrast to the 40–50 % decrease in concentration of opiate receptors found in the dorsal horn of the spinal cord after dorsal root section both in rats (Ninkovic et al., 1981) and monkey (Ninkovic et al., 1982).

Our findings bear relevance to both the proposed mechanism for opiate action on neurohypophysial hormone secretion, and to a consideration of the role of pituicytes in the neural lobe of the pituitary gland. Van Leeuwen (1981; and this volume) has recently reported immunohistochemical studies that have led him to suggest that enkephalinergic fibres act directly on pituicytes in the neural lobe, and this hypothesis would be supported by our data. The mechanism by which pituicytes themselves could effect hormone release is unclear. However, Tweedle and Hatton (1980) have shown that neurosecretory axons often terminate within pituicytes and that the number of enclosed axons is highest at times of low hormone demands. Alterations in ionic environment, GABA uptake, or uptake and removal of vasopressin and oxytocin by the pituicytes, might inhibit or facilitate neurohypophysial hormone release.

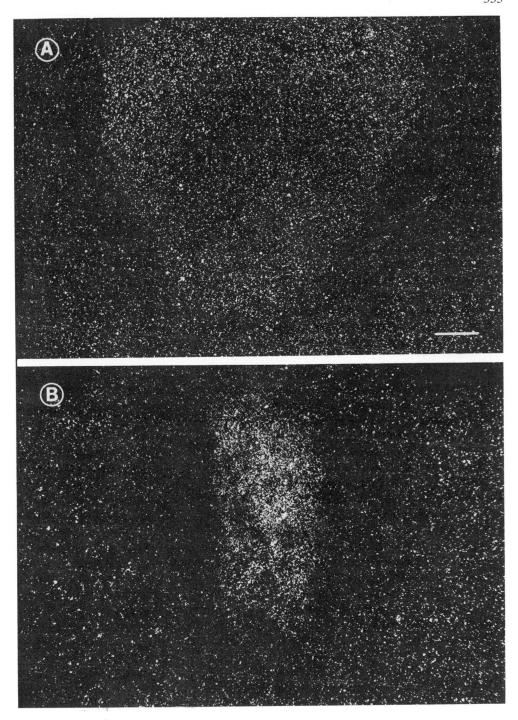

Fig. 1. Dark-field photomicrograph of the distribution of opiate receptors within the pituitary gland of a control animal (A) and after pituitary stalk transection (B). Sections are cut in a coronal plane and show the neural lobe surrounded by a rim of pars intermedia which is in turn surrounded by pars distalis. Scale bar = 150μm.

ACKNOWLEDGEMENTS

We should like to thank Dr. L.L. Iversen for his critical discussion of our work and Dr. G. Raisman for his advice on stalk transection (to S.L.). S.L. is a Wellcome Trust senior lecturer.

REFERENCES

Aziz, L.A., Forsling, M.L. and Woolfe, C.J. (1981) The effect of intracerebroventricular injections of morphine on vasopressin secretion in the rat. *J. Physiol. (Lond.)*, 311: 401–409.

Bicknell, R.J. and Leng, G. (1982) Endogenous opiates regulate oxytocin but not vasopressin secretion from the neurohypophysis. *Nature (Lond.)*, 298: 161–162.

Dellman, H.D., Stoeckel, M.E., Porte, A., Statinsky, F., Klein, M.J., Chang, N. and Adlinger, H.K. (1973) Ultrastructure of the rat neural lobe following interruption of the hypophysial stalk. *Anat. Rec.*, 175: 305.

Iversen, L.L., Iversen, S.D. and Bloom, F.E. (1980) Opiate receptors influence vasopressin release from nerve terminals in the rat neurohypophysis. *Nature (Lond.)*, 284: 350–351.

Lightman, S.L., Iversen, L.L. and Forsling, M.L. (1982) Dopamine and (D-Ala^2, D-Leu^5) enkephalin inhibit the electrically stimulated neurohypophyseal release of vasopressin in vitro: evidence for calcium-dependent opiate action. *J. Neurosci.*, 2: 78–81.

Ninkoviç, M., Hunt, S.P. and Kelly, J.S. (1981) Effect of dorsal rhizotomy on the autoradiographic distribution of opiate and neurotensin receptors and neurotensin-like immunoreactivity within the rat spinal cord. *Brain Res.*, 230: 111–119.

Ninkoviç, M., Hunt, S.P. and Gleave, J.R.W. (1982) Localisation of opiate and histamine H_1-receptors in the primate sensory ganglia and spinal cord. *Brain Res.*, 241: 197–206.

Tweedle, C.D. and Hatton, G.I. (1980) Glial cell enclosure of neurosecretory endings in the neurohypophysis of the rat. *Brain Res.*, 192: 555–559.

Van Leeuwen, F.W. (1981) Light and electron microscopical demonstration of Leu-enkephalin immunoreactivity in the rat neural lobe. *Neurosci. Lett.*, Suppl. 7: S182.

Van Wimersma Greidanus, Tj.B., Thody, T.J., Verspaget, H., De Rotte, G.A., Goedemans, H.J.H., Croiset, G. and Van Ree, J.M. (1979) Effects of morphine and β-endorphin on basal and elevated plasma levels of α-MSH and vasopressin. *Life Sci.*, 24: 570–585.

The Neurohypophysis: Structure, Function and Control, Progress in Brain Research, Vol. 60, edited by B.A. Cross and G. Leng

Evidence that Dopamine is a Neurotransmitter in the Neurointermediate Lobe of the Hypophysis

M. HOLZBAUER, E. MUSCHOLL*, K. RACKÉ* and D.F. SHARMAN

A.R.C. Institute of Animal Physiology, Babraham, Cambridge CB2 4AT (U.K.)

INTRODUCTION

Werman (1966, 1972) has noted the conditions which must be satisfied in order that a substance can be classified as a neurotransmitter. In the latter publication only three criteria are regarded as essential, the others serve only to explain how the neurotransmitter functions. The essential characteristics are:

(1) the criterion of presence of the transmitter in the tissue;

(2) the criterion of identical actions in that the response to the putative neurotransmitter when applied to the tissue must be the same as that resulting from activation of the nerve fibres which contain it; and

(3) the criterion of collectability of the transmitter. The present paper summarizes the evidence available to permit dopamine to be defined as a neurotransmitter substance in the neural and intermediate lobes of the pituitary gland.

THE PRESENCE OF DOPAMINE IN THE NEUROINTERMEDIATE LOBE

The presence of catecholamine-containing nerve fibres in the neural and intermediate lobe (NIL) of the mammalian pituitary gland has been demonstrated by fluorescence histochemical methods (see Björklund et al., 1973). With the use of chemical analytical methods the major catecholamine in the pituitary gland has been identified as dopamine (Björklund et al., 1967; Saavedra et al., 1975). Most of the investigations on dopamine (DA) in the NIL have been carried out in the rat. In this species lesion experiments have shown that the perikarya of the hypophysial DA neurones are chiefly located in the rostral part of the arcuate nucleus (Björklund et al., 1973). The catecholamine-containing nerve fibres in the NIL are characterized by dense cored vesicles 15–120 nm in diameter). In the intermediate lobe they make synaptic contacts with glandular cells; in the posterior lobe the varicosities are frequently situated in close proximity (8–12 nm gap) to the neurosecretory axons and pituicyte processes. However, postsynaptic membrane thickenings are absent (Baumgarten et al., 1972). A similar

---

* Present address: Pharmakologisches Institut der Universität, 65 Mainz, Obere Zahlbacher Str. 67, D-6500 Mainz, F.R.G.

anatomical relation involving monoamine-containing nerve fibres is seen in many brain regions (for review see Beaudet and Descarries, 1978). The quantities of DA present in the rat pituitary vary with age, strain and the conditions in which the animals are kept. In an undisturbed young adult rat the DA content of the neural lobe is of the order of 10–15 ng/mg protein, and of the intermediate lobe 20–25 ng/mg protein. DA concentrations in the pituitary glands of sheep, pig, goat, rabbit and guinea pig are of a similar order of magnitude (Holzbauer et al., 1978b).

The enzymes required for DA synthesis, tyrosine hydroxylase (TH) and DOPA-decarboxylase, have been detected in the NIL of the rat. TH activity was found in both the intermediate lobe and the neural lobe (Saavedra et al., 1975). In experiments in which TH was inhibited by injecting rats with α-methyl-p-tyrosine, a decrease in the DA content of the NIL occurred indicating the utilization of DA in this tissue (Godden et al., 1977). TH activity was further indicated by the accumulation of 3,4-dihydroxyphenylalanine (DOPA) in the NIL after inhibition of DOPA-decarboxylase in vivo (Demarest et al., 1979).

The presence of 3,4-dihydroxyphenylacetic acid (DOPAC) in the NIL (Holzbauer et al., 1978b; Annunziato and Weiner, 1980) is evidence that oxidative deamination is one of the pathways of DA catabolism in the NIL. Furthermore, injecting rats with the monoamine oxidase (MAO) inhibitor pargyline caused a significant increase in the DA content of the NIL and in the DA release from the NIL (Sharman et al., 1982). MAO activity was demonstrated in pieces of intermediate lobe and neural lobe tissue by Saavedra et al. (1975). With the use of specific MAO inhibitors, Demarest and Moore (1981) observed that type A MAO was the predominant form of the enzyme in the NIL of the rat.

An uptake mechanism for [³H]DA in the NIL was demonstrated in studies with tissue homogenates. The affinity for DA of this uptake mechanism was found to be smaller in the NIL than in the striatum (Demarest and Moore, 1979; Annunziato and Weiner, 1980).

FUNCTION OF DOPAMINE IN THE NEUROINTERMEDIATE LOBE

A participation of DA in the function of the NIL has been suggested by both in vivo and in vitro experiments.

Results of in vivo experiments have shown changes in the concentrations and turnover rates of DA in the NIL under conditions in which pituitary hormone release was increased over an extended period. Thus, water deprivation in rats followed by sodium loading, a procedure which leads to a massive release of vasopressin and oxytocin (Jones and Pickering, 1969) and also affects intermediate lobe hormones (e.g. Howe and Thody, 1970), resulted in an increase in the DA content of the NIL (Holzbauer et al., 1978b, 1980; Torda et al., 1978; Alper et al., 1980). After separation of the two tissues, a rise in the DA concentration was seen in the intermediate as well as in the neural lobe (Holzbauer et al., 1980). Alper et al. (1980) observed in dehydrated rats an increased accumulation of L-DOPA in the NIL following inhibition of the enzyme DOPA-decarboxylase, which reflects an increase in the synthesis rate of DA. The changes in the rate of DA synthesis in the NIL during dehydration were found to be related to changes in plasma sodium concentrations (Alper et al., 1982). These authors suggested that tuberohypophysial DA neurones may be regulated, at least in part, by sodium- or osmoreceptors.

In lactating rats where the secretion of oxytocin from the neural lobe is increased (Lincoln et al., 1973), the DA content of the NIL was decreased and the turnover of DA in the NIL was increased (Holzbauer et al., 1978a, b).

A functional link between the DA-containing neuronal cell bodies in the rostral arcuate nucleus and the activity of neurosecretory axons in the posterior lobe of the pituitary gland has been demonstrated by Passo et al. (1981). These authors observed a depression of multi-unit electrical activity recorded from the neurosecretory axons in the NIL following electrical stimulation of the rostral arcuate nucleus. This inhibitory response was prevented by pimozide, a DA receptor blocking drug, applied locally to the neurohypophysis. Superfusion of the neurohypophysis with DA also inhibited the electrical activity in the neurosecretory axons.

Results of in vitro experiments have provided evidence that DA, when applied locally to the NIL, can modify the release of hormones from this tissue.

DA was reported to inhibit the release of oxytocin induced by ouabain (Vizi and Volbekas, 1980). These authors also observed that when rats were pretreated with α-methyl-p-tyrosine, which reduces the DA content in the NIL (Holzbauer et al., 1978b), the basal release of oxytocin from the NIL, incubated in vitro, was greater than in controls. The release of oxytocin evoked by electrical stimulation of the NIL in vitro was found to be decreased when DA was present in the incubation medium (Barnes and Dyball, 1982). The same concentration of DA did not alter the release of oxytocin induced by high potassium concentrations.

Vasopressin release evoked by electrical stimulation of the pituitary stalk was decreased by DA and DA agonists. This effect was antagonized by sulpiride (Lightman et al., 1982; Racké et al., 1982a) which indicates the involvement of D_2 receptors (Kebabian and Calne, 1979). Similar to the observations made on oxytocin release, DA and the DA agonist apomorphine did not alter the vasopressin release induced by high potassium concentrations (Racké et al., 1982a). Furthermore, the inhibition of electrically evoked vasopressin release by the DA agonist 6,7-ADTN (2-amino-6, 7-dihydroxy-1,2,3,4-tetrahydronaphthalene) could not be prevented by increasing the calcium concentration in the incubation medium (Lightman et al., 1982). Thus the inhibitory effect of DA on hormone release from the neural lobe may be due to a decrease of the excitability of neurosecretory axons rather than to an effect on stimulus–secretion coupling. This interpretation is supported by the in vivo results of Passo et al. (1981) that DA has a direct inhibitory effect on multi-unit electrical activity of neurosecretory axons in the neural lobe.

Ahn et al. (1979) demonstrated the presence in the NIL of a DA receptor-linked adenylate cyclase (D_1 receptor according to the classification of Kebabian and Calne, 1979). Recent results of Racké et al. (1982c) suggested that activation of this D_1 receptor may facilitate the electrically evoked vasopressin release. The benzazepine derivative SKF 82526, a potent agonist at the D_1 receptor, caused an increase in vasopressin release which was antagonized by the DA antagonist flupenthixol. The DA antagonist sulpiride, which is specific for the D_2 receptor, had no effect on the stimulatory action of SKF 82526. That activation of the adenylate cyclase in the NIL may facilitate the evoked vasopressin release was further supported by studies with forskolin. Forskolin, a drug which directly activates adenylate cyclase in intact neuronal tissue (Seamon et al., 1981), increased the evoked vasopressin release from the NIL (Racké et al., 1982b).

An action of DA in the intermediate lobe was suggested by in vitro experiments which have shown that DA and DA agonists can inhibit the release of proopiocortin-derived peptides. This has been demonstrated for ACTH-like peptides (Fischer and Moriarty, 1977; Rosa et al., 1980), β-endorphin (Rosa et al., 1980; Vermes et al., 1980b) and α-MSH (Bower et al., 1974; Munemura et al., 1980). The latter authors obtained evidence that the DA receptor involved was of the D_2 type.

Douglas and Taraskevich (1978) demonstrated that DA suppresses the generation of action potentials in cells cultured from the intermediate lobe. Evidence was also provided that endogenous DA released in the isolated NIL by increased potassium concentrations inhibited the secretion of α-MSH and β-endorphin in this tissue (Tilders et al., 1979; Vermes et al., 1980a). As the spontaneous release of peptides from isolated intermediate lobe cells proceeds at a high rate, DA may exert a tonic inhibition on the secretion of peptides from this tissue in vivo (see Rosa et al., 1980). This assumption is supported by experiments which showed that acute treatment of rats with the DA antagonist haloperidol increased the plasma concentration of immunoreactive α-MSH and β-endorphin (Usategui et al., 1976; Penny and Thody, 1978; Giraud et al., 1980; Höllt and Bergmann, 1982).

The presence of short portal vessels linking the NIL with the anterior lobe of the pituitary gland suggests that substances released in the NIL might be involved in the function of the anterior lobe. This could be the case with DA because Peters et al. (1981) have observed that after removal of the NIL in anaesthetized rats there was an increase in circulating prolactin which could be counteracted by the injection of DA.

DETECTION OF DOPAMINE RELEASE

A method using high performance liquid chromatography and electrochemical detection developed by Keller et al. (1976) for the estimation of catecholamines has proved sensitive enough to enable us to study the release of DA from the NIL. Initially, the release of DA from four rat NILs cut into 1 mm^3 pieces and incubated in a small volume (40 μl) of Krebs-bicarbonate solution was studied using a high potassium concentration to depolarize the DA-containing neurones. The DA release (about 300 pg/10 min per NIL; $[K^+] = 47.0$ mM, $[Ca^{2+}] = 2.5$ mM) was calcium dependent and was facilitated by increasing the calcium concentration in the Krebs solution (Holzbauer et al., 1981; Sharman et al., 1982).

Recently, experiments have been carried out in which DA release from single rat NILs was evoked by electrical stimulation of the pituitary stalk (Holzbauer et al., 1982). Fig. 1 shows the overflow of DA from the NIL of rats pretreated with pargyline. The DA overflow elicited by the stimulation (parameters given on the diagram) was about 40 fg/pulse. When stimulation was carried out in the presence of tetraethylammonium (TEA, 10 mM), a treatment which prolongs the duration of action potentials, the DA overflow was nearly doubled. DA overflow was abolished by the addition of tetrodotoxin (TTX), indicating that the release of DA was in response to propagated action potentials. There was also an increase of DA overflow when the DA-uptake inhibiting drug GBR 12921 (Van der Zee et al., 1980) was included in the incubation medium.

The overflow of DA evoked by propagated action potentials from NILs of rats not treated with pargyline was very low. In the presence of TEA or of GBR 12921 about 30 fg DA/pulse were released into the incubation medium, which was less then 50% of the amount released in the pargyline-treated rats. This demonstrated the importance of MAO in inactivating DA released from neurones in the NIL.

When the voltage and pulse length of the electrical stimulation were increased (1 msec, 50 V, 10 Hz, 8–12 mA) without changing the rest of the experimental protocol, there was a five-fold increase in the DA overflow per pulse from the NILs of pargyline-treated rats. This increased release was doubled in the presence of TEA (10 mM) and was completely inhibited when the incubation medium contained no calcium and included EGTA (2 mM) to chelate the calcium present in the tissue. The DA overflow resulting from this increased stimulation was, however, only partially inhibited by TTX, which indicates that there was direct electrical depolarization of the nerve terminals (field stimulation).

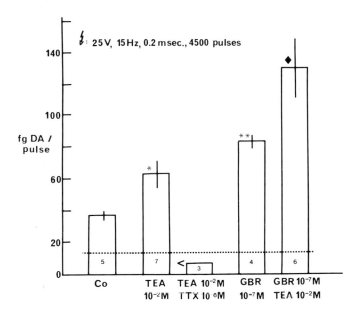

Fig. 1. DA overflow from the isolated NIL of the rat hypophysis evoked by electrical stimulation of the pituitary stalk. The preparation was incubated in 40 μl Krebs solution. The rats were pretreated with pargyline (50 mg/kg, i.p., 1 h) and pargyline (1μM) was present in the Krebs solution. ⨍, Electrical stimulation applied 5 times for 1 min with 1 min intervals. Height of columns, mean DA overflow (expressed as fg/pulse ± S.E.M.) during the stimulation period and the following two 10-min periods. The basal DA release (dotted line) was below the limit of the estimation method. Abbreviations: GBR, GBR 12921, 1,(2-diphenylmethoxy)-ethyl-4-(-3-phenyl-2 propenyl)-piperazine; TEA, tetraethylammonium chloride; TTX, tetrodotoxin. Numbers at bottom of columns show numbers of observations. Significance of difference from controls (Co): *$P < 0.05$; **$P < 0.01$; and from the TEA group: ♦$P < 0.05$ (multiple comparison procedure, Dunnett, 1964).

The experiments on the electrically stimulated NIL also provided an opportunity to obtain some information on the DA synthesis which took place in the tissue during the experiment. When the amount of DA present in the NIL at the end of the experiment was added to the amount of DA released into the bath during the experiment, it was observed in several experimental groups that this sum ("total DA of the NIL") was larger than the DA content of non-stimulated NIL tissue. The increase in the "total DA of the NIL" from pargyline-pretreated rats incubated in the presence of pargyline can be assumed to be due to an increase in DA synthesis. From Fig. 2 it can be seen that a substantial increase in the "total DA of the NIL" occurred after electrical stimulation of the stalk in the presence of TEA when MAO was inhibited. TEA added to the incubation medium of non-stimulated NILs did not increase their DA content. An increase of the "total DA of the NIL" in the presence of TEA also occurred during field stimulation, provided calcium was present in the incubation medium. Thus, the effect of TEA may be the result of increased calcium influx as a consequence of prolonged action potentials. A calcium-dependent increase in catecholamine biosynthesis has been described for both central and peripheral nervous tissues and was attributed to an increased activity of the rate-limiting enzyme tyrosine hydroxylase (Nagatsu et al., 1964; Weiner, 1970). An increase in "total DA of the NIL" also occurred when re-uptake was inhibited by the addition of GBR 12921. GBR 12921 was without effect on the DA content of NILs which were not electrically stimulated. It appears that DA, which is returned to the neurone after it has been released, inhibits DA synthesis.

362

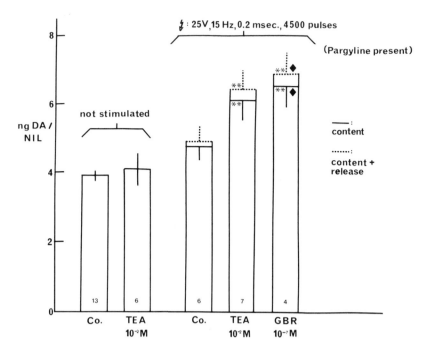

Fig. 2. Sum of the amount of DA contained in the NIL after electrical stimulation of the pituitary stalk plus the amount of DA released into the bath ("total DA of the NIL"). Release results and stimulation conditions given in Fig. 1. Height of columns, mean values; bars pointing downwards, S.E.M. of the DA content; bars pointing upwards, S.E.M. of the "total DA of the NIL". Significance of differences from unstimulated NIL: ** $P < 0.01$; and from stimulated control (Co.): ◆ $P < 0.05$, (multiple comparison procedure, Dunnett, 1964). Abbreviations as in Fig. 1.

SUMMARY

Recent results have shown that DA is released in the NIL by propagated action potentials induced by electrical stimulation of the pituitary stalk; that the released DA is inactivated by MAO and that there is a DA re-uptake mechanism in the NIL which contributes to the inactivation of the released DA. They have also shown that DA synthesis occurs in the isolated NIL and that the rate of synthesis may be related to the degree of activation of the neurones.

These findings, taken together with the neurophysiological and neuroendocrinological observations discussed above, provide convincing evidence that DA is a neurotransmitter substance in the NIL of the pituitary gland.

REFERENCES

Ahn, H.S., Feldman, S.C. and Makman, M.H. (1979) Posterior pituitary adenylate cyclase: stimulation by dopamine and other agents. *Brain Res.*, 166: 422–425.
Alper, R.H., Demarest, K.T. and Moore, K.E. (1980) Dehydration selectively increases dopamine synthesis in tuberohypophyseal dopaminergic neurones. *Neuroendocrinology*, 31: 112–115.
Alper, R.H., Demarest, K.T. and Moore, K.E. (1982) Changes in the rate of dopamine synthesis in the posterior pituitary during dehydration and rehydration: relationship to plasma sodium concentrations. *Neuroendocrinology*, 34: 252–257.

Annunziato, L. and Weiner, R.I. (1980) Characteristics of dopamine uptake and 3,4-dihydroxyphenylacetic acid (DOPAC) formation in the dopaminergic terminals of the neurointermediate lobe of the pituitary gland. *Neuroendocrinology, 31*: 8–12.

Barnes, P.R.J. and Dyball, R.E.J. (1982) Inhibition of neurohypophyseal hormone release by dopamine in the rat. *J. Physiol. (Lond.), 327*: 85–86P.

Baumgarten, H.G., Björklund, A., Holstein, A.F. and Nobin, A. (1972) Organization and ultrastructural identification of the catecholamine nerve terminals in the neural lobe and pars intermedia of the rat pituitary. *Z. Zellforsch., 126*: 483–517.

Beaudet, A. and Descarries, L. (1978) The monoamine innervation of rat cerebral cortex: synaptic and non synaptic axon terminals. *Neuroscience, 3*: 851–860.

Björklund, A., Falck, B. and Rosengren, E. (1967) Monoamines in the pituitary gland of the pig. *Life Sci., 6*: 2103–2110.

Björklund, A., Moore, R.Y., Nobin, A. and Stenevi, V. (1973) The organization of the tuberohypophyseal and reticulo-infundibular catecholamine neuron system in the rat brain. *Brain Res., 51*: 171–191.

Bower, A., Hadley, M.E. and Hruby, V.J. (1974) Biogenic amines and control of melanophore stimulating hormone release. *Science, 184*: 70–72.

Demarest, K.T. and Moore, K.E. (1979) Lack of high affinity transport system for dopamine in the median eminence and posterior pituitary. *Brain Res., 171*: 545–551.

Demarest, K.T. and Moore, K.E. (1981) Type A monoamine oxidase catalyzes the intraneuronal deamination of dopamine within nigrostriatal, mesolimbic tuberoinfundibular and tuberohypophyseal neurones in the rat. *J. Neural Transm., 52*: 175–187.

Demarest, K.T., Alper, R.H. and Moore, K.E. (1979) DOPA accumulation is a measure of dopamine synthesis in the median eminence and posterior pituitary. *J. Neural Transm., 46*: 183–193.

Douglas, W.W. and Taraskevich, P.S. (1978) Action potentials in gland cells of rat pituitary pars intermedia: inhibition by dopamine, an inhibitor of MSH secretion. *J. Physiol. (Lond.), 285*: 171–184.

Dunnett, C.W. (1964) New tables for multiple comparisons with a control. *Biometrics, 20*: 482–491.

Fischer, J.L. and Moriarty, C.M. (1977) Control of bioactive corticotropin release from the neurointermediate lobe of the rat pituitary in vitro. *Endocrinology, 100*: 1047–1054.

Giraud, P., Lissitzky, I.C., Conte-Devolx, B., Gillioz, P. and Oliver, C. (1980) Influence of haloperidol on ACTH and β-endorphin secretion in the rat. *Europ. J. Pharmacol., 62*: 215–217.

Godden, U., Holzbauer, M. and Sharman, D.F. (1977) Dopamine utilization in the posterior pituitary gland of the rat. *Brit. J. Pharmacol., 59*: 478–479P.

Höllt, V. and Bergmann, M. (1982) Effects of acute and chronic haloperidol treatment on the concentrations of immunoreactive β-endorphin in plasma, pituitary and brain of rats. *Neuropharmacology, 21*: 147–154.

Holzbauer, M., Sharman, D.F. and Godden, U. (1978a) Effect of lactation on the DA content of the rat hypophysis *J. Endocr., 77*: 57–58P.

Holzbauer, M., Sharman, D.F. and Godden, U. (1978b) Observations on the function of the dopaminergic nerves innervating the pituitary gland. *Neuroscience, 3*: 1251–1262.

Holzbauer, M., Sharman, D.F., Godden, U., Mann, S.P. and Stephens, D.B. (1980) Effect of water and salt intake on pituitary catecholamines in the rat and domestic pig. *Neuroscience, 5*: 1959–1968.

Holzbauer, M., Holzer, P. and Sharman, D.F. (1981) Release of endogenous dopamine from the neuro-intermediate lobe of the rat hypophysis in vitro. *Brit. J. Pharmacol., 73*: 265P

Holzbauer, M., Muscholl, E., Racké, K. and Sharman, D.F. (1982) Release of endogenous dopamine from single neuro-intermediate lobes of the rat hypophysis in vitro following electrical stimulation of the stalk. *J. Physiol. (Lond.), 332*: 88–89P.

Howe, A. and Thody, A.J. (1970) The effect of ingestion of hypertonic saline on the melanocyte stimulating hormone content and histology of the pars intermedia of the rat pituitary gland. *J. Endocr., 46*: 201–208.

Jones, C.W. and Pickering, B.T. (1969) Comparison of the effect of water deprivation and sodium chloride imbibition on the hormone content of the neurohypophysis of the rat. *J. Physiol. (Lond.), 203*: 449–458.

Kebabian, J.W. and Calne, D.B. (1979) Multiple receptors for dopamine. *Nature (Lond.), 277*: 93–96.

Keller, R., Oke, A., Mefford, I. and Adams, R.N. (1976) Liquid chromatographic analysis of catecholamines. Routine assay for regional brain mapping. *Life Sci., 19*: 995–1004.

Lightman, S.L., Iversen, L.L. and Forsling, M. (1982) Dopamine and [D-Ala^2, D-Leu^5]enkephalin inhibit the electrically stimulated neurohypophyseal release of vasopressin in vitro: evidence for calcium dependent opiate action. *J. Neurosci., 2*: 78–81.

Lincoln, D.W., Hill, A. and Wakerley, J.B. (1973) The milk-ejection reflex of the rat: an intermediate function not abolished by surgical levels of anaesthesia. *J. Endocr., 57*: 459–476.

Munemura, M., Cote, T.E., Tsuruta, K., Eskay, R.L. and Kebabian, J.W. (1980) The dopamine receptor in the intermediate lobe of the rat pituitary gland: pharmacological characterization. *Endocrinology,* 107: 1676–1683.

Nagatsu, T., Levitt, M. and Udenfriend, S. (1964) Tyrosine hydroxylase: the initial step in norepinephrine biosynthesis. *J. biol. Chem.,* 239: 2910–2917.

Passo, S.S., Thornborough, J.R. and Ferris, C.F. (1981) A functional analysis of dopaminergic innervation of the neurohypophysis. *Amer. J. Physiol.,* 241: E186–E190.

Penny, R.J. and Thody, A.J. (1978) An improved radioimmunoassay for α-melanocyte-stimulating hormone (α-MSH) in the rat: serum and pituitary α-MSH levels after drugs which modify catecholaminergic neurotransmission. *Neuroendocrinology,* 25: 193–203.

Peters, L.L., Hoefer, M.T. and Ben-Jonathan, N. (1981) The posterior pituitary: regulation of anterior pituitary prolactin secretion. *Science,* 213: 659–661.

Racké, K., Ritzel, H., Trapp, B. and Muscholl, E. (1982a) Dopaminergic modulation of evoked vasopressin release from the isolated neurohypophysis of the rat. Possible involvement of endogenous opioids. *Naunyn-Schmiedeberg's Arch. Pharmacol.,* 319: 56–65.

Racké, K., Rothländer, M. and Muscholl, E. (1982b) Isoprenaline and forskolin increase evoked vasopressin release from rat pituitary. *Europ. J. Pharmacol.,* 82: 97–100.

Racké, K., Rothländer, M. and Trapp, B. (1982c) Effects of the dopaminergic drug SKF82526 and of forskolin on the electrically evoked vasopressin release from the isolated neurointermediate lobe (NIL). *Naunyn-Schmiedeberg's Arch. Pharmacol.,* 319: R74.

Rosa, P.A., Policastro, P. and Herbert, E.A. (1980) A cellular basis for the differences in the regulation of synthesis and secretion of ACTH/endorphin peptides in anterior and intermediate lobes of the pituitary. *J. exp. Biol.,* 89: 215–237.

Saavedra, J.M., Palkovits, M., Kizer, J.S., Brownstein, M. and Zivin, J.A. (1975) Distribution of biogenic amines and related enzymes in the rat pituitary gland. *J. Neurochem.,* 25: 257–260.

Seamon, K.B., Padgett, W. and Daly, J.W. (1981) Forskolin: unique diterpene activator of adenylate cyclase in membranes and in intact cells. *Proc. nat. Acad. Sci., U.S.A.,* 78: 3363–3367.

Sharman, D.F., Holzer, P. and Holzbauer, M. (1982) In vitro release of endogenous catecholamines from the neural and intermediate lobe of the hypophysis. *Neuroendocrinology,* 34: 175–179.

Tilders, F.J.H., Van der Woude, H.A., Swaab, D.F. and Mulder, A.H. (1979) Identification of MSH release-inhibiting elements in the neurointermediate lobe of the rat. *Brain Res.,* 171: 425–435.

Torda, T., Lichardus, B., Kvetňanský, R. and Ponec, J. (1978) Posterior pituitary dopamine and noradrenaline content: effect of thirst, ethanol and saline load. *Endokrinologie,* 72: 334–338.

Usategui, R., Olivier, C., Vaudry, H., Lombardi, J. Rozenberg, J. and Mourre, A.M. (1976) Immunoreactive α-MSH and ACTH levels in rat plasma and pituitary. *Endocrinology,* 98: 189–196.

Van der Zee, P., Koger, H.S., Gootjes, J. and Hespe, W. (1980) Aryl-1,4-dialk(en)ylpiperazines as selective and very potent inhibitors of dopamine uptake. *Europ. J. Chem., Chim. Ther.,* 15: 363–370.

Vermes, I., Mulder, G.H. and Smelik, P.G. (1980a) Opposite effects of K^+-induced depolarisation on endorphin/lipotropin secretion by anterior and intermediate lobes of the rat pituitary. *Europ. J. Pharmacol.,* 63: 89–90.

Vermes, I., Mulder, G.H., Smelik, P.G. and Tilders, F.J.H. (1980b) Differential control of β-endorphin/β-lipotropin secretion from anterior and intermediate lobes of the rat pituitary gland in vitro. *Life Sci.,* 27: 1761–1768.

Vizi, E.S. and Volbekas, V. (1980) Inhibition by dopamine of oxytocin release from isolated posterior lobe of the hypophysis of the rat, disinhibitory effect of β-endorphin/enkephalin. *Neuroendocrinology,* 31: 46–52.

Weiner, N. (1970) Regulation of norepinephrine biosynthesis. *Ann. Rev. Pharmacol.,* 10: 273–290.

Werman, R. (1966) Criteria for identification of a central nervous system transmitter. *Comp. Biochem. Physiol.,* 18: 745–766.

Werman, R. (1972) Amino acids as central neurotransmitters. *Res. Publ. Ass. nerv. ment. Dis.,* 50: 147–180.

Receptor Mechanisms

The Neurohypophysis: Structure, Function and Control, Progress in Brain Research, Vol. 60, edited by B.A. Cross and G. Leng
© *1983 Elsevier Science Publishers B.V.*

Design of Potent and Selective In Vivo Antagonists of the Neurohypophysial Peptides

M. MANNING and W.H. SAWYER[1]

Department of Biochemistry, Medical College of Ohio, Toledo, OH 43699 and [1]Department of Pharmacology, College of Physicians and Surgeons, Columbia University, New York, NY 10032 (U.S.A.)

INTRODUCTION *

The design and synthesis of effective in vivo antagonists of the oxytocic, vasopressor and antidiuretic responses to oxytocin and arginine-vasopressin have been long-standing goals of structure–activity studies on these peptides since the original synthesis of oxytocin and arginine-vasopressin by du Vigneaud and associates nearly 30 years ago (du Vigneaud et al., 1954a, b). Significant progress towards reaching these goals has been made since the Key Biscayne Conference six years ago. To put this progress in proper perspective, it is worthwhile to look back briefly at the status of structure–activity studies on neurohypophysial peptides as we summarized them at that conference (Manning and Sawyer, 1977). Our presentation dealt almost exclusively with the design and synthesis of potent and selectively acting agonistic analogues of oxytocin and vasopressin. Our discussion of antagonists was indeed sparse by comparison. Although promising leads to useful oxytocic and vasopressor antagonists had been uncovered in the early 1960s, (Law and du Vigneaud, 1960; Berankova et al., 1961; Cash and Smith, 1963; Smyth, 1967; Schultz and du Vigneaud, 1966; Krejci et al., 1967; Bisset and Clark, 1968; Chimiak et al., 1968; Bisset et al., 1970), these had not been followed up with anything like the vigour used in pursuing the design of agonists. For example, although we had embarked on a modest programme of antagonist design in the early 1970s, by 1976 we had only one oxytocic antagonist and two vasopressor antagonists to show for our efforts (Manning et al., 1975; Manning and Sawyer, 1977). The oxytocic antagonist was [1-deaminopenicillamine,4-threonine]oxytocin (dPTOT). The vasopressor antagonists were [1-deamino,4-valine,8-D-arginine]vasopressin (dVDAVP) (Manning et al., 1973; Sawyer et al., 1974) and [1-deaminopenicillamine,4-valine,8-D-arginine]vasopressin (dPVDAVP). While dPTOT and dPVDAVP were the most potent antagonists reported up to then, by today's standards they are relatively weak. Since 1976, progress in the design of neurohypophysial hormone antago-

---

* Abbreviations: AVP, arginine-vasopressin; LVP, lysine-vasopressin; OT, oxytocin; OVT, ornithine-vasotocin. Amino acid substitutions in the above are designated by the recommended IUPAC abbreviations. Unnatural amino acids are designated as: Orn, ornithine; Tyr(Me), O-methyltyrosine; Tyr(Et), O-ethyltyrosine. Other abbreviations used in designating analogues: D, substitution of an 8-D-arginine; d, "deamino" (substitution of $1\text{-}\beta\text{-mercaptopropionic acid}$); dP, substitution of a 1-deaminopenicillamine [$1\text{-}(\beta\text{-mercapto-}\beta,\beta\text{-dimethylpropionic acid})$]; dEt$_2$, substitution of a $1\text{-}(\beta\text{-mercapto-}\beta,\beta\text{-diethylpropionic acid})$; d(CH$_2$)$_5$, substitution of a $1\text{-}(\beta\text{-mercapto-}\beta,\beta\text{-cyclopentamethylenepropionic acid})$; T, substitution of a 4-threonine; V, substitution of a 4-valine.

[367]

nists has been dramatic, particularly with the discovery just two years ago of the first reported antagonists of antidiuretic responses to exogenous and endogenous AVP (Sawyer et al., 1981a; Manning et al., 1981a). Well over 150 new antagonists have been synthesized during this period.

Since the original antidiuretic antagonists were discovered, further significant progress has been made towards: (a) increasing anti-antidiuretic potency and selectivity, and (b) obtaining a detailed profile of the structural features required for antagonists (Manning et al., 1982a, b). For more in-depth reviews of the structure–activity relationships of the neurohypophysial hormones, see Manning et al. (1981b) and Sawyer et al. (1981b). For an overview of the current status of the AVP antagonists, see Manning and Sawyer (1982).

Perhaps the most exciting fallout from the progress made in designing potent oxytocin and vasopressin antagonists, one which we find most gratifying, is the widespread use of many of these antagonists, particularly the AVP vasopressor antagonists, in studies by other investigators of the known and putative roles of AVP in the periphery and in the CNS (for a brief summary, see Manning and Sawyer, 1982). We will discuss some of these uses following a presentation of the highlights of our findings on neurohypophysial peptide antagonists over the past six years.

LACK OF SPECIFICITY OF PRESENTLY AVAILABLE ANTAGONISTS

As will become apparent further on, designation of the currently available antagonists as oxytocic, vasopressor and antidiuretic antagonists is indeed arbitrary. All the reported oxytocic and vasopressor antagonists antagonize both uterine and vascular responses to oxytocin and AVP, and all the known antidiuretic antagonists also antagonize vasopressor responses to AVP and oxytocic responses to oxytocin. However, many of the more recent antagonists in each category exhibit considerably enhanced selectivities with respect to their antagonistic potencies at uterine, vascular and renal tubular receptors (Manning et al., 1982b).

GENERAL APPROACH TO ANTAGONIST DESIGN

The approach to antagonist design we have taken over the past nine years (Manning et al., 1975, 1981b; Sawyer et al., 1981b) has relied heavily on: (1) the wealth of structure–activity data on oxytocin and AVP analogues (Berde and Boissonnas, 1968) from many laboratories — particularly du Vigneauds, and our own, and, where appropriate, structure–activity data on analogues of other peptides (Rudinger, 1971); (2) judicious application of the additivity principle, i.e. combining in a single molecule those individual modifications which (a) lead to enhancement of in vivo agonist or antagonistic potency and/or selectivity at specific receptors and/or (b) lead to prolonged duration of action. This approach has produced many excellent new lead compounds with antioxytocic, antivasopressor and anti-antidiuretic activities.

The importance of work from du Vigneaud's laboratory to the recent upsurge in design of effective neurohypophysial peptide antagonists is perhaps best illustrated by the key roles played by the β,β-dialkyl modifications at position 1 which he introduced in the period 1966–1975. These modifications, i.e. the β,β-dimethyl$((CH_3)_2)$, the β,β-diethyl $((C_2H_5)_2$ and the β,β-cyclopentamethylene$(CH_2)_5$, when incorporated in [1-deamino]oxytocin (dOT) (Hope et al., 1962) to give dPOT (Schultz and du Vigneaud, 1966), dEt$_2$OT (Vavrek et al., 1972) and d$(CH_2)_5$OT (Nestor et al., 1975b), respectively, were reported to produce (a) increases in in vitro oxytocic antagonism and (b) diminishments in vasopressor antagonism, which correlated with the increase in size of the β,β-dialkyl substituents. Since 1976 these modifications have, in our hands, proved to be of exceptional value in the design of potent in vivo antagonists of uterine, vascular and renal tubular responses to oxytocin and vasopressin.

SOLID PHASE SYNTHESIS AND MULTIPLE BIOASSAYS HAVE FACILITATED ANTAGONIST DESIGN

Synthesis

The antagonists were synthesized by the solid phase method (Merrifield, 1963) by previously described procedures (Manning et al., 1981b). The speed and efficiency of the Merrifield solid phase method have been of inestimable value in the design and synthesis of these peptide antagonists. With this method, a skilled peptide chemist can synthesize 25–30 highly purified analogues per year. This increased rate of output has greatly facilitated the design of antagonists by permitting (a) the expeditious follow-up of new clues and (b) the rapid completion of promising series of analogues.

Bioassays

These include oxytocic assays on isolated rat uteri and rat uteri in situ, milk-ejection assays (Sawyer et al., 1980), vasopressor assays in phenoxybenzamine-treated rats under urethane anaesthesia (Dekanski, 1952), and antidiuretic assays in rats under ethanol anaesthesia (Sawyer, 1958). Agonistic activities are expressed in units/mg. Antagonistic potencies are measured and expressed as pA_2s (Schild, 1947) and as "effective doses". In vitro pA_2s are the negative logs of the "effective" concentrations of antagonists. An effective dose is defined as the dose (in nmol/kg) that reduces the response seen from 2x units of agonist (vasopressin or oxytocin) to the response with 1x units of agonist in the rat. Estimated in vivo pA_2 values represent the negative logarithms of the effective doses divided by the estimated volume of distribution 67 ml/kg (Dyckes et al., 1974), and are of course based on rather arbitrary assumptions concerning transport, metabolism, distribution, storage and elimination. Inhibition of antidiuretic responses is tested by injecting the USP posterior pituitary reference standard 20 min after injection of the antagonist to allow for the recovery of the initial antidiuretic responses to some antagonists.

HIGHLIGHTS OF NEW FINDINGS ON ANTAGONIST DESIGN

Oxytocin antagonists

Thr^4 substitution offered early promise (Table I)

As indicated in the Introduction, dPOT (pA_2(in vitro) = 6.94), dEt$_2$OT (pA_2(in vitro) = 7.24) and d(CH$_2$)$_5$OT (pA_2(in vitro) = 7.43), all first synthesized in du Vigneaud's laboratory, have proved to be extremely valuable lead compounds for the design of potent in vivo antagonists of oxytocin.

Our most potent antagonist in 1976 was dPTOT, which had an in vitro (no Mg^{2+}) pA_2 of 7.52 (Manning et al., 1978) and was later found to be a mixed agonist/antagonist in vivo (pA$_2$ = 6.31) (Sawyer et al., 1980). This was designed by substituting Thr for Gln at position 4 in dPOT, which has the following structure:

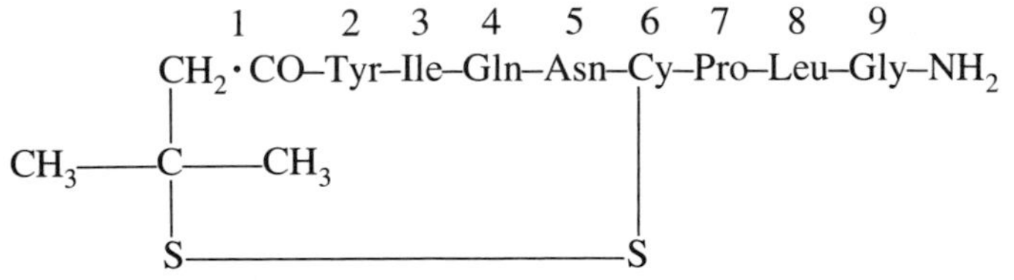

$$CH_2 \cdot CO\text{--}Tyr\text{--}Ile\text{--}Gln\text{--}Asn\text{--}Cy\text{--}Pro\text{--}Leu\text{--}Gly\text{--}NH_2$$

positions labeled 1 2 3 4 5 6 7 8 9

dPOT

The subsequent substitution of Thr^4 in dEt$_2$OT and d(CH$_2$)$_5$OT resulted in substantial increases in in vitro and in vivo anti-oxytocic potencies. Thus, dEt$_2$TOT and d(CH$_2$)$_5$TOT exhibit in vivo anti-oxytocic pA$_2$ values of 6.47 and 6.94 respectively (Lowbridge et al., 1979) (Table I).

TABLE I

4-THREONINE SUBSTITUTION IN [1-(β-MERCAPTO-β,β-DIALKYLPROPIONIC ACID)]OXYTOCIN ANALOGUES ENHANCES ANTI-OXYTOCIC POTENCIES

(From Lowbridge et al., 1979.)

Analogue	Anti-oxytocic (in vitro) pA$_2$[a]		Anti-oxytocic (in vivo)	Antivasopressor
	No Mg^{2+}	0.5 mM Mg^{2+}	pA$_2$[a]	pA$_2$[a]
dPOT	7.14 (6.94)[c]	5.63[b]	mixed[b]	6.27[c]
dPTOT	7.52	6.23	6.31[b]	6.67
d(Et$_2$)OT	7.55 (7.24)[c]	6.82	6.20	6.83[a]
d(Et$_2$)TOT	7.72	7.36	6.47	6.30
d(CH$_2$)$_5$OT	7.61 (7.43)[c]	7.15	6.65	weak[c]
d(CH$_2$)$_5$TOT	7.91	7.81	6.94	5.86

[a] The pA$_2$ is the negative logarithm of the molar concentration of antagonist that reduces the response to 2x units of agonist to equal the response to 1x units in the absence of antagonist (Schild, 1947). In vivo "pA$_2$" values are estimated by assuming an arbitrary volume of distribution of the antagonists which allows one to estimate molar concentrations.

[b] These analogues had mixed agonistic and antagonistic properties on these assays.

[c] From Nestor et al. (1975).

Tyr(Me)^2, Orn^8 in dialkyl-oxytocins enhance oxytocic antagonism (Table II)

The Thr^4 substitution in dPOT, dEt$_2$OT and d(CH$_2$)$_5$OT, although initially promising, was later superceded by two other substitutions — one old (Tyr(Me)^2) and the other new (Orn^8) in the design of oxytocin antagonists. As far back as 1960, du Vigneaud and associates had shown that the substitution of Tyr(Me) at position 2 in óxytocin resulted in a compound (Tyr(Me)^{2}oxytocin) (Law and du Vigneaud, 1960) that was a weak antagonist of vasopressor responses to AVP. Rudinger and colleagues subsequently showed that this could act as an oxytocic agonist or a weak antagonist of oxytocin in vitro depending on the ionic milieu and the hormonal status of the rats (Berankova et al., 1961). During the 1960s, much effort was expended by the Rudinger group in characterizing the antagonistic properties of O-alkyl tyrosine-substituted oxytocins on the rat uterus in assays carried out under different in vitro and in vivo conditions (for review, see Rudinger et al., 1972). Although no really potent in vivo antagonists emerged from these studies, some promising leads were uncovered. In 1968 Bisset and Rudinger and their colleagues, exploiting clues from the in vitro inhibitory properties of [Tyr(Me)^2]oxytocin with those from earlier findings on the effects of N-carbamylation at position 1 (Bisset et al., 1964), together with those of Smyth on the effects of combining N and O-carbamyl substitutions at positions 1 and 2 in oxytocin (Smyth 1967), reported that car-bamylation of the NH$_2$-group of [Tyr(Me)^2]oxytocin resulted in the first effective in vivo antagonist of uterine responses to oxytocin (Bisset and Clark, 1968; Chimiak et al., 1968; Bisset et al., 1970). Although this antagonist was rather weak both in vitro and in vivo (pA$_2$(in vitro) = 6.9), the additive approach used in its design offered real promise for the design of more potent oxytocic antagonists. For some inexplicable reason, however, apart from a study of the inhibitory properties of a series of N-acylated analogues of [Tyr(Me)^2]oxytocin (Kro-jidlo et al., 1975), virtually no further use was made of the Tyr(Me)^2 substitution in antagonist design until we "rediscovered" it so to speak just a few years ago and found it to be a very effective modification for the design of antagonists. The Orn^8 substitution was uncovered rather serendipidously (Sawyer et al., 1980) during the course of one of our early attempts to design an antidiuretic antagonist (Manning et al., 1975) by modifying a selective pressor agonist (Huguenin 1964).

Both Tyr(Me)^2 and Orn^8 have proved to be highly valuable substitutions alone and in combination for the design of potent and effective in vivo oxytocic antagonists. (Subsequently, the Tyr(Me)^2 substitution also fulfilled its earlier promise in the design of vasopressor antagonists (Law and du Vigneaud, 1960) and has played a key role in the discovery of antidiuretic antagonists, see below.) Space considerations do not permit a complete elabora-tion of the many potent antagonists which have resulted from these substitutions in dPOT, dEt$_2$OT and d(CH$_2$)$_5$OT. Suffice it to say that the two most potent in vivo oxytocic antagonists reported to date incorporate both of these substitutions. These are dEt$_2$Tyr(Me)OVT (pA$_2$ = 7.35) and d(CH$_2$)$_5$Tyr (Me)OVT (pA$_2$ = 7.37) (Bankowski et al., 1980) (Table II). The latter has the following structure:

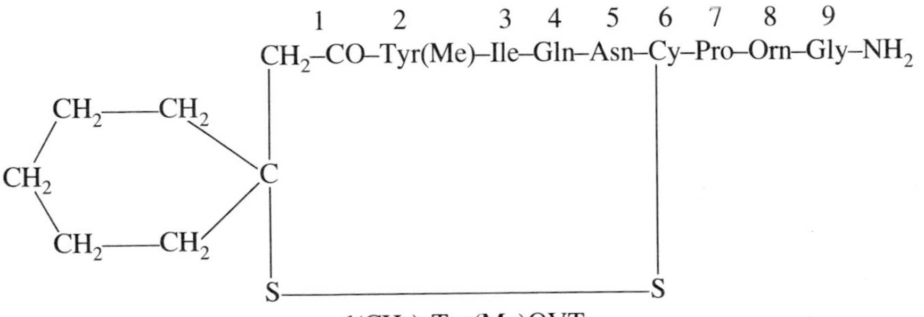

$$\begin{array}{ccccccccc} 1 & 2 & 3 & 4 & 5 & 6 & 7 & 8 & 9 \end{array}$$

CH$_2$–CO–Tyr(Me)–Ile–Gln–Asn–Cy–Pro–Orn–Gly–NH$_2$

d(CH$_2$)$_5$Tyr(Me)OVT

Its full chemical name is: [1-(β-mercapto-β,β-cyclopentamethylenepropionic acid),2-(O-methyl)tyrosine,8-ornithine]vasotocin.

TABLE II

Tyr(Me)[2] AND Orn[8] SUBSTITUTIONS IN 1-β,β-DIALKYL OXYTOCIN ANALOGUES ENHANCE
ANTI-OXYTOCIC AND ANTIVASOPRESSOR POTENCIES

Analogue	Anti-oxytocic			Antivasopressor		Ref.[c]
	in vitro (no Mg^{2+}) pA$_2$	in vivo ED[a] (nmol/kg)	pA$_2$[b]	ED[a] (nmol/kg)	pA$_2$[b]	
dPOT	7.14	mixed agonist/antagonist			6.27	1
Tyr(Me)OT	mixed	agonist		weak antagonist		2,3
dPTyr(Me)OT	7.76	13	6.86	1.8	7.59	4
dPTyr(Me)OVT	7.70	6	7.15	1.8	7.62	1
d(Et$_2$)Tyr(Me)OVT	8.91	3	7.35	0.1	8.02	5
d(CH$_2$)$_5$Tyr(Me)OVT	8.52	4	7.37	0.7	7.96	5

[a] The "effective dose". This is the estimated dose that would reduce the response to 2x units of oxytocin or AVP to
equal the response to 1x units administered before the antagonist.

[b] The in vivo pA$_2$ values are estimated as the negative log of the "effective dose" divided by an assumed volume of
distribution of 67 ml/kg (Dyckes et al., 1974).

[c] References: 1 Sawyer et al. (1980)
2 Krejci et al. (1967)
3 Law and du Vigneaud (1960)
4 Lowbridge et al. (1979)
5 Bankowski et al. (1980)

Vasopressor antagonists (Table III)

Our first vasopressor antagonist was the highly potent and selective antidiuretic peptide
[1-deamino,4-valine,8-D-arginine]vasopressin (dVDAVP) (Manning et al., 1973; Sawyer et
al., 1974) (antidiuretic activity = 1230 U/mg; antivasopressor pA$_2$ = 7.03 (Manning et al.,
1977)). As alluded to in the Introduction, the incorporation of the β,β-dimethyl ((CH$_3$)$_2$) group
at position 1 in this peptide gave rise to dPVDAVP (antivasopressor pA$_2$ = 7.82; antidiuretic
activity = 123 U/mg) (Manning et al., 1977), which was then the most potent known vasopressor antagonist. In the meantime, du Vigneaud and colleagues had reported that dEt$_2$LVP
had an antivasopressor pA$_2$ of 7.15 (Dyckes et al., 1974). As we shall see below, further
appropriate modifications of dVDAVP produced, on the one hand, highly potent and selective
vasopressor antagonists and, on the other, albeit rather circuitously, the first reported antagonists of the antidiuretic responses to AVP. Again space considerations do not permit a full
discussion of the vasopressor antagonists developed to date and of the structure–activity
insights gained from these.

Effects of β,β-dialkyl substituents on antivasopressor potencies — surprising findings

Following the discovery of dPVDAVP (we had first synthesized this in 1973) and the
reported properties of dEt$_2$LVP (Dyckes et al., 1974), we synthesized d(CH$_2$)$_5$VDAVP
(Lowbridge et al., 1978). This compound exhibited reduced antivasopressor potency
(pA$_2$ = 7.6, Table III). This was consistent with the trend for antivasopressor potencies of
oxytocin antagonists reported by du Vigneaud and colleagues (Nestor et al., 1975b) (See
Table I). It thus appeared that the β,β-dimethyl substitution would be more useful than either
the β,β-diethyl or the β,β-cyclopentamethylene in the design of vasopressor antagonists.

TABLE III

ADDITIVE EFFECTS OF SUBSTITUTIONS IN THE 1- AND 2-POSITIONS OF dVDAVP AND dAVP ON
ANTIVASOPRESSOR, ANTI-OXYTOCIC AND ANTIDIURETIC ACTIVITIES

Analogue	Antivasopressor activity $pA_2{}^a$	Anti-oxytocic activity (in vitro) no Mg^{2+} $pA_2{}^{a,b}$	Antidiuretic activity (U/mg)	Ref.[d]
dVDAVP	7.03	agonist	1230	1,2
dPVDAVP	7.83	7.23	123	2
d(CH$_2$)$_5$VDAVP	7.68	6.62	0.10[c]	3
dTyr(Me)VDAVP	7.01	7.99	⪝ 2000	4
dPTyr(Me)VDAVP	7.83	7.5	3.2	4
d(CH$_2$)$_5$Tyr(Me)VDAVP	8.44	7.93	inhibits	5
dAVP	agonist	agonist	1745	6
dPAVP	7.45	6.93	42	7
d(CH$_2$)$_5$AVP	8.35	8.15	0.03	8
dTyr(Me)AVP	agonist	7.41	⪝ 830	9
dPTyr(Me)AVP	7.96	7.61	3.5	7
d(CH$_2$)$_5$Tyr(Me)AVP	8.62	8.13	0.31	8

[a] For definitions of pA_2, see footnotes to Tables I and II.
[b] Values from Kruszynski et al. (1980) and unpublished.
[c] Also acts as partial agonist (Sawyer et al., 1981b unpublished).
[d] References: 1 Sawyer et al. (1974a)
                2 Manning et al. (1977)
                3 Lowbridge et al. (1978)
                4 Bankowski, Manning, Sawyer (unpublished)
                5 Manning et al. (1981a)
                6 Manning et al. (1981b)
                7 Bankowski et al. (1978)
                8 Kruszynski et al. (1980)
                9 Manning and Sawyer (unpublished)

Fortunately this assumption proved to be invalid. We subsequently found that the relative effectiveness of the β,β-dimethyl, β,β-diethyl and the β,β-cyclopentamethylene groupings depends entirely on which peptides they are incorporated into. Thus, we found that the incorporation of the β,β-dimethyl grouping in 1-deamino-AVP (dAVP) (Huguenin and Boissonnas, 1966) resulted in a peptide, dPAVP, with an antivasopressor pA_2 of only 7.45 (Bankowski et al., 1978) — a drastic reduction from that of dPVDAVP ($pA_2 = 7.82$). We were subsequently truly delighted to find that the incorporation of the (CH$_2$)$_5$ grouping in dAVP resulted in a peptide, d(CH$_2$)$_5$AVP, with an antivasopressor pA_2 of 8.3 (Kruszynski et al., 1980) — a dramatic increase from that of dPAVP and in striking contrast to the effects of this substitution in dVDAVP which had, as we have seen, resulted in the diminished antivasopressor potency exhibited by d(CH$_2$)$_5$VDAVP. The incorporation of Tyr(Me) at position 2 in d(CH$_2$)$_5$AVP led to a further increase in antivasopressor potency. The resulting peptide, d(CH$_2$)$_5$Tyr(Me)AVP, is the most potent vasopressor antagonist reported to date (Kruszynski et al., 1980) (Table III). Its full chemical name is: [1-(β-mercapto-β,β-cyclopentamethylene-nepropionic acid), 2-O-methyltyrosine]arginine-vasopressin. This antagonist has the following structure:

$$
\begin{array}{c}
\overset{1}{}\quad\overset{2}{}\quad\overset{3}{}\quad\overset{4}{}\quad\overset{5}{}\quad\overset{6}{}\quad\overset{7}{}\quad\overset{8}{}\quad\overset{9}{}
\end{array}
$$

1   2   3 4 5 6 7 8 9

CH₂–CO–Tyr(Me)–Phe–Gln–Asn–Cy–Pro–Arg–Gly–NH₂

```
   CH₂——CH₂
  /        \
CH₂         C
  \        /|
   CH₂——CH₂ |
            S ——————————————— S
```

d(CH₂)₅Tyr(Me)AVP

This antagonist has an antivasopressor pA_2 of 8.67 and is a weak antidiuretic agonist (0.31 units/mg). It is, however, an anti-oxytocic in vivo ($pA_2 = 6.62$). Details of the many vasopressor antagonists which we have looked at are presented in separate publications (Sawyer et al., 1981b; Manning et al., 1981b, 1982c).

Antidiuretic antagonists

This area has seen the most dramatic progress since the Key Biscayne Conference. In 1976 there were absolutely no clues to the design of competitive renal tubular AVP receptor antagonists. What appeared to be promising leads, i.e. [4-leucine]oxytocin (Chan et al., 1968) and [4-phenylalanine]oxytocin (Nestor et al., 1975a) did not appear to be effective antagonists of endogenous AVP and the mechanisms by which they reversed antidiuresis in response to exogenous AVP were not clear (Chan and du Vigneaud, 1970; Chan 1976).

This total lack of success in unearthing a clue to the design of antidiuretic antagonists, despite over 25 years of intensive study in many laboratories throughout the world, sparked gloomy fears that perhaps there was some underlying biological reason frustrating all efforts to attain this goal. Indeed in public and private discussions following our presentation at the Key Biscayne Conference serious doubts along these lines were expressed by Serg Jard. This pessimistic view was based on his findings of an abundance of spare renal tubular receptors for AVP — a mere fraction of which, when occupied, can elicit a maximal antidiuretic response in vivo (Jard et al., 1977). Fortunately these grim forebodings proved to be unwarranted.

Key clues. By a happy twist, Serg Jard in a collaboration initiated at the Key Biscayne Conference, helped to provide one of three key clues which ultimately led to the discovery of the first known effective in vivo antidiuretic antagonists. In our initial attempts to design such antagonists, we had synthesized dPVDAVP. As we have seen, this peptide was still a very potent antidiuretic agonist. We had subsequently hoped to convert this into an antidiuretic antagonist by replacing the β,β-dimethyl grouping at position 1 with the larger β,β-cyclopentamethylene grouping. The resulting compound, d(CH₂)₅VDAVP, was not an antidiuretic antagonist in vivo. It did, however, exhibit a dramatic reduction in antidiuretic activity — from 123 units/mg to 0.10 units/mg (Table III). Since it had an antivasopressor pA_2 of 7.6, it was thus a highly selective vasopressor antagonist (Lowbridge et al., 1978). Examination of the properties of d(CH₂)VDAVP in in vitro assay systems by Serg Jard yielded the first clue to the design of an in vivo antidiuretic antagonist. d(CH₂)₅VDAVP was found to be a potent in vitro antagonist of [³H]LVP binding and LVP-stimulated adenylate cyclase activation in medullopapillary membranes from rat kidneys (Butlen et al., 1978). The second clue was the discovery that d(CH₂)₅VDAVP, although not an antagonist in vivo, is indeed a partial antidiuretic agonist in vivo (Sawyer et al., 1981b; and unpublished). The third clue to the design of antidiuretic antagonists came from the work of Larsson et al. (1978) on the effects of O-alkyl-tyrosine substitution on the antidiuretic activity of [1-deamino-lysine]vasopressin. The resulting analogues exhibited inconsistent non-dose-related inhibition of the antidiuresis caused by the infusion of LVP in hydrated rats. Thus the combination of these three clues: the in vitro AVP antagonism of $d(CH_2)_5VDAVP$, its partial antidiuretic agonism in vivo, and the promising effects of O-alkyl-tyrosine substitution, were the remaining key pointers in the long pathway to the discovery of the first known antagonists of exogenous and endogenous AVP.

The first antidiuretic antagonists

The first four antidiuretic antagonists (Sawyer et al., 1981a; Manning et al., 1981a) were thus designed by incorporating Tyr(Me) and Tyr(Et) substituents in place of L-Tyr at position 2 in $d(CH_2)_5VDAVP$ (Lowbridge et al., 1978) and in its L-Arg isomer $d(CH_2)_5VAVP$ (Manning et al., 1982c) (Table IV). The most potent of these was the Tyr(Et), L-Arg compund, $d(CH_2)_5Tyr (Et)VAVP$, which has the following structure:

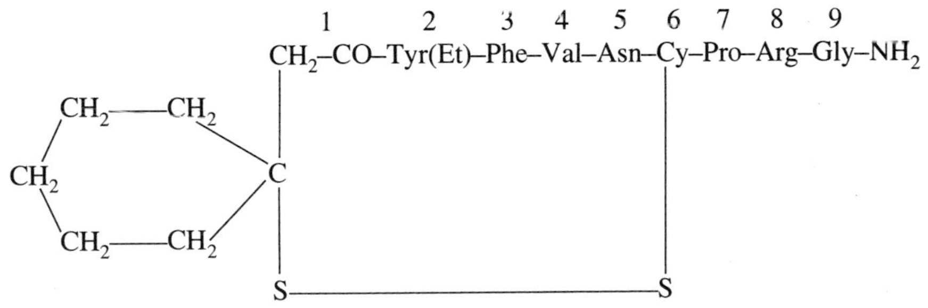

$$1 \quad 2 \quad 3 \quad 4 \quad 5 \quad 6 \quad 7 \quad 8 \quad 9$$
$$CH_2–CO–Tyr(Et)–Phe–Val–Asn–Cy–Pro–Arg–Gly–NH_2$$

d(CH_2)_5Tyr(Et)VAVP

$d(CH_2)_5Tyr(Et)VAVP$ has an anti-antidiuretic effective dose of 1.9 nmol/kg, which is equivalent to a pA_2 value of 7.57. These early antidiuretic antagonists all possessed transient antidiuretic agonistic activity and possessed potent antivasopressor (Table IV) and anti-oxytocic properties (unpublished). Increasing the size of the alkyl substituents on the tyrosine to n-propyl, isopropyl (Manning et al., 1981a) or n-butyl (unpublished) did not lead to increased potency or selectivity.

TABLE IV

THE FIRST FOUR ANTAGONISTS OF ANTIDIURETIC RESPONSES TO ARGININE-VASOPRESSIN (AVP)[a]

No.	Antagonists	Anti-antidiuretic		Antivasopressor	
		effective dose[b] (nmol/kg)	pA_2[b]	effective dose[b] (nmol/kg)	pA_2[b]
1.	$d(CH_2)_5Tyr(Me)VDAVP$	15	6.68	0.28	8.44
2.	$d(CH_2)_5Tyr(Et)VDAVP$	5.7	7.10	0.34	8.31
3.	$d(CH_2)_5Tyr(Me)VAVP$	3.1	7.35	0.29	8.32
4.	$d(CH_2)_5Tyr(Et)VAVP$	1.9	7.57	0.49	8.16

[a] From Sawyer et al. (1981a) and Manning et al. (1981a).

[b] For definitions of effective dose and pA_2, see footnotes to Tables I and II.

Design of more potent and more selective antidiuretic antagonists

Following the discovery of the initial lead compounds d(CH$_2$)$_5$Tyr (Alk)VYVP (Alk = Me, Et, iPr, nPr; Y = L or D-Arg), selected modifications of these compounds have led to significant progress towards designing more potent and highly selective antidiuretic antagonists devoid of antidiuretic agonism.

In brief, some of the key findings, subsequent to our initial discovery, are as follows.

(1) D-Tyr(alk) substitution in d(CH$_2$)$_5$Tyr(alk)VAVP leads to enhanced anti-antidiuretic potencies (Manning et al., 1982a) (Table V).

(2) D-Tyr substitution alone at position 2 in d(CH$_2$)$_5$VAVP and d(CH$_2$)$_5$VDAVP turned these weak antidiuretic agonists/vasopressor antagonists into antidiuretic antagonists (Manning et al., 1982a) (Table VI).

TABLE V

D-Tyr(alk)[2] SUBSTITUTION ENHANCES ANTI-ANTIDIURETIC POTENCIES

(From Manning et al., 1982a).

No.	Antagonists	Anti-antidiuretic		
		Effective dose[a] *(nmol/kg)*	*pA$_2$*[b]	*pA$_2$*[a,b]
1.	d(CH$_2$)$_5$D-Tyr(Me)VDAVP	4.9	7.19	(6.68)
2.	d(CH$_2$)$_5$D-Tyr(Et)VDAVP	1.8	7.59	(7.10)
3.	d(CH$_2$)$_5$D-Tyr(Me)VAVP	1.2	7.77	(7.35)
4.	d(CH$_2$)$_5$D-Tyr(Et)VAVP	1.1	7.81	(7.57)

[a] For definitions of effective dose and pA$_2$, see footnotes to Tables I and II.
[b] Values for each of the corresponding O-alkylated L-tyrosine antagonists (from Table IV).

TABLE VI

UNALKYLATED D-Tyr[2] ANALOGUES OF TWO WEAK ANTIDIURETIC AGONISTS ARE POTENT ANTIDIURETIC ANTAGONISTS

(From Manning et al., 1982a).

Peptide	Anti-antidiuretic		Antivasopressor	
	effective dose[a] *(nmol/kg)*	*pA$_2$*[a]	*effective dose*[a] *(nmol/kg)*	*pA$_2$*[a]
d(CH$_2$)$_5$VDAVP	agonist		1.50	7.68
d(CH$_2$)$_5$D-TyrVDAVP	6.3	7.03	0.60	8.05
d(CH$_2$)$_5$VAVP	agonist		0.76	7.97
d(CH$_2$)$_5$D-TyrVAVP	2.2	7.51	0.29	8.41

[a] For definitions of effective dose and pA$_2$, see footnotes to Tables I and II.

(3) The finding that alkylation of the tyrosine (L or D) in d(CH$_2$)$_5$Tyr(alk)AVP is unnecessary for antidiuretic antagonism led to a series of more potent antidiuretic antagonists devoid of antidiuretic agonism: d(CH$_2$)$_5$X[2]VAVP where X = D-Phe, D-Ile, D-Leu, D-Val (Manning et al., 1982b). These antagonists also exhibit enhanced anti-antidiuretic/antivasopressor selec-

tivities and antidiuretic/anti-oxytocic selectivities relative to $d(CH_2)_5D$-TyrVAVP (Table VII).

(4) The most potent reported antidiuretic antagonists contain D-Phe and D-Ile at position 2, i.e. $d(CH_2)_5$D-Phe^2-VAVP and $d(CH_2)_5$D-Ile^{2}VAVP. Their anti-antidiuretic effective doses are 0.67 and 0.70 nmol/kg and the corresponding pA_2 values are 8.07 and 7.98, respectively (Manning et al., 1982b) (Table VII). Both of these have been used as lead compounds in subsequent modifications (unpublished).

TABLE VII

MORE SELECTIVE ANTAGONISTS OF ANTIDIURETIC RESPONSES TO AVP AND RELATED PEPTIDES

(From Manning et al., 1982b).

No.	Peptide	Anti-antidiuretic		Antivasopressor	
		Effective dose[a] (nmol/kg)	pA_2[a]	Effective dose[a] (nmol/kg)	pA_2[a]
1.	$d(CH_2)_5$VAVP	agonist	—	0.76	7.97
2.	$d(CH_2)_5$D-TyrVAVP	2.2	7.51	0.29	8.41
3.	$d(CH_2)_5$D-TyrVDAVP	6.3	7.03	0.60	8.05
4.	$d(CH_2)_5$D-PheVAVP	0.67[b]	8.06	0.58	8.06
5.	$d(CH_2)_5$D-PheVDAVP	6.9	7.07	0.73	7.98
6.	$d(CH_2)_5$D-IleVAVP	0.70[b,c]	7.98	8.2	6.94
7.	$d(CH_2)_5$D-LeuVAVP	1.2[b,c]	7.79	26	6.45
8.	$d(CH_2)_5$D-ValVAVP	2.3[b,c]	7.48	27	6.41
9.	$d(CH_2)_5$D-AlaVAVP	agonist	—	172	5.79
10.	$d(CH_2)_5$GlyVAVP	agonist	—	agonist	—
11.	$d(CH_2)_5$D-ArgVAVP	> 90	< 5.9	⪝ 260	⪝ 5.4

[a] For definitions of effective dose and pA_2, see footnotes to Tables I and II.

[b] No evident agonistic activity.

[c] Exhibit enhanced anti-antidiuretic/antivasopressor and antidiuretic/anti-oxytocic selectivities.

POTENTIAL USEFULNESS OF OXYTOCIN AND VASOPRESSIN ANTAGONISTS

As pointed out in the Introduction, many of these antagonists are proving to be very useful as pharmacological tools in other studies. They may also have clinical potential (Manning and Sawyer, 1982).

Selective oxytocic antagonists

Effective in vivo antagonists of the oxytocic and milk-ejecting responses of oxytocin are of value as pharmacological probes of the actions of both oxytocin and vasopressin. In addition, such antagonists could be of value for the control of the onset and of the terminal stages of labour.

Selective vasopressor antagonists

Vasopressor antagonists from these laboratories have been used in various studies seeking to clarify the roles of vasopressin in regulating blood pressure in normal and pathophysiological states and in memory processing (Le Moal et al., 1981). For a state of the art review on the role of vasopressin in normal and abnormal blood pressure regulation, see Johnson et al. (1981). Vasopressin is the most potent vasopressor substance known, yet it has long been believed to serve a role in cardiovascular regulation only when released in massive quantities after severe blood loss (e.g., see Rocha-e-silva and Rosenberg, 1969). Evidence that vasopressin makes a significant contribution to the maintenance of blood pressure after hypotensive (Cowley et al., 1980) and non-hypotensive haemorrhage in dogs (Schwartz and Reid, 1981) and during mild dehydration in rats (Aisenbrey et al., 1981; Andrews and Brenner, 1981), was obtained through use of antagonists of the vasopressor responses to vasopressin. These studies, together with others cited in Manning et al. (1982c), clearly show a significant function for vasopressin in maintaining blood pressure during hypovolaemia. Although controversy surrounds the role of vasopressin in different forms of hypertension in animals and humans (Johnson et al., 1981; Lohmeier et al., 1981), injections of an antagonist of vasopressor responses to vasopressin have been shown to reduce blood pressure acutely in rats with deoxycorticosterone–salt hypertension (Crofton et al., 1979; Mento et al., 1982) and in rabbits with hypertension following lesioning of noradrenaline-containing neurones in the caudal ventrolateral medulla oblongata (Blessing et al., 1982). Should a clear involvement of vasopressin in either the pathogenesis or maintenance of hypertension in humans be shown, the development of potent and selective vasopressor antagonists completely devoid of antidiuretic and oxytocic agonistic or antagonistic activities as diagnostic tools or therapeutic agents would be warranted.

Selective antidiuretic antagonists

Vasopressin renal tubular receptor antagonists could be of value (a) as pharmacological tools for studying the contribution of vasopressin to water retention in normal and pathophysiological states, and (b) as therapeutic agents for the treatment of hyponatraemia secondary to the syndrome of inappropriate secretion of antidiuretic hormone (SIADH or the Schwartz–Bartter syndrome) (Bartter and Schwartz, 1967). In addition, such antagonists could be useful for the treatment of vasopressin-stimulated water retention that may arise in other clinical situations (Bichet et al., 1982; Ishikawa and Schrier, 1982). Existing methods for the treatment of vasopressin-induced water retention have many shortcomings (Zerbe et al., 1981). Thus the development of a satisfactory receptor antagonist would fill a long-standing therapeutic need.

SUMMARY AND CONCLUSIONS

Much progress has been made since the last Neurohypophysis Conference in the design of potent and effective antagonists of the uterine, vascular and renal tubular responses to oxytocin and vasopressin, and many of these are proving to be very useful in other studies (Manning and Sawyer, 1982). It is important to note, however, that this field is still very much in its infancy. It is at a similar stage of development as the study of structure–activity relationships on AVP and oxytocin agonists was 25 years ago. This is particularly true for the antidiuretic antagonists, which were first discovered only two years ago! Thus, it will take many more years to obtain an accurate profile of the optimal and minimal side-chain structures at positions 1–9 in each antagonistic type required for specific inhibition of AVP and oxytocin binding to renal tubular, vascular, uterine receptors and to other, e.g. CNS isoreceptors. Also, as mentioned in the Introduction, all of the antagonists developed to date lack absolute specificity. In certain clinical situations, these multiple antagonistic properties could produce non-desirable side-effects. Certainly for pharmacological and receptor studies, highly selective antagonists are of much greater value than multiple site antagonists. Thus the search for potent and selective antagonists in each category must continue in the hope of attaining therapeutically useful antagonists devoid of possible unwanted side-effects and which, in addition, might be active following oral administration. To end on a heuristic note, the elucidation of new roles for oxytocin and vasopressin in other tissues, e.g. brain, may endow these and future antagonists with significance and uses far beyond any present day expectations.

ACKNOWLEDGEMENTS

Work from these laboratories cited in this review was supported by Research Grants from the National Institutes of Health, GM-25280, AMO1940, HL 12738. We are deeply indebted to our many colleagues who participated during the past six years in the development of these antagonists: Dr. John Lowbridge, Dr. Andras Turan, Dr. Marian Kruszinski, Dr. Krzysztof Bankowski, Dr. Bernard Lammek, Dr. Zbigniew Grzonka, Dr. Aleksander Kolodziejczyk, Dr. Wieslaw Klis, Dr. Aleksandra Olma, Dr. Jaya Halder, Janny Seto and Becky Wo. We thank Ms. Beverly Lockwood for invaluable assistance in the preparation of this manuscript.

REFERENCES

Aisenbrey, G.A., Handelman, W.A., Arnold, P., Manning, M. and Schrier, R.W. (1981) Vascular effects of arginine vasopressin during fluid deprivation in the rat. *J. clin. Invest.*, 67: 961–968.

Andrews, C.E., Jr and Brenner, B.M. (1981) Relative contributions of arginine vasopressin and angiotensin II to maintenance of systemic arterial pressure in the anesthetized water-deprived rat. *Circulat. Res.*, 48: 254–258.

Bankowski, K., Manning, M., Haldar, J. and Sawyer, W.H. (1978) Design of potent antagonists of the vasopressor response to arginine-vasopressin. *J. med. Chem.*, 21: 850–853.

Bankowski, K., Manning, M., Seto, J., Haldar, J. and Sawyer, W.H. (1980) Design and synthesis of potent in vivo antagonists of oxytocin. *Int. J. Peptide Prot. Res.*, 16: 382–391.

Bartter, F.C. and Schwartz, W.B. (1967) The syndrome of inappropriate secretion of antidiuretic hormone. *Amer. J. Med.* 42: 790–806.

Berankova, Z., Rychlik, I., Jost, K., Rudinger, J. and Sorm, F. (1961) Inhibition of the uterus-contracting effect of oxytocin by O-methyl-oxytocin. *Coll. Czech. Chem. Commun.*, 26: 2673–2675.

Berde, B. and Boissonnas, R.A. (1968) Basic pharmacological properties of synthetic analogues and homologues of the neurohypophysial hormones. In B. Berde (Ed.), *Handbook of Experimental Pharmacology, Vol. 23*, Springer-Verlag, Berlin, pp. 802–870.

Bichet, D., Szatalowicz, V., Chaimovitz, C. and Schrier, R.W. (1982) Role of vasopressin in abnormal water excretion in cirrhotic patients. *Ann. intern. Med.*, 96: 413–417.

Bisset, G.W. and Clark, B.J. (1968) Synthetic 1-N-carbamyl-hemicystine-2-O-methyltyrosine-oxytocin (N-carbamyl-O-methyl-oxytocin): a specific antagonist to the actions of oxytocin and vasopressin on the uterus and mammary gland. *Nature (Lond.)*, 218: 197–199.

Bisset, G.W., Poisner, A.M. and Smyth, D.G. (1964) 1-N-carbamyl-oxytocin — a new analogue with inhibitory properties towards oxytocin and vasopressin. *J. Physiol. (Lond.)*, 170: 12–13.

Bisset, G.W., Clark, B.J., Krejci, I., Polacek, I. and Rudinger, J. (1970) Some pharmacological properties of a synthetic oxytocin analogue [1-N-carbamoyl-hemicystine-2-O-methyl-tyrosine]oxytocin (carbamoyl-methyloxytocin), an antagonist to the neurohypophysial hormones. *Brit. J. Pharmacol.*, 40: 342–360.

Blessing, W.W., Sved, A.F. and Reis, D.J. (1982) Destruction of noradrenergic neurons in rabbit brainstem elevates plasma vasopressin, causing hypertension. *Science*, 217: 661–663.

Butlen, D., Guillon, G., Rajerison, R.M., Jard, S., Sawyer, W.H. and Manning, M. (1978) Structural requirements for activation of vasopressin-sensitive adenylate cyclase and hormone binding: effects of highly potent antidiuretic analogues and competitive inhibitors. *Molec. Pharmacol.*, 14: 1006–1017.

Cash, W.D. and Smith, BL.L. (1963) Synthesis and biological properties of 1-acetyl-8-lysine-vasopressin. *J. biol. Chem.*, 238: 994–997.

Chan, W.Y. (1976) An investigation of the natriuretic, antidiuretic and oxytocic actions of neurohypophysial hormones and related peptides: delineation of separate mechanisms of action and assessment of molecular requirements. *J. Pharmacol. exp. Ther.*, 196: 746–757.

Chan, W.Y. and du Vigneaud, V. (1970) Natriuretic, diuretic and antiarginine-vasopressin (ADH) effects of two analogs of oxytocin: [4-leucine]-oxytocin and [2,4-diisoleucine]-oxytocin. *J. Pharmacol. exp. Ther.*, 174: 541–549.

Chan, W.Y., Hruby, V.J., Flouret, G. and du Vigneaud, V. (1968) [4-Leucine]-oxytocin: natriuretic, diuretic and antivasopressin polypeptide. *Science*, 161: 280–281.

Chimiak, A., Eisler, K., Jost, K. and Rudinger, J. (1968) Unambiguous syntheses of N-carbamyl-oxytocin and N-carbamyl-2-O-methyltyrosine-oxytocin. *Coll. Czech. Chem. Commun.*, 33: 2918–2926.

Cowley, A.W., Jr., Switzer, S.J. and Guinn, M.M. (1980) Evidence and quantification of the vasopressin arterial pressure control system in the dog. *Circulat. Res.*, 46: 58–67.

Crofton, J.T., Share, L., Shade, R.E., Lee-Kwon, W.J., Manning, M. and Sawyer, W.H. (1979) The importance of vasopressin in the development and maintenance of DOC-salt hypertension in the rat. *Hypertension*, 1: 31–38.

Dekanski, J. (1952) The quantitative assay of vasopressin. *Pharmacology*, 7: 567–572.

du Vigneaud, V., Ressler, C., Swan, J.M., Katsoyannis, P.G. and Roberts, C.W. (1954a) Synthesis of oxytocin. *J. Amer. Chem. Soc.*, 76: 3115–3121.

du Vigneaud, V., Gish, D.T. and Katsoyannis, P.G. (1954b) A synthetic preparation possessing biological properties associated with arginine vasopressin. *J. Amer. Chem. Soc.*, 76: 4751–4752.

Dyckes, D.F., Nestor, J.J., Jr., Ferger, M.F. and du Vigneaud, V. (1974) [1-β-Mercapto-β,β-diethylpropionic acid]-8-lysine-vasopressin, a potent inhibitor of 8-lysine-vasopressin and of oxytocin. *J. med. Chem.*, 17: 250–252.

Hope, D.B., Murti, V.V.S. and du Vignaud, V. (1962) A highly potent analogue of oxytocin, desamino-oxytocin. *J. biol. Chem.*, 237: 1563–1566.

Huguenin, R.L. (1964) Synthèse de la Phe[2]-Orn[8]-vasopressine et de la Phe[2]-Orn[8]-oxytocine, deux analogues de la vasopressine doues d'une activité pressorique sélective. *Helv. Chim. Acta*, 47: 1934–1941.

Huguenin, R.L. and Boissonnas, R.A. (1966) Synthèse de la desamino-Arg-vasopressine et de la desamino-Phe[2]-Arg[8]-vasopressine, deux analogues possédant une activité antidiuretique plus léevée et plus sélective que celle des vasopressines naturelles. *Helv. chim. Acta*, 49: 695–705.

Ishikawa, S. and Schrier, R.W. (1982) Effect of arginine vasopressin antagonist on renal water retention in glucocorticoid and mineralocorticoid deficient rats. *Kidney Int.*, 22: 587–593.

Jard, S., Butlen, D., Rajerison, R. and Roy, C. (1977) The vasopressin-sensitive adenylate cyclase from the mammalian kidney. In A.M. Moses and L. Share (Eds.), *Neurohypophysis*, Karger, Basel, pp. 211–219.

Johnston, C.I., Newman, M. and Woods, R. (1981) Role of vasopressin in cardiovascular homeostasis and hypertension. *Clin. Sci.*, 61: 129–139.

Krejci, I., Polacek, I. and Rudinger, J. (1967) The action of 2-O-methyl-tyrosine-oxytocin on the rat and rabbit uterus: effect of some experimental conditions on change from agonism to antagonism. *Brit. J. Pharmacol., Chemother.* 30: 506–517.

Krojidlo, M., Barth, T., Servitova, L., Dobrovsky, K., Jost, K. and Sorm, F. (1975) Synthesis and inhibitory properties of oxytocin analogues modified in the amino-terminal region of the molecule. *Coll. Czech. Chem. Commun.*, 40: 2708–2717.

Kruszynski, M., Lammek, B., Manning, M., Seto, J., Haldar, J. and Sawyer, W.H. (1980) [1-(β-mercapto-β,β-cyclopentamethylenepropionic acid), 2-(O-methyl-tyrosine]-arginine-vasopressin and [1-(β-Mercapto-β,β-cyclopentamethylenepropionic acid)arginine-vasopressin, two highly potent antagonists of the vasopressor response to arginine-vasopressin. *J. med. Chem.*, 23: 364–368.

Larsson, L.E., Lindeberg, G., Melin, P. and Pliska, V. (1978) Synthesis of O-alkylated lysine-vasopressins, inhibitors of the antidiuretic response to lysine-vasopressin. *J. med. Chem.*, 21: 352–356.

Law, H.D. and du Vigneaud, V. (1960) Synthesis of 2-p-methoxy-phenylalanine oxytocin (O-methyl-oxytocin) and some observations on its pharmacological behavior. *J. Amér. Chem. Soc.*, 82: 4579–4581.

Le Moal, M., Koob, G.F., Koda, L.Y., Bloom, F.E., Manning, M. and Sawyer, W.H. (1981) Vasopressor receptor antagonist prevents behavioural effects of vasopressin. *Nature (Lond.)*, 291: 491–493.

Lohmeier, T.E., Smith, M.J., Cowley, A.W., Jr., Manning, R.D., Jr. and Guyton, A.C. (1981) Is vasopressin an important hypertensive hormone? *Hypertension*, 3: 416–425.

Lowbridge, J., Manning, M., Haldar, J. and Sawyer, W.H. (1978) [1-(β-Mercapto-β,β-cyclopentamethylenepropanoic acid),4-valine,8-D-arginine]-vasopressin, a potent and selective inhibitor of the vasopressor response to arginine vasopressin. *J. med. Chem.*, 21: 313–315.

Lowbridge, J., Manning, M., Seto, J., Haldar, J. and Sawyer, W.H. (1979) Synthetic antagonists of in vivo responses by the rat uterus to oxytocin. *J. med. Chem.*, 22: 565–569.

Manning, M. and Sawyer, W.H. (1977) Structure–activity studies on oxytocin and vasopressin 1954–1976; from empiricism to design. In A. Moses (Ed.), *Conference on the Neurohypophysis*, Karger, Basel, pp. 9–21.

Manning, M. and Sawyer, W.H. (1982) Antagonists of vasopressor and antidiuretic responses to arginine vasopressin. *Ann. intern. Med.*, 96: 520–522.

Manning, M., Balaspiri, L., Acosta, M. and Sawyer, W.H. (1973) Solid-phase synthesis of [1-deamino,4-valine,8-D-arginine]vasopressin (dVDAVP), a highly potent and specific antidiuretic agent possessing protracted effects. *J. med. Chem.*, 16: 975–978.

Manning, M., Lowbridge, J. and Sawyer, W.H. (1975) Towards the design of neurohypophysial peptides possessing selectively enhanced and inhibitory properties. In R. Walter and J. Meienhofer (Eds.), *Peptides, Chemistry, Structure and Biology*, Ann Arbor Science, p. 737.

Manning, M., Lowbridge, J., Stier, C.T., Jr., Haldar, J. and Sawyer, W.H. (1977) [1-Deaminopenicillamine,4-valine]-8-D-arginine vasopressin, a highly potent inhibitor of the vasopressor response to arginine vasopressin. *J. med. Chem.*, 20: 1228–1230.

Manning, M., Lowbridge, J., Seto, J., Haldar, J. and Sawyer, W.H. (1978) [1-Deamino-penicillamine,4-threonine]oxytocin, a potent inhibitor of oxytocin. *J. med. Chem.*, 21: 179–182.

Manning, M., Lammek, B., Kolodziejczyk, A., Seto, J. and Sawyer, W.H. (1981a) Synthetic antagonists of in vivo antidiuretic and vasopressor responses to arginine vasopressin. *J. med. Chem.*, 24: 701–706.

Manning, M., Grzonka, Z. and Sawyer, W.H. (1981b) Synthesis of posterior pituitary hormones and hormone analogues. In C. Beardwell and G. Robertson (Eds.), *The Pituitary*, Butterworth, U.K., pp. 265–296.

Manning, M., Olma, A., Klis, W.A., Kolodziejczyk, A.M., Seto, J. and Sawyer, W.H. (1982a) Design of more potent antagonists of the antidiuretic responses to arginine vasopressin. *J. med. Chem.*, 25: 45–50.

Manning, M., Klis, W.A., Olma, A., Seto, J. and Sawyer, W.H. (1982b) Design of more potent and selective antagonists of the antidiuretic responses to arginine vasopressin. *J. med. Chem.*, 25: 414–419.

Manning, M., Lammek, B., Kruszynski, M., Seto, J. and Sawyer, W.H. (1982c) Design of potent and selective antagonists of the vasopressor responses to arginine vasopressin. *J. med. Chem.*, 25: 408–414.

Mento, P.R., Wang, H.H. and Sawyer, W.H. (1982) Relative contributions of arginine vasopressin (AVP) and the sympathetic nervous system in maintaining DOC–salt hypertension in rats. *Fed. Proc.*, 41: 1230.

Merrifield, R.B. (1963) Solid phase synthesis I. The synthesis of a tetrapeptide. *J. Amer. Chem. Soc.*, 85: 2149–2154.

Nestor, J.J., Jr., Ferger, M.R. and Chan, W.Y. (1975a) [4-Phenylalanine]oxytocin, an inhibitor of the antidiuretic effect of 8-arginine-vasopressin. *J. med. Chem.*, 18: 1022–1024.

Nestor, J.J., Jr., Ferger, M.F. and du Vigneaud, V. (1975b) [1-β-Mercapto-β,β-pentamethylene-propionic acid]oxytocin, a potent inhibitor of oxytocin. *J. med. Chem.*, 18: 284–287.

Rocha-e-Silva, M., Jr. and Rosenberg, M. (1969) The release of vasopressin in response to haemorrage and its role in the mechanism of blood pressure regulation. *J. Physiol. (Lond.)*, 202: 535–557.

Rudinger, J. (1971) The design of peptide hormone analogs. In E.J. Ariens (Ed.), *Drug Design*, Academic Press, New York, pp. 319–419.

Rudinger, J., Pliška, V. and Krejci, I. (1972) Oxytocin analogs in the analysis of some phases of hormone action. *Rec. Progr. Hormone Res.*, 28: 131–172.

Sawyer, W.H. (1958) Differences in antidiuretic responses of rats to the intravenous administration of lysine and arginine vasopressins. *Endocrinology*, 63: 694–698.

Sawyer, W.H., Acosta, M., Balaspiri, L., Judd, J. and Manning, M. (1974) Structural changes in the arginine vasopressin molecule that enhance antidiuretic activity and specificity. *Endocrinology*, 94: 1106.

Sawyer, W.H., Haldar, J., Gazis, D., Seto, J., Bankowski, K., Lowbridge, J., Turan, A. and Manning, M. (1980) The design of effective in vivo antagonists of rat uterus and milk-ejection responses to oxytocin. *Endocrinology*, 106: 81–91.

Sawyer, W.H., Pang, P.K.T., Seto, J., McEnroe, M., Lammek, B. and Manning, M. (1981a) Vasopressin analogs that antagonize antidiuretic responses by rats to the antidiuretic responses by rats to the antidiuretic hormone. *Science*, 212: 49–51.

Sawyer, W.H., Grzonka, Z. and Manning, M. (1981b) Neurohypophyseal peptides: Design of tissue-specific agonists and antagonists. *Molec. cell. Endocr.*, 22: 117–134.

Schild, H.O. (1947) pA, a new scale of the measurement of drug antagonism. *Brit. J. Pharmacol. Chemother.*, 2: 189–206.

Schulz, H. and du Vigneaud, V. (1966) Synthesis of 1-L-penicillamine-oxytocin, 1-D-penicillamine-oxytocin, and 1-deaminopenicillamine, potent inhibitors of the oxytocic response of oxytocin. *J. med. Chem.*, 9: 647–650.

Schwartz, J. and Reid, I.A. (1981) Effect of vasopressin blockade on blood pressure regulation during hemorrhage in conscious dogs. *Endocrinology*, 109: 1178–1780.

Smyth, D.G. (1967) Carbamylation of amino and tyrosine hydroxyl groups. Preparation of an inhibitor of oxytocin with no intrinsic activity on the isolated uterus. *J. biol. Chem.*, 242: 1579–1591.

Vavrek, R.J., Ferger, M.F., Ashled, A.G., Rich, D.H., Blomquist, A.T. and du Vigneaud, V. (1972) Synthesis of three oxytocin analogs related to [1-deaminopenicillamine]oxytocin possessing antioxytocic activity. *J. med. Chem.*, 15: 123–126.

Zerbe, R.L., Baylin, P.H. and Robertson, G.L. (1981) Vasopressin function in clinical disorders of water balance. In C. Beardwell and G.L. Robertson (Eds.), *The Pituitary*, Butterworths Int. Med. Rev., London, pp. 297–329.

The Neurohypophysis: Structure, Function and Control, Progress in Brain Research, Vol. 60, edited by B.A. Cross and G. Leng
© *1983 Elsevier Science Publishers B.V.*

Vasopressin: Mechanisms of Receptor Activation

S. JARD

Centre CNRS-INSERM de Pharmacologie-Endocrinologie, rue de la Cardonille, B.P. 5055, 34033 Montpellier Cedex (France)

INTRODUCTION

Besides its well known roles in the regulation of body fluid osmolality and blood pressure, vasopressin exerts a large variety of biological effects. Among these are: increased glycogenolysis and neoglucogenesis by liver cells (Hems and Whitton, 1973), increased corticotropin release by the adenohypophysis (Gillies et al., 1978), platelet aggregation (Haslam and Rosson, 1972), mitogenic effects on several cell types (Hunt et al., 1977; Miller et al., 1977; Whitfield et al., 1970; Rozengurt et al., 1979), increased firing rate of several neuronal groups in the brain (Mühlethaler et al., 1982), and several effects on animal behaviour (De Wied and Bohus, 1978; De Wied and Versteeg, 1979). It is clearly established (Sawyer et al., 1974) that structural modifications of the vasopressin molecule affect its biological activities in a differential manner depending on the target tissue considered. In addition, vasopressin acts either through cyclic AMP-dependent (antidiuretic effect) or cyclic AMP-independent, calcium-dependent (vasopressor and glycogenolytic effects, among others) mechanisms (for review see Jard and Bockaert, 1975; De Wulf et al., 1980). Therefore, it can be concluded that, in mammals, there are at least two types of vasopressin receptors (vasopressin isoreceptors). The subdivision of vasopressin receptors into two classes (V_1 and V_2 vasopressin receptors) was formally introduced by Michell et al. (1979) on the basis of the different nature of the effectors to which these receptors are coupled: adenylate cyclase (V_2-receptors) or the effector responsible for an increase in calcium entry into the cell and(or) mobilization of cellular calcium stores.

The purpose of the present article is to review the available pharmacological and biochemical data on vasopressin receptors in mammals. The discussion will be restricted to those receptors for which binding data are presently available.

KINETICS OF VASOPRESSIN BINDING TO VASOPRESSIN RECEPTORS

Specific vasopressin binding sites which could be identified to vasopressin receptors involved in vasopressin-induced adenylate cyclase activation have been characterized on membranes prepared from porcine (Bockaert et al., 1973; Roy et al., 1975a, b), bovine (Hechter et al., 1978), rat (Rajerison et al., 1974; Butlen et al., 1978) and human kidneys (Guillon et al., 1982). In all cases [^{3}H]vasopressin binding was found to be time-dependent, reversible and saturable. Scatchard plots derived from the determination of the dose-dependency for hormone binding at equilibrium did not show any clear deviation from linearity. This indicates that there is no cooperativity in hormonal binding. This conclusion was confirmed by the similarity of the dissociation constants as evaluated independently from equilibrium saturation and kinetic data. The apparent homogeneity in the population of vasopressin binding sites present in membrane preparations derived from the medullopapillary portion of the kidney suggests that vasopressin receptors from collecting ducts and ascending limbs of the loops of Henlé, the two segments of the nephron containing a vasopressin-sensitive adenylate cyclase (Imbert et al., 1975a, b), have similar properties with respect to the kinetics of hormonal binding. As indicated in Table I, the determined dissociation constants (K_d) for vasopressin binding to renal vasopressin receptors are somewhat different depending on the mammalian species considered, ranging from 0.4 nM in the rat to 10–20 nM in the pig. In contrast to the data obtained on membrane preparations, binding studies on intact LLC-PK1 cells * showed a marked heterogeneity in the population of vasopressin binding sites present on these cells as revealed by curvilinear Scatchard plots of the equilibrium dose–binding relationship (Roy and Ausiello, 1981). A precise analysis of the kinetics of vasopressin binding to LLC-PK1 cells, including determination of the rate of formation and dissociation of hormone–receptor complexes, led Roy and Ausiello to conclude that neither negative cooperativity nor binding to two or more independent populations of binding sites could adequately account for the kinetics of hormonal binding to LLC-PK1 cells. The experimental data could be fitted with a model involving a hormone-induced change in receptor affinity. The authors (Roy et al., 1981) provided convincing evidence suggesting that this change in receptor affinity reflects a rapid desensitization of vasopressin-sensitive adenylate cyclase activity. Thus, receptor transition was not apparent in purified membranes from LLC-PK1 cells or EDTA-treated cells, two preparations in which rapid desensitization of vasopressin-sensitive adenylate cyclase activity did not occur. For all the above-mentioned biological preparations numerous correlations between hormone binding and adenylate cyclase activation could be demonstrated (for review see Jard et al., 1975). These correlations clearly demonstrate that the specific vasopressin binding sites detected on kidney membrane fractions and LLC-PK1 cells are the hormonal receptors involved in adenylate cyclase activation.

TABLE I

KINETICS OF VASOPRESSIN BINDING TO RENAL MEDULLOPAPILLARY MEMBRANES

Species	Equilibrium dissociation constant (nM)	Binding capacity pmol/mg protein	Reference
Ox	1.4–4[a]	1.3–4	Hechter et al. (1978)
Pig	10–20[b]	1.0	Bockaert et al. (1973)
Rat	0.4 ± 0.1[a]	0.22 ± 0.02	Rajerison et al. (1974)
Human	4.0[a]	0.5–0.8	Guillon et al. (1982)

[a] Value for arginine-vasopressin.
[b] Value for lysine-vasopressin.

* LLC-PK1 cells are an established pig kidney cell line which maintains characteristics of polar epithelial cells and responds to vasopressin by an increased cAMP production and subsequent activation of cAMP-dependent protein kinase (Mills et al., 1979; Ausiello et al., 1980).

TABLE II

KINETICS OF VASOPRESSIN BINDING TO LIVER AND VASCULAR VASOPRESSIN RECEPTORS

All values refer to arginine-vasopressin.

Receptor source	Equilibrium dissociation constant (nM)	Binding capacity pmol/mg protein or fmol/10^6 cells	Reference
Isolated rat hepatocytes	8	320	Cantau et al. (1980)
Rat liver membranes	3	0.8	Cantau et al. (1980)
Rat aortic myocytes in culture	12	40	Penit et al. (1982)

Extrarenal vasopressin receptors have been characterized on isolated rat hepatocytes and purified liver membranes (Cantau et al., 1980), and on rat aortic smooth muscle cells in primary culture (Penit et al., 1983). On isolated hepatocytes and purified liver membranes vasopressin binds to an apparently homogeneous population of sites. The apparent dissociation constants for [^{3}H]vasopressin binding to isolated cells and purified membranes are different: 8 and 3 nM, respectively. As will be discussed later, this difference probably reflects the effects of "agonist-specific" modulators of receptor function operating in intact cells. The dissociation constant of 3 nM determined on purified rat liver membranes is about ten times higher than that determined on kidney membranes from the same species (compare data from Tables I and II). The maximal vasopressin binding capacity of isolated hepatocytes was 320 fmol/10^6 cells, a figure about three times higher than those found on LLC-PK1 cells. The vasopressin binding sites detected on isolated hepatocytes were identified to the receptors involved in phosphorylase activation on the following grounds: (1) [^{3}H]vasopressin binding was inhibited by vasopressin structural analogues which were shown to inhibit vasopressin-induced phosphorylase activation. A close correspondence was found between the K_d values for the binding of these analogues to hepatocytes and the corresponding inhibition constants (K_i); and (2) the same order of potency was found when the activities of a series of vasopressin analogues were measured by their abilities either to promote phosphorylase activation or to inhibit [^{3}H]vasopressin binding. However, the apparent dissociation constants (K_d) were found to be 5–50 times higher than the corresponding phosphorylase activation constants (K_a).

The specific vasopressin binding sites detected on rat aortic myocytes maintained in primary culture had a similar affinity for vasopressin to that of vasopressin receptors on isolated hepatocytes (Table II). The maximal binding capacity of myocytes (40 fmol/10^6 cells) was about eight times less than that of hepatocytes. For a series of five antivasopressor peptides, the determined pK_d* values for binding to aortic myocytes were almost identical to the corresponding pA_2* values for inhibition of the vasopressor response to vasopressin in vivo. For a series of 15 vasoactive vasopressin analogues a clear correlation could be demonstrated between their respective vasopressor activities and the corresponding K_d values for binding to aortic myocytes. Together these data suggest that the vasopressin binding sites on aortic myocytes in primary culture belong to the main class of vasopressin receptors involved in the vasopressor response to vasopressin.

---

* pK_d is the negative logarithm of the binding dissociation constant (K_d); pA_2 is the negative logarithm of the molar concentration of antagonist that reduces the response to 2 x units of agonist to equal the response to 1 x unit in the absence of antagonist.

MODULATORS OF VASOPRESSIN RECEPTOR FUNCTION: COMPARATIVE STUDIES WITH RENAL AND EXTRARENAL VASOPRESSIN RECEPTORS

The kinetics of vasopressin binding to renal and extrarenal vasopressin receptors is affected by magnesium ions and triphosphonucleotides. As shown in Fig. 1, binding of [³H]vasopressin to LLC-PK1 cells and to purified liver membranes exhibits an absolute requirement for the presence of magnesium ions in the incubation medium. The effect of reducing the magnesium concentration is to reduce receptor affinity. On liver membranes it could be shown that the magnesium effect is agonist-specific. Receptor affinity for vasopressin and several analogues active in promoting phosphorylase activation is reduced when magnesium concentration is decreased while, under the same conditions, receptor affinity for antagonists of the glycogenolytic response is unchanged. The corresponding data for renal vasopressin receptors have

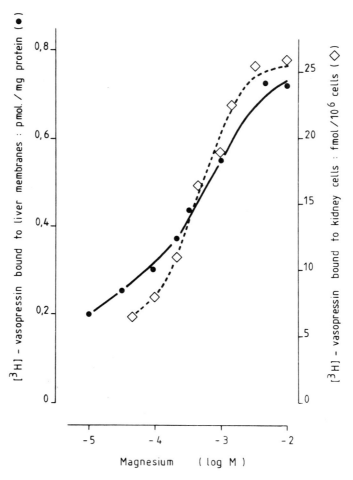

Fig. 1. Effect of Mg²⁺ on [³H]vasopressin binding to LLC-PK1 cells and rat liver membranes. LLC-PK1 cells (◊) and rat liver membranes (●) were incubated in the presence of the indicated amounts of magnesium together with 3.3 nM (◊) or 0.5 nM (●) [³H]vasopressin. For both LLC-PK1 cells and liver membranes the [³H]vasopressin concentrations used represented about one-third of the corresponding K_d values. The observed changes in the amount of hormone bound reflect changes in receptor affinity. Data on LLC-PK1 cells are taken from Roy and Ausiello (1981). Details on the vasopressin binding assay on liver membranes are given in Cantau et al. (1980).

not been collected. The dose-dependencies determined on liver membranes and LLC-PK1 cells are similar, with an apparent K_m value for magnesium of about 0.5 mM. These data suggest that magnesium ions act at the external border of the membrane.

Kidney and liver vasopressin receptors are sensitive to triphosphonucleotides. The nucleotide effect results in an increased dissociation rate of hormone–receptor complexes and a corresponding increase in the equilibrium dissociation constant. The nucleotide effects on kidney and hepatic vasopressin receptors could be clearly distinguished on the basis of their dose-dependencies and specificities (Fig. 2). ATP and GTP are equally active on liver membranes, with an apparent K_m value of 0.5 mM. It is likely that hydrolysis of ATP or GTP is involved in their effects. Thus, 5'-guanylylimidodiphosphate (Gpp(NH)p) and 5'-adenylylimidodiphosphate are inactive. In contrast, Gpp(NH)p is almost as active as GTP on renal vasopressin receptors with an apparent K_m value in the micromolar range. ATP is far less active than GTP or Gpp(NH)p. Furthermore, in the experiments shown in Fig. 2, one can hardly exclude that the ATP effect observed in the millimolar range is not due to small amounts of GTP contaminating the ATP preparation used. On both liver and kidney membranes the nucleotide effect was found to be agonist-specific.

The agonist-specific character of the magnesium and nucleotide effects on renal and extrarenal vasopressin receptors could indicate that these agents are involved in the transduction mechanisms triggered by these receptors. Alternatively, magnesium and triphosphonucleotides could be involved in the desensitization of vasopressin receptors. Indeed, it has been clearly established that desensitization of membrane receptors for hormones and neurotransmitters is induced by the binding of agonists but not by the binding of antagonists. Anyway, the above-described data indicate clearly that renal and hepatic vasopressin receptors differ with respect to their sensitivities to triphosphonucleotides.

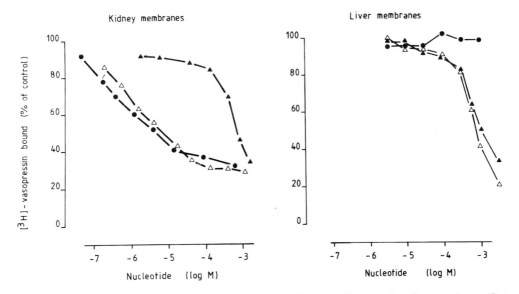

Fig. 2. Effects of triphosphonucleotides on [³H]vasopressin binding to rat kidney and rat liver membranes. Rat kidney membranes (left panel) and rat liver membranes (right panel) were incubated in the presence of [³H]vasopressin and the indicated amounts of ATP (▲), GTP (△) or 5'-guanylylimidodiphosphate (●). The [³H]vasopressin concentrations used were adjusted to equal about one-third of the K_d value. The observed changes in the amount of bound hormone mainly reflect changes in receptor affinity. Data on rat kidney membranes are taken from Rajerison (1979).

For experimental details on the vasopressin binding assays see Rajerison (1979) and Cantau et al. (1980).

388

PHYSICOCHEMICAL PROPERTIES AND RECOGNITION PATTERNS OF RENAL AND EXTRARENAL VASOPRESSIN RECEPTORS

Vasopressin receptors from kidney and liver membranes can be solubilized in an active form under the influence of non-ionic detergents (Roy et al., 1975c; Guillon et al., 1980). Determination of the hydrodynamic properties of rat kidney and rat liver receptors indicated (Guillon et al., 1981) that these two receptors are hydrophobic and highly asymmetrical proteins of similar sizes (Table III). Kidney and liver vasopressin receptors could not be

TABLE III

MOLECULAR PARAMETERS OF SOLUBILIZED VASOPRESSIN RECEPTORS

Experimental data are taken from Guillon et al. (1980)

	Liver receptor	Kidney receptor
Stokes radius (nm)	5.4 + 0.1 (5)	5.6 + 0.1 (7)
Apparent sedimentation coefficient in		
H_2O gradient, Sapp (S)	3.7 + 0.1 (6)	3.5 + 0.2 (6)
D_2O gradient, Sapp (S)	3.4 + 0.1 (6)	3.0 + 0.1 (6)
Standard sedimentation coefficient, S_2OW (S)	3.7	3.7
Partial specific volume (ml/g)	0.75 + 0.01 (10)	0.78 + 0.02 (14)
Frictional ratio, F/F_o	1.81	1.77
Apparent molecular weight, M_r	92,000	101,000
Detergent bound (mg/mg protein)	0.09	0.22
Molecular weight of the protein moiety, M_r	83,000	80,000

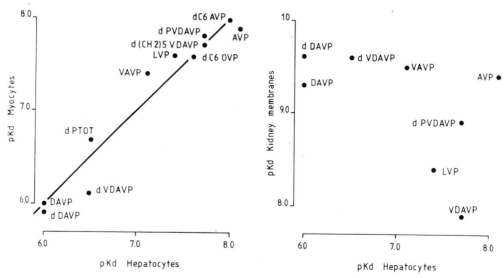

Fig. 3. Recognition patterns of vasopressin receptors from rat kidney membranes, isolated hepatocytes and aortic myocytes. The figure was constructed from published data by Butlen et al. (1978), Cantau et al. (1980) and Penit et al. (1982). Abbreviations: AVP, arginine-vasopressin; LVP, lysine-vasopressin; DAVP, [8-D-arginine]vasopressin; VAVP, [4-valine]arginine-vasopressin; VDAVP, [4-valine, 8-D-arginine]vasopressin; dC6AVP, deamino-6-carba-arginine-vasopressin; dC6OVP, deamino-6-carba-8-ornithine-vasopressin; dVDAVP, deamino-[4-valine, 8-D-arginine]vasopressin; d(CH2)5-VDAVP, [1-(β-mercapto-β, β-cyclopentamethylenepropionic acid),4-valine,8-D-arginine]vasopressin; dPTOT, 1-deminopenicillamine-[4-threonine]oxytocin; dPVDAVP, 1-deaminopenicillamine-[4-valine,8-D-arginine]vasopressin.

distinguished on the basis of any of the hydrodynamic parameters which can be determined by classical biochemical methods.

Pharmacological studies using a large series of vasopressin structural analogues revealed (Fig. 3) the existence of striking similarities in the respective recognition patterns of vasopressin receptors from rat hepatocytes and rat aortic myocytes. Marked differences could be demonstrated between the recognition patterns of hepatic and aortic receptors on the one hand, and renal receptors on the other hand. As recognized from pharmacological studies in vivo (for review see Manning and Sawyer, 1977), substitution of D-arginine for L-arginine in position 8 and(or) substitution of valine for asparagine in position 4, affect the affinity of the vasopressin molecule for renal and extrarenal receptors in a clearly differential manner.

TRANSDUCTION MECHANISMS TRIGGERED BY VASOPRESSIN RECEPTORS

The molecular mechanisms involved in renal adenylate cyclase activation by vasopressin are probably similar to those which operate in the most extensively studied systems such as the glucagon-sensitive adenylate cyclase from liver or the β-adrenergic receptor-coupled enzyme from turkey erythrocytes (for review see Levitsky, 1982). Hormone-sensitive adenylate cyclases are composed of three distinct molecular entities: a receptor unit (R), a catalytic unit (C), and a coupling unit frequently denominated nucleotide regulatory unit (N). According to current views (see Levitski, 1982), both hormone binding to R and GTP binding to N are required to induce activation of C. The active state of the system decays concomitantly with the hydrolysis of GTP to GDP and P_i at the N regulatory site. Replenishment of N with GTP and the continued presence of hormone at the receptor ensures the ability of the system to reacquire its active cAMP producing state. This "on–off" cycle accounts for most of the properties of hormone-dependent adenylate cyclases. In the case of vasopressin-sensitive adenylate cyclase, it could be demonstrated that: (1) vasopressin receptors and adenylate cyclase are distinct molecular entities which can be physically separated by various biochemical methods (Guillon et al., 1981); (2) the guanylnucleotide binding component involved in adenylate cyclase activation by sodium fluoride and guanylnucleotides has been indirectly identified in renal membranes (Guillon et al., 1981); and (3) GTP and the non-hydrolysable GTP analogue 5′-guanylylimidodiphate, markedly increase the sensitivity of rat (Rajerison, 1979) and human (Guillon et al., 1982) kidney adenylate cyclase to stimulation by vasopressin. Several models of receptors to adenylate coupling have been proposed. The more frequently discussed models are the so-called "collision coupling" model and the shuttle-ternary activation model. According to the first model (Tolkovsky and Levitski, 1978), the hormone–receptor complex makes a transient encounter with the adenylate cyclase complex viewed as a fairly stable complex formed between the catalytic unit and the N component (1). The intermediary $HR.N_{GTP}C$ complex does not accumulate.

$$HR + N_{GTP}C \rightleftharpoons HRN_{GTP}C \rightarrow HR + N_{GTP}C'$$
$$N_{GTP}C' \rightarrow NC + GDP + P_i \tag{1}$$

in which C′ and C represent the activated and non-activated forms of the catalytic unit, respectively.

The collision coupling model contains the implicit assumption that one hormone–receptor complex can activate more than one adenylate cyclase molecule, as suggested by Jard et al. (1975) in the case of vasopressin-sensitive adenylate cyclase. In the shuttle ternary activation model it is assumed that the hormone–receptor complex can form a fairly stable complex with the N regulatory component according to the following scheme:

$$HR + N_{GTP} \rightleftharpoons HRN_{GTP} \rightarrow R + N'_{GTP} + H$$
$$N'_{GTP} + C \rightarrow N'_{GTP}C' \tag{2}$$

This model offers the advantage of accounting for the existence of two affinity states of the receptor and the role of guanylnucleotides in the interconversion between these two states. A precise analysis of the kinetics of adenylate cyclase activation by vasopressin allowing to select the most adequate model has not been performed yet. Anyway, the abovementioned models do not predict that for all hormonal concentrations the fractional enzyme activation is identical to the fractional receptor occupancy. They can account for the observation that renal adenylate cyclase activation is a saturable function of receptor occupancy. Half-maximal adenylate cyclase activation is obtained for a fractional receptor occupancy less than 0.5. The non-linearity in the coupling of hormone binding to response, as estimated by the ratio of vasopressin concentrations leading to half-maximal binding and half-maximal adenylate cyclase activation, varies somewhat depedending on the mammalian species considered: 40, 5, 5 and 1.2, for porcine (Jard et al., 1975), bovine (Hechter et al., 1978), rat (Butlen et al., 1978) and human (Guillon et al., 1982) renal adenylate cyclases, respectively. These differences might reflect species differences in the relative number of interacting R, N, and C units. Although marked amplification of the hormonal signal occurs at the cyclic AMP production step, it is clear that vasopressin concentrations eliciting half-maximal adenylate cyclase activation are much higher that hormonal concentrations needed to elicit half-maximal increase in water permeability of isolated collecting ducts (Grantham and Burg, 1966) or half-maximal antidiuretic response in vivo. These observations suggest that an additional amplification of the hormonal signal also occurs at steps beyond the cyclic AMP production step. This conclusion is supported by the observation that vasopressin structural analogues which behave as partial agonists of low intrinsic activity at the adenylate cyclase activation step are able to induce a full antidiuretic response in vivo (Butlen et al., 1978).

The primary involvement of changes in cell calcium fluxes in the glycogenolytic response to vasopressin stimulation of isolated hepatocytes has been convincingly established (for review see De Wulf et al., 1980). There is also much evidence that a rise in cytosolic calcium concentration is also the initiator of the contraction of vascular smooth muscle in response to vasopressin stimulation. Conversely it has been established that vasopressin receptors in liver and vascular smooth muscle cells are neither positively nor negatively coupled to adenylate cyclase.

In rat hepatocytes (Kirk et al., 1977) and rat aorta (Takhar and Kirk, 1981) vasopressin increases the incorporation of ^{32}P into phosphatidylinositol. Stimulated phosphatidylinositol breakdown followed by compensatory resynthesis is a response of a wide variety of cells to many hormones and neurotransmitters acting through cyclic-AMP independent mechanisms. Michell and collaborators (Michell et al., 1979; Billah and Michell, 1979) have developed the view that phosphatidylinositol breakdown might be a reaction intrinsic to the same unitary mechanism whereby these hormones bring about calcium mobilization in their target cells.

Several arguments support the proposal by Michell and collaborators that a causal relationship between hormone-induced increase in phosphatidylinositol breakdown and calcium mobilization are as follows: (1) the phosphatidylinositol response appears to occur independently of hormone-induced changes in cytosolic calcium concentration (Billah and Michell, 1979). Thus, phosphatidylinositol breakdown and labelling are resistant at least partially to calcium elimination from the incubation medium, a situation in which phosphorylase activation by vasopressin is abolished. Furthermore, admission of calcium into hepatocytes with the ionophore A23187 does not elicit the phosphatidylinositol response (Billah and Michell, 1979); (2) stimulation of phosphatidylinositol breakdown by vasopressin is rapid. The effect is clearly detectable within 1–2 min after addition of vasopressin (Kirk et al., 1977; Tolbert et al., 1980); (3) studies by Kirk et al. (1981), using vasopressin structural analogues, indicate that dose–response curves for phosphorylase activation and for enhanced phosphatidylinositol metabolism are parallel suggesting that the same receptor population is responsible for triggering both responses; (4) comparison of the dose-dependencies for the four different detectable effects of vasopressin on isolated hepatocytes, namely binding of the hormone to the receptor (Cantau et al., 1980), increase in phosphatidylinositol turnover (Kirk et al., 1981), increase in calcium fluxes and the final glycogenolytic response, indicate that the A_{50} value for the phosphatidylinositol effect is almost identical to the dissociation constant for vasopressin binding to hepatocytes. On the other hand, vasopressin-induced increase in ^{45}Ca uptake can be detected upon exposure of hepatocytes to 0.1 nM vasopressin; phosphorylase activation is detectable for about ten times less than concentration. These results are compatible with the supposed sequence of events: hormone binding to the receptor, increase in phosphatidylinositol turnover, rise in cytosolic calcium concentration with subsequent triggering of the calcium-dependent mechanisms of phosphorylase activation. They also suggest that a marked amplification exists between the primary signal in hormone action and the final biological response, and that the larger part of this amplification occurs between the phosphatidylinositol breakdown step and calcium mobilization. Parallel determinations of K_d values for the binding of vasopressin structural analogues to rat hepatocytes and of K_a values for phosphorylase activation, showed (Cantau et al., 1980) that the ratios K_d/K_a, an estimate of the amplification of the hormonal signal, were not identical for all analogues tested. Furthermore, the additive character of several amino acid substitutions was clearly apparent. Thus (Table IV), substitution of D-arginine for L-arginine led to a 2.5-fold decrease in the K_d/K_a ratio as compared to that observed for arginine-vasopressin. Deamination of [8-D-arginine]vasopressin led to a further 5-fold decrease in the K_d/K_a ratio. The same structural modifications introduced in [4-valine]arginine-vasopressin led to deamino-[4-valine, 8-D-arginine]vasopressin, an antagonist of vasopressin-induced phosphorylase activation for which the K_d/K_i ratio was equal to unity.

TABLE IV

EFFECTS OF STRUCTURAL MODIFICATIONS OF THE VASOPRESSIN MOLECULE ON THE RELATION OF BINDING TO PHOSPHORYLASE ACTIVATION IN RAT HEPATOCYTES

The K_d/K_a value is an estimate of the amplification of the hormonal signal. It is maximal for arginine-vasopressin. It equals unity for the competitive antagonist deamino-[4-valine,8-D-arginine]vasopressin. Intermediate values observed for several analogues might indicate that these analogues are partial agonists at an early step of the hormonal action. Experimental data are from Cantau et al. (1980).

Peptide	K_d/K_a	Magnitude of the phosphorylase response (% of arginine-vasopressin-induced response)
Arginine-vasopressin	50	100
[8-D-Arginine]vasopressin	20	100
Deamino-[8-D-arginine]vasopressin	4	100
[4-Valine]arginine-vasopressin	50	100
[4-Valine, 8-D-arginine]vasopressin	2	100
Deamino-[4-valine, 8-D-arginine]vasopressin	1	0

392

These data suggest that [8-D-arginine]vasopressin, deamino-[8-D-arginine]vasopressin and [4-valine, 8-D-arginine]vasopressin behave like partial agonists at the primary step of vasopressin action on isolated hepatocytes. In line with Michell's hypothesis, it would be of great interest to compare the magnitude of the maximal effect of these analogues on phosphatidylinositol breakdown with that of vasopressin.

The nature of the effector molecule to which hepatic and vascular vasopressin receptors are coupled is not known. By analogy with hormone-responsive adenylate cyclases, it is possible that several receptors triggering calcium-dependent responses in the same cell are coupled to the same pool of effector molecules. In line with such a view is the recent demonstration by Breant et al. (1981) of a heterologous desensitization of the glycogenolytic response in rat liver cells induced by occupation by an agonist of one of three independent receptors which activate the calcium-dependent pathway for phosphorylase activation namely, vasopressin, angiotensin and α-adrenergic receptors.

SUMMARY

Vasopressin receptors have been characterized on renal membranes from several mammalian species and on two extrarenal vasopressin-sensitive cell types in the rat, namely isolated hepatocytes and aortic smooth muscle cells in primary culture. On all biological preparations so far tested vasopressin binds to a single class of sites. The dissociation constant for vasopressin binding to renal receptors varies depending on the mammalian species considered, from 0.4 nM in the rat to 10–20 nM in the pig. In the rat, the affinities of hepatic and vascular vasopressin receptors for vasopressin are similar and about ten times lower than the affinity of kidney receptors. Renal and extrarenal vasopressin receptors have similar hydrodynamic properties. They can be distinguished on the following grounds. (1) Renal vasopressin receptors are coupled to adenylate cyclase. Hepatic and vascular receptors have no direct functional relationship with adenylate cyclase. A primary involvement of a rise of cytosolic calcium in the biological responses triggered by these receptors has been established. In isolated hepatocytes and aorta, vasopressin stimulates phosphatidylinositol breakdown. Available experimental data are compatible with the existence of a causal relationship between vasopressin-induced phosphatidylinositol breakdown and the increase in cytosolic calcium. (2) Kidney and liver vasopressin receptors are affected by triphosphonucleotides. The nucleotide effect results in a reduction in receptor affinity for agonists but not for antagonists. On kidney receptors, the nucleotide effect is specific for guanylnucleotides; it is observable in a micromolar range and does not involve GTP hydrolysis. On liver receptors ATP and GTP are equally active in a millimolar range. Non-hydrolysable ATP and GTP analogues are inactive. (3) Hepatic and aortic vasopressin receptors in the rat have almost identical recognition patterns. This recognition pattern is clearly different from that of kidney receptors.

In all vasopressin-sensitive cells so far tested the dissociation constant for vasopressin binding to the receptors is much higher than the hormonal concentration eliciting half-maximal biological response. This suggests that a marked amplification occurs at steps beyond adenylate cyclase activation (renal receptors) or activation of the primary effector involved in calcium mobilization (hepatic and vascular receptors).

REFERENCES

Ausiello, D.A., Hall, D.H. and Dayer, J.M. (1980) Modulation of cyclic AMP-dependent protein kinase by vasopressin and calcitonin in cultured porcine renal LLC-PK1 cells. *Biochem J.*, 186: 773–780.

Billah, M.M. and Michell, R.H. (1979) Phosphatidylinositol metabolism in rat hepatocytes stimulated by glycoge-nolytic hormones. Effects of angiotensin, vasopressin, adrenaline, ionophore A23187 and calcium-ion deprivation. *Biochem. J.*, 182: 661–668.

Bockaert, J., Roy, C., Rajerison, R. and Jard, S. (1973) Specific binding of (^{3}H)-lysine-vasopressin to pig kidney plasma membranes. *J. biol. Chem.*, 249: 5922–5931.

Breant, B., Keppens, S. and De Wulf, H. (1981) Heterologous desensitization of the cyclic-AMP-independent glycogenolytic response in rat liver cells. *Biochem. J.*, 200: 509–514.

Butlen, D., Guillon, G., Rajerison, R.M., Jard, S., Sawyer, W.H. and Manning, M. (1978) Structural requirements for activation of vasopressin-sensitive adenylate cyclase, hormone binding, and antidiuretic action: effects of highly potent analogues and competitive inhibitors. *Molec. Pharmacol.*, 14: 1006–1017.

Cantau, B., Keppens, S., De Wulf, H. and Jard, S. (1980) (^{3}H)-Vasopressin binding to isolated rat hepatocytes and liver membranes: regulation by GTP and relation to glycogenphosphorylase activation. *J. Receptor Res.*, 1: 137–168.

De Wied, D. and Bohus, B. (1978) The modulation of memory processes by vasotocin, the evolutionarily oldest neurosecretory principle. In M.A. Corner, R.E. Baker, N.E. van de Poll, D.F. Swaab and H.B.M. Uylings (Eds.), *Maturation of the Nervous System, Progress in Brain Research, Vol. 48*, Elsevier/North-Holland, Elsevier, pp. 327–336.

De Wied, D. and Versteeg, D.H.G. (1979) Neurohypophyseal principles and memory. *Fed. Proc.*, 38: 2348–2354.

De Wulf, H., Keppens, S., Vandenheede, J.R., Haustraete, F., Proost, C. and Carton, H. (1980) Cyclic AMP-inde-pendent regulation of liver glycogenolysis. In J. Nunez and J. Dumont (Eds.), *Hormone and Cell Regulation*, North-Holland Publ., Amsterdam.

Gillies, G., Van Wimersma Greidanus, Tj.B. and Lowry, P.J. (1978) Characterization of rat stalk eminence vasopressin and its involvement in adrenocorticotropin release. *Endocrinology*, 103: 528–534.

Grantham, J.J. and Burg, M.B. (1966) Effect of vasopressin and cyclic AMP on permeability of isolated collecting tubules. *Amer. J. Physiol.*, 211: 255–259.

Guillon, G., Couraud, P.O., Butlen, D., Cantau, B. and Jard, S. (1980) Size of vasopressin receptors from rat liver and kidney. *Europ. J. Biochem.*, 111: 287–294.

Guillon, G., Cantau, B. and Jard, S. (1981) Effects of thiol-protecting reagents on the size of solubilized adenylate cyclase and on its ability to be stimulated by guanylnucleotides and fluoride. *Europ. J. Biochem.*, 117: 401–406.

Guillon, G., Butlen, D., Cantau,, B., Barth, T. and Jard, S. (1982) Kinetic and pharmalogical characterization of vasopressin membrane receptors from human kidney medulla: relation to adenylate cyclase activation. *Europ. J. Pharmacol.*, 85: 291–304.

Haslam, R.J. and Rosson, G.M. (1972) Aggregation of human blood platelets by vasopressin. *Amer. J. Physiol.*, 233: 958–967.

Hechter, O., Terada, S., Nakahara, T. and Flouret, G. (1978) Neurohypophyseal hormone-responsive renal adenylate cyclase. II. Relationship between hormonal occupancy of neurohypophyseal hormone receptor sites and adenylate cyclase activation. *J. biol. Chem.*, 253: 3219–3229.

Hems, D.A. and Whitton, P.D. (1973) Stimulation by vasopressin of glycogen breakdown and glucogenesis in the perfused rat liver. *Biochem. J.*, 136 705–709.

Hunt, N.H., Perris, A.D. and Sandford, P.A. (1977) Role of vasopressin in the mitotic response of rat bone marrow cells to hemorrhage. *J. Endocr.*, 72: 5–16.

Imbert, M., Chabardes, D., Montegut, M., Clique, A. and Morel, F. (1975a) Vasopressin dependent adenylate cyclase in single segments of rabbit kidney tubule. *Pflügers Arch.*, 357: 173–186.

Imbert, M., Chabardes, D., Montegut, M., Clique, A. and Morel, F. (1975b) Présence d'une adényl cyclase stimulée par la vasopressine dans la branche ascendante des anses du néphron de rein de lapin. *C.R. Acad. Sci. (Paris)*, 280: 2129–2132.

Jard, S. and Bockaert, J. (1975) Stimulus–response coupling in neurohypophysial peptide target cells. *Physiol. Rev.*, 55: 489–536.

Jard, S., Roy, C., Barth, T., Rajerison, R. and Bockaert, J. (1975) Antidiuretic hormone-sensitive kidney adenylate cyclase. *Advanc. Cyclic Nucleotides Res.*, 5: 31–52.

Kirk, C.J., Verrinder, T.R. and Hems, D.A. (1977) Rapid stimulation by vasopressin and adrenaline of inorganic phosphate incorporation into phosphatidylinositol in isolated hepatocytes. *FEBS Lett.*, 83: 267–271.

Kirk, C.J., Michell, R.H. and D.A. Hems (1981) Phosphatylinositol metabolism in rat hepatocytes stimulated by vasopressin. *Biochem. J.*, 194: 155–165.

Levitski, A. (1982) Activation and inhibition of adenylate cyclase by hormones: mechanistic aspects. *Trends Pharmacol. Sci.*, 3: 203–208.

Manning, M. and Sawyer, W.H. (1977) Structure–activity studies on oxytocin and vasopressin 1954–1976; from empiricism to design. In A. Moses (Ed.), *Proc. Conference on the Neurohypophysis*, Karger, Basel, pp. 9–21.

Michell, R.H., Kirk, C.J. and Billah, M.M. (1979) Hormonal stimulation of phosphatidylinositol breakdown, with particular reference to the hepatic effects of vasopressin. *Biochem. Soc. Trans.*, 7: 861–865.

Miler, R.P., Husain, F., Svensson, M. and Lohin, S. (1977) Enhancement of ^{3}H-methylthymidine incorporation and replication of rat chondrocytes grown in tissue culture by plasma tissue extracts and vasopressin. *Endocrinology*, 100: 1365–1375.

Mills, J.W., MacKnight, A.D.C., Dayer, J.M. and Ausiello, D.A. (1979) Localization of [^{3}H]ouabain-sensitive Na pump sites in cultured pig kidney cells. *Amer. J. Physiol.*, 236: C157–C162.

Mühlethaler, M., Dreyfuss, J.J. and Gäwiler, B.H. (1982) Vasopressin causes excitation of hippocampal neurons. *Nature (Lond.)*, 296: 749–751.

Penit, J., Faure, M. and Jard, S. (1983) Vasopressin and angiotensin II receptors in rat aorta smooth muscle cells in culture. *Amer. J. Physiol.*, 244: E72–E83.

Rajerison, R.M. (1979) *Aspects moléculaires de la Régulation de la Sensibilité à l'Hormone Antidiurétique de l'Adényl Cyclase de Reins de Mammifères.* Thèse de Doctorat d'Etat, Université Pierre et Marie Curie, Paris.

Rajerison, R., Marchetti, J., Roy, C., Bockaert, J. and Jard, S. (1974) The vasopressin-sensitive adenylate cyclase of the rat kidney: effect of adrenalectomy and corticostroids on hormonal receptor–enzyme coupling. *J. biol. Chem.*, 249: 6390–6400.

Roy, C. and Ausiello, D.A. (1981) Characterization of (8-lysine)-vasopressin binding sites on a pig kidney cell line (LLC-PK1). *J. biol. Chem.*, 256: 3415–3422.

Roy, C., Barth, T. and Jard, S. (1975a) Vasopressin-sensitive kidney adenylate cyclase. Structural requirements for attachment to the receptor and enzyme activation. Studies with oxytocin analogues. *J. biol. Chem.*, 250: 3157–3168.

Roy, C., Barth, T. and Jard, S. (1975b) Vasopressin-sensitive kidney adenylate cyclase. Structural requirements for attachment to the receptor and enzyme activation. Studies with vasopressin structural analogues. *J. biol. Chem.*, 250: 3149–3156.

Roy, C., Rajerison, R., Bockaert, J. and Jard, S. (1975c) Solubilization of the 8-lysine vasopressin receptor and adenylate cyclase from pig kidney plasma membranes. *J. biol. Chem.*, 250: 7885–7893.

Roy, C., Hall, D., Karish, M. and Ausiello, D.A. (1981) Relationship of (8-lysine)-vasopressin receptor transition to receptor functional properties in a pig kidney cell line (LLC-PK1). *J. biol. Chem.*, 256: 3423–3427.

Rozengurt, E., Legg, A. and Curd Pettican, P. (1979) Vasopressin stimulation of mouse 3T3 cell growth. *Proc. nat. Acad. Sci. (U.S.A.)*, 76: 1284–1287.

Sawyer, W.H., Acosta, M., Balaspiri, L., Judd, J. and Manning, M. (1974) Structural changes in the arginine vasopressin molecule that enhance antidiuretic activity and specificity. *Endocrinology*, 94: 1106–1115.

Takhar, A.P.S. and Kirk, C.J. (1981) Stimulation of inorganic phosphate incorporation in rat thoracic aorta mediated through V1-vasopressin receptors. *Biochem. J.*, 194: 167–172.

Tolbert, M.E.M., White, A.C., Aspry, K., Cutts, J. and Fain, J.N. (1980) Stimulation by vasopressin and alpha-catecholamines of phosphatidylinositol formation in isolated rat liver parenchymal cells. *J. biol. Chem.*, 255: 1938–1944.

Tolkovsky, A.M. and Levitski, A. (1978) Mode of coupling between the beta-adrenergic receptor and adenylate cyclase in turkey erythrocytes. *Biochemistry*, 17: 3811–3817.

Whitfield, J.P., MacManus, J.P. and Gillan, D.J. (1970) The possible mediation by cyclic AMP of the stimulation of thymocyte proliferation by vasopressin and the inhibition of this mitogenic action by thyrocalcitonin. *J. Cell Physiol.*, 76: 65–76.

The Neurohypophysis: Structure, Function and Control, Progress in Brain Research, Vol. 60, edited by B.A. Cross and G. Leng

Critical Differences Between Species in the In Vivo and In Vitro Renal Responses to Antidiuretic Hormone Antagonists

F.L. STASSEN*, W. BRYAN, M. GROSS, B. KAVANAGH, D. SHUE, L. SULAT, V.D. WIEBELHAUS, N. YIM[1] and L.B. KINTER

*Smith Kline & French Laboratories,
Department of Pharmacology and Department of [1]Medicinal Chemistry,
Philadelphia, PA 19101 (U.S.A.)*

INTRODUCTION

Vasopressin analogues are invaluable tools to study the roles of vasopressin in health and disease, and to elucidate mechanisms of vasopressin action. Recently described vasopressin antagonists (Manning et al., 1981; Sawyer et al., 1981) could also be of therapeutic use as specific and effective agents for the treatment of the syndrome of inappropriate secretion of antidiuretic hormone (SIADH) and hypertension (Cowley et al., 1980; Gross et al., 1981; Schrier and Ishikawa, 1981).

Until recently, most of the vasopressin antagonists reported were potent antipressor agents but did not have diuretic (anti-antidiuretic or "aquaretic"**) activity (Dyckes et al., 1974; Kruszynski et al., 1980; Lowbridge et al., 1978; Manning et al., 1977, 1982c). A major breakthrough was achieved when Sawyer et al. (1981) and Manning et al. (1981) reported in vivo diuretic activity associated with a series of analogues having O-alkyltyrosine substitutions at position two (Larsson et al., 1978) of $d(CH_2)_5VDAVP$*** (Butlen et al., 1978; Lowbridge et al., 1978). These analogues reversed the antidiuretic activity of vasopressin in water-loaded, ethanol-anaesthetized rats and caused diuresis in normally hydrated, conscious rats (Sawyer et al., 1981). Subsequently, we demonstrated that these molecules were potent vasopressin receptor antagonists; they were specific competitive inhibitors of vasopressin binding and adenylate cyclase activation in membranes from pig renal medulla (Stassen et al., 1982a, b).

In addition we reported that one of these compounds, $d(CH_2)_5D$-TyrVAVP (SK&F 100885), inhibited vasopressin stimulation of adenylate cyclase in membranes prepared from human renal medulla (Stassen et al., 1982b). These results suggest that such vasopressin antagonists may be diuretics (or aquaretics) in man. On the other hand, Kinter et al. (1982) have reported that another analogue, $d(CH_2)_5Tyr(Et)VAVP$ (SK&F 100398), a potent diuretic in rats, was only weakly diuretic in conscious dogs. These data indicate that critical species differences in sensitivity to vasopressin antagonists may exist.

---

* Author for correspondence at: Smith Kline & French Laboratories, Department of Pharmacology, P.O. Box 7929, Philadelphia, PA 19101, U.S.A.
** The term "aquaretic" was originally coined by Alvin E. Strack at SK&F Laboratories to denote compounds that selectively promote water excretion.
*** For peptide definitions see under *Peptides* in the Materials and Methods section.

To elucidate the mechanism underlying such species differences we have studied the vasopressin antagonist SK&F 100398 in vitro and in vivo using both rat and dog models. In addition, we have also compared d(CH$_2$)$_5$D-PheVAVP (SK&F 101071), the most potent anti-ADH antagonist reported to date in the same systems (Manning et al., 1982a, b).

MATERIALS AND METHODS

Renal medullary membranes and adenylate cyclase assay

The sources of the reagents, the methods for the preparation of renal medullary membranes, and the assay of adenylate cyclase activity, have been published elsewhere (Stassen et al., 1982b). Briefly, the renal medulla was dissected and homogenized in Tris buffer (pH 7.5) containing 0.25 M sucrose. The 300 g pellet was discarded and the 1200 g fraction was extensively washed in Tris buffer (pH 7.5) without sucrose. In this membrane preparation adenylate cyclase activity was determined by measuring the amount of [^{32}P]cAMP formed from [α-^{32}P]ATP. Agonist activity was determined by measuring cAMP formed in the presence of the drug alone; antagonist activity was assayed in the presence of vasopressin plus the drug.

Hydropenic rats

Male Sprague–Dawley rats (150–250 g body weight; Charles River Labs.) were deprived of food and water for 18 h. Vasopressin antagonists were administered intraperitoneally (0–100 μg per rat). Urine volume and osmolality were determined at hourly intervals. For potency comparison the diuretic activity of a peptide was expressed as the ED$_{10}$ or ED$_{300}$, where the ED$_{10}$ is the dose (μg/kg) required to increase urine flow to 10 ml/kg/4 h, and the ED$_{300}$ is the dose (μg/kg) required to decrease urine osmolality from hydropenic levels (> 1000 mOsm/kg H$_2$O) to 300 mOsm/kg H$_2$O.

Hydropenic dogs

Trained mongrel dogs were deprived of food and water for 18 h. A standard renal clearance protocol was executed. Saline was infused at 0.5 ml/min for the duration of the experiment and urine was collected via a bladder catheter for three consecutive 20 min periods. Subsequently, a bolus of 20 μg/kg SK&F 101071 was administered i.v. followed by an infusion of 2 μg/kg/min for 60 min. Control dogs received the same volumes of saline. Osmolality and volume were determined on urine collected over three consecutive 20 min periods.

Water-loaded dogs

Trained mongrel dogs were prepared with chronic fistulas and allowed at least two weeks of recovery before the experiments. Dogs were fasted overnight and then given oral water loads of 5.0% and 2.5% of body weight 2 and 1 h, respectively, before an infusion of water (0.05% of body weight per min) was started via a gastric fistula. Urine was collected continuously via a bladder catheter at 10 min intervals. After a stable hydrated state was obtained, a bolus of vasopressin (0.9 ng/kg) was administered i.v. A modest antidiuretic response was obtained. The hydration state was maintained by adjusting the infusion rate into the gastric fistula to match renal water loss. The urine flow rate returned to the pre-vasopressin level within 50 min. In control dogs the experiment was repeated twice more (see Fig. 2). In experimental animals the vasopressin analog SK & F 101071 (9 μg/kg) was administered i.v. and urine was collected for three 10-min periods. Subsequently, a second dose of SK&F 101071 (9 μg/kg) was given, followed 10 min later by a vasopressin challenge (0.9 ng/kg). Urine was collected for three 10-min periods.

Peptides

An initial sample of the vasopressin analogue [1-(β-mercapto-β,β-cyclopentamethyl-enepropionic acid),2-(O-methyl)tyrosine,4-valine]arginine-vasopressin (d(CH$_2$)$_5$Tyr(Me) VAVP; SK&F 100501) was kindly provided by Prof. M. Manning. [1-(β-mercapto-β, β-cyclopentamethylenepropionic acid),2-(O-ethyl)tyrosine,4-valine]arginine-vasopressin (d(CH$_2$)$_5$Tyr(Et)VAVP; SK&F 100398), [1-(β-mercapto-β,β-cyclopentamethylenepropionic acid), 2-D-tyrosine,4-valine]arginine-vasopressin (d(CH$_2$)$_5$D-TyrVAVP; SK&F 100885), and [1-(β-mercapto-β,β-cyclopentamethylenepropionic acid),2-D-phenylalanine, 4-valine]arginine-vasopressin (d(CH$_2$)$_5$D-PheVAVP; SK&F 101071) were prepared at SK&F Laboratories along with SK&F 100501. SK&F 100398, 100885 and 101071 were also synthesized for us by Peninsula Laboratories. The peptides were dissolved in saline or 0.1% bovine serum albumin (BSA) for animal and membrane studies, respectively.

RESULTS

In vivo studies

Administration of the vasopressin analogues listed in Table I to conscious hydropenic rats resulted in dose-dependent increases in urine volume and decreases in urine osmolality. Insignificant changes in urinary solute excretion were observed. We also found that these molecules were potent, competitive antagonists of adenylate cyclase activation by vasopressin in membranes of rat renal medulla (Table I).

TABLE I

POTENCY OF INHIBITORS OF ADENYLATE CYCLASE ACTIVATION AND ANTIDIURETIC ACTIVITY IN THE RAT

Values are mean + S.E.M. Numbers of determinations are shown in brackets.

Vasopressin analogue	Inhibition of adenylate cyclase activation K_i $(\times 10^9 \, M^{-1})$	Anti-ADH activity	
		Urine volume ED_{10} $(\mu g/kg)$	Urine osmolality ED_{300} $(\mu g/kg)$
d(CH$_2$)$_5$D-PheVAVP SK&F 101071	5.3 ± 0.6 (3)	23.0 ± 4.0 (9)	23.7 ± 3.2 (9)
d(CH$_2$)$_5$D-TyrVAVP SK&F 100885	5.1 ± 1.1 (4)	38.0 ± 6.0 (6)	31.8 ± 5.4 (7)
d(CH$_2$)$_5$Tyr(Me)VAVP SK&F 100501	6.9 ± 2.3 (2)	54.0 ± 19.0 (3)	65.5 ± 19.0 (4)
d(CH$_2$)$_5$Tyr(Et)VAVP SK&F 100398	6.3 ± 0.3 (4)	38.0 ± 7.0 (4)	57.8 ± 21.3 (4)

398

In contrast to the hydropenic rat, administration of large doses of SK&F 101071 to the hydropenic dog was not associated with changes in urine volume and osmolality (Fig. 1). Also, glomerular filtration rate, renal blood flow and sodium excretion remained unchanged. Doses lower than 140 μg/kg total were also ineffective (data not shown). It is notable that plasma vasopressin levels (measured by a radioimmunoassay) were similar in our hydropenic rat and dog models (4–10 pg/ml plasma).

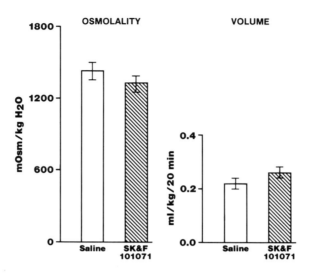

Fig. 1. Effect of SK&F 101071 on urine volume and osmolality of hydropenic dogs. Average urine volume and osmolality were determined of three consecutive 20-min collections. Mean values ± S.E.M. for five dogs are presented. A bolus of 20 μg/kg SK&F 101071 was administered i.v. followed by an infusion of 2 μg/kg/min.

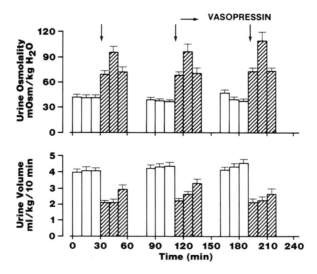

Fig. 2. Effect of vasopressin on urine volume and osmolality of water-loaded conscious dogs. Mean values ± S.E.M. for 15 dogs are presented. Vasopressin (0.3 mU Pitressin/kg) was administered i.v. at the times indicated.

SK&F 101071 was also tested against exogenous vasopressin in a water-loaded, conscious dog preparation. Fig. 2 illustrates that vasopressin administered to this dog preparation reproducibly increased urine osmolality and decreased volume. Within 50 min these parameters returned to pre-vasopressin levels. Tachyphylaxis was not observed and the same responses were obtained upon repeated vasopressin administration. SK&F 101071 injected in a 10,000-fold molar excess at 40 and 10 min before the injection of vasopressin did not prevent the changes in urine volume and osmolality (Fig. 3). Lower doses were also ineffective. Kinter et al. (1982) have reported similar results for SK&F 100398.

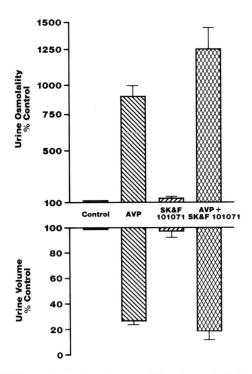

Fig. 3. Effect of SK&F 101071 on urine volume and osmolality of water-loaded, conscious dogs. Volume and osmolality of urine collected over three 10-min periods were determined. Mean peak values ± S.E.M. for four dogs are presented. Columns, from left to right, are: vehicle; 0.9 ng/kg AVP; 9 μg/kg SK&F 101071; 0.9 ng/kg AVP preceded by 9 μg/kg SK&F 101071 at 10 and 40 min.

In vitro studies

SK&F 101071 and 100398 were potent, competitive inhibitors of vasopressin-stimulated adenylate cyclase in dog renal membranes (Table II). The potencies for dog and rat renal receptors were similar; the potencies for pig renal receptors were lower.

SK&F 101071 and 100398 were also tested for activation of basal adenylate cyclase activity. Both molecules partially stimulated adenylate cyclase in membranes of dog renal medulla (Table III). In contrast, no significant activation of rat and pig adenylate cyclase was observed.

TABLE II

INHIBITION OF THE ACTIVATION BY VASOPRESSIN OF ADENYLATE CYCLASE IN DOG, RAT AND PIG RENAL MEMBRANES

Values are mean ± S.E.M. Numbers of determinations are shown in brackets.

Vasopressin analogue	Inhibition of adenylate cyclase activation ($K_i \times 10^9$ M^{-1})		
	Dog	Rat	Pig
d(CH$_2$)$_5$D-PheVAVP SK&F 101071	6.2 ± 1.1 (3)	5.3 ± 0.6 (3)	47.0 ± 1.0 (4)
d(CH$_2$)$_5$Tyr(Et)VAVP SK&F 100398	4.8 ± 0.2 (2)	6.3 ± 0.3 (4)	32.0 ± 1.0 (4)

TABLE III

EFFECT OF VASOPRESSIN ANALOGUES ON BASAL ADENYLATE CYCLASE ACTIVITY

For dog and pig the analogues were tested from 10^{-4} to 10^{-7} M; for rat at 10^{-4} and 10^{-5} M.

Vasopressin analogue	Maximal stimulation of basal adenylate cyclase activity (Δ%)		
	Dog	Rat	Pig
d(CH$_2$)$_5$D-PheVAVP SK&F 101071	33.6[a]	−4.8	−5.0
d(CH$_2$)$_5$Tyr(Et)VAVP SK&F 100398	16.5[a]	−1.9	8.4

[a] Significantly different from control ($P < 0.05$).

DISCUSSION

The vasopressin analogues SK&F 101071, 100885, 100501 and 100398 have previously been reported to inhibit the antidiuretic activity of exogenous vasopressin in ethanol-anaesthetized, water-loaded rats. In our hydropenic rat model these novel diuretic agents also caused increases in urine volume and decreases in urine osmolality (Table I). To elucidate the molecular mechanism of action we studied the effects of these molecules on adenylate cyclase activity of the renal medulla. We found that the diuretic activity was associated with potent and competitive inhibition of adenylate cyclase activation by vasopressin (Table I). Therefore, the diuretic activity of these vasopressin analogues is most likely the result of inhibition of the antidiuretic hormone at the receptors of the renal collecting duct. Inhibition of the pressor activity of vasopressin on the renal vasculature does not seem to play an important role in the diuretic activity, because vasopressin analogues with potent antipressor activity but no diuretic activity have been reported.

In the dog, it was previously reported that SK&F 100398, a potent aquaretic in rats, was a poor aquaretic in a hydropenic model and failed to block the effects of vasopressin in the water-loaded animal. In the present studies SK&F 101071, the most potent aquaretic in rats reported to date, also did not affect water excretion in hydropenic and water-loaded dog models

(Figs. 1 and 3). This could be explained by the absence of vasopressin antagonism at the renal medullary receptor. However, we found that SK&F 100398 and 101071 were potent inhibitors of adenylate cyclase activation by vasopressin in dog medullary membranes (Table II). Plasma vasopressin concentrations in our hydropenic animals were not excessively high and do not explain the observed species specifity of these analogues. It is possible that the analogues were metabolized much more quickly in the dog than in the rat. This also does not appear to be the case. Bioassays of vasopressin antagonist activity in dog plasma measured in hydropenic rats indicated that sufficient concentrations of the analogue were present in the circulation (unpublished results).

On the other hand, the results from the water-loaded dog suggested weak agonist activity in vivo (Fig. 3). This observation was substantiated by in vitro experiments demonstrating significant activation of adenylate cyclase by SK&F 101071 and 100398 in dog tissue, but not in rat and pig tissues (Table III). It is possible that under these experimental conditions net agonist activity prevailed in the dog. The sensitivity for agonist activity varies between species. In the rat, based on in vivo data, Manning et al. (1982a) demonstrated that SK&F 101071 was virtually devoid of agonist activity. We demonstrated directly the absence of agonist activity of SK&F 101071 and 100398 for rat renal adenylate cyclase (Table III).

The conventional diuretics such as furosemide and chlorothiazide act primarily through interference with renal electrolyte handling and are termed saluretics. The vasopressin analogues appear to act on the antidiuretic hormone receptors that regulate the water permeability of collecting duct epithelia. Unlike conventional diuretics, vasopressin antagonists do not appear to be associated with large increases in solute excretion. Thus the mechanisms of action of conventional diuretics and vasopressin antagonists are fundamentally different. To distinguish clearly these two classes of diuretics, we propose the term "aquaretics" for the vasopressin analogues as distinguished from saluretics for the conventional diuretics.

In conclusion, the diuretic activity of the recently described vasopressin analogues is associated with inhibition of vasopressin activation of adenylate cyclase, probably at the level of vasopressin receptors located on renal collecting tubules. Furthermore, a vasopressin analogue may only be an aquaretic in vivo if the molecule, in addition to being a potent inhibitor of adenylate cyclase activation by vasopressin, does not activate basal adenylate cyclase in vitro and is thus not also a partial agonist. Preliminary data of in vitro studies with membranes prepared from human renal medulla indicate that SK&F 101071 is a potent antagonist of vasopressin-stimulated adenylate cyclase and devoid of agonist activity. SK&F 101071 and similar compounds may therefore be aquaretics in man and merit further study.

SUMMARY

A series of vasopressin analogues with diuretic activity in rats was recently discovered by Sawyer et al. (1981). We have demonstrated that the diuretic activity of these analogues is associated with potent inhibition of adenylate cyclase activation by vasopressin in renal medullary membranes. Our laboratories have also reported that, in contrast to the rat, the analogue $d(CH_2)_5Tyr(Et)VAVP$ was only poorly active in the dog. To elucidate the mechanism of such species differences we studied this analogue and $d(CH_2)_5D$-PheVAVP, the most potent antagonist reported to date, in rat and dog models both in vivo and in vitro. In the rat, we found that these molecules were both potent inhibitors of vasopressin-stimulated adenylate cyclase and potent diuretic agents. Insignificant changes in urinary solute excretion were observed. In the dog, little or no diuretic activity was observed at doses up to $140\,\mu g/kg$.

Surprisingly, both analogues were potent inhibitors of adenylate cyclase activation by vasopressin in dog renal tissue. However, the low diuretic potency in the dog could be explained by the activation of basal adenylate cyclase activity of dog renal membranes. Such activation was detected in dog renal membranes but was not found in rat membranes. We conclude that diuretic activity of vasopressin analogues in vivo is associated with: (1) potent inhibition of adenylate cyclase activation by vasopressin, and (2) with the absence of agonist activity in vitro. Critical differences in the sensitivity of renal vasopressin receptors for antagonists exist between species. We propose that the specific water losing activity as caused by vasopressin antagonists be termed "aquaretic" activity, as distinguished from the saluretic activity of conventional diuretics.

ACKNOWLEDGEMENTS

We thank Drs. Maurice Manning and Wilbur H. Sawyer for supplying us with a sample of SK&F 100501, and for the preliminary disclosure to us of the structures of SK&F 100501, 100398 and 101071. The continuing support of Drs. B. Berkowitz and W. Huffman is gratefully acknowledged. We thank Frank Brennan, Robert Erickson, William Mann, Joan Silvestri, Genevieve Sosnowski and James Stefankiewicz for their expert technical assistance, and Carole Cosmas for secretarial assistance.

REFERENCES

Butlen, D., Guillon, G., Rajerison, R.M., Jard, S., Sawyer, W.H. and Manning, M. (1978) Structural requirements for activation of vasopressin-sensitive adenylate cyclase, hormone binding, and antidiuretic actions: effects of highly potent analogs and competitive inhibitors. *Molec. Pharmacol.,* 14: 1006–1017.

Cowley, A.W., Jr., Smith, M.J. Jr., Manning, R.D., Jr. and Hockel, G.M. (1980) Hypertensive and hypotensive roles of other hormones: vasopressin, prostaglandin, and kallikrein-kinin systems. In A.C. Guyton (Ed.), *Arterial Pressure and Hypertension,* W.B. Saunders, Philadelphia, pp. 225–235.

Dyckes, D.F., Nestor, J.J., Jr., Ferger, M.F. and duVigneaud, V. (1974) [1-β-Mercapto-β,β-diethylpropionic acid]-8-lysine vasopressin, a potent inhibitor of 8-lysine vasopressin and of oxytocin. *J. med. Chem.,* 17: 250–251.

Gross, P.A., Horwitz, L., Schrier, R.W. and Anderson, R.J. (1981) Mechanism of hypertensive effect of water retention. In *Proc. 14th Annual Meeting of the American Society of Nephrology,* 57A.

Kinter, L., Sosnowski, G., Mann, W., Shue, D., Gross, M., Brennan, F. and Wiebelhaus, V. (1982) Apparent in vivo species specificity of the vasopressin antagonist, SK&F 100398. *Fed. Proc.,* 41: 1367.

Kruszynski, M., Lammek, D., Manning, M., Seto, J., Haldar, J. and Sawyer, W.H. (1980) [1-(β-Mercapto-β,β-cyclopentamethylenepropionic acid), 2-(O-methyl)tyrosine]arginine-vasopressin and [1-(β-mercapto-β,β-cyclopentamethylenepropionic acid)]arginine-vasopressin, two highly potent antagonists of the vasopressor response to arginine-vasopressin. *J. med. Chem.,* 23: 364–368.

Larsson, L.-E., Lindeberg, G., Melin, P. and Pliška, V. (1978) Synthesis of O-alkylated lysine-vasopressins, inhibitors of the antidiuretic response to lysine-vasopressin. *J. med. Chem.,* 21: 352–356.

Lowbridge, J., Manning, M., Haldar, J. and Sawyer, W.H. (1978) [1-(β-Mercapto-β,β-cyclopentamethylenepropionic acid),4-valine, 8-D-arginine]-vasopressin, a potent and selective inhibitor of the vasopressor response to arginine-vasopressin. *J. med. Chem.,* 21: 313–315.

Manning, M., Lowbridge, J., Stier, C.T., Jr., Haldar, J. and Sawyer, W.H. (1977) [1-Deaminopenicillamine, 4-valine]8-D-arginine-vasopressin, a highly potent inhibitor of the vasopressor response to arginine-vasopressin. *J. med. Chem.,* 20: 1228–1230.

Manning, M., Lammek, B., Kolodziejczyk, A.M., Seto, J. and Sawyer, W.H. (1981) Synthetic antagonists of in vivo antidiuretic and vasopressor responses to arginine vasopressin. *J. med. Chem.,* 24: 701–706.

Manning, M., Klis, W.A., Olma, A., Seto, J. and Sawyer, W.H. (1982a) Design of more potent and selective antagonists of the antidiuretic responses to arginine-vasopressin devoid of antidiuretic agonism. *J. med. Chem.,* 25: 414–419.

Manning, M., Olma, A., Klis, W.A., Kolodziejczyk, M., Seto, J. and Sawyer, W.H. (1982b) Design of more potent antagonists of the antidiuretic responses to arginine-vasopressin. *J. med. Chem.,* 25: 45–50.

Manning, M., Lammek, B., Kruszynski, M., Seto, J. and Sawyer, W.H. (1982c) Design of potent and selective antagonists of the vasopressor responses to arginine-vasopressin. *J. med. Chem.,* 25: 408–414.

Sawyer, W.H., Pang, P.K.T., Seto, J., McEnroe, M., Lammek, B. and Manning, M. (1981) Vasopressin analogs that antagonize antidiuretic responses by rats to the antidiuretic hormone. *Science,* 212: 49–51.

Schrier, R. and Ishikawa, S. (1981) Effect of arginine vasopressin (AVP) antagonist on renal water excretion in glucocorticoid deficient rats. In *Proc. 14th Annual Meeting of the American Society of Nephrology,* 138A.

Stassen, F., Erickson, R., Huffman, W., Stefankiewicz, J., Sulat, L. and Wiebelhaus, V. (1982a) Characterization of novel vasopressin antagonists for vasopressin binding and adenylate cyclase activation in animal and human kidney. *Fed. Proc.,* 41: 1723.

Stassen, F., Erickson, R., Huffman, W., Stefankiewicz, J., Sulat, L. and Wiebelhaus, V. (1982b) Molecular mechanisms of antidiuretic antagonists: analysis of the effects on vasopressin binding and adenylate cyclase activation in animal and human kidney. *J. Pharmacol. exp. Ther.,* 223: 50–54.

The Neurohypophysis: Structure, Function and Control, Progress in Brain Research, Vol. 60, edited by B.A. Cross and G. Leng

Is Vasopressin-Stimulated Inositol Lipid Breakdown Intrinsic to the Mechanism of Ca^{2+}-Mobilization at V_1 Vasopressin Receptors?

C.J. KIRK, J.A. CREBA, P.T. HAWKINS and R.H. MICHELL

Department of Biochemistry, University of Birmingham, P.O. Box 363, Birmingham B15 2TT (U.K.)

INTRODUCTION

In addition to its recently proposed role as a neurotransmitter in the central nervous system (Buijs et al., 1978), vasopressin has three well documented effects in mammals: it causes contraction in vascular smooth muscle (see Altura and Altura, 1977, for a review), it influences hepatic metabolism (e.g. stimulating glycogen degradation; see Hems, 1977), and it stimulates water retention in the kidney tubule (Jaenike, 1961). Studies with synthetic analogues of vasopressin indicate that the ligand-selectivity of the vasopressin receptors found in the liver and vasculature (V_1-receptors) is quite different to that of renal vasopressin receptors (V_2-receptors, Michell et al., 1979). Nevertheless, early attempts to fathom the mechanism of vasopressin receptors were confined to the renal V_2-receptor, which has been shown to activate a membrane-bound adenylate cyclase (see Jard and Bockaert, 1975, for a review).

The likelihood that extra-renal effects of vasopressin are not mediated by receptors coupled to adenylate cyclase emerged in 1974, when Kirk and Hems reported that the glycogenolytic effect of vasopressin in rat liver is not accompanied by an increase in the intracellular concentration of cyclic AMP. A role for Ca^{2+} in the mechanism whereby vasopressin stimulates liver and smooth muscle was suggested by the observations that aortic contraction and hepatic glycogenolysis are diminished in Ca^{2+}-free media (Altura and Altura, 1976; Stubbs et al., 1976) and that the latter effect can be mimicked by the Ca^{2+} ionophore A23187 (Keppens et al., 1977). It seems probable that calmodulin mediates the mechanism whereby an increase in intracellular Ca^{2+} concentration provokes smooth muscle contraction (Adelstein and Eisenberg, 1980) and hepatic glycogen phosphorylase activation (Chrisman et al., 1980), but the way in which activation of V_1-receptors at the plasma membrane increases the intracellular concentration of Ca^{2+} in these tissues remains a mystery.

A ROLE FOR INOSITOL LIPIDS IN V_1-RECEPTOR FUNCTION?

In 1975, Michell first noted that hormones and neurotransmitters which utilize Ca^{2+} as their intracellular messenger also share the ability to provoke a diminution in the cellular concentration of phosphatidylinositol (PtdIns), a quantitatively minor membrane phospholipid. The disappearance of PtdIns in many stimulated tissues, unlike the ultimate physiological responses to such stimulation, is not a consequence of intracellular Ca^{2+} mobilization and it

406

appears to be closely coupled to receptor occupation. These characteristics have led to the proposal that inositol lipid breakdown may have a general role in stimulus–response coupling at Ca^{2+}-mobilizing receptors (Michell, 1975; Michell and Kirk, 1981; Michell et al., 1981).

In addition to PtdIns, eukaryotic cells contain two other inositol lipids: phosphatidylinositol-4-phosphate (PtdIns4P) and phosphatidylinositol-4,5-bis-phosphate (PtdIns4,5P$_2$). In liver, these are quantitatively very minor lipids, each comprising about 1 % of the total cellular inositol lipid pool, and indirect evidence suggests that they may be primarily located at the plasma membrane (Kirk et al., 1981a). The known routes by which the three inositol lipids are metabolised in a number of tissues are shown in Fig. 1.

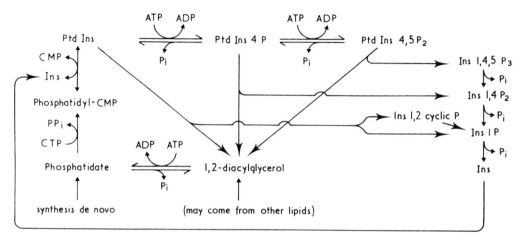

Fig. 1. The metabolism of inositol lipids. The pathways shown are based on an assemblage of information from many tissues; in no single cell type have all the reactions shown been identified. Further information and original sources may be found in Downes and Michell (1982a). Abbreviations: PtdIns, 1-(3-*sn*-phosphatidyl)-L-*myo*-inositol; PtdIns4P, 1-(3-*sn*-phosphatidyl)-L-*myo*-inositol-4-phosphate; PtdIns4,5P$_2$, 1-(3-*sn*-phosphatidyl)-L-*myo*-inositol-4,5-bisphosphate; Ins, inositol; Ins 1P, Inositol-1-phosphate; Ins 1,2-cyclic P, inositol-1,2-cyclic monophosphate; Ins 1,4P$_2$, inositol-1,4-bisphosphate; Ins 1,4,5P$_3$, inositol-1,4,5-trisphosphate.

We have studied the influence of V_1 vasopressin receptor stimulation upon the [^{32}P]PtdIns4,5P$_2$ concentration of hepatocytes in which the monoester phosphate groups of the PtdIns4,5P$_2$ pool have been labelled to equilibrium with ^{32}P$_i$ (Kirk et al., 1981a). Vasopressin provokes a very rapid diminution in the concentration of [^{32}P]PtdIns4,5P$_2$ in these cells (Fig. 2a). Of the cellular complement of this lipid 20 % disappears within 30 sec of hormone treatment, and a maximum decrease in PtdIns4,5P$_2$ concentration (about 30 %) occurs within 1 min. After about 2 min of hormonal stimulation, the radioactivity in PtdIns4,5P$_2$ starts to return towards its prestimulation level, and recent experiments in which we have studied the radioactivity of the individual phosphate groups of PtdIns4,5P$_2$ suggest that this re-labelling represents resynthesis of the lipid towards control levels (P.T. Hawkins, unpublished results). The most rapid phase of PtdIns4,5P$_2$ disappearance coincides with the period during which the Ca^{2+}-mediated activation of glycogen phosphorylase is maximal in the liver cell (Fig. 2b). In contrast, the vasopressin-stimulated diminution in PtdIns concentration in hepatocytes proceeds at an approximately linear rate for 15 min, by which time about 10 % of the hepatic complement of this lipid has disappeared (Fig. 2a; Kirk et al., 1981b).

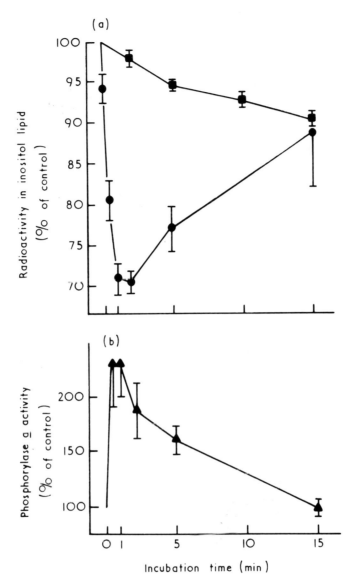

Fig. 2. Time courses of inositol lipid disappearance and glycogen phosphorylase activation in vasopressin-treated rat hepatocytes. a: the disappearance of inositol lipids was assayed as the decrease in [³H]PtdIns in hepatocytes labelled to equilibrium with [³H]inositol in vivo (■; see Kirk et al., 1981b), or as the loss of ³²P from [³²P]PtdIns4,5P₂ in which the monoester phosphate groups were labelled to equilibrium in vitro (●, see text). b: glycogen phosphorylase a activity (▲) was assayed as described by Kirk et al. (1979). 0.23 μM Arg⁸-vasopressin was added to hepatocyte suspensions at time 0. Results are means ± S.E.M. from 3–6 separate hepatocyte preparations.

Unlike vasopressin-induced hepatic phosphorylase activation, PtdIns4,5P₂ disappearance is not abolished in the presence of extracellular EGTA (Kirk et al., 1981a). This suggests that it is not a consequence of intracellular Ca²⁺ mobilization. The concentration dependence of vasopressin-induced PtdIns4,5P₂ disappearance is very similar to that of V₁ vasopressin receptor occupation in hepatocytes, and the concentration of vasopressin which half-

408

maximally stimulates these events is about 50 times that required to cause half-maximal phosphorylase activation (Fig. 3; Kirk et al., 1981a). Ligand selectivity studies and experiments with specific V_1-receptor antagonists confirm that phosphorylase activation and effects upon inositol lipid metabolism are both mediated by V_1-receptors in hepatocytes (Kirk et al., 1979, 1981b; Keppens and De Wulf, 1979). Thus the diminution of PtdIns4,5P$_2$ concentration in these cells appears to be closely coupled to V_1-receptor occupation, whilst the mobilization of sufficient Ca^{2+} within the cell to provoke glycogen phosphorylase activation requires occupation of only a small fraction of V_1-receptors.

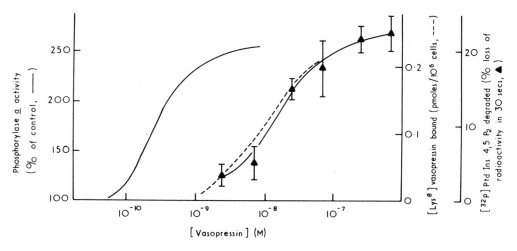

Fig. 3. The relationship between V_1-receptor occupation and hepatic responses to vasopressin. Sources of data are as follows: occupation of V_1-receptors by Lys[8]-vasopressin (----), Cantau et al. (1980, with permission of Marcel Dekker, New York); glycogen phosphorylase activation (——), Kirk et al. (1979). The disappearance of PtdIns4,5P$_2$ (▲) was assayed 30 sec after addition of hormone as described for Fig. 2 (results are means ± S.E.M. from 3–6 separate hepatocyte preparations).

In the experiments described above, we also observed that V_1-receptor stimulation provokes the disappearance of [^{32}P]PtdIns4P: the characteristics of this response are similar to those of vasopressin-induced PtdIns4,5P$_2$ disappearance. However, we would wish to interpret the data concerning PtdIns4P with some caution, since our separation and assay techniques for this lipid do not yield a product as free from contamination as do those for PtdIns4,5P$_2$.

These characteristics of the vasopressin-stimulated depletion of hepatic PtdIns4P and PtdIns4,5P$_2$ in liver are similar to those reported for ligand-stimulated PtdIns disappearance in a variety of tissues (Michell and Kirk, 1981). They are compatible with the notion that vasopressin-stimulated inositol lipid breakdown may have a role in the mechanism whereby V_1-receptor activation provokes Ca^{2+}-mobilization in stimulated cells (Kirk et al., 1981a; Michell et al., 1981).

UNSOLVED PROBLEMS AND FUTURE DIRECTIONS

Recent studies in our own and other laboratories have suggested that PtdIns4,5P$_2$ disappearance may be a more general accompaniment of ligand-stimulated PtdIns metabolism, at least in parotid (L.M. Jones and C.J. Kirk, unpublished results; C.P. Downes, personal communication; Weiss et al., 1982), platelets (Billah and Laptina, 1982) and the blowfly salivary gland (M.J. Berridge, personal communication). It is, therefore, pertinent to pose a number of questions regarding vasopressin-stimulated inositol phospholipid breakdown. (1) Does a single mechanism underlie the reduced concentrations of these three lipids following hormone treatment? (2) If so, what is the primary metabolic event which initiates lipid breakdown? (3) In what way might this primary event be involved in the mechanism whereby vasopressin (and other Ca^{2+}-mobilizing ligands) increases the concentration of Ca^{2+} in the cytosol of stimulated cells?

To consider this last question briefly, there have been a number of suggestions as to how inositol lipid breakdown might be coupled to Ca^{2+}-mobilization in stimulated cells. These have included a putative Ca^{2+}-ionophoric role for the phosphatidic acid which is synthesized from diacylglycerol produced by inositol lipid breakdown (Salmon and Honeyman, 1980; Putney et al., 1980; Barritt et al., 1981) and the notion that a local alteration in the membrane lipid environment may cause a conformational change in a Ca^{2+} binding or "gating" protein (Michell, 1975). We do not intend to speculate further upon these ideas in the present article since we believe that elucidation of the role of inositol lipid degradation will not be achieved until we know the answers to questions (1) and (2) above.

Although the proportions of cellular PtdIns and PtdIns4,5P$_2$ that disappear during hormone stimulation are different (Fig. 2a), the initial rate of lipid depletion is very similar in each case (about 0.2 nmol/g dry wt per sec: Michell et al., 1981; Kirk et al., 1981a). We have therefore suggested that the disappearance of all three inositol lipids may be a consequence of a single initiating reaction; i.e. vasopressin-induced breakdown of one of these lipids may be followed by its resynthesis, thus depleting the liver cell of other inositol lipids (Kirk et al., 1981a; Michell et al., 1981).

In prelabelled hepatocytes vasopressin provokes a rapid loss of radioactivity (either [^{3}H]inositol or ^{32}P$_i$) from the inositol phosphate headgroups of all three inositol lipids. Inositol lipid breakdown via a phosphomonoesterase attack upon PtdIns4P or PtdIns4,5P$_2$ therefore seems unlikely, since this should lead to an accumulation of radioactivity in other inositol lipids. Our method for separating the three inositol lipids involves their deacylation by alkaline methanolysis followed by separation of the released glycerophosphoryl esters by ion exchange chromatography (Downes and Michell, 1981). If vasopressin-stimulated inositol lipid breakdown was a consequence of deacylation by a phospholipase A, this would not influence the products of alkaline methanolysis. Hence a phospholipase A-mediated attack would not be detected by our method and we conclude that the hormone stimulated reaction must involve a phosphodiesterase. This enzyme is probably a phospholipase C, since animal cells have active inositol-lipid specific phospholipases C, but rather little phospholipase D activity (Downes and Michell, 1981, 1982; Irvine et al., 1982).

The water-soluble product of phospholipase C attack on each of the inositol lipids is different (Fig. 1). Hence it should be possible to define the hormone-stimulated reaction in inositol lipid breakdown by identifying these water-soluble products. As yet we have not achieved this in vasopressin-stimulated hepatocytes, but previous studies in acetylcholine-stimulated synaptosomes (Durell and Garland, 1969) and recent experiments with the blowfly salivary gland (M. Berridge, personal communication) suggest that these products may include inositol bisphosphate and/or inositol trisphosphate. In view of the existence of a very active inositol trisphosphate phosphomonoesterase, at least in erythrocytes (Downes et al., 1982), we feel that the hormone-stimulated reaction which initiates inositol lipid breakdown in liver (and perhaps other tissues) is likely to be a phospholipase C-mediated attack on PtdIns4P or PtdIns4,5P$_2$. Future experiments must seek unequivocally to identify this hormone-stimulated event, investigate its control and elucidate its relationship with hormone-stimulated Ca^{2+} mobilization in the cytosol of stimulated cells.

In our opening sentence, we alluded to the suggestion that vasopressin might be a neurotransmitter in the CNS. It is interesting to note that V$_1$-receptors have recently been identified in hippocampal neurones of the rat (Mühlethaler et al., 1982) and recent studies in a colleagues laboratory have indicated that vasopressin stimulates the accumulation of inositol phosphates in rat hippocampal slices (L.R. Stephens and S. Logan, personal communication) and rat sympathetic ganglia (S. Hardy, E.A. Bone, P. Fretton, R.H. Michell and C.J. Kirk, unpublished observations). So it seems likely that information on the mechanism of action of V$_1$-receptors in peripheral tissues may also help us to understand the actions of vasopressin in the CNS.

ACKNOWLEDGEMENT

We thank the Medical Research Council (U.K.) for financial support.

REFERENCES

Adelstein, R.S. and Eisenberg, E. (1980) Regulation and kinetics of the actin–myosin–ATP interaction. *Ann. Rev. Biochem.*, 49: 921–956.

Altura, B.M. and Altura, B.T. (1976) Magnesium withdrawal and contraction of arterial smooth muscle: effects of EDTA, EGTA and divalent cations. *Proc. Soc. exp. Biol. Med.*, 151: 752–765.

Altura, B.M. and Altura, B.T. (1977) Vascular smooth muscle and neurohypophysial hormones. *Fed. Proc.*, 36: 1853–1860.

Barritt, G.J., Dalton, K.A. and Whiting, J.A. (1981) Evidence that phosphatidic acid stimulates the uptake of calcium by liver cells but not calcium release from mitochondria. *FEBS Lett.*, 125: 137–140.

Billah, M.M. and Lapetina, E.G. (1982) Rapid decrease in triphosphatidylinositol in thrombin stimulated platelets. *J. biol. Chem.*, 257: 12705–12708.

Buijs, R.M., Swaab, D.F., Dogterom, J. and Van Leeuwen, F.W. (1978) Intra- and extrahypothalamic vasopressin and oxytocin pathways in the rat. *Cell. Tiss. Res.*, 186: 423–433.

Cantau, B., Keppens, S., De Wulf, H. and Jard, S. (1980) (^{3}H)-Vasopressin binding to isolated rat hepatocytes and liver membranes: regulation by GTP and relation to glycogen phosphorylase activation. *J. Receptor Res.*, 1:137–168.

Chrisman, T.D., Vandenheede, J.R., Khandewal, R.L., Gella, F.J., Upton, J.D. and Krebs, E.G. (1980) Purification and regulatory properties of liver phosphorylase kinase. *Advanc. Enz. Regul.*, 18: 145–159.

Downes, C.P. and Michell, R.H. (1981) The polyphosphoinositide phosphodiesterase of erythrocyte membranes. *Biochem. J.*, 198: 133–140.

Downes, C.P. and Michell, R.H. (1982) Phosphatidylinositol 4-phosphate and phosphatidylinositol 4,5 bisphosphate: lipids in search of a function. *Cell Calcium*, 3: 467–502.

Downes, C.P., Mussat, M.C. and Michell, R.H. (1982) The inositol trisphosphate phosphomonoesterase of the human erythrocyte membrane. *Biochem. J.*, 203: 169–177.

Durell, J. and Garland, J.T. (1969) Acetylcholine-stimulated phosphodiesteratic cleavage of polyphosphoinositides: hypothetical role in membrane depolarisation. *Ann. N.Y. Acad. Sci.*, 165: 743–754.

Hems, D.A. (1977) Short-term hormonal control of hepatic carbohydrate and lipid metabolism. *FEBS Lett.*, 80: 237–245.

Irvine, R.F., Dawson, R.M.C. and Freinkel, N. (1982) Stimulated phosphatidylinositol turnover — a brief appraisal. In N. Freinkel (Ed.), *Contemporary Metabolism, Vol. 2*, Plenum Press, New York, in press.

Jaenike, J.R. (1961) The influence of vasopressin on the permeability of the mammalian collecting duct to urea. *J. clin. Invest.*, 40: 144–151.

Jard, S. and Bockaert, J. (1975) Stimulus–response coupling in neurohypophysial peptide target cells. *Physiol. Rev.*, 55: 489–536.

Keppens, S. and De Wulf, H. (1979) The nature of the hepatic receptors involved in vasopressin-induced glycogenolysis. *Biochem. biophys. Acta*, 588: 63–69.

Keppens, S., Vandenheede, J.R. and De Wulf, H. (1977) On the role of calcium as second messenger in liver for the hormonally induced activation of glycogen phosphorylase. *Biochem. biophys. Acta*, 496: 448–457.

Kirk, C.J. and Hems, D.A. (1974) Hepatic action of vasopressin: lack of a role for adenosine 3′,5′-cyclic monophosphate. *FEBS Lett.*, 47: 128–131.

Kirk, C.J., Rodrigues, L.M. and Hems, D.A. (1979) The influence of vasopressin and related peptides on glycogen phosphorylase activity and phosphatidylinositol metabolism in hepatocytes. *Biochem. J.*, 178: 493–496.

Kirk, C.J., Creba, J.A., Downes, C.P. and Michell, R.H. (1981a) Hormone-stimulated metabolism of inositol lipids and its relationship to hepatic receptor function. *Biochem. Soc. Trans.*, 9: 377–379.

Kirk, C.J., Michell, R.H. and Hems, D.A. (1981b) Phosphatidylinositol metabolism in rat hepatocytes stimulated by vasopressin. *Biochem. J.*, 194: 155–165.

Michell, R.H. (1975) Inositol phospholipids and cell surface receptor function. *Biochem. biophys. Acta*, 415: 81–147.

Michell, R.H. and Kirk, C.J. (1981) Why is phosphatidylinositol degraded in response to stimulation of certain receptors? *Trends Pharmacol. Sci.*, 2: 86–89.

Michell, R.H., Kirk, C.J. and Billah, M.M. (1979) Hormonal stimulation of phosphatidylinositol breakdown, with particular reference to the hepatic effects of vasopressin. *Biochem. Soc. Trans.*, 7: 861–865.

Michell, R.H., Kirk, C.J., Jones, L.M., Downes, C.P. and Creba, J.A. (1981) The stimulation of inositol lipid metabolism that accompanies calcium mobilization in stimulated cells: defined characteristics and unanswered questions. *Phil. Trans. Roy Soc. B*, 296: 123–137.

Mühlethaler, M., Dreifuss, J.J. and Gähwiler, B.H. (1982) Vasopressin excites hippocampal neurones. *Nature (Lond.)*, 296: 749–751.

Putney, J.W., Jr., Weiss, S.J., Van De Walle, C.M. and Haddas, R.A. (1980) Is phosphatidic acid a calcium ionophore under neurohumoral control? *Nature (Lond.)*, 284: 345–347.

Salmon, D.M. and Honeyman, T.W. (1980) Proposed mechanism of cholinergic action in smooth muscle. *Nature (Lond.)*, 284: 344–345.

Stubbs, M., Kirk, C.J. and Hems, D.A. (1976) Role of extracellular calcium in the action of vasopressin on hepatic glycogenolysis. *FEBS Lett*, 69: 199–202.

Weiss, S.J., McKinney, J.S. and Putney, J.W. (1982) Receptor mediated net breakdown of phosphatidylinositol-4,5-bisphosphate in parotid acinar cells. *Biochem. J.*, 206: 555–560.

Neurohypophysial Hormones in Cardiovascular Regulation

The Neurohypophysis: Structure, Function and Control, Progress in Brain Research, Vol. 60, edited by B.A. Cross and G. Leng

Vasopressin Vascular and Reflex Effects — A Theoretical Analysis

A.W. COWLEY, Jr. and B.J. BARBER

Department of Physiology, Medical College of Wisconsin, 8701 Watertown Plank Road, Milwaukee, WI 53226
(U.S.A.)

INTRODUCTION

The role of vasopressin (AVP) in cardiovascular function has not been appreciated until recently. Although we have just begun to evaluate quantitatively the role of AVP in the regulation of the cardiovascular system, some essential points reviewed below are relatively well established. The first is evidence for the participation of AVP in the short-term regulation of arterial pressure by its direct vascular actions. The second is evidence for AVP interaction with the central nervous system baroreceptor reflex pathways.

DIRECT VASCULAR ACTIONS OF AVP

The physiological range of plasma AVP levels is now clearly defined. Plasma AVP concentrations range between 0.3 pg/ml, with water overhydration in amounts averaging 20 ml/kg body weight, to levels between 20 and 30 pg/ml with 48-h water restriction. Plasma AVP levels during surgical procedures and hypotensive haemorrhage may increase to levels exceeding 600 pg/ml. There is now clear evidence that the vascoconstrictor actions of AVP occur in both man and animals at plasma levels associated with endogenous secretion rates (Cowley, 1982).

Arterial pressure does not increase substantially in normal unanaesthetized dogs until plasma levels of AVP are reached which are well above the normal range indicated by the shaded zone in Fig. 1 (Cowley et al., 1974, 1980). The threshold plasma AVP concentration needed to raise mean arterial pressure by more than 5 mm Hg exceeded plasma AVP levels of 42 pg/ml, nearly twice that needed to achieve maximum antidiuretic activity. In contrast, in unanaesthetized dogs which had undergone denervation of sinoaortic baroreceptors, the threshold sensitivity to AVP was decreased nearly 11-fold and the overall pressor sensitivity was enhanced 60–100-fold above normal, as indicated by a shift to the left and an increased slope of the dose–response curve. An even greater enhancement of pressure sensitivity was observed in dogs in which the spinal cord was anaesthetized with alcohol, and all CNS structures above the foramen magnum ablated. In this situation the dose–response relationship was displaced to the left of normal by a factor of 8000 at doses required to increase pressure by 50 mm Hg (Cowley et al., 1974). Comparable increases in vascular sensitivity to AVP have been observed in human subjects lacking baroreceptor reflex responses (Mohring et al., 1980).

[415]

AVP administration to unanaesthetized dogs which raised plasma levels to 15–20 pg/ml raised the total peripheral resistance more than 20 % despite nearly no change of mean arterial blood pressure (Fig. 2) (Montani et al., 1980). In situ microcirculatory techniques have also demonstrated that physiological amounts of AVP can cause significant alterations of both vascular diameter and elasticity (Altura et al., 1965; Monos et al., 1978). These studies, and those from our own laboratory comparing vasoconstrictor actions of various humoral agents, indicate that the direct vascular actions of AVP represent the most potent circulating vasoconstrictor hormone yet studied (Cowley, 1982).

ABILITY OF AVP TO SERVE AS A SHORT-TERM CONTROLLER OF ARTERIAL PRESSURE

The relative importance of endogenously released AVP in the short-term stabilization of arterial pressure has been demonstrated in dogs in which the sympathetic nervous system and renin–angiotensin system were abolished in order to study the independent actions of the vasopressin control system (Cowley et al., 1980). When arterial pressure was lowered rapidly to 50 mm Hg, a prompt recovery to 90 mm Hg was observed within 3 to 4 min. Arterial pressure then stabilized at a level of 85 mm Hg over the next 30 min. This represented a 72 % steady-state fractional compensation of arterial pressure. The response was abolished in the absence of the pituitary gland or when a specific competitive antagonist to AVP vascular effects was injected (dPVDAVP). These results, together with other recent studies, demonstrate that AVP can serve as an independent and rapid controller of arterial pressure during hypovolaemic conditions (Aisenbrey et al., 1981; Andrews and Brenner, 1981; Laycock et al., 1979; Schwartz and Reid, 1981).

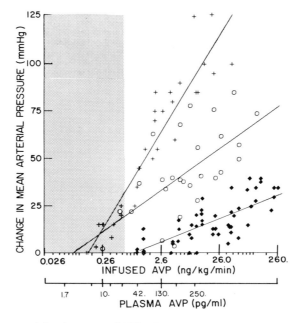

Fig. 1. Relationship between infused amounts of AVP, plasma AVP concentrations, and changes in mean arterial pressure, during three conditions of autonomic reflex activity: normal conscious dogs (solid diamonds, n = 7), conscious sinoaortic baroreceptor-denervated dogs (open circles, n = 6), and dogs with total CNS ablation (crosses, n = 5). (From Cowley, 1982, with permission.)

AVP INTERACTIONS WITH AUTONOMIC REFLEX SYSTEMS

The evidence which first suggested that AVP could influence autonomic reflex pathways is shown in Fig. 1. In these studies, the enhancement of AVP pressor activity in the absence of baroreflexes or with total CNS ablation, was found to be substantially greater than the enhancement of pressor sensitivity observed with other vasoconstrictor agents. For example, angiotensin II and noradrenaline exhibit a 4–5-fold increase in pressor sensitivity following baroreceptor denervation compared to an 80–100-fold increase in pressor sensitivity exhibited by AVP (Cowley et al., 1974; Cowley and DeClue, 1976). These observations suggest that under normal conditions AVP enhances the ability of the autonomic reflex mechanisms to offset changes of arterial pressure.

Studies of Montani et al. (1980) demonstrated that elevations of plasma AVP within the physiological range (1–20 pg/ml) in normal conscious dogs resulted in a lowering of cardiac output so that arterial pressure remained nearly unchanged despite substantial increases of total peripheral resistance. In conscious baroreceptor denervated dogs, comparable elevations of AVP were associated with only slight decreases of cardiac output, and arterial pressure was substantially elevated. These data indicated that AVP was exerting a potent action on the baroreflex pathways.

More direct evidence for AVP interaction with baroreceptor reflexes has been reported in preliminary form from our laboratory (Cowley et al., 1982). Utilizing an open-loop isolated carotid sinus preparation in anaesthetized dogs, elevations of plasma AVP within the physiological range significantly enhanced baroreceptor reflex gain. When plasma AVP concentrations were increased in dogs from control levels of 7 pg/ml to 50 pg/ml, more than a 2-fold increase in the maximum strength of the reflex control system was observed. Enhancement of the feedback gain of the baroreflexes, however, was apparent only when intrasinus pressure was decreased below its normal operating point. Between intrasinus pressures of 50–105 mm Hg, the changes of total peripheral resistance were three times greater at elevated levels of AVP than at normal levels. In addition, elevations of plasma AVP substantially lowered cardiac output at all levels of intrasinus pressure between 40 and 160 mm Hg. The latter response, although not a change in the reflex responsiveness per se, resulted in attenuation of the expected rise of arterial pressure from AVP infusion, thereby mimicking an increase in the reflex gain at elevated levels of AVP. The precise mechanisms whereby AVP modulates autonomic reflex activity remain to be determined.

ANALYSIS OF MECHANISMS WHEREBY AVP COULD INFLUENCE CARDIOVASCULAR SYSTEM

The studies cited above have resulted in several observations for which explanations are not obvious. One problem is that AVP influences specific vascular beds differently (Ericsson, 1971; Schmid et al., 1974; Liard et al., 1982). In some tissues and organs, AVP results in a relative decrease in flow which is greater than the relative fall in cardiac output. This is the case for skeletal muscle, skin, fat and pancreas, where flow is reduced by about 30%. In other tissues, the relative decrease in flow is nearly equal to the relative cardiac output decrease. This is seen in the gastrointestinal tract, the myocardium and brain. Finally, in another group of organs there is no fall in flow at all, notably, the liver and the kidney.

These complex responses coupled with AVP baroreflex interactions have made it necessary to use a fairly detailed model of the cardiovascular system to explain observed changes. To

418

simplify and facilitate the reasoning process, we constructed a mathematical model of the known physical properties of the cardiovascular system. An effort was then made to predict the data that would result from the earlier experiments using various hypotheses. A variety of possible mechanisms could be examined in this way without the need to reason repeatedly through complex interactions in the physical system. The differential equations were programmed in DETRAN and solved on a PDP 11-44, FPS 100 digital computer using predictor-corrector techniques.

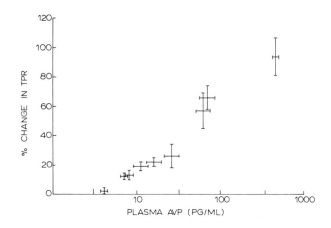

Fig. 2. Composite graph of the influence of changes of plasma AVP on total peripheral resistance determined in dogs. (From Montani et al., 1980; Cowley et al., 1982, with permission.)

The analysis was separated into a physical system representing the functional components affected by AVP (controlled subsystem seen in Fig. 3), and a neurohumoral system (controlling subsystem). The physical system contained a heart–lung and vascular system. The heart–lung was represented as a two-sided heart governed by the filling equations described by Grodins (1959), with the left and right hearts separated by a pulmonary bed with arterial and venous compliance segments (Benekin and Dewit, 1967; Coleman et al., 1974). The vascular portions of the system consisted of three parallel flow beds whose flow originated from a common arterial segment with compliance (aorta) and terminated in a common venous compliant segment (vena cava). Each of the three parallel flow regions was chosen to represent major functional regions of blood flow upon which AVP could exert differential actions. Two of the flow beds were described in terms of an arterial inflow resistance (Ra), a compliance (C), and a venous outflow resistance (Rv). One represented a region with a highly compliant venous system (C_G), such as the visceral circulation and the skin, and received about 30% of the cardiac output. A second represented a region with a relatively low venous compliance (C_M), such as the skeletal muscle at rest, and received about 15% of the cardiac output. The third region was assigned about 50% of the cardiac output and represented those regions such as the kidneys, brain and heart, which exhibit a high degree of blood flow autoregulation. Flow was assumed to be constant in this bed with an equivalent resistance calculated as the perfusion pressure divided by the flow. This was in contrast to the other two parallel flow beds where arterial and venous resistance, unstressed volume, and venous compliance were designed to be strongly influenced by neural and endocrine factors which could be varied in this model. Renal excretory and capillary exchange functions were not considered in this analysis.

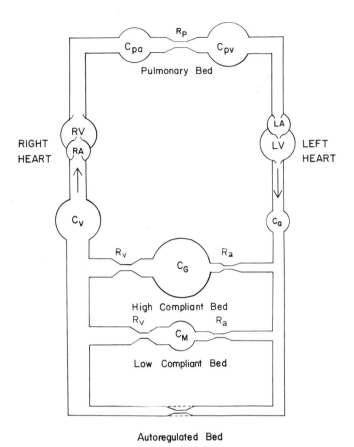

Autoregulated Bed

Fig. 3. Schematic representation of the circulation with parallel systemic flow channels.
Abbreviations: LA, left atrium; LV, left ventricle; RA, right atrium; RV, right ventricle; C_{pa} and C_{pv}, compliance of pulmonary artery (vein); C_a, C_v, C_G and C_M, arterial, vena cava, gut and muscle compliances; R_a and R_v, arterial and venous resistances.

ANALYSIS OF AVP INFLUENCE ON CARDIAC OUTPUT

An initial goal was to account for the unexpectedly small influence of AVP upon cardiac output in the baroreceptor denervated state during graded increases in total peripheral resistance (TPR) brought about by increasing concentrations of plasma AVP. The present analysis indicated that the parallel flow bed systems were hydraulically capable of exhibiting an increased TPR with virtually no decrease in cardiac output; in fact, cardiac output could even increase. Such responses were possible only if one of the parallel beds had a greater vascular compliance than the other. If AVP was assigned twice the potency on arterial resistance in the highly compliant flow bed, then the resulting decrease of intravascular pressures in the compliant bed transferred volume to other high flow segments of the circulation (Fig. 4A). Total peripheral resistance and arterial pressure increased nearly 50% above control levels with less than a 7% decrease of cardiac output as plasma AVP rose to levels of 20 pg/ml. Hydraulic behaviour of this type has been demonstrated in dogs by several investigators (Krogh, 1912; Caldini et al., 1974). Since AVP exerts its greatest vasoconstrictor actions in vascular beds of high compliance such as portions of the splanchnic circulation and the skin, the constancy of cardiac output which is predicted by the present analysis could be a natural consequence of these actions.

A second interesting feature also became apparent in this analysis. As arterial pressure was elevated from AVP vasoconstrictor actions, the overperfusion of the autoregulating flow region resulted in vasoconstriction to maintain a constant blood flow within that region. This enhanced the elevation of arterial pressure to a level even greater than would be predicted by AVP vasoconstrictor actions alone. As AVP exerts minimum vasoconstrictor actions on either the kidney or the brain, these potently autoregulating beds may indirectly enhance changes in TPR induced by circulating AVP.

We next considered the effects of increasing plasma AVP concentrations in the presence of intact baroreceptor reflexes. We first restricted our analysis to predictions of what would occur if the baroreceptors buffered arterial pressure changes in response to AVP solely by controlling arterial resistance to the high and low compliance beds and heart rate. In this case control of arterial pressure with AVP infusion could be controlled only by cancelling in effect the arterial vasoconstrictor actions of AVP. Although pressure was well controlled, as observed experimentally, cardiac output remained nearly unchanged in contrast to the substantial decrease seen in normal dogs. Reflex control was then programmed to control not only arterial resistance equally to the high and low compliance parallel flow regions, but the venous unstressed volume was also reflexly controlled predominantly to the high compliance region (5:1) as well as the heart rate. In this case (Fig. 4B) AVP infusion resulted initially in a direct vasoconstriction of arterial resistance vessels, again with a predominant effect on the region of greatest compliance. The associated rise of arterial pressure stimulated the baroreceptors which lowered heart rate and TPR reflexly to offset the rise of pressure. In so doing, however, cardiac output decreased substantially as plasma AVP levels rose from 4 to 20 pg/ml. Thus, as seen experimentally, arterial pressure rose only minimally despite the large increase in total peripheral resistance.

Thus the analysis indicated that arterial pressure cannot be controlled solely by arterial dilatation. The predictions could be improved considerably if it was assumed that alterations occurred in venous compliance or unstressed volume in the high compliant regions of the system. In this situation, as arterial pressure tended to rise with AVP infusion, there would be a reflex relaxation of capacitance vessels with the resultant removal of blood from the circulation by pooling in the high compliance region. This would decrease cardiac output and buffer the rise of arterial pressure. It was noted that heart rate was also reflexly controlled, but this factor had little effect on cardiac output unless heart rate was driven to levels of less than 30 beats/min.

In brief, the present analysis indicated that most of the arterial pressure regulation with AVP infusion can be explained by reflex control of venous compliance or unstressed volume. The extent to which cardiac output was altered by AVP was dependent on the relative degree of arterial vasoconstriction between the compliant and non-compliant parallel flow beds.

However, not all of the observed actions of AVP were accounted for. In particular, the predicted rise in TPR was less than that seen in normal animals with comparable AVP concentrations. It appears that some mechanism exists whereby the reflex buffering of arterial resistance with AVP infusion is attenuated so that TPR rises to a higher level than would be predicted if the baroreceptors were attempting to offset the rise in resistance. While equations were found which could predict such behaviour, they differed significantly from the classical single set point control theory and went beyond our present understanding of the autonomic nervous system.

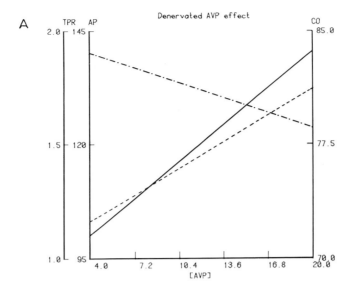

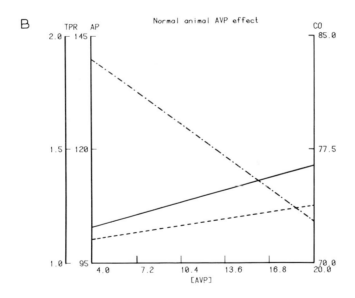

Fig. 4. Relationship between plasma AVP levels (AVP) and the changes in total peripheral resistance (TPR), mean arterial pressure (AP) and cardiac output (CO) in baroreceptor-denervated state (A) and in the normal state (B). CO represented by dash-dot line, AP by solid line and TPR by dashed line.

ANALYSIS OF HAEMORRHAGE

The behaviour of the system in response to haemorrhage yielded results similar to those observed experimentally. Fig. 5 represents the response of the system to the rapid withdrawal

422

of blood and projects the consequences of the overlapping control of arterial pressure by the baroreceptor reflexes and AVP. First, the response in the absence of any neural or humoral control is shown. Following removal of 300 ml of blood in 30 sec, arterial pressure fell from 100 to 55 mm Hg but recovered to only 60 mm Hg (an 11 % recovery). TPR decreased due to the vasodilatation in the autoregulatory segment of the system. Next, the influence of baroreceptors was analyzed using the same degree of control used in Fig. 4A. In this case, arterial pressure stabilized at a level of 85 mm Hg within 1 min (a 67 % recovery), primarily as a result of reflex reduction of the unstressed volume of the veins of the high compliant bed and in the vena cava, which helped restore cardiac output and redistributed 216 ml of blood into the other regions of the circulation. Total peripheral resistance remained nearly unchanged due to the offsetting effects of autoregulated vasodilatation of the autoregulating bed and the reflex-induced increased resistance in the neurally controlled beds.

The third response analysis included both the direct vascular effects of AVP using the vascular effects described in Fig. 3 together with the two-fold enhancement of reflex gain between 50 and 100 mm Hg (Cowley et al., 1980, 1982). In response to the same haemorr-hage, arterial pressure fell only to 92 mm Hg over a period of 4 min (an 85 % recovery). In addition to direct effects of AVP on arterial resistance, enhancement of reflex venous constriction in the high compliant bed with transfer of 230 ml of blood out of this region contributed substantially to the recovery of pressure. With AVP direct vascular effects alone, a 73 % recovery of arterial pressure was obtained.

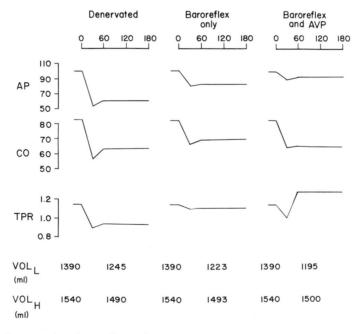

Fig. 5. Predicted responses based on cardiovascular model in response to an equivalent haemorrhage in the absence of neural–endocrine control, with baroreflex control only, and with baroreflex enhancement by AVP together with direct AVP vascular effects. Changes in mean arterial pressure (AP), cardiac output (CO), and total peripheral resistance (TPR), volume of blood in the low compliant region (VOL$_L$), and volume of blood in the high compliant region (VOL$_H$), are indicated in the figure.

Thus, with all of the control systems operating together, arterial pressure recovered to 85% of its control value. Even in the absence of other well-known control mechanisms, such as the renin–angiotensin system and other stretch receptor reflex mechanisms from both the aortic arch and low pressure receptors in the heart, the present analysis coupled with experimental observations indicates that the carotid baroreceptor reflexes and vasopressin could influence the hydraulics of a parallel flow bed system to provide good control of arterial blood pressure during both hypovolaemic states and during normovolaemic states with elevated AVP levels.

ACKNOWLEDGEMENT

Supported in part by U.S. Public Health Service Grants HL 27285 and HL 29587.

REFERENCES

Aisenbrey, F., Handleman, W.A., Arnold, P., Manning, M. and Schrier, R. (1981) Vascular effects of arginine vasopressin during fluid deprivation in the rat. *J. clin. Invest.,* 67: 961–968.

Altura, B.M., Hershey, S.G. and Zweifach, B.W. (1965) Effects of a synthetic analogue of vasopressin on vascular smooth muscle. *Proc. Soc. exp. Biol. Med.,* 119: 258–261.

Andrews, C.E., Jr. and Brenner, B.M. (1981) Relative contributions of arginine vasopressin and angiotensin II to maintenance of systemic arterial pressure in the anesthetized water-deprived rat. *Circulat Res.,* 48: 254–258.

Beneken, J.E.W. and Dewit, B. (1967) A physical approach to hemodynamic aspects of the human cardiovascular system. In A.C. Guyton and E.B. Reeve (Eds.), *Physical Basis of Circulatory Transport: Regulation and Exchange,* W.B. Saunders, Philadelphia, pp. 1–45.

Caldini, P., Permutt, S., Waddell, J.A and Riley, R.L. (1974) The effect of epinephrine on pressure, flow, and volume relationships in the systemic circulation of dogs. *Circulat. Res.,* 34: 606–623.

Coleman, T.G., Manning, R.D., Norman, R.A. and Guyton, A.C. (1974) Control of cardiac output by regional blood flow distribution. *Ann. Biomed. Engng.,* 2: 149–163.

Cowley, A.W., Jr. (1982) Vasopressin and cardiovascular regulation. In A.C. Guyton and J.E. Hall (Eds.), *Cardiovascular Physiology IV. International Review of Physiology,* University Park Press, Baltimore, MD, pp. 189–242.

Cowley, A.W., Jr. and De Clue, J.W. (1976) Quantification of baroreceptor influence on arterial pressure changes seen in primary angiotensin-induced hypertension in dogs. *Circulat. Res.* 39: 779–787.

Cowley, A.W., Monos, E. and Guyton, A.C. (1974) Interaction of vasopressin and the baroreceptor reflex system in the regulation of arterial blood pressure in the dog. *Circulat. Res.,* 34: 505–514.

Cowley, A.W., Jr., Switzer, S.J. and Guinn, M.M. (1980) Evidence and quantification of the vasopressin arterial pressure control system in the dog. *Circulat. Res.,* 46: 58–67.

Cowley, A.W., Jr., Merrill, C.D., Quillen, D.W., Jr. and Skelton, M.M. (1982) Vasopressin enhancement of carotid baroreceptor reflex sensitivity. *Fed. Proc.,* 41: 1116.

Ericsson, B.F. (1971) Effect of vasopressin on the distribution of cardiac output and organ blood flow in the anesthetized dog. *Acta chir. scand.,* 137: 729–738.

Grodins, F.S. (1959) Integrative cardiovascular physiology: a mathematical synthesis of cardiac and blood vessel hemodynamics. *Quart. Rev. Biol.,* 34: 93–116.

Krogh, A. (1912) The regulation of the supply of blood to the right heart (with a description of a new circulation model). *Scand. Arch. Physiol.,* 27: 227–248.

Laycock, J.F., Penn, W., Shirley, D.G. and Walter, S.J. (1979) The role of vasopressin in blood pressure regulation immediately following acute haemorrhage in the rat. *J. Physiol. (Lond.),* 296: 267–275.

Liard, J.F., Deriaz, O., Schelling, P. and Thibonnier, M. (1982) Cardiac output distribution during vasopressin infusion or dehydration in conscious dogs. *Amer. J. Physiol.,* 243: 663–669.

Mohring, J., Glanzer, K., Maciel, J.A., Jr., Dusing, R., Kramer, H.J., Arbogast, R. and Koch-Weser, J. (1980) Greatly enhanced pressor response to antidiuretic hormone in patients with impaired cardiovascular reflexes due to idiopathic orthostatic hypotension. *J. Cardiovasc. Pharmacol.,* 2: 367–376.

Monos, E., Cox, R.H. and Peterson, L.H. (1978) Direct effect of physiological doses of arginine vasopressin on the arterial wall in vivo. *Amer. J. Physiol.,* 234: H167–H172.

424

Montani, J.P., Liard, J.F., Schoun, J. and Mohring, J. (1980) Hemodynamic effects of exogenous and endogenous vasopressin at low plasma concentrations in conscious dogs. *Circulat. Res.,* 47: 346–355.

Schmid, P.G., Abboud, F.M., Wendling, M.G., Ramberg, E.S., Mark, A.L., Heistad, D.D. and Eckstein, J.W. (1974) Regional vascular effects of vasopressin: Plasma levels and circulatory responses. *Amer. J. Physiol.,* 227: 998–1004.

Schwartz, J. and Reid, I.A. (1981) Effect of vasopressin blockade on blood pressure regulation during hemorrhage in conscious dogs. *Endocrinology,* 109: 1778–1780.

The Neurohypophysis: Structure, Function and Control, Progress in Brain Research, Vol. 60, edited by B.A. Cross and G. Leng

Centrally Acting Humoral Factors in the Control of Vasopressin Release

L. SHARE

Department of Physiology and Biophysics, University of Tennessee Center for the Health Sciences, Memphis TN 38163 (U.S.A.)

INTRODUCTION

The major physiological stimuli for vasopressin release are reductions in arterial blood pressure and blood volume and an increase in plasma osmolality. Changes in blood volume and pressure are sensed by receptors in the cardiovascular system (Share and Grosvenor, 1974), and vasopressin release is modified by neural pathways coursing through the central nervous system to the supraoptic and paraventricular nuclei of the anterior hypothalamus. There is also evidence that osmoreceptors, that sense changes in plasma osmolality, are separated from the magnocellular neurosecretory cells of the anterior hypothalamus by at least one synapse (Bridges and Thorn, 1970; Sladek, 1980). It is evident, then, that vasopressin secretion is under neural control. Consequently, neurotransmitters and neuromodulators, acting either at synapses in the central neural pathways that control vasopressin release or directly on the neurosecretory neurones, can affect vasopressin secretion. This review will focus upon recent studies of the central actions of catecholamines, prostaglandins, and vasopressin itself, on vasopressin release.

NORADRENALINE

The heavy noradrenergic innervation of vasopressin neurones in the supraoptic and paraventricular nuclei (Sladek et al., 1980) suggests that noradrenaline has an important function as a neurotransmitter in the control of vasopressin secretion. Reports of the central actions of noradrenaline on the release of vasopressin have been controversial. There have been a number of reports that vasopressin release is stimulated by the central application of noradrenaline (Bhargava et al., 1972; Bridges et al., 1976; Hisada et al., 1977; Hoffman et al., 1977; Milton and Paterson, 1974; Kühn, 1974; Olsson, 1970; Urano and Kobayashi, 1978; Vandeputte-Van Messom and Peeters, 1975). On the other hand, Beal and Bligh (1980) suggested that centrally administered noradrenaline inhibited vasopressin release, and Moss et al. (1971) and Barker et al. (1971) observed that direct application of noradrenaline to neurosecretory cells in the supraoptic and paraventricular nuclei inhibited their electrical activity, indicating, presumably, an inhibition of secretion. This controversy could be due largely to methodological problems. Only Bhargava et al. (1972) and Milton and Paterson (1974) measured plasma levels of vasopressin; in the other studies, changes in urine flow were used as an index of changes in the plasma vasopressin concentration. As

[425]

426

intracerebroventricular (i.c.v.) injection of vasopressin lowers blood pressure (e.g. Kobinger, 1978), the reduction in urine flow following central administration of noradrenaline could be due to the reduction in blood pressure rather than to an increase in the plasma vasopressin concentration. In many of the experiments cited above, arterial blood pressure was not measured.

To clarify the role of noradrenaline in the control of vasopressin release, the following experiments (Kimura et al., 1981a) were carried out in dogs, sedated with morphine and anaesthetized with a mixture of chloralose and urethane, in which a cannula was placed in a lateral cerebral ventricle. Vasopressin was measured with a sensitive and specific radioimmunoassay (Crofton et al., 1978, 1980), and arterial blood pressure and heart rate were monitored. The i.c.v. infusion of noradrenaline at 0.7 μg/kg per min for 20 min resulted in a sustained fall in mean arterial blood pressure. This fall in blood pressure, which ordinarily would result in an increased release of vasopressin (Share and Grosvenor, 1974), was accompanied by a profound fall in the plasma vasopressin concentration (Fig. 1) that continued for 55 min after the infusion of noradrenaline was stopped, and that reached a level that was only 11 % of the pre-infusion value. Although noradrenaline is considered to have predominantly α-adrenergic activity centrally, with little β-adrenergic effect, the responses to i.c.v. clonidine, a relatively pure α-adrenergic agonist, were also determined. The effects of clonidine on mean arterial blood pressure and the plasma vasopressin concentration (Fig. 1) were virtually identical to those of noradrenaline.

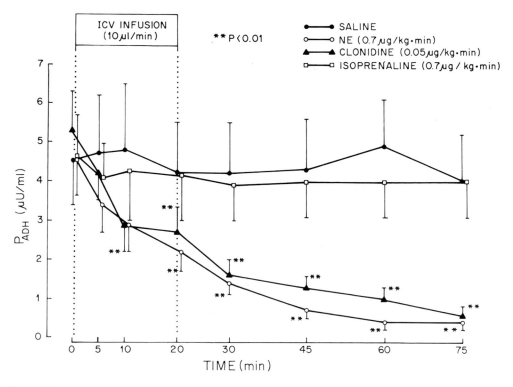

Fig. 1. Effects of i.c.v. infusion of noradrenaline, clonidine, and isoprenaline on the plasma vasopressin concentration. (From Kimura et al., 1981a.) Asterisks indicate significant differences from zero time.

To confirm that the inhibition of vasopressin secretion by noradrenaline was due to its α-adrenergic activity, the effects of pretreatment with the α-adrenoreceptor antagonist phenoxybenzamine were determined. Phenoxybenzamine, at a dose of 100 μg/kg, was injected i.c.v. 90 min before the start of the i.c.v. infusion of noradrenaline or its saline vehicle. Treatment with phenoxybenzamine alone was without effect on mean arterial blood pressure, but produced a small reduction in plasma vasopressin (Fig. 2). Although phenoxybenzamine completely blocked the effect of i.c.v. noradrenaline on blood pressure, it inhibited the effect of noradrenaline on vasopressin release by only approximately 50% (Fig. 2). The reason for the failure of phenoxybenzamine to block completely the effect of noradrenaline on vasopressin secretion is not certain.

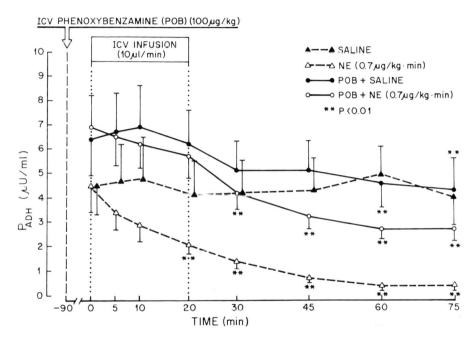

Fig. 2. Effects of pretreatment with phenoxybenzamine i.c.v. on the changes in plasma vasopressin concentrations in response to i.c.v. noradrenaline. (From Kimura et al., 1981a.) Asterisks indicate significant differences from zero time.

Further evidence that the central actions of noradrenaline on the secretion of vasopressin are due to its α-adrenergic activity is found in the observation that the i.c.v. infusion of the β-adrenergic agonist isoprenaline, at 0.7 μg/kg per min for 20 min, was without effect on the plasma vasopressin concentration (Fig. 1).

Thus, in the anaesthetized dog, the central action of noradrenaline is to inhibit vasopressin release, and this action is due to α-adrenergic activity. The data, however, do not make it possible to distinguish between activation of α_1- and α_2-adrenoreceptors. In view of the heavy noradrenergic innervation of the magnocellular vasopressin neurones of the anterior hypothalamus, it is likely that this is the primary site of action of noradrenaline to inhibit vasopressin release. This view is supported by the observation by Armstrong et al. (1982) that noradrenaline inhibited the release of vasopressin from the hypothalamo-neurohypophysial complex in vitro. Physiologically, inhibition of vasopressin secretion results from activation of arterial baroreceptors and left atrial stretch receptors (Share and Grosvenor, 1974). It is, then, reasonable to conjecture that the noradrenergic neurones that innervate vasopressin perikarya in the supraoptic and paraventricular nuclei are the rostral terminations of this pathway.

DOPAMINE

Dopamine neurones project to the supraoptic and paraventricular nuclei, the median eminence, and the posterior pituitary (Palkovits, 1981), but the role of these neurones in the control of vasopressin secretion is highly controversial. There are reports that dopamine increases (Bridges et al., 1976; Milton and Paterson, 1973; Urano and Kobayashi, 1978), decreases (Barker et al., 1971; Forsling et al., 1981; Johnston et al., 1975; Lightman and Forsling, 1980; Passo et al., 1981; Wolny et al., 1974), or has little or no effect on (Bhargava et al., 1972; Hoffman et al., 1977; Olsson, 1970) vasopressin secretion. These reports are based upon in vitro and in vivo studies, and in most of the latter, plasma vasopressin levels were not measured (the exceptions are the reports by Bhargava et al. (1972) and Lightman and Forsling (1980)).

We therefore studied the effects of dopamine, administered centrally, on vasopressin secretion under carefully controlled conditions (Kimura et al., 1981b). Dogs were anaesthetized and prepared in the manner described above for the study of i.c.v. noradrenaline. The infusion of dopamine i.c.v. at $1.25\,\mu g$/kg per min for 20 min resulted in a small transient reduction in mean arterial blood pressure. The plasma vasopressin concentration, however, fell 44 %, beginning 25 min after the end of the dopamine infusion (Fig. 3). The findings were quite different when bromocriptine mesylate, a specific dopamine agonist, was infused i.c.v. at $0.25\,\mu g$/kg per min for 20 min. There was a larger sustained fall in mean arterial blood pressure, which did not begin until after the bromocriptine infusion was completed, and a marked increase in the plasma vasopressin concentration (Fig. 3). As the increase in plasma vasopressin occurred before the fall in blood pressure, the increased secretion of vasopressin was due to a central action of the bromocriptine, rather than as a consequence of the fall in blood pressure.

There are several explanations for the apparently paradoxical findings that dopamine and its specific agonist, bromocriptine, had opposite effects. The inhibition of vasopressin release by dopamine could have been due to its inherent α-adrenergic activity (e.g. Goldberg et al., 1978) or to its conversion to noradrenaline (Glowinski and Iversen, 1966), and, as we have shown (Kimura et al., 1981a), α-adrenergic agonists act centrally to inhibit the release of vasopressin. Although bromocriptine has some α-adrenergic antagonistic activity, it seems more likely that the stimulation of vasopressin release by bromocriptine was due primarily to its dopaminergic agonistic activity. These findings may also partly explain the diverse reports of the effects of dopamine on vasopressin release. Thus, the specific experimental conditions may determine whether the α-adrenergic or dopaminergic activity of exogenous dopamine predominates, and therefore, whether vasopressin secretion is inhibited or stimulated. As there are three dopamine pathways within the hypothalamus (Palkovits, 1981), it is also possible that dopamine neurones inhibit the release of vasopressin at one site, e.g. the posterior pituitary (Forsling et al., 1981; Passo et al., 1981), and stimulate the release of vasopressin at another site, perhaps the perikarya of the vasopressin cells.

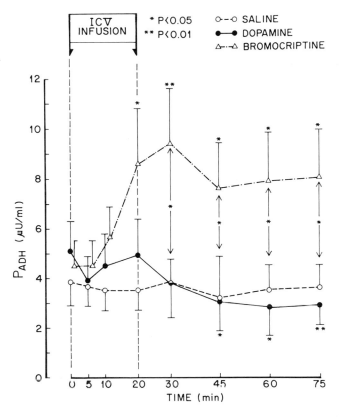

Fig. 3. Effects of i.c.v. dopamine and bromocriptine on plasma vasopresssin concentrations. (From Kimura et al., 1981b.) Asterisks above or below the lines indicate significant differences from zero time; asterisks between the lines indicate significant differences between the bromocriptine-treated and time-control groups.

The physiological significance of the hypothalamic and neurohypophysial dopamine pathways in the control of vasopressin secretion is conjectural. Dehydration results in an increased dopamine content of the posterior pituitary (Alper et al., 1980; Holzbauer et al., 1978), which suggests that dopamine pathways may be involved in the osmotic control of vasopressin secretion. Brooks and Claybaugh (1982) found that the dopamine antagonist haloperidol blocked the stimulation of vasopressin release by angiotensin II, and suggested that dopamine may be involved in angiotensin-mediated vasopressin secretion.

PROSTAGLANDINS

The evidence indicates that centrally generated prostaglandins can serve as humoral mediators in the control of vasopressin secretion. Yamamoto et al. (1976) found that perfusion of the cerebral ventricles in the anaesthetized dog with artificial CSF containing prostaglandin (PG) E_2 resulted in a marked, sustained increase in plasma vasopressin (Fig. 4). Consistent with this observation are the reports that prostaglandins of the E series, given centrally

430

(Andersson and Leksell, 1975; Leksell, 1978) or into a common carotid artery (Vilhardt and Hedqvist, 1970), inhibit a water diuresis. It has also been reported that $PGF_{2\alpha}$, PGH_2 and arachidonic acid decrease urine flow when given centrally (Leksell, 1978; Fujimoto et al., 1980). Fujimoto and Hisada (1978) observed that, in the ethanol-anaesthetized rat, PGE_2 i.c.v. caused first a diuresis and then an antidiuresis, but this report is difficult to interpret in the absence of measurement of the plasma vasopressin levels.

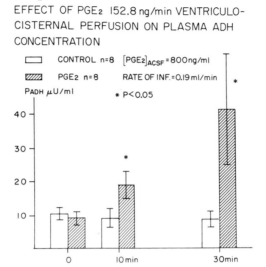

Fig. 4. Effect of ventriculocisternal perfusion with PGE_2 on the plasma vasopressin concentration. (From Yamamoto et al., 1976.) Asterisks above the bars indicate significant differences from zero time.

The demonstration that exogenous, centrally administered prostaglandins affect vasopressin release does not necessarily indicate that endogenous brain prostaglandins participate in the control of vasopressin secretion. There is, however, evidence that this may indeed be the case. First, PGE_1 i.c.v. and hypertonic NaCl i.c.v. interact synergistically in inhibiting a water diuresis in the conscious goat (Andersson and Leksell, 1975). Second, the stimulation of vasopressin release by i.c.v angiotensin II was blunted by blockade of prostaglandin biosynthesis by i.c.v. indomethacin (Fig. 5; Yamamoto et al., 1978). However, the most convincing demonstration that brain prostaglandins have a role in the control of vasopressin release is found in the report by Hoffman et al. (1982). These investigators found that, in the dog, the stimulation of vasopressin release by i.v. infusion of hypertonic NaCl was almost completely blocked by the central administration of indomethacin (Fig. 6). Centrally administered indomethacin alone was without effect on basal plasma vasopressin levels (Yamamoto et al., 1978; Hoffman et al., 1982). These data suggest that brain prostaglandins of the E series play an important role in the osmotic control of vasopressin release, perhaps as modulators of input from osmoreceptors to neurosecretory cells. This locus of action for the prostaglandins is supported by the work of Ishikawa et al. (1981) with explants of the hypothalamo-neurohypophysial complex in organ culture. The addition of PGE_2 to the incubation medium increased the release of vasopressin into the incubation medium; the addition of indomethacin to the incubation medium reduced substantially the ability of angiotensin II and hypertonic saline to stimulate the release of vasopressin into the medium.

Whether brain prostaglandins participate in other components of the control of vasopressin release remains to be determined.

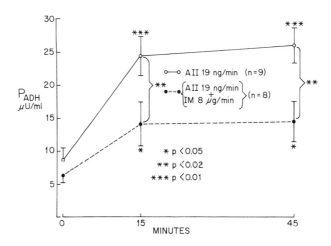

Fig. 5. Effect of central administration of indomethacin (IM) on the increased plasma vasopressin concentration in response to central administration of angiotensin II (AII). (From Yamamoto et al., 1978.) Asterisks above or below the lines indicate significant differences from zero time; asterisks between the lines indicate significant differences between the groups.

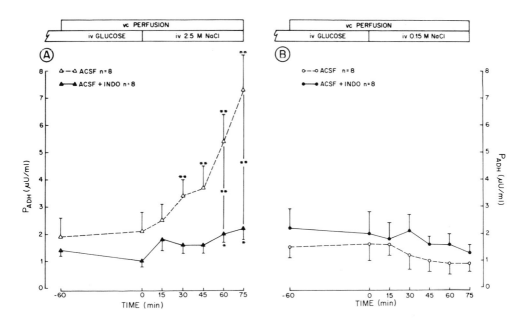

Fig. 6. Effects of ventriculocisternal (vc) perfusion with indomethacin (INDO) on the changes in plasma vasopressin concentrations in response to the i.v. infusion of: A, 2.5 M NaCl, and B, 0.15 M NaCl. (From Hoffman et al., 1982.) Asterisks above or below the lines indicate significant differences from zero time; asterisks between the lines indicate significant differences between the groups.

VASOPRESSIN

There is reason to believe that vasopressin can act centrally to inhibit its release from the posterior pituitary into the peripheral circulation. Bhargava et al. (1977) reported that the i.c.v. injection of Pitressin in anaesthetized dogs resulted in a reduction in the concentration of vasopressin in blood. There is some concern about this work, however. First, very large doses of vasopressin were necessary; the i.c.v. bolus injection of 10 mU of Pitressin produced only a 10 % reduction in the blood vasopressin concentration. Second, the Pitressin was dissolved in 0.9 % NaCl and administered in relatively large volumes (up to 0.5 ml). Finally, the Pitressin was probably a mixture of arginine- and lysine-vasopressins. Somewhat similar findings have been obtained by Nashold et al. (1963), who found that the i.c.v. injection of huge doses (10–15 U) of lysine-vasopressin increased urine flow in cats. As there was an accompanying increase in osmolar clearance, it is not certain that the increased urine flow was due to a fall in plasma vasopressin.

Because of these problems we (Wang et al., 1982a) re-examined the effects of the central administration of vasopressin on vasopressin release. In anaesthetized dogs, pure synthetic arginine-vasopressin dissolved in artificial CSF was infused i.c.v. at rates of 10, 20 and 50 μU/min (10 μl/min) for 90 min. Concentrations of vasopressin in plasma and CSF were monitored during the 90 min infusion and for 120 min thereafter. The concentration of vasopressin in CSF increased slowly during the vasopressin infusion, and decreased slowly after the end of the infusion, with a half-life of roughly 1–2 h. The maximum vasopressin levels achieved in the CSF were 32 ± 5, 83 ± 5, and 131 ± 13 μU/ml for infusion rates of 10, 20 and 50 μU/min, respectively. There was little or no effect on mean arterial blood pressure and heart rate, but there were slow progressive reductions in plasma vasopressin concentrations, which continued for a considerable time after the vasopressin infusion was discontinued (Fig. 7).

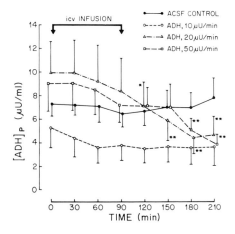

Fig. 7. Effect of i.c.v. vasopressin on the plasma vasopressin concentration. (From Wang et al., 1982a.) Asterisks indicate significant differences from zero time.

The maximum CSF vasopressin concentration obtained when vasopressin was infused i.c.v. at 10 μU/min was similar to that found in CSF after severe haemorrhage (Wang et al., 1981) or the i.c.v. infusion of hypertonic artificial CSF (Wang et al., 1982b). Furthermore, if the vasopressin diffused from the CSF to a site of action removed from the borders of the cerebral ventricles, the concentration at that site would have been relatively low. Thus, the concentrations of vasopressin in CSF achieved in these experiments are physiologically reasonable. These data suggest, then, that centrally released vasopressin may act under physiological or pathophysiological conditions to inhibit the release of vasopressin into the peripheral circulation.

The available data do not answer the question of whether centrally released vasopressin is transported to its site of action via the CSF, or whether it is released at its site of action from the axonal endings of vasopressin cells. In view of the sluggish turnover of vasopressin in CSF, the latter seems to be more likely. The central site of action for vasopressin is also not certain. Vasopressin could act directly on the neurosecretory cells in the anterior hypothalamus, as it has been shown that the microelectrophoretic application of vasopressin to cells in the supraoptic nucleus inhibits the electrical activity of these cells (Nicoll and Barker, 1971). Vasopressin may also act at brain centres remote from the anterior hypothalamus, and these centres could, in turn, inhibit the neurosecretory cells in the paraventricular and supraoptic nuclei. There is an anatomical and functional basis for this route of action. Parvocellular vasopressin neurones project from the anterior hypothalamus to centres in the medulla concerned with blood pressure regulation (e.g. Sofroniew and Schrell, 1981) and which are, presumably, way-stations in the neural pathway which subserves baroreceptor control of vasopressin release. In addition, centrally administered vasopressin affects the activity of catecholamine neurones in several brain regions which have neural projections to the anterior hypothalamus (Tanaka et al., 1977).

SUMMARY AND CONCLUSIONS

Thus, noradrenaline, dopamine, prostaglandins of the E series and vasopressin itself, can act centrally to affect the release of vasopressin from the posterior pituitary into the circulating blood. In addition, there is evidence that other centrally acting humoral agents, e.g. acetylcholine, angiotensin II and the opioids, also influence vasopressin secretion. The failure to review the data relating to these latter agents reflects a limitation of space rather than a lack of importance. These agents may act as neurotransmitters at synapses on the neurosecretory cells in the supraoptic and paraventricular nuclei, or at interneuronal synapses in the neural systems that control vasopressin release. Some of these agents, e.g. the prostaglandins, may act as neuromodulators, modifying the response to a stimulus of some element in the neural control system for vasopressin release. A given agent, e.g. dopamine, may act in several different neural pathways that innervate the supraoptic and paraventricular nuclei and the neurohypophysis. Thus, the effects of such an agent, when it is administered centrally, could vary according to the experimental conditions. Considerable work remains to be done to identify the humoral agents that act centrally on vasopressin release, and to characterize carefully their actions, their sites of action, and their role in the control of vasopressin secretion.

REFERENCES

Alper, R.H., Demarest, K.T. and Moore, K.E. (1980) Dehydration selectively increases dopamine synthesis in tuberohypophyseal dopaminergic neurons. *Neuroendocrinology*, 31: 112–115.

Andersson, B. and Leksell, L.G. (1975) Effects on fluid balance of intraventricular infusions of prostaglandin E_1. *Acta physiol. scand.*, 93: 286–288.

434

Armstrong, W.E., Sladek, C.D. and Sladek, J.R. (1982) Characterization of noradrenergic control of vasopressin release by the organ-cultured rat hypothalamo-neurohypophyseal system. *Endocrinology*, 111: 273–279.

Barker, J.L., Crayton, J.W. and Nicoll, R.A. (1971) Noradrenaline and acetylcholine responses of supraoptic neurosecretory cells. *J. Physiol. (Lond.)*, 218: 19–32.

Beal, A.M. and Bligh, J. (1980) Diuretic effect of intraventricular and intravenous infusions of noradrenaline in conscious sheep. *Quart. J. exp. Physiol.*, 65: 321–333.

Bhargava, K.P., Kulshrestha, V.K. and Srivastava, Y.P. (1972) Central cholinergic and adrenergic mechanisms in the release of antidiuretic hormone. *Brit. J. Pharmacol.*, 44: 617–627.

Bhargava, K.P., Kulshrestha, V.K. and Srivastava, Y.P. (1977) Central mechanism of vasopressin-induced changes in antidiuretic hormone release. *Brit. J. Pharmacol.*, 60: 77–81.

Bridges, T.E. and Thorn, N.A. (1970) The effect of autonomic blocking agents on vasopressin release in vivo induced by osmoreceptor stimulation. *J. Endocr.*, 48: 265–276.

Bridges, T.E., Hillhouse, E.W. and Jones, M.T. (1976) The effect of dopamine on neurohypophysial hormone release in vivo and from the rat neural lobe and hypothalamus in vitro. *J. Physiol. (Lond.)*, 260: 647–666.

Brooks, D.P. and Claybaugh, J.R. (1982) Role of dopamine in the angiotensin II-induced vasopressin release in the conscious dehydrated dog. *J. Endocr.*, in press.

Crofton, J.T., Share, L., Shade, R.E., Allen, C. and Tarnowski, D. (1978) Vasopressin in the rat with spontaneous hypertension. *Amer. J. Physiol.*, 235: H361–H366.

Crofton, J.T., Share, L., Wang, B.C. and Shade, R.E. (1980) Pressor responsiveness to vasopressin in the rat with DOC-salt hypertension. *Hypertension*, 2: 424–431

Forsling, M.L., Iversen, L.L. and Lightman, S.L. (1981) Dopamine and enkephalin directly inhibit vasopressin release from the neurohypophysis. *J. Physiol. (Lond.)*, 319: 66.

Fujimoto, S. and Hisada, S. (1978) Effects of centrally affecting drugs on the diuretic and antidiuretic actions of intracerebroventricular prostaglandin E_2. *Jap. J. Pharmacol.*, 28: 49–56.

Fujimoto, S., Tsushima, H. and Mori, M. (1980) Antidiuretic and thermogenic effects of intracerebroventricular prostaglandin H_2 in ethanol-anaesthetized rats. *Experientia*, 36: 209–211.

Glowinski, J. and Iversen, L. (1966) Regional studies of catecholamines in the rat brain — I. The disposition of [^{3}H]norepinephrine, [^{3}H]dopamine and [^{3}H]dopa in various regions of the brain. *J. Neurochem.*, 13: 655–669.

Goldberg, L.I., Volkman, P.H. and Kohli, J.D. (1978) A comparison of the vascular dopamine receptor with other dopamine receptors. *Ann. Rev. Pharmacol. Toxicol.*, 18: 57–79.

Hisada, S., Fujimoto, S., Kamiya, T., Endo, Y. and Tsushima, H. (1977) Antidiuresis of centrally administered amines and peptides and release of antidiuretic hormone from isolated rat neurohypophysis. *Jap. J. Pharmacol.*, 27: 153–161.

Hoffman, P.K., Share, L., Crofton, J.T. and Shade, R.E. (1982) The effect of intracerebroventricular indomethacin on osmotically stimulated vasopressin release. *Neuroendocrinology*, 34: 132–139.

Hoffman, W.E., Phillips, M.I. and Schmid, P. (1977) The role of catecholamines in central antidiuretic and pressor mechanisms. *Neuropharmacology*, 16: 563–569.

Holzbauer, M., Sharman, D.F. and Godden, U. (1978) Observations on the function of the dopaminergic nerves innervating the pituitary gland. *Neuroscience*, 3: 1251–1262.

Ishikawa, S., Toshikazu, S. and Yoshida, S. (1981) The effect of prostaglandins on the release of arginine vasopressin from the guinea pig hypothalamo-neurohypophyseal complex in organ culture. *Endocrinology*, 108: 193–198.

Johnston, C.I., Hutchinson, J.S., Morris, B.J. and Dax, E.M. (1975) Release and clearance of neurophysins and posterior pituitary hormones. *Ann. N.Y. Acad. Sci.*, 248: 272–280.

Kimura, T., Share, L., Wang, B.C. and Crofton, J.T. (1981a) The role of central adrenoreceptors in the control of vasopressin release and blood pressure. *Endocrinology*, 108: 1829–1836.

Kimura, T., Share, L., Wang, B.C. and Crofton, J.T. (1981b) Central effects of dopamine and bromocriptine on vasopressin release and blood pressure. *Neuroendocrinology*, 33: 347–351.

Kobinger, W. (1978) Central α-adrenergic systems as targets for hypotensive drugs. *Rev. Physiol. Biochem. Pharmacol.*, 81: 39–100.

Kühn, E.R. (1974) Cholinergic and adrenergic release mechanism for vasopressin in the male rat: a study with injections of neurotransmitters and blocking agents into the third ventricle. *Neuroendocrinology*, 16: 255–264.

Leksell, L.G. (1978) Effects on fluid balance induced by non-febrile intracerebroventricular infusions of PGE_2, $PGF_{2\alpha}$, and arachidonic acid in the goat. *Acta physiol. scand.*, 104: 225–231.

Lightman, S.L. and Forsling, M. (1980) Evidence for dopamine as an inhibitor of vasoprotein release in man. *Clin. Endocr.*, 12: 39–46.

Milton, A.S. and Paterson, A.T. (1973) Intracranial injections of 6-hydroxydopamine (6-OH-DA) in cats: effects on the release of antidiuretic hormone. *Brain Res.*, 61: 423–427.

Milton, A.S. and Paterson, A.T. (1974) A microinjection study of the control of antidiuretic hormone release by the supraoptic nucleus of the hypothalamus in the cat. *J. Physiol. (Lond.)*, 241: 607–628.

Moss, R.L., Dyball, R.E.J. and Cross, B.A. (1971) Responses of antidromically identified supraoptic and paraventricular units to acetylcholine, noradrenaline and glutamate applied iontophoretically. *Brain Res.*, 35: 573–575.

Nashold, B.S., Mannarino, E.M. and Robinson, R.R. (1963) Effect of posterior pituitary polypeptides on the flow of urine after injection in lateral ventricle of the brain of a cat. *Nature (Lond.)*, 197: 293.

Nicoll, R.A. and Barker, J. (1971) The pharmacology of recurrent inhibition in the supraoptic neurosecretory system. *Brain Res.*, 35: 501–511.

Olsson, K. (1970) Effects on water diuresis of infusions of transmitter substances into the 3rd ventricle. *Acta physiol. scand.*, 79: 133–135.

Palkovits, M. (1981) Catecholamines in the hypothalamus: an anatomical review. *Neuroendocrinology*, 33: 123–128.

Passo, S.S., Thornborough, J.R. and Ferris, C.F. (1981) A functional analysis of dopaminergic innervation of the neurohypophysis. *Amer. J. Physiol.*, 241: E186–E190.

Share, L. and Grosvenor, C.E. (1974) The neurohypophysis. In S.M. McCann (Ed.), *Physiology, Series One, Vol. 5, Endocrine Physiology*, Butterworths, London, pp. 1–30.

Sladek, C. (1980) Osmotic control of vasopressin release: role of acetylcholine and angiotensin. In S. Yoshida, L. Share and K. Yagi (Eds.), *Antidiuretic Hormone*, Japan Scientific Societies Press, Tokyo, pp. 117–132.

Sladek, J.R., McNeill, T.H., Khachaturian, H. and Zimmerman, E.A. (1980) Chemical neuroanatomy of monoamine-neuropeptide interactions in the hypothalamic magnocellular system. In S. Yoshida, L. Share and K. Yagi (Eds.), *Antidiuretic Hormone*, Japan Scientific Societies Press, Tokyo, pp. 3–17.

Sofroniew, M.V. and Schrell, U. (1981) Evidence for a direct projection from oxytocin and vasopressin neurons in the hypothalamic paraventricular nucleus to the medulla oblongata: immunohistochemical visualization of both the horseradish peroxidase transported and the peptide produced by the same neurons. *Neurosci. Lett.* 22: 211–217.

Tanaka, M., Versteeg, D.H.G. and De Wied, D. (1977) Regional effects of vasopressin on rat brain catecholamine metabolism. *Neurosci. Lett.*, 4: 321–325.

Urano, A. and Kobayashi, H. (1978) Effects of noradrenaline and dopamine injected into the supraoptic nucleus on urine flow rate in hydrated rats. *Exp. Neurol.*, 60: 140–150.

Vandeputte-Van Messom, G. and Peeters, G. (1975) Effect of intraventricular administration of noradrenaline on water diuresis in goats. *J. Endocr.*, 66: 375–383.

Vilhardt, H. and Hedqvist, P. (1970) A possible role of prostaglandin E_2 in the regulation of vasopressin secretion in rats. *Life Sci.*, 9: 825–830.

Wang, B.C., Share, L., Crofton, J.T. and Kimura, T. (1981) Changes in vasopressin concentration in plasma and cerebrospinal fluid in response to hemorrhage in anesthetized dogs. *Neuroendocrinology*, 33: 61–66.

Wang, B.C., Share, L. and Crofton, J.T. (1982a) Central infusion of vasopressin decreased the plasma vasopressin concentration in dogs. *Amer. J. Physiol.*, in press.

Wang, B.C., Share, L., Crofton, J.T. and Kimura, T. (1982b) Effect of intravenous and intracerebroventricular infusion of hypertonic solutions on plasma and cerebrospinal fluid vasopressin concentrations. *Neuroendocrinology*, 34: 215–221.

Wolny, H.L., Plech, A. and Herman, Z.S. (1974) Diuretic effects of intraventricularly injected noradrenaline and dopamine in rats. *Experientia*, 30: 1062–1063.

Yamamoto, M., Share, L. and Shade, R.E. (1976) Vasopressin release during ventriculo-cisternal perfusion with prostaglandin E_2 in the dog. *J. Endocr.*, 71: 325–331.

Yamamoto, M., Share, L. and Shade, R.E. (1978) Effect of ventriculo-cisternal perfusion with angiotensin II and indomethacin on the plasma vasopressin concentration. *Neuroendocrinology*, 25: 166–173.

The Neurohypophysis: Structure, Function and Control, Progress in Brain Research, Vol. 60, edited by B.A. Cross and G. Leng'
© *1983 Elsevier Science Publishers B.V.*

Anatomical Reciprocity Between Magnocellular Peptides and Noradrenaline in Putative Cardiovascular Pathways

J.R. SLADEK, Jr.* and C.D. SLADEK

Departments of Anatomy and Neurology, and the Center for Brain Research, University of Rochester, School of Medicine Rochester, NY (U.S.A)

INTRODUCTION

Changes in blood pressure and blood volume are accompanied by appropriate changes in plasma vasopressin concentration. For example, a fall in blood pressure results in the release of vasopressin (see Share, 1974). Noradrenaline has been implicated in the mediation of the response by vasopressin neurones to changes in cardiovascular status. Pharmacological blockade of central noradrenaline neurones blocks the response to decreased blood volume (Miller et al., 1979). Moreover, destruction of the central noradrenaline-containing neurones of the A1 group in the caudal, ventrolateral medulla, results in increased plasma vasopressin levels and hypertension (Blessing et al., 1982).

Noradrenaline neurones of the A1 and A2 medullary groups contribute, via the ventral noradrenergic pathway, to a massive innervation of the hypothalamus (Ungerstedt 1971). In 1965, Fuxe demonstrated an extremely dense catecholamine innervation of the supraoptic (SON) and paraventricular (PVN) nuclei, and with Hökfelt focused attention on a role for noradrenaline in the control of water balance by the observation of changes in fluorescence intensity of terminals in the SON following dehydration (Fuxe and Hökfelt, 1967). Concurrently, Vandesande and Dierickyx (1975) demonstrated the relative position of vasopressin and oxytocin neurones in the rat SON and PVN which supported the probability of a noradrenergic innervation of vasopressin neurones due to their prevalence in ventral and caudal portions of the SON. This relationship was confirmed with the development of a simultaneous visualization technique for neuropeptides and monoamines (Sladek et al., 1978). It is now clear that the noradrenergic innervation pattern favours vasopressin over oxytocin neurones; in the rat SON by about 4:1 (Sladek et al., 1980a). Moreover, there appears to be some degree of phylogenetic homology in the rhesus monkey, especially in the SON (Sladek et al., 1980b, Sladek and Zimmerman, 1982).

Sawchenko and Swanson (1981) demonstrated that this noradrenergic innervation of vasopressin neurones arises predominantly from the A1 group. These neurones in turn receive a massive projection from the area which receives information from the glossopharyngeal and vagal nerves, the nucleus tractus solitarius and dorsal motor nucleus of the vagus (Sawchenko and Swanson, 1981). Thus, the morphological substrate exists for regulatory signals from the

---

* Address for reprints: John R. Sladek, Jr., Department of Anatomy — Box 603, University of Rochester School of Medicine, 601 Elmwood Avenue, Rochester, NY 14642, U.S.A.

cardiovascular volume and baroreceptors to be transmitted to the vasopressin neurones by way of the noradrenergic afferents from the A1 neurones.

The possibility of a reciprocal pathway between the magnocellular neurosecretory neurones and the noradrenaline neurones arises from the finding of a descending pathway from the PVN to the brainstem and spinal cord (Conrad and Pfaff, 1976; Swanson, 1977; Nilaver et al., 1980; Sofroniew and Schrell, 1981). Oxytocin and vasopressin fibres descend through the brainstem and spinal cord, and are found in virtually all regions of the brainstem which contain noradrenaline perikarya; namely, the A1, A2, A5, A6 and A7 groups. Although many of these fibres appear in juxtaposition to neuronal perikarya, and often are seen in a pericellular array, it is not possible to conclude that they are in a position, morphologically, to contact the noradrenergic neurones because of the rather heterogeneous, and often diffuse, distribution of these neurones amongst the non-aminergic neurones located in the same regions. Thus, the present study addressed the question of potential reciprocity between noradrenergic neurones of the brainstem, and oxytocin and vasopressin neurones of the hypothalamus.

METHODS

Male, Fischer 344 rats (3–6 months old) were examined for the simultaneous demonstration of monoamines and neuropeptides as described previously (Sladek et al., 1978). Basically, this involves the preparation of tissue blocks for the generation of formaldehyde-induced histofluorescence of catecholamines and the indoleamine, serotonin, according to the method of Falck and Hillarp (Falck et al., 1962). Brains are removed following decapitation, freeze-dried, p-formaldehyde vapour-perfused and paraffin-embedded. Serial sections are cut at $6\,\mu$m. Every tenth section is stained with cresyl violet and Luxol fast blue for identification of appropriate neuroanatomical levels. The remaining sections are analyzed for monoamine–neuropeptide interactions. The position of catecholamine groups is verified by the examination of selected sections for precursory fluorescence microscopy so that sections containing the appropriate catecholamine group can be chosen for peptide immunohistochemistry; these sections are rehydrated, placed on glass slides and are stained with the peroxidase–antiperoxidase (PAP) technique for neurophysin. Most staining for the present examination utilized an anti-rat neurophysin which recognizes both oxytocin- and vasopressin-associated neurophysins and was provided by Dr. Alan Robinson. Additionally, selected medullary sections were stained with selective neurophysin antisera commercially obtained from California Medicinal.

Histological sections are then examined in a fluorescence microscope which is optically linked to an identical microscope with a comparator bridge. Two adjacent sections, one stained for neurophysin and the other unstained, but maintaining strong catecholamine histofluorescence, are examined simultaneously. The relative position of neurophysin- and catecholamine-containing neurones is then determined as described in detail elsewhere (McNeill and Sladek, 1980).

RESULTS

The examination of sections prepared for Falck–Hillarp histofluorescence revealed the occurrence of catecholamine-containing neurones (presumably noradrenergic) within the previously identified A1, A2, A5, A6 and A7 groups. Briefly, the A1 group was situated heterogeneously in the ventrolateral, caudal medulla. These neurones are characteristically multipolar and display prominent, catecholamine-filled dendrites (Fig. 1). The A2 neurones

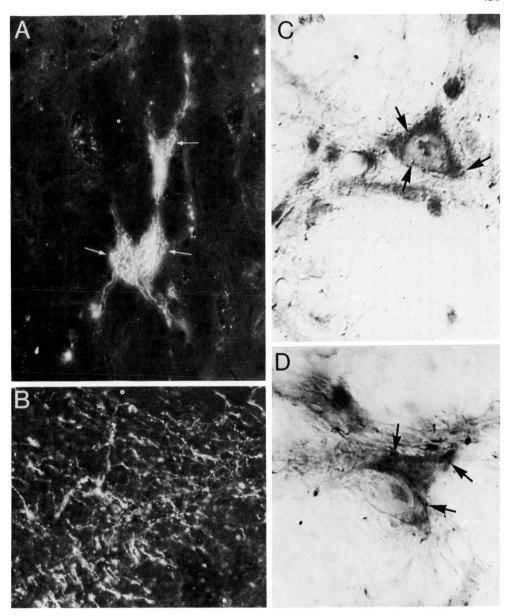

Fig. 1. A: the A1 region of the ventrolateral medulla is characterized by the presence of noradrenaline-containing neurones (arrows) which yield an intense formaldehyde-induced fluorescence indicative of catecholamines. Varicosities often were seen in apposition to proximal dendrites. B: this region of the ventrolateral medulla also contains a dense network of neurophysin-positive fibres as depicted with dark-field illumation. C and D: at higher magnification, neurophysin-positive varicosities are seen in apposition to neurones situated in the ventrolateral medulla seen to advantage with Normarski optics. Neuronal cell bodies have been stained with cresyl violet to aid their identification. At this level of analysis it is not possible to identify these neurones unequivocally as noradrenergic. A × 330; B × 170; C × 415; D × 415.

440

are reasonably evenly distributed among the perikarya of the nucleus of the solitary tract and the adjacent dorsal motor vagal nucleus. The A5 and A7 groups appeared as more widespread groups in the ventrolateral pontine reticular formation; A7 being more rostrally placed. Group A6 is the well known locus coeruleus which is comprised of a dense cluster of primarily noradrenergic perikarya.

Neurophysin-containing fibres and varicosities were observed within the anatomical confines of each of the above-mentioned noradrenaline-containing groups (Fig. 1). Comparator bridge analysis revealed varicosity-perikaryal juxtapositions within each group; in general, neurophysin-positive varicosities appeared adjacent to noradrenaline-containing perikarya and dendrites. This was most apparent in the A1 group where a majority of fluorescent perikarya appeared to be contacted. Varicosities often were seen adjacent to proximal dendritic shafts (Fig. 2) over distances approximately 2–3 times the diameter of the noradrenaline perikarya when such dendrites coursed parallel to the plane (frontal) of the section. The noradrenaline neurones of the A2 region appeared contacted to a lesser extent both in terms of contacts per perikaryon and the percentage of neurones contacted. The smaller size of these neurones in comparison with the A1 neurones coupled with the relative lack of fluorescent dendrites did not permit the routine visualization of neurophysin-positive varicosities in apposition to noradrenaline-containing dendrites. The A5 and A7 groups displayed appositions less frequently than the A1 and A2 groups. This distinction was difficult to make with certainty in the A6 region, because the dense packing of noradrenergic perikarya and dendrites made it difficult to assign a neurophysin varicosity to a single noradrenergic element.

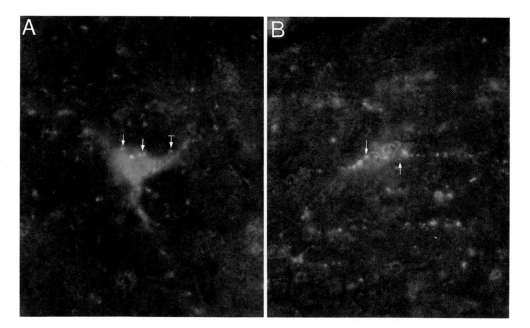

Fig. 2. These comparator bridge photomicrographs depict neurophysin-containing varicosities (arrows) in apparent juxtaposition to perikarya and proximal dentrites (⊢→) of catecholaminergic neurones of the caudal medulla. Neurones in groups A1 (A) and A2 (B) are illustrated. A and B × 300.

Analysis of the above phenomena with the use of vasopressin- and oxytocin-specific neurophysin antisera on sections of caudal medulla revealed positive staining for each respective peptide in the A1 and A2 groups. Comparator bridge analysis extended the observation to include varicosity-perikaryal juxtaposition between each peptidergic fibre type and noradrenaline neurones in each medullary group. It is not possible at present to assign a relative percentage of oxytocin versus vasopressin contact as stereological analysis is still being performed.

DISCUSSION

The occurrence of neurophysin-positive varicosities in juxtaposition to noradrenaline-containing perikarya of the A1 and A2 medullary groups raises the possibility of a reciprocal link between aminergic and peptidergic neurones. This pathway may modulate the release of vasopressin in response to alterations in peripheral blood pressure. A possible route of information would begin with the transfer of information from baroreceptors in the carotid arch and atrial wall through glossopharyngeal and vagal afferents which terminate centrally on neuronal perikarya of the dorsal motor vagal nucleus and the solitary nucleus. Some of these central neurones synthesize noradrenaline as a transmitter and send ascending axons through the ventral noradrenergic bundle (Ungerstedt, 1971) to terminate in the PVN (Sawchenko and Swanson, 1981). In addition, non-catecholaminergic cells of the dorsal motor vagal and solitary nuclei project to the A1 neurones in the ventrolateral medulla. These neurones also send ascending axons through the ventral noradrenergic bundle (Ungerstedt, 1971) to terminate on the vasopressin neurones and, to a lesser extent, oxytocin neurones of the SON and PVN (Sladek et al., 1980b). Thus, noradrenaline could be involved in the cardiovascular regulation of vasopressin release.

The descending component of this reciprocal circuit consists of neurophysin fibres projecting to the medullary catecholamine neurones. The PVN sends afferent pathways to a number of central loci including the caudal medulla (Nilaver et al., 1980) where vasopressin and oxytocin fibres appear to ramify throughout the A1 and A2 regions; the present results draw attention to the higher incidence of neurophysin catecholamine juxtapositions in the A1 than the A2 region. This reciprocal connection between the A1 noradrenaline neurones and the magnocellular peptidergic neurones could serve as a short-loop feedback system modulating the release of vasopressin in response to cardiovascular signals. The PVN projection to the A2 neurones, which has been described morphologically (Sofroniew and Schrell, 1981) and electrophysiologically (Yamashita et al., this volume) may participate in the central regulation of blood pressure and heart rate (Matsuguchi et al., 1982).

Stimulation of the baro- and atrial receptors by increases in blood pressure or blood volume inhibits vasopressin release (see Share, 1974). Thus, the ascending limb of the reciprocal circuit may utilize an inhibitory transmitter. An inhibitory effect of noradrenaline on vasopressin release is supported by several in vivo and in vitro studies. Kimura et al. (1981) demonstrated a decrease in vasopressin release following injection of noradrenaline into the lateral ventricle of dogs. Antidromically identified neurones of the SON were shown electrophysiologically to be inhibited by the iontophoretic application of noradrenaline (Barker et al., 1971), and both basal and acetylcholine-stimulated vasopressin release from organ cultured hypothalamo-neurohypophysial explants is attenuated by noradrenaline (Armstrong et al., 1982; Sladek et al., 1982). Furthermore, ablation of the A1 noradrenergic neurones results in an increase in plasma vasopressin and blood pressure (Blessing et al., 1982). Thus, all of these data are consistent with an involvement of the noradrenergic innervation of the vasopressin neurones in the cardiovascular control of vasopressin release.

442

From a morphological perspective the present data suggest that varicosities which contain magnocellular peptides are in a position to contact noradrenaline perikarya and dendrites. It is not certain that these varicosities make synaptic contacts with their putative targets, as immunoelectron microscopy would be necessary to provide appropriate data. Nevertheless, Yamashita et al. (this volume) have provided electrophysiological evidence for a monosynaptic pathway from the PVN to the A2 region of the medulla, but it is not known whether this pathway is peptidergic. Also it should be recalled that the descending connections from the PVN continue caudally to terminate at spinal cord levels, thus an alternative interpretation is that peptide-containing varicosities within brainstem nuclei may wholly of in part represent fibres of passage, en route to the spinal cord. However, the high density of fibres in the A1 and A2 regions and the particularly high incidence of varicosity-perikaryal appositions upon noradrenergic neurones of the A1 region favour the interpretation of a functional interaction between these two classes of chemically identified neurones.

ACKNOWLEDGEMENTS

This work was supported by USPHS Grants HL 28172 (C.D.S.), NS 15816 (J.R.S.), AG 00847 (J.R.S.) and Career Development Award NS 00259 (C.D.S.). The authors thank B. Blanchard and J. Fields for skilled technical assistance.

REFERENCES

Armstrong, W.E., Sladek, C.D. and Sladek, J.R., Jr. (1982) Characterization of noradrenergic control of vasopressin release by the organ-cultured rat hypothalamo-neuropophyseal system. *Endocrinology,* 111: 273–279.

Barker, J.L., Crayton, J.W. and Nicoll, R.A. (1971) Noradrenaline and acetylcholine responses of supraoptic neurosecretory cells. *J. Physiol. (Lond.),* 218: 19–32.

Blessing, W.W., Sved, A.F. and Reis, D.J. (1982) Destruction of noradrenergic neurons in rabbit brainstem elevates plasma vasopressin, causing hypertension. *Science,* 217: 661–663.

Conrad, L.C.A. and Pfaff, D.W. (1976) Efferents from medial basal forebrain and hypothalamus in the rat. II. An autoradiographic study of the anterior hypothalamus. *J. comp. Neurol.,* 169: 221–261.

Falck, B., Hillarp, N.-A., Thieme, G. and Torp, A. (1962) Fluorescence of catecholamines and related compounds condensed with formaldehyde. *J. Histochem. Cytochem.,* 10: 348–354.

Fuxe, K. (1965) Evidence for the existence of monoamine neurons in the central nervous system. IV. The distribution of monoamine nerve terminals in the central nervous system. *Acta physiol. scand.,* Suppl. 64: 39–85.

Fuxe, K. and Hökfelt, T. (1967) The influence of central catecholamine neurons on hormone secretion from the anterior and posterior pituitary. In F. Stutinsky (Ed.), *Neurosecretion,* Springer-Verlag, Berlin, pp. 166–176.

Kimura, T., Share, L., Wang, B.C. and Crofton, J.R. (1981) The role of central adrenoreceptors in the control of vasopressin release and blood pressure. *Endocrinology,* 108: 1829–1836.

Matsuguchi, A., Sharabi, F.M., Gordon, F.J., Johnson, A.K. and Schmid, P.G. (1982) Blood pressure and heart rate responses to vasopressin microinjection into the nucleus tractus solitarius region of the rat. *J. Neuropharmacol.,* in press.

McNeill, T.H. and Sladek, J.R., Jr (1980) Simultaneous monoamine histofluorescence and neuropeptide immunocytochemistry. V. A detailed methodology. *Brain Res. Bull.,* 5: 599–608.

Miller, T.R., Handleman, W.A., Arnold, P.E., MacDonald, K.M., Molinoff, P.B. and Schrier, R.W. (1979) Effect of central catecholamine depletion on the osmotic and nonosmotic stimulation of vasopressin (antidiuretic hormone) in the rat. *J. clin. Invest.,* 64: 1599–1607.

Nilaver, G., Zimmerman, E.A., Wilkins, J., Michaels, J., Hoffman, D. and Silverman, A.J. (1980) Magnocellular hypothalamic projections to the lower brain stem and spinal cord of the rat. *Neuroendocrinology,* 30: 150–158.

Sawchenko, P. and Swanson, L.W. (1981) Central noradrenergic pathways for the integration of hypothalamic neuroendocrine and autonomic responses. *Science,* 214: 685–687.

Share, L. (1974) Blood pressure, blood volume, and the release of vasopressin. In E. Knobil and W.H. Sawyer (Eds.),

Handbook of Physiology; Section 7: Endocrinology, Vol. 4: The Pituitary Gland and Its Neuroendocrine Control, Part 1, Williams and Wilkins, Baltimore, MD, pp. 243–256.

Sladek, C.D., Armstrong, W.E. and Sladek, J.R., Jr. (1982) Norepinephrine control of vasopressin release. In Y. Ibata and E.A. Zimmerman (Eds.), *Structure and Function of Peptidergic and Aminergic Neurons,* J. Wiley and Sons, New York.

Sladek, J.R., Jr. and Zimmerman, E.A. (1982) Simultaneous monoamine histofluorescence and neuropeptide immunocytochemistry VI. Catecholamine innervation of vasopressin and oxytocin neurons in the rhesus monkey hypothalamus. *Brain Res. Bull.,* 9: 431–440.

Sladek, J.R., Jr., Sladek, C.D., McNeill, T.H. and Wood, J.G. (1978) New sites of monoamine localization in the endocrine hypothalamus as revealed by new methodological approaches. In D.E. Scott, G.P. Kozlowski and A. Weindl (Eds.), *Neural Hormones and Reproduction,* Brain–Endocrine Interaction III, Karger, Basel, pp. 154–171.

Sladek, J.R., Jr., Khachaturian, H., Hoffman, G.E. and Scholer, J. (1980a) Aging of central endocrine neurons and their aminergic afferents. *Peptides,* 1, Suppl. 1: 141–157.

Sladek, J.R., Jr., McNeill, T.H., Khachaturian, H. and Zimmerman, E.A. (1980b) Chemical neuroanatomy of monoamine-neuropeptide interactions in the hypothalamic magnocellular system. In S. Yoshida, L. Share and K. Yagi (Eds.), *Antidiuretic Hormone,* Japan Societies Press, Tokyo, pp. 3–17.

Sofroniew, M.V. and Schrell, U. (1981) Evidence for a direct projection from oxytocin and vasopressin neurons in hypothalamic paraventricular nucleus to the medulla oblongata: immunohistochemical visualization of both the horseradish peroxidase transported and the peptide produced by the same neurons. *Neurosci. Lett.,* 22: 211–217.

Swanson, L.W. (1977) Immunohistochemical evidence for a neurophysin-containing autonomic pathway arising in the paraventricular nucleus of the hypothalamus. *Brain Res.,* 128: 346–353.

Ungerstedt, U. (1971) Stereotaxic mapping of the monoamine pathways in the rat brain. *Acta physiol. scand.,* Suppl., 367: 1–48.

Vandesande, R. and Dierickyx, K. (1975) Identification of the vasopressin producing and of the oxytocin producing neurons in the hypothalamic magnocellular neurosecretory system of the rat. *Cell Tiss. Res.,* 164: 153–162.

The Neurohypophysis: Structure, Function and Control, Progress in Brain Research, Vol. 60, edited by B.A. Cross and G. Leng
© 1983 Elsevier Science Publishers B.V.

Neurohypophysial Hormones and Central Cardiovascular Control

B. BOHUS*, C.A.M. VERSTEEG, W. DE JONG, K. CRANSBERG AND J.G. KOOY

Rudolf Magnus Institute for Pharmacology, University of Utrecht, Vondellaan 6, 3521 GD Utrecht (The Netherlands)

INTRODUCTION

More than 80 years ago Oliver and Schäfer (1895) first described the existence of a substance with vasoactive properties from the posterior pituitary. The principle was later named vasopressin. The physiological importance of vasopressin as antidiuretic hormone has long been accepted, but its role in cardiovascular regulation is still not clear. It is likely that the circulating vasopressin serves an important function during haemorrhage by its potent systemic vasoconstrictor action (Cowley et al., 1980).

An action of a posterior pituitary extract on the brain was first described by Cushing in 1932. He found that pituitrin injection into the lateral cerebral ventricle in patients suffering from brain tumour resulted in peripheral vasodilatation, profuse sweating, salivation, fall in body temperature and lowered metabolic rate. He postulated that parasympathetic mechanisms were activated by the extract. Years later Nashold et al. (1962) reinvestigated this question in the cat and found that lysine[8]-vasopressin (LVP) and also oxytocin decrease blood pressure (BP) upon intracerebroventricular (i.c.v.) administration at low doses (0.2–0.5 IU), and increase BP at higher doses (1–1.5 IU). Subsequently, Nashold et al. (1963) reported a "diuretic" action of i.c.v. vasopressin in the cat. This effect was clearly dissimilar to the classical peripheral actions of the peptide.

The concept that the brain is not only the source but also one of the target organs of the neurohypophysial hormones has been confirmed by extensive behavioural, electrophysiological and neurochemical observations (De Wied and Versteeg, 1979; Kovàcs et al., 1979; Bohus et al., 1982a; Koob and Bloom, 1982; De Wied, this volume). Furthermore, an extensive network of peptidergic systems arising from the hypothalamic neurosecretory nuclei and terminating in limbic-, mid- and hindbrain areas and the spinal cord has been discovered (see Swaab, 1980; Sofroniew and Weindl, 1981).

This paper summarizes some evidence for the involvement of neurohypophysial hormones in the modulation of central cardiovascular control mechanisms. It is hypothesized that dysfunctions of these central peptidergic systems may be of an aetiological significance in the development of neurogenic hypertension.

---

* New address for all correspondence: Department of Animal Physiology, University of Groningen, P.O. Box 14, 9750 AA Haren (Gn), The Netherlands

PERIPHERAL PEPTIDE ADMINISTRATION AND CENTRALLY INDUCED CARDIOVASCULAR RESPONSES

Behavioural observations on posterior lobectomized or intact rats (De Wied, 1965; De Wied and Bohus, 1966) suggested that a peptide or peptides in Pitressin has long-term actions related to memory processes. It was subsequently found that vasopressin is the active principle for these long-term effects (Bohus, 1971; De Wied, 1971). Similar long-term alterations in behaviour may be induced by increasing the arousal level following learning, in particular in the ascending reticular activating system. Bloch (1970) found that electrical stimulation of the mesencephalic reticular formation (MRF) of the rat shortly after learning facilitates memory processes. To investigate the possibility that vasopressin affects arousal, the action of the peptide on cortical electrical activity was investigated in relation to brainstem stimulation. As psychophysiological studies such as classical cardiac conditioning and concurrent measurements of cardiac and behavioural responses in the rat in fearful conditions showed effects of vasopressin on autonomic responses (Bohus, 1975), the BP and heart rate changes accompanying cortical arousal were also studied. Electrical stimulation of the MRF resulted in an increase of BP and decrease of heart rate in urethane-anaesthetized rats. The effect of i.v. LVP on these responses was surprising. The peptide increased the current threshold of the effect on BP (Bohus, 1974), and also reduced the pressor response evoked by electrical stimulation of the posterior hypothalamus, a well-defined pressor area in the brain. The action of LVP on the pressor response was maximal after 60 min — long after disappearance of the peripheral vasoactive effect of the peptide. Desglycin-amide[9]-LVP (DGLVP), a vasopressin analogue with practically no antidiuretic and pressor activities, but which is as behaviourally active as LVP (De Wied et al., 1972), produced a similar inhibition of the hypothalamically induced pressor response (Bohus, 1974). The relatively long latency of action, probably due to the uptake of the peptides in the brain, and the activity of DGLVP, suggest that vasopressin and its analogue affect BP control by a direct action on the brain.

ACUTE NEUROGENIC HYPERTENSIVE RESPONSES: AN EXPERIMENTAL MODEL IN THE RAT

Electrical stimulation of the MRF in urethane-anaesthetized rats raises systolic and diastolic BP and decreases heart rate. The magnitude of these responses depends upon the frequency of the stimulation. Increasing the stimulation frequency from 10 Hz to 90 Hz at the same stimulus intensity results in a monotonic increase in systolic and diastolic BP and a decrease in heart rate. The increase in systolic BP is linear and steep between 30 and 70 Hz. The increments in diastolic BP are less than those in systolic BP, and the slope of the curve is flatter. The bradycardia response is linear between 10 and 90 Hz (Fig. 1; Versteeg et al., 1982a, b). To standardize the neurogenic hypertensive response, the current intensity that induced a systolic BP increase of 50 mm Hg was determined and served as the basic pressor response. Subsequently the same stimulus intensity was used for the other stimulation frequencies. To evoke the basic pressor response a current intensity of 40–100 μA was used when the stimulation electrodes were located in the medial MRF or in the vicinity of the cuneiform nucleus. The maximal increase in the systolic BP and decrease in heart rate during the 5-sec stimulations served as the measure of the pressor and heart rate responses. Following a random series of stimulations, the peptides or vehicle were injected into a cerebral ventricle (or locally in the brain). The stimulation series was repeated 20, 40 and 60 min later, and the differences between the magnitudes of the responses before and after the treatments (Δ pressor and heart rate responses) were determined. The methodological details have been published elsewhere (Versteeg et al., 1982a, b).

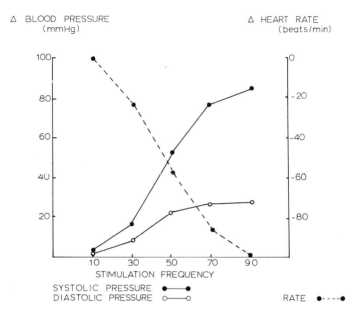

Fig. 1. Cardiovascular responses to the electrical stimulation of the MRF in the rat: frequency-dependent increases of systolic BP and decrease in heart rate. The intensity of stimulation was selected to induce a systolic BP increase of 50 mm Hg at 50 Hz frequency.

The original observations on cortical and limbic arousal following MRF stimulation suggested that the reticular formation is part of an ascending activating system (Moruzzi and Magoun, 1949). Autonomic responses evoked by MRF stimulation, however, may be the result of excitation of cell bodies or fibres of ascending or descending neuronal systems. To determine how the pressor responses upon MRF stimulation are organized, the effects of transections in the brainstem on the neurogenic blood pressure response were investigated (Kooy, Versteeg and Bohus, unpublished). Transections placed cranially or caudally from the stimulation sites were performed with a microknife, shortly before the stimulation. Ipsilateral cuts caudal from the stimulation site, which disconnected the descending pathways, reduced the pressor response (Table I), whereas control caudal cuts placed more dorsally had practically no effect on the response. Cuts placed cranially from the stimulation sites which disconnected ascending neuronal systems reduced the response by about 50 %, in particular at the lower stimulation frequencies. The pressor response was also diminished following dorso-cranial cuts. These findings suggest that a substantial part of the pressor response is mediated through higher brain structures. Furthermore, the neural pathways involved in the pressor response are ipsilateral. Contralateral transection caudal to the stimulation site had no effect on the pressor response. These findings suggest that modulation of the acute hypertensive response evoked by MRF stimulation may occur both cranially (e.g. in the diencephalon or limbic forebrain) and caudally to the stimulation site.

TABLE I

THE EFFECT OF TRANSECTIONS OF THE BRAINSTEM ON THE MAGNITUDE OF PRESSOR RESPONSES
INDUCED BY THE ELECTRICAL STIMULATION OF THE MRF IN URETHANE-ANAESTHETIZED RATS

Site of transection[a]	Δ Pressor response[b] at stimulation frequencies[c] of:		
	30 Hz	50 Hz	70 Hz
Ipsilateral			
Caudal Experimental	11.8±2.0[d, e]	21.0±4.7[e]	28.3±4.4[e]
Control	80.0±6.7	85.5±3.5	79.9±4.5
Cranial Experimental	42.2±6.6	48.8±6.3	72.2±5.7
Control	51.0±4.0	68.5±5.1	84.0±5.6

[a] Relative to the stimulation site.

[b] In percentage of the preoperative systolic blood pressure increase.

[c] Frequency of stimulation with fixed intensity

[d] Mean ± S.E.M.

[e] Significance of difference between experimental and control rats: $P < 0.05$ (t-test, two-tailed).

ATTENUATION OF THE ACUTE NEUROGENIC PRESSOR RESPONSES BY
ADMINISTRATION OF ARGININE[8]-VASOPRESSIN AND RELATED PEPTIDES INTO
A LATERAL CEREBRAL VENTRICLE

Arginine[8]-vasopressin (AVP) attenuates the centrally evoked pressor and bradycardia
responses following injection into a lateral cerebral ventricle of urethane-anaesthetized rats
(Versteeg et al., 1979a, 1982a) by up to approximately 40% for 60 min following a single
injection. The attenuation of the pressor response is dose-dependent in the range 3–25 ng (Fig.
2). The dose–response curve is almost linear at the stimulation frequency of 70 Hz, but 12.5 ng

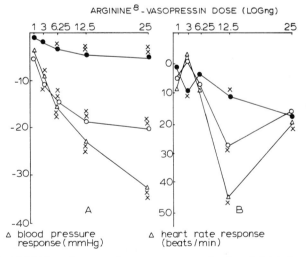

Fig. 2. Dose-dependent inhibition of neurogenic pressor responses by the administration of AVP into a lateral
cerebral ventricle. Frequencies of the stimulation of the MRF were: ●, 30 Hz; ○, 50 Hz; Δ, 70 Hz. Δ values (axes)
represent the difference in the magnitude of the response before and 20 min after peptide administration. Significance
of differences (*$P < 0.05$; **$P < 0.001$) was calculated by means of the multiple comparison test of Dunnett. (From
Versteeg et al., 1982a.)

is almost maximally effective at both 50 and 30 Hz. This phenomenon is probably related to characteristics of the peptide rather than to the pretreatment magnitude of the pressor responses. However, the reduction of the bradycardia response to AVP fails to show a clear dose–response relation (Fig. 2). A dose of 12.5 ng appears to be the most effective at the stimulation frequencies of 50 and 70 Hz. The higher dose (25 ng) is less effective and does not always significantly reduce the heart rate response.

Fragments of AVP such as AVP_{1-6} or AVP_{7-9} but also DGLVP are practically devoid of classical endocrine activities. These fragments have a potent inhibitory action on the pressor responses but fail to reduce the heart rate response (Versteeg et al., 1982b) (Table II).

TABLE II

THE COMPARATIVE EFFECTS OF NEUROHYPOPHYSIAL HORMONES AND THEIR FRAGMENTS IN REDUCING THE MAGNITUDE OF A NEUROGENIC PRESSOR RESPONSE

The peptides were injected in a dose of 25 ng both in one lateral or the 4th ventricle. The inhibitory effect of the most effective natural neurohypophysial hormone (AVP_{1-9} in the lateral and OXT_{1-9} in the 4th ventricle) was considered as 100.

Cys–Tyr– X –Gln–Ans–Cys–Pro– Y –Gly–NH_2
 1   2   3   4   5   6   7   8   9

Peptide	Position	X	Y	Relative potency	
				lateral ventricle	4th ventricle
Arginine-vasopressin	(AVP_{1-9})	Phe	Arg	100.0	25.2
Pressinamide	(AVP_{1-6})	Phe	-	80.6	N.D.
Prolyl-argynyl-glycinamide	(AVP_{7-9})	-	Arg	112.1	87.8
Oxytocin	(OXT_{1-9})	Ile	Leu	73.9	100.0
Tocinamide	(OXT_{1-6})	Ile	-	36.3	N.D.
Prolyl-leucyl-glycinamide	(OXT_{7-9})	-	Lcu	84.8	113.9

These findings suggest that modulation of an acute neurogenic pressor response as evoked by MRF stimulation is a central action of AVP or related peptides. This effect is unrelated to the classical vasoactive properties of AVP. Furthermore, the differential action of AVP and fragments on the pressor and heart rate responses suggests that different mechanisms are involved in these responses. It may be that an action on the bradycardia response to AVP requires the whole molecule. This is in contrast with the BP effects, where structure–activity studies (Table II) suggest the presence of two active sites in the AVP molecule: one related to the covalent ring structure (AVP_{1-6}) and one to the C-terminal linear tripeptide residue (AVP_{7-9}). Structure–activity studies also show that the central cardiovascular action of AVP is not specific: oxytocin also has some inhibitory activity (Table II), but is much less potent than AVP. The tocinoid ring structure of oxytocin (OXT_{1-6}) has very low activity, but the C-terminal tripeptide residue OXT_{7-9} (prolyl-lcucyl-glycinamidc) appears to bc highly active. Fig. 3 shows that OXT_{7-9} reduces the magnitude of the neurogenic pressor response in the dose range of 6–25 ng. The higher dose of 50 ng is no more effective than 25 ng. The slope of the dose–response curve is rather steep and the degree of reduction is remarkably similar at both 50 and 70 Hz stimulation frequencies. This characteristic of action of the tripeptide is dissimilar to that of AVP and suggests that the two peptides may affect different brain mechanisms.

450

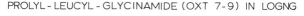

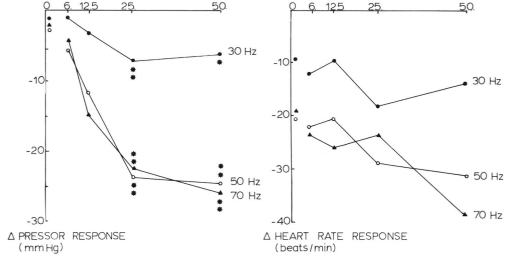

Fig. 3. Inhibition of neurogenic pressor responses by the administration of OXT₇₋₉ into a lateral cerebral ventricle. For explanations see Fig. 2.

These observations suggest that centrally available vasopressin or related peptides may be modulators of cardiovascular regulation. However, none of the peptides affected BP or heart rate in anaesthetized rats after administration into the lateral cerebral ventricle. These observations contrast with the finding of Pittman et al. (1982), who reported BP increase with short latency upon injection of AVP in doses of 25–5000 ng into a lateral cerebral ventricle. The reason for this discrepancy is not yet clear.

Alterations in central levels of vasopressin are followed by changes in the activity of noradrenergic systems in the brain (Tanaka et al., 1977; Versteeg et al., 1978, 1979b). Noradrenaline is believed to be an inhibitory transmitter in the central regulation of the cardiovascular system (Chalmers, 1975; De Jong et al., 1975a). Interactions between AVP and noradrenaline in the brain may also be involved in the modulation of centrally evoked BP changes.

Modulation of noradrenergic transmission in the dorsal noradrenergic bundle is involved in the effect of AVP on memory processes (Kovàcs et al., 1979). The dentate gyri of the dorsal hippocampus appear to be important for the peptide–noradrenaline interaction. Local injection of AVP in the dentate area facilitates memory storage and increases noradrenaline turnover in situ (Kovàcs et al., 1979).

THE HIPPOCAMPUS AND THE MODULATION OF THE NEUROGENIC PRESSOR RESPONSES BY NEUROHYPOPHYSIAL PEPTIDES

The inhibitory action of AVP but not of OXT₇₋₉ (PLG) on pressor responses evoked by MRF stimulation involves hippocampal mechanism (Versteeg et al., unpublished; Bohus et al., 1982b). Bilateral destruction of the dorsal hippocampus in the rat prevents the action of AVP administered into one lateral cerebral ventricle on the pressor response (Fig. 4). The reduction of the BP responses by OXT₇₋₉ is affected only slightly by lesioning the dorsal hippocampus.

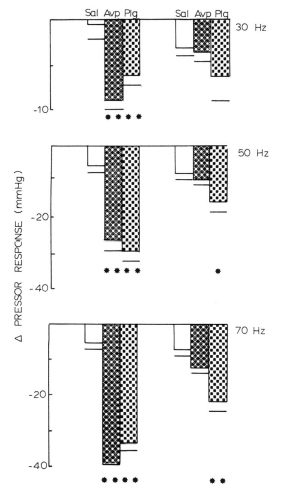

Fig. 4. Inhibitory effect of ΛVP, but not of prolyl-leucyl-glycinamide (Plg; OXT$_{l-9}$) on neurogenic pressor responses was prevented by bilateral destruction of the dorsal hippocampus (right panel). The peptides were administered into a lateral cerebral ventricle in a dose of 25 ng. Further abbreviations see Fig. 2.

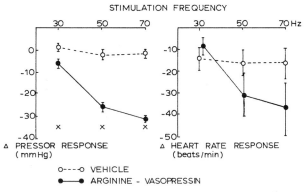

Fig. 5. Inhibition of neurogenic pressor responses by bilateral microinjection of AVP into the dentate area of the dorsal hippocampus. Abbreviations as in Fig. 2.

Accordingly, the absence of action of AVP in hippocampal-lesioned rats cannot be ascribed to an effect of the lesion on cerebroventricular circulation or on the penetration of the peptides into the brain tissue. Subsequent observations indicated that AVP acts within the hippocampus. Microinjection of the peptide into the dentate areas of the dorsal hippocampus in a dose of 1 ng (an ineffective dose intraventricularly) results in a marked reduction of the pressor response (Fig. 5).

These observations suggest that modulation of behavioural and cardiovascular responses by AVP may take place in the same (or related) locations in the hippocampus and probably involve a similar mode of action. Modulation of the hippocampal output by the peptide may then, in parallel but probably separately, affect brain mechanisms involved in the expression of behaviour and cardiovascular responses.

ACTION OF NEUROHYPOPHYSIAL HORMONE FRAGMENTS AT LOWER BRAINSTEM LEVEL

Administration of oxytocin, OXT_{7-9} and AVP_{7-9} into the 4th ventricle results in a marked diminution of the pressor response evoked by MRF stimulation. However, AVP appears to be practically inactive by this route of administration. As shown in Table II, OXT_{7-9} is the most active peptide in suppressing the pressor response (Versteeg et al., unpublished). The dose–response curve for OXT_{7-9} upon 4th ventricular injection is similar to that following lateral ventricular injection (Fig. 3). The curve is linear in the dose-range of 6–25 ng, but with a rather steep slope. Additionally, the dose of 50 ng is no more effective than 25 ng. OXT_{7-9} fails to affect the bradycardia response to stimulation.

These observations, together with the findings in rats with lesions to the dorsal hippocampus, suggest that oxytocin and related peptides act in the vicinity of the 4th ventricle to reduce the pressor responses. The ineffectiveness of AVP by this route of administration reinforces the notion that AVP acts primarily in the hippocampus. That AVP_{7-9} is active following 4th ventricular administration may be explained in different ways. Receptors for neurohypophysial peptides and/or for their biologically active fragments may not distinguish between Leu-(OXT_{7-9}) and Arg-(AVP_{7-9}) in position 8 of the molecules. Alternatively, the enzymes that metabolize AVP into active fragments may be absent in the vicinity of the 4th ventricle.

Subsequent observations reinforced the notion that oxytocin and related peptides affect neurogenic pressor responses through brainstem mechanisms. Microinjection of OXT_{7-9} into the dorsal raphe nucleus reduces the pressor response (Table III). The dorsal raphe nucleus is rich in oxytocin innervation (Sofroniew and Weindl, 1981) and has been implicated in cardiovascular regulation (Adair et al., 1977; Cabot et al., 1979). This nucleus contains cell bodies of serotonergic neurones whose axons terminate in the forebrain and the spinal cord. A role of this transmitter in cardiovascular regulation has already been suggested (De Jong et al., 1975b; Baum and Shropshire, 1975). However the dorsal raphe may not be the only site of action of neurohypophysial hormones in the (lower) brainstem. Fibres containing neurohypophysial hormone terminate in areas such as the nucleus tractus solitarius, the dorsal nuclei of the vagus nerve or the lateral reticular nuclei in the medulla oblongata (Sofroniew and Weindl, 1981), which are involved in the regulation of the cardiovascular system. Furthermore, interaction of vasopressin with noradrenergic transmission in these areas (Tanaka et al., 1977) may be important in the control of BP in conditions which may differ from the one studied in this series of experiments.

TABLE III

THE EFFECT OF MICROINJECTION OF OXT_{7-9} INTO THE DORSAL RAPHE NUCLEUS ON THE MAGNITUDE OF PRESSOR RESPONSES INDUCED BY THE STIMULATION OF THE MRF

Stimulation frequency in Hz[a]	Pressor response[b] in mm Hg	
	OXT_{7-9}	vehicle
30	-11.7 ± 1.6[c]	-9.0 ± 1.4
50	-33.2 ± 2.0[d]	-22.5 ± 2.5
70	-56.7 ± 1.4[e]	-43.8 ± 2.5

[a] The stimulation intensity that induced a pressor response of 50 mm Hg at 50 Hz was determined for each rat and used for the subsequent stimulations.

[b] The difference in the magnitude of the pressor response before and 30 min after peptide (1 ng) or vehicle administration.

[c] Mean $\pm$ S.E.M. of 8 observations.

[d] $P < 0.01$ (t-test, two-tailed).

[e] $P < 0.05$.

NEUROGENIC PRESSOR AND BRADYCARDIA RESPONSES IN RATS WITH HEREDITARY HYPOTHALAMIC DIABETES INSIPIDUS

Suppression of neurogenic hypertensive responses by AVP and related peptides may be a protective mechanism against over-response of the cardiovascular system to "stressful" stimuli. The physiological significance of a vasopressin system in the brain as a "protective" mechanism has been investigated in Brattleboro rats (Bohus, Versteeg, Ransom and De Jong, unpublished), homozygous for diabetes insipidus (DI rats), which are unable to synthesize vasopressin. The heterozygous variants of the Brattleboro strain have a partial deficit in the synthesis and release of vasopressin (Valtin and Schroder, 1964). A homozygous normal variant appears to be normal as far as the water intake and urine output are concerned. In these experiments the magnitude of the pressor and bradycardia responses was investigated using brain stimulations with either variable intensity (1–12 V) and fixed frequency (50 Hz), or variable frequency (10–300 Hz) and fixed intensity (200 μA). The rats were anaesthetized with urethane and the stimulation electrodes were inserted into the MRF, posterior hypothalamus and the posterior thalamic parafascicular nucleus.

The pressor and heart rate responses following MRF stimulations were larger in heterozygous rats than in either DI or homozygous normal littermates (Fig. 6). DI rats showed responses that were practically indistinguishable from those of the homozygous normal rats. Similar results were produced by posterior hypothalamic and parafascicular thalamic stimulations.

These observations suggest that the total absence of vasopressin does not alter neurogenic hypertensive responses. However, partial deficits of vasopressin synthesis and release as occur in heterozygous Brattleboro rats are associated with exaggerated pressor and bradycardiac responses.

We have also attempted to cause acute changes in the central vasopressin state by neutralizing the endogenous AVP with i.c.v. injections of specific antiserum against AVP. This approach was useful in behavioural (Van Wimersma Greidanus et al., 1975), electrophysiological (Urban and De Wied, 1978) and neurochemical studies (Versteeg et al., 1979b) in

454

non-anaesthetized rats, but not in our urethane-narcotized rats. I.c.v. administration of control rabbit serum even in an amount of 1 μl results in a profound diminution of the pressor and heart rate responses to MRF stimulations, probably due to changes in CSF or brain osmolality (Versteeg and Bohus, unpublished). The near normal responsiveness of DI rats to MRF or other brain stimulations may be related to a compensatory action of centrally available oxytocin or related peptides. An increased synthesis and release, and increased brain concentration of oxytocin was found in DI rats in comparison to their heterozygous littermates (Valtin et al., 1965; Dogterom et al., 1977, 1978).

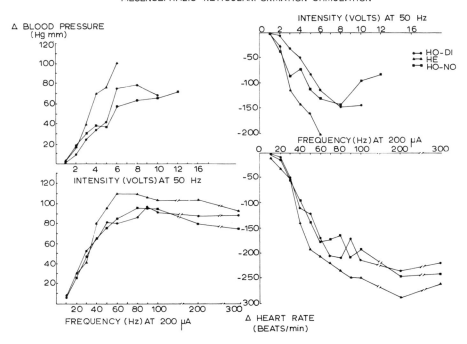

Fig. 6. The effects of intensity and frequency-dependent stimulations of the MRF on the systolic BP and heart rate in Brattleboro rats. HO-DI, homozygous rats suffering from hereditary hypothalamic diabetes insipidus; HE, heterozygous littermates; HO-NO, homozygous normal variant.

CONCLUDING REMARKS

Vasopressin and oxytocin, or fragments of these peptides, profoundly affect cardiovascular control mechanisms related to hypertensive responses of brain origin. Dysfunctions of these central peptide systems may have an aetiological significance in neurogenic hypertensions. This hypothesis is supported by a number of recent findings. Changes in brain vasopressin concentration have been reported in a stroke-prone substrain of spontaneously hypertensive rats (SHR; Lang et al., 1981), in SHR rats following stress (Negro-Vilar and Saavedra, 1980) and in the forebrain of hypertension-prone and -resistant Sabra strain of rats (Feuerstein et al.,

1981). These findings, together with our observations reviewed here, are consonant with the notion that neurogenic hypertension involves neuropeptide dysfunction with or without interaction with brain noradrenergic or adrenergic systems (e.g. Yamori et al., 1970; Versteeg et al., 1976; Saavedra et al., 1978; Wijnen et al., 1980). If this notion is correct, then neurohypophysial hormones, particularly analogues and fragments of them, may become important in the treatment of neurogenic hypertension.

REFERENCES

Adair, J.S., Hamilton, B.L., Scappaticci, K.A., Helke, C.J. and Gillis, R.A. (1977) Cardiovascular responses to electrical stimulation of the medullary raphe area of the cat. *Brain Res.,* 128: 141–145.

Baum, T. and Shropshire, A.T. (1975) Inhibition of efferent sympathetic nerve activity by 5-hydroxytryptophan and centrally administered 5-hydroxytryptamine. *Neuropharmacology,* 14: 227–233.

Bloch, V. (1970) Facts and hypotheses concerning memory consolidation processes. *Brain Res.,* 24: 561–575.

Bohus, B. (1971) Effect of hypophyseal peptides on memory functions in rats. In G. Adam and J. Szentàgothai (Eds.) *The Biology of Memory,* Publishing House of the Hungarian Academy of Sciences, Budapest, pp. 93–100.

Bohus, B. (1974) The influence of pituitary peptides on brain centers controlling autonomic responses. In D.F. Swaab and J.P. Schadé (Eds.), *Integrative Hypothalamic Activity, Progress in Brain Research, Vol. 41,* Elsevier, Amsterdam, pp. 175–183.

Bohus, B. (1975) Pituitary peptides and adaptive autonomic responses. In W.H. Gispen, Tj. B. van Wimersma Greidanus, B. Bohus and D. de Wied (Eds.), *Hormones, Homeostasis and the Brain, Progress in Brain Research, Vol. 42,* Elsevier, Amsterdam, pp. 275–283.

Bohus, B., Conti, L., Kovàcs, G.L. and Versteeg, D.H.G. (1982a) Modulation of memory processes by neuropeptides: interaction with neurotransmitter systems. In C. Ajmone Marsan and H. Matthies (Eds.), *Neuronal Plasticity and Memory Formation,* Raven, New York, pp. 75–87.

Bohus, B., Versteeg, C.A.M. and De Jong, W. (1982b) Vasopressin and central blood pressure control in the rat. In W. Rascher, D. Clugh and S. Ganten (Eds.), *Hypertensive Mechanisms,* Schattauer Verlag, Stuttgart, pp. 592–596.

Buijs, R.M., Swaab, D.F., Dogterom, J. and Van Leeuwen, F.W. (1978) Intra- and extrahypothalamic vasopressin and oxytocin pathways in the rat. *Cell. Tiss. Res.,* 186: 423–433.

Cabot, J.B., Wild, J.M. and Cohen, D.H. (1979) Raphe inhibition of sympathetic preganglionic neurons. *Science,* 203: 184–186.

Chalmers, J.P. (1975) Brain amines and models of experimental hypertension. *Circulat. Res.,* 36: 469–480.

Cowley, A.W., Jr., Switzer, S. and Guinn, M.M. (1980) Evidence and quantification of the vasopressin arterial pressure control in the dog. *Circulat. Res.,* 46: 58–67.

Cushing, H. (1932) Posterior–pituitary hormone and parasympathetic apparatus. In *Papers Relating to the Pituitary Body, Hypothalamus and Parasympathetic Nervous System,* C.C. Thomas, Springfield, pp. 59–111.

De Jong, W., Zandberg, P. and Bohus, B. (1975a) Central inhibitory noradrenergic cardiocascular control. In W.H. Gispen, Tj. B. van Wimersma Greidanus, B. Bohus and D. de Wied (Eds.); *Hormones, Homeostasis and the Brain, Progress in Brain Research, Vol. 42,* Elsevier, Amsterdam, pp. 285–298.

De Jong, W., Nijkamp, F.P. and Bohus, B. (1975b) Role of noradrenaline and serotonin in the central control of blood pressure in normotensive and spontaneously hypertensive rats. *Arch. int. Pharmacodyn.,* 213: 272–284.

De Wied, D. (1965) The influence of the posterior and intermediate lobe of the pituitary and pituitary peptides on the maintenance of a conditioned avoidance response in rats. *Int. J. Neuropharmacol.,* 4: 157–167.

De Wied, D. (1971) Long term effect of vasopressin on the maintenance of a conditioned avoidance response in rats. *Nature (Lond.),* 232: 58–60.

De Wied, D. and Bohus, B. (1966) Long term and short term effects on retention of a conditioned avoidance response in rats by treatment with long acting Pitressin and α-MSH. *Nature (Lond.),* 212: 1484–1486.

De Wied, D. and Versteeg, D.H.G. (1979) Neurohypophyseal principles and memory. *Fed. Proc.,* 38: 2348–2354.

De Wied, D., Greven, H.M., Lande, S. and Witter, A. (1972) Dissociation of the behavioural and endocrine effects of lysine vasopressin by tryptic digestion. *Brit. J. Pharmacol.,* 45: 118–122.

De Wied, D., Bohus, B. and Van Wimersma Greidanus, Tj. B. (1975) Memory deficit in rats with hereditary diabetes insipidus. *Brain Res.,* 85: 152–156.

Dogterom, J., Van Wimersma Greidanus, Tj. B. and Swaab, D.F. (1977) Evidence for the release of vasopressin and oxytocin into cerebrospinal fluid: measurements in plasma and CSF of intact and hypophysectomized rats. *Neuroendocrinology,* 24: 108–118.

456

Dogterom, J., Snijdewint, F.G.M. and Buijs, R.M. (1978) The distribution of vasopressin and oxytocin in the rat brain. *Neurosci. Lett.,* 9: 341–346.

Feuerstein, G., Zerbe, R.L., Ben-Ishay, D., Kopin, I.J. and Jacobowitz, D.M. (1981) Catecholamines and vasopressin in forebrain nuclei of hypertension prone and resistant rats. *Brain Res. Bull.,* 7: 671–676.

Gillies, G. and Lowry, P.J. (1979) The relationship between vasopressin and corticotropin-releasing factor. In M.T. Jones, B. Gillham, M.F. Dallman and S. Chattopadhyay (Eds.), *Interaction within the Brain–Pituitary–Adrenocortical System,* Academic Press, London, pp. 51–61.

Koob, G.F. and Bloom, F.E. (1982) Behavioral effects of neuropeptides: endorphins and vasopressin. *Ann. Rev. Physiol.,* 44: 571–582.

Kovàcs, G.L., Bohus, B. and Versteeg, D.H.G. (1979) The effects of vasopressin on memory processes: the role of noradrenergic neurotransmission. *Neuroscience,* 4: 1529–1537.

Lang, R.E., Rascher, W., Unger, Th. and Ganten, D. (1981) Reduced content of vasopressin in the brain of spontaneously hypertensive as compared to normotensive rats. *Neurosci. Lett.,* 23: 199–202.

Le Moal, M., Koob, G.F., Koda, L.Y., Bloom, F.E., Manning, M., Sawyer, W.H. and Rivier, J. (1981) Vasopressor receptor antagonist prevents behavioural effects of vasopressin. *Nature (Lond.),* 291: 491–493.

Mialhe, C., Lutz-Butcher, B., Briaud, B., Schleiffer, R. and Koch, B. (1979) Corticotropin-releasing factor (CRF) and vasopressin in the regulation of corticotropin (ACTH) secretion. In M.T. Jones, B. Gillham, M.F. Dallman and S. Chattopadhyay (Eds.), *Interaction within the Brain–Pituitary–Adrenocortical System,* Academic Press, London, pp. 63–74.

Moruzzi, G. and Magoun, H.W. (1949) Brain stem reticular formation and activation of the EEG. *Electroenceph. clin. Neurophysiol.,* 1: 455–473.

Nashold, B.S., Jr., Mannarino, E. and Wunderlich, M. (1962) Pressor–depressor blood pressure responses in the cat after intraventricular injection of drugs. *Nature (Lond.),* 193: 1297–1298.

Nashold, B.S., Jr., Mannarino, E.M. and Robinson, R.R. (1963) Effect of posterior pituitary polypeptides on the flow of urine after injection in lateral ventricle of the brain of a cat. *Nature (Lond.),* 194: 293.

Negro-Vilar, A. and Saavedra, J.M. (1980) Changes in brain somatostatin and vasopressin levels after stress in spontaneously hypertensive and Wistar-Kyoto rats. *Brain Res. Bull.,* 5: 353–358.

Oliver, G. and Schäfer, E.A. (1895) On the physiological action of extracts of pituitary body and certain other glandular organs. *J. Physiol. (Lond.),* 18: 277–279.

Pittman, Q.J., Lawrence, D. and McLean, L. (1982) Central effects of arginine vasopressin on blood pressure in rats. *Endocrinology,* 110: 1058–1060.

Rodriguez, E.M. (1976) The cerebrospinal fluid as a pathway in neuroendocrine integration. *J. Endocr.,* 71: 407–437.

Saavedra, J.M., Grobecker, H. and Axelrod, J. (1978) Changes in central catecholaminergic neurons in spontaneously (genetic) hypertensive rats. *Circulat. Res.,* 42: 529–534.

Sofroniew, M.V. and Weindl, A. (1981) Central nervous system distribution of vasopressin, oxytocin, and neurophysin. In J.L. Martinez, Jr., R.A. Jensen, R.B. Messing, H. Rigter and J.L. McGaugh (Eds.), *Endogenous Peptides and Learning and Memory Processes,* Academic Press, New York, pp. 327–369.

Sterba, G. (1974) Ascending neurosecretory pathways of the peptidergic type. In F. Knowles and L. Vollrath (Eds.), *Neurosecretion — The Final Neuroendocrine Pathway,* Springer, Berlin, pp. 38–47.

Swaab, D.F. (1980) Neurohypophysial hormones and their distribution in the brain. In D. de Wied and P.A. van Keep (Eds.), *Hormones and the Brain,* MTP Press, Lancaster, pp. 87–100.

Tanaka, M., De Kloet, E.R., De Wied, D. and Versteeg, D.H.G. (1977) Arginine[8]-vasopressin affects catecholamine metabolism in specific brain nuclei. *Life Sci.,* 20: 1799–1808.

Urban, I. and De Wied, D. (1978) Neuropeptides: effects on paradoxical sleep and theta rhythm in rats. *Pharmacol. Biochem. Behav.,* 8: 51–59.

Valtin, H. and Schroeder, H.A. (1964) Familial hypothalamic diabetes insipidus in rats (Brattleboro strain). *Amer. J. Physiol.,* 206: 425–430.

Valtin, H., Sawyer, W.H. and Sokol, H.W. (1965) Neurohypophyseal principles in rats homozygous and heterozygous for hypothalamic diabetes insipidus (Brattleboro strain). *Endocrinology,* 77: 701–706.

Van Wimersma Greidanus, Tj. B., Dogterom, J. and De Wied, D. (1975) Intraventricular administration of anti-vasopressin serum inhibits memory in rats. *Life Sci.,* 16: 637–644.

Versteeg, C.A.M., Bohus, B. and De Jong, W. (1982a) Attenuation by arginine- and desglycinamide-lysine-vasopressin of a centrally evoked pressor response. *J. Auton. Nerv. Syst.,* 6: 253–262.

Versteeg, C.A.M., Bohus, B. and De Jong, W. (1982b) Inhibition of centrally-evoked pressor responses by neurohypophyseal peptides and their fragments. *Neuropharmacology,* 21: 1359–1364.

Versteeg, D.H.G., Palkovits, M., Van der Gugten, J., Wijnen, H.J.L.M., Smeets, G.W.M. and De Jong, W. (1976) Catecholamine content of individual brain region of spontaneously hypertensive rats. *Brain Res.,* 112: 429–434.

Versteeg, D.H.G., Tanaka, M. and De Kloet, E.R. (1978) Catecholamine concentration and turnover in discrete regions of the brain of the homozygous Brattleboro rat deficient in vasopressin. *Endocrinology,* 103: 1654–1661.

Versteeg, C.A.M., Bohus, B. and De Jong, W. (1979a) Inhibitory effects of neuropeptides on centrally evoked pressor responses. In Y. Yamori, W. Loevenberg and E.D. Freis (Eds.), *Prophylactic Approach to Hypertensive Disease,* Raven, New York, pp. 329–335.

Versteeg, D.H.G., De Kloet, E.R., Van Wimersma Greidanus, Tj. B. and De Wied, D. (1979b) Vasopressin modulates the activity of catecholamine containing neurons in specific brain regions. *Neurosci. Lett.,* 11: 69–73.

Wijnen, H.J.L.M., Spierenburg, H.A., De Kloet, E.R., De Jong, W. and Versteeg, D.H.G. (1980) Decrease in noradrenergic activity in hypothalamic nuclei during the development of spontaneous hypertension. *Brain Res.,* 184: 153–162.

Yamori, Y., Lovenberg, W. and Sjoerdsma, A. (1970) Norepinephrine metabolism in brain stem of spontaneous hypertensive rats. *Science,* 170: 1673–1686.

The Neurohypophysis: Structure, Function and Control, Progress in Brain Research, Vol. 60, edited by B.A. Cross and G. Leng
© *1983 Elsevier Science Publishers B.V.*

Role of Neurones in the Supraoptic and Paraventricular Nuclei in Cardiovascular Control

H. YAMASHITA, H. KANNAN, K. INENAGA and K. KOIZUMI[1]

Departments of Physiology, University of Occupational and Environmental Health, School of Medicine, Kitakyushu (Japan) and [1]State University of New York, Downstate Medical Center, Brooklyn, NY 11203 (U.S.A.)

INTRODUCTION

Recent studies have shown that neurosecretory neurones in the supraoptic (SON) and paraventricular nuclei (PVN) are strongly influenced by baro-, chemo- and atrial receptors (Kannan and Yagi, 1978; Koizumi and Yamashita, 1978; Yamashita, 1977; Yamashita and Koizumi, 1979; Yamashita et al., 1979). As these neurones release vasopressin and oxytocin from the neurohypophysis and as a number of studies indicate that vasopressin (and probably oxytocin as well) is involved in cardiovascular control (Gauer, 1978; Gauer and Henry, 1976; Robertson, 1977; Share, 1976), there may be a close relationship between these neurones and the autonomic system. How, and to what extent, the SON and PVN are involved in regulation of the autonomic system, particularly cardiovascular functions, is not yet clarified.

Recent morphological studies have revealed neural connections between these hypothalamic nuclei and the regions concerned with sympathetic and vagal activity. Electrophysiological studies have also shown that there may be specific pathways from the SON and PVN to the medulla and the spinal cord through which these neurones may participate in control of the cardiovascular system.

INFLUENCES EXERTED BY RECEPTORS IN THE CARDIOVASCULAR SYSTEM ON THE HYPOTHALAMIC NEUROSECRETORY NEURONES

Changes in blood pressure, blood volume and body position, which alter the distribution of the blood in the circulatory system, all influence the level of vasopressin in plasma. These changes in the hormone level are exerted through baroreceptors and "volume receptors" or receptors situated in the low pressure region in the circulatory system.

Excitation of baroreceptors in the carotid sinus inhibits the activity of "identified" neurosecretory neurones in the SON and PVN in cats (Fig. 1A) (Yamashita, 1977; Yamashita and Koizumi, 1979). Using the "isolated" carotid sinus preparation we found that the threshold for this inhibition was fairly low, i.e. 60–70 mm Hg (Fig. 1B), the level at which the activity of myelinated afferents in the carotid sinus nerve begins to increase. With stronger stimuli (i.e. high carotid sinus pressure) the magnitude of the inhibitory action could be graded and it reached its maximum at a sinus pressure of 110–120 mm Hg, when neurosecretory neurones ceased to fire. This level of sinus pressure was similar to the level at which the maximum discharge of the myelinated sinus afferents occurred, though it was still below threshold for

[459]

460

exciting unmyelinated afferents (Kirchheim, 1976). The magnitude of inhibition of neurosecretory neurone activity seemed to parallel the degree of depressor response caused by excitation of baroreceptors. Stimulation of the aortic baroreceptors also inhibited neurosecretory cells in the SON and PVN.

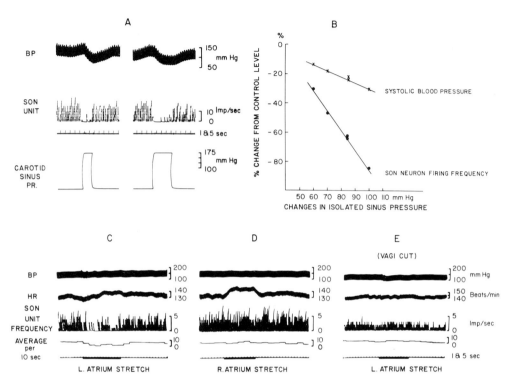

Fig. 1. Changes produced in SON neurones by activation of receptors in the cardiovascular system. A: stimulation of baroreceptors by an increase in pressure in the isolated carotid sinus. From top to bottom, systemic blood pressure (BP), integrated record of firing frequencies of a SON neurone (Unit), and pressure in the isolated carotid sinus (Sinus Pr.). B: effects of changing pressure in the isolated carotid sinus on single SON neurone activity and the depressor response. Percentage changes in response were plotted against stimulus intensities. (A and B are from two different experiments in cats). C–E: effects of atrial stretch on SON neurone activity, blood pressure (BP) and heart rate (HR). Experiments in dogs. Note differences in responses by stimulation of left (L) or right (R) atrium. The effects on both HR and SON neurone activity were abolished after section of the vagi bilaterally at the neck.

The use of occlusion of both carotid arteries to "unload" the sinus baroreceptors, or electrical stimulation of carotid sinus and aortic nerves, confirmed these findings. Carotid occlusion excited neurosecretory cells, while stimulation of baroreceptor afferents inhibited them. However, these two manoeuvres, though simpler to apply than more physiological stimuli, had to be carried out carefully to avoid exciting chemoreceptors situated in the same area or chemoreceptor afferents. We found that excitation of chemoreceptors caused strong activation of neurosecretory neurones (Yamashita, 1977).

The inhibition of SON neurones by activation of sinus baroreceptors has also been observed in rats. It was found that 90% of SON neurones in cats (Yamashita and Koizumi, 1979) and 30% in rats (Kannan and Yagi, 1978) were thus affected by baroreceptor stimulation.

Activation of atrial receptors which produce cardiovascular responses as well as changes in the autonomic nerve activity (Koizumi et al., 1975; Kollai et al., 1978), affected both SON and PVN neurones (Koizumi and Yamashita, 1978; Koizumi et al., 1979) (Fig. 1C–E). Mechanical stretch of the left atrium inhibited most neurosecretory cells in the SON and PVN. However stimulation of the right atrial receptors, though it caused cardiovascular reactions, had no inhibitory effect on these neurones. As the right and left atria play different roles in controlling cardiac function, and as excitation of the receptors in the two atria produce different recorded responses from cardiac vagal and sympathetic nerves (Kollai et al., 1978), it is understandable that their actions on neurosecretory neurones should also differ.

PATHWAYS MEDIATING CARDIOVASCULAR RESPONSES FROM NEURONES IN THE PVN AND SON

Morphological studies have revealed "direct" connections between the PVN and the medulla and spinal cord (Hosoya and Matsushita, 1979; Loewy, 1981; Loewy and McKeller, 1980; Saper, 1979; Saper et al., 1976; Swanson and Kuypers, 1980). However, the functional significance of such connections has not been studied. We have investigated this problem with electrophysiological techniques.

First, we studied the afferent connections from baro- and chemoreceptors to the SON and PVN. As shown by a number of investigators, afferent impulses from these receptors travelling via the carotid sinus nerve or aortic nerve first reach relay neurones in the region of the nucleus tractus solitarius (NTS). It has been reported (Nakai et al., 1982) that stimulation of NTS releases vasopressin from the neurohypophysis. We found two afferent pathways between NTS and neurosecretory neurones in the SON in cats; a "fast" or short latency, and a "slow" or long latency pathway. The inhibitory effect on neurosecretory neurones in the SON was exerted mostly through the "fast" pathway, while the excitatory effect on SON neurones was conveyed mostly by the "slow" pathway (Kannan and Koizumi, 1981).

More recently "direct" *efferent* connections have been investigated between PVN neurones and certain areas in the dorsomedial medulla which are particularly concerned with cardiovascular control. For this purpose, responses of neurones in the PVN to stimulation of the dorsomedial medulla were recorded in rats. Of 415 neurones tested, 66 were antidromically activated, indicating that axons of these neurones terminate in the dorsal medulla. A small proportion of these neurones (7 out of 51; 14%) were inhibited by baroreceptor activation. Only two of the 66 neurones whose axons terminated in the dorsomedial medulla were found to project to the neurohypophysis as well, and they were affected by baroreceptor stimulation. This study also enabled us to locate the site of axon terminals in the medulla (Fig. 2C) (Kannan and Yamashita 1982a; see also Zerihun and Harris, 1981). All areas in the dorsal medulla where axons of PVN neurones were found to terminate produced a clear depressor response upon weak stimulation with repetitive pulses (50 Hz). The areas included the dorsal vagal nucleus, NTS and adjacent sites.

The threshold of medullary stimulation for activating PVN neurones antidromically ranged between 10 and 290 μA, with a mean latency of 38.5 msec (n = 66, S.D. $\pm$ 9.8 msec) (Fig. 2B; Kannan and Yamashita, 1982b). This indicates that the axons from the PVN to the medulla are unmyelinated (estimated average speed of conduction, 0.4 m/sec). Stimulation of the PVN produced both excitation and inhibition of neurones in the dorsal vagal nucleus and NTS (Fig. 2D). Seventy-six neurones were excited orthodromically with latencies of 35–60 msec. These latencies were similar to those of antidromically evoked action potentials

462

recorded from PVN neurones following medullary stimulation. Twenty-two neurones were inhibited after a shorter latency by stimulation of the PVN.

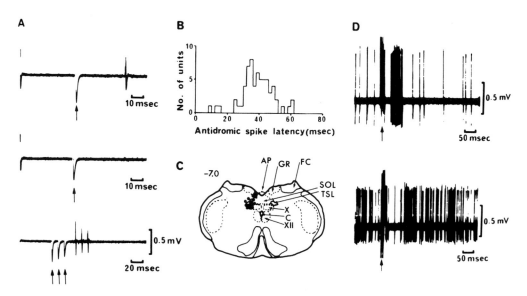

Fig. 2. Efferent connections between the PVN and dorsomedial medulla in rats. A: antidromic action potentials recorded from a PVN neurone following stimulation (indicated by an arrow) of the dorsomedial medulla. In upper and middle traces the oscilloscope sweeps were triggered by spontaneous action potentials (seen at the left end of the traces). Stimuli applied to the medulla with 44 msec delay after the spontaneous action potentials evoked antidromic action potentials (upper trace). With the delay less than 41 msec action potentials evoked by the stimuli were extinguished by collision with the spontaneous action potentials (middle trace). Both pictures are 5 superimposed oscilloscope tracings. In the bottom trace 3 stimulating pulses at 100 Hz were applied to the medulla. Three action potentials evoked indicate that this PVN neurone can follow this high frequency stimulation. The threshold for evoking the antidromic spike was 0.14 mA. B: distribution of latencies of antidromically evoked action potentials recorded from PVN neurones following stimulation of the dorsomedial medulla. C: sites of stimulation (marked by ●) in the dorsomedial medulla which evoked antidromic action potentials in PVN neurones. The number −7.0 indicates stereotaxic transverse coordinate according to the atlas of Pellegrino et al. (1979). Abbreviations: AP, area postrema; C, canalis centralis; FC, fasciculus cuneatus; SOL, nucleus tractus solitarius; TSL, tractus solitarius; X, nucleus nervi vagi; XII, nucleus nervi hypoglossi. D: excitatory (upper) and inhibitory (lower trace) responses of neurones in the dorsomedial medulla orthodromically evoked by stimulation of the PVN. Each picture represents 10 superimposed oscilloscope tracings. All stimuli (3 pulses at 200 Hz, 0.3 mA, 0.5 msec) were given at arrows. Note that latencies of excitatory responses were similar to those shown in B. The latency of inhibition was shorter than that of excitation.

Morphological studies in rats (Hosoya and Matsushita, 1979; Swanson and Kuypers, 1980) have shown that the PVN neurones which project to the medulla are mainly parvocellular cells and are situated in regions other than those where most magnocellular cells are located.

Possible functional connections between neurones in the PVN, SON and sympathetic preganglionic neurones in the spinal cord were also investigated (Koizumi et al., 1983; Ciriello and Calaresu, 1980). With the use of a microelectrode and a stimulus strength below 50 μA, a "map" of the hypothalamus showing the sites of effective stimulation was constructed. Stimulation of certain regions in the vicinity of PVN produced strong pressor response (Fig. 3A). In other experiments, stimulation of these regions was shown to influence the activity of sympathetic preganglionic neurones recorded from the thoracic white ramus (T2 or T3 WR). Stimulation of certain areas in the PVN region, particularly in its dorsal part (3–5

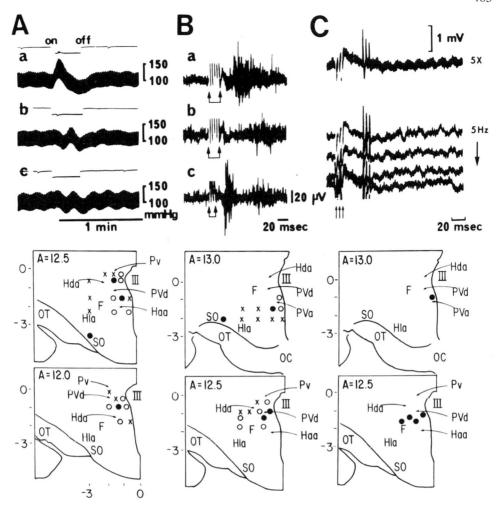

Fig. 3. Efferent connections between PVN and intermediolateral cell column of the spinal cord (T2–T3) in cats. A: upper panels (a–c) show blood pressure changes caused by stimulation (50 µA, 0.5 msec at 50 Hz, marked by on, off signs) of the areas marked in the lower panel. ●, Clear pressor response, as shown in a; o, moderate pressor responses, as b; ×, none or weak responses, as c. B: upper panels (a–c) show sympathetic preganglionic discharges recorded from T2 white ramus following stimulation of the hypothalamus (between arrows; 3–5 pulses, 0.5 msec at 200 Hz; intensity, 50 µA in a and b, 20 µA in c). All recordings are 5 superimposed oscilloscope tracings. Lower panels show stimulation sites in the hypothalamus. ●, stimulation caused sympathetic discharges after less than 50 msec latency, as shown in a and c; o, stimulation caused some discharges with a latency of 70–90 msec, as b; ×, none or very weak response. C: upper panel shows a PVN neurone antidromically activated by stimulation of ipsilateral intermediolateral cell column of the thoracic spinal cord (60 µA, 0.5 msec at 200 Hz, arrows). The neurone responded with a fixed latency and with three spikes to three stimulating pulses. The top is 5 superimposed tracings, the next four tracings are successive records of responses following stimulation (3 pulses) given at 5 Hz. Stimulation of the neurohypophysis did not excite this neurone antidromically. Lower panels show recording sites of neurones antidromically activated by stimulation of the cord. Abbreviations: F, fornix; Haa, anterior hypothalamic area; Hda, dorsal hypothalamic area; Hla, lateral hypothalamic area; OT, optic tract; OC, optic chiasm; PVa, paraventricular nucleus, anterior component; PVd, paraventricular nucleus, dorsal component; Pv, parvocellular nucleus; SO, supraoptic nucleus. A = 12.0, 12.5 and 13.0 indicate stereotaxic frontal coordinates (Bleier, 1961).

pulses at 200 Hz, 0.5 msec) evoked a discharge in the white ramus after a latency of less than 50 msec (Fig. 3B) with a threshold of 20–30 μA. In addition, stimulation of a region just outside the histological boundaries of SON evoked a distinct sympathetic discharge with very low current intensity (threshold 10 μA, see Fig. 3Bc).

Thus neurones in or near the PVN (and SON) may be involved in cardiovascular reactions. However, it is well known that stimulation of many other areas in the hypothalamus excites sympathetic neurones (Koizumi and Kollai, 1981). Therefore the response discussed above may not be conveyed through monosynaptic pathways from PVN to the sympathetic pregang-lionic neurones. To find whether any PVN neurone projects to the sympathetic neurone pool in the spinal cord, an attempt was made to record antidromically activated neurones in the PVN following stimulation of the spinal cord. Of 294 neurones studied (239 in the PVN, 49 in the SON and six in other hypothalamic areas) five were activated antidromically in response to stimulation of the intermediolateral cell column of the thoracic cord (Fig. 3C). Another nine cells may also be included in this category, though the evidence for antidromic activation was not very ·strong. Of these antidromically excited neurones (five definite, nine doubtful), two were found to send their axons to the neurohypophysis but eight others were excited orthodro-mically by the pituitary stalk stimulation (Pittman et al., 1981), i.e. they responded to the stimulus with varied latencies. The remaining four neurones did not respond to stimulation of the neurohypophysis. All 14 neurones showed spontaneous activity and some of them could belong to the parvocellular group.

DISCUSSION

For maintenance of homeostasis, neural and humoral systems must co-operate. To un-derstand control of the cardiovascular function, the study of interactions between the endocrine and the autonomic nervous sytems becomes quite important.

Recent discovery and re-discovery of roles played by vasopressin in various functions has provided much new information. Vasopressin may act directly on central neurones, thus participating in regulation of the blood pressure (Brody, 1981; Matsuguchi et al., 1980). In the periphery the hormone not only acts on blood vessels but also alters vascular responsiveness to vasoconstrictors, such as noradrenaline (Altura and Altura, 1977; Brody 1981). Some studies suggest involvement of vasopressin in hypertension (Berecek et al., 1980; Crofton et al., 1978, 1979).

Morphological studies have revealed both a "direct" connection between neurones in the PVN and the medulla and the spinal cord, and vasopressin- and oxytocin-containing fibres which extend from the hypothalamus to the medulla and the spinal cord (Swanson, 1977; Buijs, 1978; Swanson and McKeller, 1979; Nilaver et al., 1980; Sofroniew, 1980; Swanson and Hartman, 1980; Sofroniew and Schrell, 1981; Weindl and Sofroniew, 1980). However, the results of both morphological and electrophysiological studies must be interpreted with caution. The mere finding that some neurones in SON and PVN send axons to specific regions in the medulla and the spinal cord concerned with autonomic control of the cardiovascular system does not necessarily indicate functional significance. It is not known whether neurones in the SON and PVN play any unique role in cardiovascular control. The hypothalamus is concerned with integration of various behavioural reactions which often include changes in cardiovascular responses. There are many different areas in the hypothalamus which, upon stimulation, influence the activity of sympathetic and vagal efferent nerves (Koizumi and Kollai, 1981). Many of these responses are thought to be evoked through polysynaptic pathways from the hypothalamus to vagal and preganglionic sympathetic neurones, relaying at medulla and other regions in the CNS. The fact that rather few neurones in the PVN send axons to the medulla or to the cord can be interpreted in two ways. One is that these fibres, though few and slow conducting, subserve their specific function by releasing hormone or transmitter at their terminals. The other interpretation is that these fibres do not have any unique function other than being a part of many other fibres projecting from the hypothalamus to the various areas through polysynaptic paths. Some experimental results suggest the former possibility. Small injections of vasopressin into the NTS affect blood pressure and heart rate (Matsuguchi et al., 1980) and oxytocin has a direct action on medullary neurones (Morris et al., 1980), although the majority of PVN neurones projecting to the medulla or the cord are not magnocellular, and may not contain oxytocin or vasopressin. Whether these neurones are functionally related to neurosecretory neurones of the neurohypophysis is not known. As *most* neurones projecting to different regions (medulla, cord, neural lobe, median eminence, etc.) are thought to be separate cells (Kannan and Yamashita, 1982a; Swanson et al., 1980; Zerihun and Harris, 1981), relationships between these neurones must be clarified.

Other studies indicate the importance of noradrenergic input to the SON and PVN neurones which is thought to regulate vasopressin release from the nuclei. Lesions of the locus coeruleus abolish the response of cells in the SON to baroreceptor stimulation without affecting the autonomic reactions of baroreceptor reflex or the response of the neurones to chemoreceptors (Banks and Harris, 1982). Lesions of the A_1 area in the medulla, which is known to contain noradrenergic neurones, result in an increase in vasopressin in the blood. Hypertension caused by A_1 lesions in rabbits is considered to be due, at least partly, to the loss of continuous inhibitory influence from the A_1 area to the SON and PVN through catecholaminergic pathways (Blessing et al., 1982, 1983). There is anatomical evidence for such connections (Sawchenko and Swanson, 1981, 1982a; Swanson et al., 1981). In addition, a recent report suggests an involvement of a PVN-adrenergic system in a non-cardiovascular function (Sawchenko et al., 1981).

SUMMARY

Our recent electrophysiological studies have shown that receptors in the cardiovascular system (baro-, chemo- and atrial receptors) influence neurosecretory neurones in the SON and PVN. In anaesthetized cats and rats, excitation of baro- and atrial receptors (high and low pressure receptors) inhibits the activity of neurosecretory neurones while activation of chemoreceptors excites them. Our studies of the afferent projections to SON and PVN from regions in the medulla where most afferents from receptors in the cardiovascular system project, have revealed that there are both "fast" and "slow" pathways. Results of our work on efferent projections from PVN and SON neurones indicate that a few of these neurones send axons directly to the medullary regions which are specifically concerned with cardiovascular functions, and to the vicinity of sympathetic preganglionic neurones in the thoracic spinal cord. Some of these neurones are magnocellular neurosecretory cells. These results, together with recent morphological and physiological evidence, suggest that the hypothalamo-neurohypophysial system contributes significantly to control of autonomic functions and that further study in this field is much needed.

466

ACKNOWLEDGEMENTS

The work presented in this paper was supported in part by Grants 56370007 and 57570056 from the Japanese Ministry of Education and by USPHS Grant NS-00847 and NSF Grant INT 8006323.

REFERENCES

Altura, B.M. and Altura, B.T. (1977) Vascular smooth muscle and neurohypophyseal hormones. *Fed. Proc.*, 36: 1853–1860.

Banks, D. and Harris, M.C. (1982) Involvement of the locus coeruleus in the inhibition of supraoptic neurones during baroreceptor stimulation in rats. *Neuroscience*, 7, Suppl.: S16–S17.

Berecek, K.H., Murray, R.D., Brody, M.J. and Gross, F. (1980) Vasopressin (VP) and vascular reactivity in the development of desoxycorticosterone hypertension in rats with hereditary diabetes insipidus (DI). *Circulation*, 62: 111–124.

Bleier, R. (1961) *The Hypothalamus of the Cat,* Johns Hopkins Press, Baltimore, MD.

Blessing, W.W., Jaeger, C. B., Ruggiero, D.A. and Reis, D.J. (1982) Hypothalamic projections of medullary catecholamine neurons in the rabbit: a combined catecholamine fluorescence and HRP transport study. *Brain Res. Bull.*, 9: 279–286.

Blessing, W.W., Sved, A.F. and Reis, D.J. (1983) Elevated plasma vasopressin contributes to fulminating hypertension produced by acute lesions of A1 catecholamine neurons in rabbit medulla. *Clin. Sci.*, in press.

Brody, M.J. (1981) New developments in our knowledge of blood pressure regulation. *Fed. Proc.*, 40: 2257–2261.

Buijs, L.M. (1978) Intra- and extrahypothalamic vasopressin and oxytocin pathways in the rat. *Cell Tiss. Res.*, 192: 423–435.

Ciriello, J. and Calaresu, F.R. (1980) Role of paraventricular and supraoptic nuclei in central cardiovascular regulation in the cat. *Amer. J. Physiol.*, 239: R137–142.

Crofton, J.T., Share, L., Shade, R.E., Allen, C. and Tarnowski, D. (1978) Vasopressin in the rat with spontaneous hypertension. *Amer. J. Physiol.*, 235: H361–366.

Crofton, J.T., Share, L., Shade, R.E., Ler-Kwon, W.J., Manning, M. and Sawyer, W.H. (1979) The importance of vasopressin in the development and maintenance of DOC–salt hypertension in the rat. *Hypertension*, 1: 31–38.

Gauer, O.H. (1978) Role of cardiac mechanoreceptors in the control of central plasma volume. In C.B. Jorgensen and E. Skadhange (Eds.), *Osmotic and Volume Regulation*, Munksgaard, Copenhagen, pp. 229–247.

Gauer, O.H. and Henry, J.P. (1976) Neurohormonal control of plasma volume. In A.C. Guyton and A.W. Cowley (Eds.), *Cardiovascular Physiology II, Int. Review of Physiology*, Vol. 9, Univ. Park Press, Baltimore, ND, pp. 145–190.

Hosoya, Y. and Matsushita, M. (1979) Identification and distribution of the spinal and hypophyseal projection neurons in the paraventricular nucleus of the rat. A light and electron microscopic study with the horseradish peroxidase method. *Exp. Brain Res.*, 35: 315–331.

Kannan, H. and Koizumi, K. (1981) Pathways between the nucleus tractus solitarius and neurosecretory neurons of the supraoptic nucleus: electrophysiological studies. *Brain Res.*, 213: 17–28.

Kannan, H. and Yagi, K. (1978) Supraoptic neurosecretory neurons: evidence for the existence of converging inputs both from carotid baroreceptors and osmoreceptors. *Brain Res.*, 145: 385–390.

Kannan, H. and Yamashita, H. (1982a) Electrophysiological studies of the hypothalamic paraventricular neurons projecting to the dorsomedial medulla. *J. Physiol. Soc. Japan*, 44: 177–178.

Kannan, H. and Yamashita, H. (1982b) Paraventricular nucleus neurons projecting to the dorsomedial medulla receive synaptic input from carotid baroreceptors in rats, *Neurosci. Lett.*, Suppl. 9: S 3.

Kirchheim, H.R. (1976) Systemic arterial baroreceptor reflexes. *Physiol. Rev.*, 56: 100–176.

Koizumi, K. and Kollai, M. (1981) Control of reciprocal and non-reciprocal actions of vagal and sympathetic efferents: study of centrally induced reactions. *J. auton. Nerv. Syst.*, 3: 483–501.

Koizumi, K. and Yamashita, H. (1978) Influence of atrial stretch receptors on hypothalamic neurosecretory neurons. *J. Physiol. (Lond.)*, 285: 341–358.

Koizumi, K., Ishikawa, T., Nishino, H. and Brooks, C.McC. (1975) Cardiac and autonomic system reactions to stretch of the atria. *Brain Res.*, 87: 247–261.

Koizumi, K., Yamashita, H., Kollai, M. and Brooks, C.McC. (1979) Differential responses in reflex action: the question of blood volume and pressure control. In C.McC. Brooks, K. Koizumi and A. Sato (Eds.), *Integrative Functions of the Autonomic Nervous System*, Univ. of Tokyo Press/Elsevier/North-Holland, Tokyo/Amsterdam, 1979, pp. 293–308.

Koizumi, K., Yamashita, H. and Inenaga, K. (1983) Electrophysiological examination of the "direct connection" between paraventricular nucleus of the hypothalamus and sympathetic preganglionic neurons. In E. Endröczi (Ed.), *Integrative Neurohumoral Mechanisms*, Elsevier Biomedical Press, Amsterdam, in press.

Kollai, M., Koizumi, K., Yamashita, H. and Brooks, C.McC. (1978) Study of cardiac sympathetic and vagal activity during reflex responses produced by stretch of the atria. *Brain Res.*, 150: 519–532.

Loewy, A.D. (1981) Descending pathways to sympathetic and parasympathetic preganglionic neurons. *J. auton. Nerv. Syst.*, 3: 265–275.

Loewy, A.D. and McKeller, S. (1980) The neuroanatomical basis of central cardiovascular control, *Fed. Proc.*, 39: 2495–2503.

Matsuguchi, H., Schmid, P.G., Gordon, F.G. and Johnson, A.K. (1980) Increase in blood pressure and heart rate after vasopressin administration by microinjection into area of nucleus tractus solitarius of rats. *Physiologist*, 23: 29.

Morris, R., Salt, T.E., Sofroniew, M.V. and Hill, R.G. (1980) Actions of microiontophoretically applied oxytocin, and immunohistochemical localization of oxytocin, vasopressin and neurophysin in the rat caudal medulla. *Neurosci. Lett.*, 18: 163–168.

Nakai, M., Yamane, Y., Umeda, Y. and Ogino, K. (1982) Vasopressin induced pressor response elicited by electrical stimulation of solitary nucleus and dorsal motor nucleus of vagus of rat. *Brain Res.*, 251: 164–168.

Nilaver, G., Zimmerman, E.A., Wilkins, J., Michaels, J., Hoffman, D. and Silverman, A.J. (1980) Magnocellular hypothalamic projections to the lower brain stem and spinal cord of the rat. Immunocytochemical evidence for predominance of the oxytocin-neurophysin system compared to the vasopressin-neurophysin system, *Neuroendocrinology*, 30: 150–158.

Pellegrino, L.J., Pellegrino, A.S. and Cushman, A.J. (1979) *A Stereotaxic Atlas of the Rat Brain,* 2nd edn., Plenum, New York.

Pittman, Q.J., Blume, H.W. and Renaud, L.P. (1981) Connections of the hypothalamic paraventricular nucleus with the neurohypophysis, median eminence, amygdala, lateral septum and midbrain periaqueductal gray: an electrophysiological study in the rat. *Brain Res.*, 215: 15–28.

Robertson, G.L. (1977) The regulation of vasopressin function in health and disease. *Rec. Progr. Hormone Res.*, 33: 333–374.

Saper, C.B. (1979) Anatomical substrates for the hypothalamic control of the autonomic nervous system. In C.McC. Brooks, K. Koizumi and A. Sato (Eds.), *Integrative Functions of the Autonomic Nervous System*, Univ. of Tokyo Press/Elsevier/North-Holland, Tokyo/Amsterdam, pp. 333–341.

Saper, C.B., Loewy, A.D., Swanson, L.W. and Cowan, W.M. (1976) Direct hypothalamo-autonomic connections. *Brain Res.*, 117: 305–312.

Sawchenko, P.E. and Swanson, L.W. (1981) Central noradrenergic pathways for the integration of hypothalamic neuroendocrine and autonomic responses. *Science*, 214: 685–687.

Sawchenko, P.E. and Swanson, L.W. (1982) The organization of noradrenergic pathways from the brainstem to the paraventricular and supraoptic nuclei in the rat. *Brain Res. Rev.*, 275–325.

Sawchenko, P.E., Gold, R.M. and Leibowitz, S.F. (1981) Evidence for vagal involvement in the eating elicited by adrenergic stimulation of the paraventricular nucleus. *Brain Res.*, 225: 249–269.

Share, L. (1976) Role of cardiovascular receptors in the control of ADH release, *Cardiology*, 61, Suppl. 1: 51–64.

Sofroniew, M.V. (1980) Projections from vasopressin, oxytocin and neurophysin neurons to neural targets in the rat and human. *J. Histochem. Cytochem.*, 28: 475–478.

Sofroniew, M.V. and Schrell, U. (1981) Evidence for a direct projection from oxytocin and vasopressin neurons in the hypothalamic paraventricular nucleus to the medulla oblongata: immunohistochemical visualization of both the horseradish peroxidase transported and the peptide produced by the same neurons. *Neurosci. Lett.*, 22: 211–217.

Swanson, L.W. (1977) Immunohistochemical evidence for a neurophysin-containing autonomic pathway arising in the paraventricular nucleus of the hypothalamus. *Brain Res.*, 128: 346–353.

Swanson, L.W. and Hartman, B.K. (1980) Biochemical specificity in central pathways related to peripheral and intracerebral homeostatic functions. *Neurosci. Lett.*, 16: 55–60.

Swanson, L.W. and Kuypers, H.G.J.M. (1980) The paraventricular nucleus of the hypothalamus: cytoarchitectonic subdivisions and organization of projections to the pituitary, dorsal vagal complex and spinal cord as demonstrated by retrograde fluorescence double-labeling methods. *J. comp. Neurol.*, 194: 555–570.

Swanson, L.W. and McKeller, S. (1979) The distribution of oxytocin- and neurophysin-stained fibers in the spinal cord of the rat and monkey. *J. comp. Neurol.*, 188: 87–106.

Swanson, L.W., Sawchenko, P.E., Wiegand, S.J. and Price, J.L. (1980) Separate neurons in the paraventricular nucleus project to the median eminence and to the medulla and spinal cord. *Brain Res.*, 198: 190–195.

Swanson, L.W., Sawchenko, P.E., Bérod, A., Hartman, B.K., Helle, K.B. and Vanorden, D.E. (1981) An immunohistochemical study of the organization of catecholaminergic cells and terminal fields in the paraventricular and supraoptic nuclei of the hypothalamus. *J. comp. Neurol.*, 196: 271–285.

Weindl, A. and Sofroniew, M.V. (1980) Immunohistochemical localization of hypothalamic peptide hormones in neural target areas. In W. Wuttke, A. Weindl, K.H. Voigt and R.-R. Dries (Eds.), *Brain and Pituitary Peptides*, Karger, Basel, pp. 97–109.

Yamashita, H. (1977) Effect of baro- and chemoreceptor activation on supraoptic nuclei neurons in the hypothalamus. *Brain Res.*, 126: 551–556.

Yamashita, H. and Koizumi, K. (1979) Influence of carotid and aortic baroreceptors on neurosecretory neurons in supraoptic nuclei. *Brain Res.*, 170: 259–277.

Yamashita, H., Koizumi, K. and Brooks, C.McC. (1979) Rhythmic patterns of discharge in hypothalamic neurosecretory neurons of cats and dogs. *Proc. nat. Acad. Sci. U.S.A.*, 76: 6684–6688.

Zerihun, L. and Harris, M. (1981) Electrophysiological identification of neurones of paraventricular nucleus sending axons to both the neurohypophysis and the medulla in the cat. *Neurosci. Lett.*, 23: 157–160.

The Neurohypophysis: Structure, Function and Control, Progress in Brain Research, Vol. 60, edited by B.A. Cross and G. Leng
© 1983 Elsevier Science Publishers B.V.

Vascular Effects of Arginine-Vasopressin, Angiotensin and Noradrenaline in Adrenal Insufficiency

S. ISHIKAWA and R.W. SCHRIER

Jichi Medical School, 3311-1 Yakushiji, Minamikawachi-Machi, Tochigi 329-04 (Japan) and Department of Medicine, University of Colorado Health Sciences Center, 4200 East Ninth Avenue, Denver, CO 80262 (U.S.A.)

INTRODUCTION

Non-osmotic release of arginine-vasopressin (AVP) is present in conscious, adrenalectomized animals with either gluco- or mineralocorticoid (Boykin et al., 1978, 1979; Linas et al., 1980; Mandell et al., 1980) deficiency. Moreover, administration of a specific inhibitor of the hydroosmotic effect of AVP profoundly improves the capacity of mineralocorticoid- or glucocorticoid-deficient animals to excrete an acute water load (Ishikawa and Schrier, 1982). It is not known, however, whether this non-osmotic release of AVP has a vascular effect in the gluco- or mineralocorticoid-deficient state. The present study was therefore undertaken to investigate this possibility. A specific inhibitor to the vascular effect of AVP was used in conscious, adrenalectomized rats with either gluco- or mineralocorticoid deficiency. As compensatory activation of the sympathetic nervous system or the renin–angiotensin system may obscure or blunt a hypotensive effect during administration of the AVP vascular inhibitor, studies using the AVP inhibitor were performed during concomitant inhibition of the renin–angiotensin system with an angiotensin II antagonist (saralasin) or blockade of the α-adrenergic nervous system with phenoxybenzamine.

COMPARISON OF GLUCOCORTICOID- AND MINERALOCORTICOID-DEFICIENT RATS

There were substantial differences between the gluco- and mineralocorticoid-deficient rats compared to hormone-replaced rats. A mean decrement in blood volume of 17% and weight loss were observed in the mineralocorticoid- but not the glucocorticoid-deficient rats. Moreover, the mean basal blood pressure was 72 ± 2 mm Hg in the mineralocorticoid-deficient compared with 110 ± 3 mm Hg in the glucocorticoid-deficient rats ($P < 0.001$); the mean basal blood pressure was 112 ± 2 mm Hg in the hormone-replaced, adrenalectomized (control) rats. As compared to glucocorticoid-deficient rats, the mineralocorticoid-deficient rats also exhibited significantly higher mean plasma renin activity (7.2 vs 40.7 ng/ml/h, $P < 0.001$), mean plasma noradrenaline concentrations (251 vs 1137 pg/ml, $P < 0.001$) and mean plasma AVP concentrations (4.8 vs 9.6 pg/ml, $P < 0.05$).

The hypotensive effect of a specific vascular antagonist, [1(β-mercapto-β,β-cyclopentamethylenepropionic acid),2-O-methyltyrosine]AVP, was then examined in the gluco- and mineralocorticoid-deficient rats. In a dose of 5 μg/kg the AVP vascular inhibitor lowered mean arterial pressure in the mineralocorticoid- (76.5 to 71.6 mm Hg, $P < 0.01$) but not glucocorticoid-deficient rats (113.2 to 111.6 mm Hg, n.s.); the vehicle for the AVP inhibitor exerted no effect on mean arterial pressure in either group. To examine whether the sympathetic nervous or renin–angiotensin systems were obscuring any vascular effect of AVP, further studies were performed during saralasin or phenoxybenzamine administration. Angiotensin II antagonism decreased mean arterial pressure (69.2 to 53.2 mm Hg, $P < 0.001$) in mineralocorticoid-deficient rats while no effect on mean arterial pressure was observed in glucocorticoid-deficient rats (110.0 to 107.2 mm Hg, n.s.). In the presence of saralasin, the AVP vascular antagonism lowered mean arterial pressure further (53.2 to 41.4 mm Hg, $P < 0.005$) in mineralocorticoid-deficient rats, but no effect of the AVP antagonist was observed in the glucocorticoid-deficient rats (106.2 to 101.8 mm Hg, n.s.).

Similar studies were then performed during α-adrenergic blockade with phenoxybenzamine. In mineralocorticoid-deficient rats, basal mean arterial pressure decreased from 82.0 to 51.0 mm Hg ($P < 0.005$) with phenoxybenzamine administration and a further significant decrease occurred to 39.0 mm Hg ($P < 0.005$) with administration of the AVP antagonist but not its vehicle. In glucocorticoid-deficient rats, α-adrenergic blockade decreased mean arterial pressure from 107.7 to 84.8 mm Hg ($P < 0.02$) and a further decrease occurred on administration of the AVP vascular antagonist from 84.8 to 78.7 mm Hg ($P < 0.05$). The decrement in mean arterial pressure during α-adrenergic blockade in glucocorticoid-deficient rats was significantly less than in mineralocorticoid-deficient rats, and was no different than that observed in hormone-replaced adrenalectomized rats. It should also be mentioned that the duration of the hypotensive effect of the AVP antagonist in mineralocorticoid-deficient rats was prolonged from 20 min to greater than 50 min in the presence of either saralasin or α-adrenergic blockade with phenoxybenzamine.

SUMMARY

Using a sensitive and potent AVP vascular antagonist, a vascular role of endogenous AVP to maintain mean arterial pressure was observed in adrenal insufficiency in the conscious rat. The effect was more readily demonstrable in the mineralocorticoid- than the glucocorticoid-deficient state. Activation of the renin–angiotensin and sympathetic nervous systems in the mineralocorticoid deficient state also contributed to the maintenance of blood pressure. In the mineralocorticoid-deficient state, antagonism of the renin–angiotensin system or α-adrenergic blockade was associated with prolongation of the hypotensive effect of the AVP vascular antagonist. Thus, AVP, angiotensin II and adrenergic stimulation all combine to support mean arterial pressure in the mineralocorticoid-deficient, conscious rat.

REFERENCES

Boykin, J., de Torrente, A., Erickson, A., Robertson, G. and Schrier, R.W. (1978) Role of plasma vasopressin in impaired water excretion of glucocorticoid deficiency. J. clin. Invest., 62: 738–744.

Boykin, J., de Torrente, A., Robertson, G.L., Erickson, A. and Schrier, R.W. (1979) Persistent plasma vasopressin levels in the hypoosmolar state associated with mineralocorticoid deficiency. Mineral Electrolyte Metab., 2: 310–315.

Ishikawa, S. and Schrier, R.W. (1982) Effect of arginine vasopressin antagonist on renal water excretion in glucocorticoid and mineralocorticoid deficient rats. *Kidney Int.*, 22: 587–593.

Linas, S.L., Berl, T., Robertson, G.L., Aisenbrey, G.A., Schrier, R.W. and Anderson, R.J. (1980) Role of vasopressin in the impaired water excretion of glucocorticoid deficiency. *Kidney Int.*, 18: 58–67.

Mandell, I.N., de Fronzo, R.A., Robertson, G.L. and Forrest, J.N., Jr. (1980) Role of plasma arginine vasopressin in the impaired water diuresis of isolated glucocorticoid deficiency in the rat. *Kidney Int.*, 17: 186–195.

Interactions of Neurohypophysial Hormones With Other Endocrine Systems

The Neurohypophysis: Structure, Function and Control, Progress in Brain Research, Vol. 60, edited by B.A. Cross and G. Leng

Interactions Between Vasopressin
and the Renin–Angiotensin System

I.A. REID, J. SCHWARTZ, L. BEN, J. MASELLI and L.C. KEIL[1]

Department of Physiology, University of California, San Francisco, San Francisco, CA 94143 and [1]Ames Research Center, Moffett Field, CA 94035 (U.S.A.)

INTRODUCTION

Vasopressin and the renin–angiotensin system interact in two major ways. Angiotensin II, the physiologically active component of the renin–angiotensin system, acts centrally to stimulate the release of vasopressin. Vasopressin, in turn, acts on the kidney to inhibit the secretion of renin. These interactions are discussed in this chapter. In addition, current concepts concerning the site and mechanism of these actions, as well as their physiological significance, are reviewed.

STIMULATION OF VASOPRESSIN SECRETION BY ANGIOTENSIN II

Angiotensin II can act on the central nervous system to increase blood pressure, stimulate drinking and increase the secretion of vasopressin and ACTH (Ramsay, 1982; Severs and Daniels-Severs, 1973). This section is concerned with the stimulatory effect of angiotensin II on vasopressin secretion. The effects of intraventricular and i.v. administration of angiotensin are discussed.

Intraventricular angiotensin II

Injection of angiotensin II into the cerebral ventricles stimulates the release of vasopressin (for review, see Share, 1979). In initial studies, changes in plasma vasopressin concentration were not measured directly but inferred from changes in renal water excretion or blood pressure. In subsequent studies, however, measurement of plasma vasopressin by bioassay or radioimmunoassay confirmed that angiotensin II stimulates vasopressin release when administered intraventricularly in rats and dogs (Share, 1979). In one study, Keil et al. (1975) investigated the effect of injecting angiotensin II into a left cerebral ventricle of conscious rats in doses of 10, 50 and 100 ng and observed increases in plasma vasopressin concentration which were related to the dose of angiotensin.

Most investigators have studied the acute effect of angiotensin II on vasopressin release. Recently, however, Sterling et al. (1980) infused angiotensin II into a lateral ventricle of rats for five days. When the rats were allowed free access to water or 0.9% saline, plasma vasopressin concentration did not increase. If, however, water intake was restricted, or if the rats were given 1.8% saline to drink, plasma vasopressin concentration increased. These findings suggest that a decrease in plasma osmolality and/or expansion of extracellular fluid volume can counteract the stimulatory effect of angiotensin II on vasopressin secretion.

Intravenous angiotensin II

Although it has been established that intraventricular angiotensin II stimulates vasopressin secretion, there is controversy concerning the effects of circulating angiotensin on vasopressin secretion. There are two major questions. Does systemically administered angiotensin II stimulate vasopressin release? What dose of angiotensin II is required to produce this effect? These questions have been investigated in the dog, rat and human.

Dog

In anaesthetized dogs, i.v. or intracarotid infusions of angiotensin II have consistently failed to stimulate vasopressin release (Cadnapaphornchai et al., 1975; Claybaugh et al., 1972; Share, 1979). However, it has been reported that intracarotid infusion of angiotensin II in anaesthetized dogs potentiates the vasopressin response to an increase in plasma osmolality (Shimizu et al., 1973).

In conscious dogs, some investigators observed increases in plasma vasopressin concentration when angiotensin II was infused i.v. in doses ranging from 5 to 20 ng/kg/min (Bonjour and Malvin, 1970; Ramsay et al., 1978). Other investigators, however, have not observed such increases (Cowley et al., 1981). In a recent study in this laboratory, the effect of i.v. and intracarotid infusion of graded doses of angiotensin II was studied in conscious dogs (Reid et al., 1982). Only the highest dose of angiotensin II, 20 ng/kg/min, which increased plasma angiotensin II concentration to an average of 449 pg/ml, increased plasma vasopressin concentration (Fig. 1). An increase in plasma vasopressin concentration was also observed with intracarotid angiotensin II but again only the highest dose, 2.5 ng/kg/min per carotid, which increased angiotensin II concentration in the cerebral circulation to an estimated 728 pg/ml, was effective (Fig. 1). Even at these high circulating angiotensin II levels, the increases in

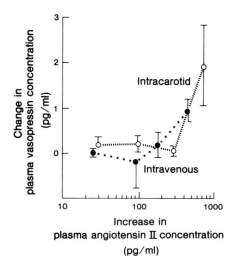

Fig. 1. Effects of i.v. and intracarotid infusion of angiotensin II on plasma vasopressin concentration in conscious dogs. Changes in plasma vasopressin concentration are plotted as a function of the measured (i.v.) or calculated (intracarotid) increases in plasma angiotensin II concentration. (From Reid et al., 1982.)

plasma vasopressin concentration were quite modest: with i.v. angiotensin II, plasma vaso-pressin concentration increased from 0.7 to 1.7 pg/ml; with intracarotid angiotensin II, the increase was from 1.6 to 3.6 pg/ml. These results indicate that circulating angiotensin II can increase vasopressin release in the dog but that high concentrations, in excess of 300 pg/ml, are required.

Rat

Knepel and Meyer (1980) studied the effect of i.v. infusion of angiotensin II in conscious rats in doses ranging from 125 to 1000 ng/kg/min. The lowest dose of angiotensin II which increased plasma vasopressin concentration was 250 ng/kg/min; this infusion increased plasma angiotensin II concentration to 1602 pg/ml. It was concluded that pharmacological doses of angiotensin II, greater than those which maximally elevate arterial pressure, are required to stimulate vasopressin release in the rat.

Human

Uhlich et al. (1975) reported that infusion of angiotensin II in doses of 3–30 ng/kg/min produced a significant increase in plasma vasopressin concentration in normal men. Padfield and Morton (1977) studied the effect of i.v. angiotensin II infusion in doses of 2, 4 and 8 ng/kg/min in normal men. There was a significant increase in plasma vasopressin only at the highest dose of angiotensin II, when plasma angiotensin II concentration was increased to 190 pg/ml. Even at this high angiotensin concentration, the increase in plasma vasopressin was small (from 5.4 to 6.4 pg/ml).

On the other hand, Hammer et al. (1980) reported that plasma vasopressin concentration failed to increase when angiotensin II was infused i.v. in healthy men at 4 ng/kg/min. Plasma vasopressin also failed to increase when angiotensin II was infused at 2–12 ng/kg/min in dialysis patients: indeed, plasma vasopressin actually showed a tendency to decrease during the angiotensin infusion.

In summary, there is still controversy concerning the effect of circulating angiotensin II on vasopressin secretion. There is increasing evidence that i.v. or intracarotid administration of angiotensin II can stimulate vasopressin secretion. However, most of the available data indicate that this stimulation only occurs with large doses of angiotensin II which increase plasma angiotensin II concentration above the normal physiological range.

Site of action

The site at which angiotensin II acts to stimulate vasopressin secretion has not been definitely established. Sites that have received particular attention include the circumven-tricular organs and the supraoptic nucleus of the hypothalamus.

Circumventricular organs

The circumventricular organs include the neurohypophysis, the subfornical organ (SFO), the organum vasculosum of the lamina terminalis (OVLT) and the area postrema. These have received considerable attention as potential sites of action of angiotensin II because they: (a) lack a blood–brain barrier; (b) contain specific angiotensin II receptors, and (c) at least in some cases, are accessible to centrally administered as well as circulating angiotensin II (Ramsay, 1982).

The area postrema can probably be excluded as a site of action of angiotensin II on vasopressin secretion because infusion of angiotensin II into the vertebral arteries, which perfuse the area postrema, does not increase vasopressin secretion (Reid et al., 1982). However, there is evidence that the neurohypophysis, SFO and OVLT may play a role. Addition of angiotensin II to rat neurohypophyses in vitro has been reported to increase vasopressin release (Gagnon et al., 1973), although this point is somewhat controversial (Gregg and Malvin, 1978). Direct injection of angiotensin II into the SFO has been reported to increase vasopressin release in rats (Simpson et al., 1979) and lesions of the SFO impair the vasopressin response to intraventricular injection of angiotensin II (Mangiapane et al., 1982). Lesions of the anteroventral region of the third ventricle, which contains the OVLT, have also been reported to reduce antidiuretic responses to intraventricular injections of angiotensin II (Bealer et al., 1979).

Supraoptic nucleus

Evidence implicating the supraoptic nucleus as a site for stimulation of vasopressin secretion by angiotensin II includes the observation that this nucleus contains angiotensin II receptors (Sakai et al., 1974) and that neurones in this nucleus can be activated by administration of angiotensin II (Akaishi et al., 1980; Nicoll and Barker, 1971). It has also been reported that vasopressin secretion is increased following injection of angiotensin II into the supraoptic nucleus of monkeys (Simmonet et al., 1979). However, the supraoptic nucleus is inside the blood–brain barrier, and could therefore be a receptor site for centrally administered angiotensin II but not for blood-borne angiotensin II.

In summary, angiotensin II may increase vasopressin release by actions at the neurohypophysis, SFO, OVLT and supraoptic nucleus. Further studies are required to establish the relative importance of these different structures.

Physiological significance

As discussed above, vasopressin release can be stimulated by centrally or peripherally administered angiotensin II. What is the physiological (or pathological) significance of this stimulatory effect? One possibility is that stimulation of vasopressin secretion represents an action of the putative brain renin–angiotensin system. However, it is not necessary to invoke the participation of such a system because vasopressin secretion can be stimulated by circulating angiotensin II formed by the renal renin–angiotensin system (Ramsay, 1982). As it has still not been demonstrated conclusively that there is a brain renin–angiotensin system (Reid, 1979), the emphasis of this section will be on circulating angiotensin II. The possible role of the renin–angiotensin system in the control of vasopressin secretion has been investigated in several situations including haemorrhage, postural changes, water deprivation, caval ligation and hypertension.

Haemorrhage

Most evidence indicates that the renin–angiotensin system plays little or no role in the vasopressin response to haemorrhage. For example, studies in dogs have shown marked increases in plasma vasopressin concentration with little change in plasma renin activity (Claybaugh and Share, 1973; Cousineau et al., 1973). Indeed, Claybaugh and Share (1972) reported that plasma vasopressin increases during haemorrhage even when changes in renin secretion are prevented. In addition, Morton et al. (1977) reported that the marked stimulation of vasopressin secretion which occurs during haemorrhagic shock in dogs is not altered by pretreatment with the converting enzyme inhibitor SQ20881.

Postural changes

Share (1979) studied the effect of ambulation and sodium depletion on plasma vasopressin concentration and renin activity in normal human subjects. Sodium deficiency increased plasma renin activity and also increased the renin secretory response to ambulation. Plasma vasopressin, however, was unchanged during sodium deficiency and ambulation.

Davies et al. (1977) studied the relationship between the release of renin and vasopressin during 85° head-up tilt in normal human subjects. Plasma renin activity and plasma vasopressin concentration both increased during tilting but the maximum increase in vasopressin concentration occurred after the maximum increase in renin activity. When the increase in renin secretion produced by tilting was blocked by administration of propranolol, the increase in plasma vasopressin was unaffected. These results indicate that the vasopressin response to tilting is not mediated via the renin–angiotensin system.

Water deprivation

Yamaguchi et al. (1980) studied the effect of intraventricular injection of the angiotensin II antagonist saralasin on the increase in plasma vasopressin produced by water deprivation in conscious rats. There was considerable scatter in the data but they reported that the "median plasma vasopressin concentration" in dehydrated rats treated with saralasin was significantly lower than the median value in dehydrated controls.

Caval ligation

The effect of intraventricular saralasin on the increase in vasopressin secretion produced by caval ligation has been investigated in dogs (Ramsay, 1982). Administration of saralasin in a dose known to block the increase in vasopressin secretion produced by i.v. angiotensin II did not modify the vasopressin response to caval ligation.

Hypertension

Several investigators have studied the effect of blockade of the renin–angiotensin system on plasma vasopressin in experimental or human hypertension. Crofton et al. (1979) reported that urinary vasopressin excretion in rats with spontaneous hypertension decreased during chronic treatment with captopril. Similarly, Thibonnier et al. (1981) reported that treatment of severely hypertensive patients with captopril produced decreases in both plasma vasopressin concentration and urinary vasopressin excretion. In neither of these studies was the mechanism of the decrease in plasma or urinary vasopressin established. The decrease may have been due to reduced stimulation of vasopressin secretion by angiotensin II. On the other hand, the decrease may simply have represented a homeostatic response to maintain a constant plasma osmolality (Crofton et al., 1979; Thibonnier et al., 1981).

Recently, we measured plasma vasopressin concentrations during the development of two-kidney, one-clip Goldblatt hypertension in dogs. Following constriction of one renal artery, plasma renin activity (Fig. 2) and plasma angiotensin II concentration both increased markedly. These increases were accompanied by a progressive increase in plasma vasopressin from the control value of 2.4 ± 0.6 pg/ml to a peak of 4.5 ± 0.2 pg/ml at 12 days ($P < 0.05$). In these hypertensive dogs, there was a significant correlation between plasma angiotensin II concentration and plasma vasopressin concentration (Fig. 3). On the other hand, acute blockade of the renin–angiotensin system with captopril or saralasin at various intervals during the development of hypertension did not reduce plasma vasopressin concentration; indeed, in some animals plasma vasopressin increased.

480

Taken together, these observations indicate that the renin–angiotensin system plays little or no role in the control of vasopressin secretion during haemorrhage, postural changes, sodium depletion or caval ligation. It may play a role during dehydration and in some forms of hypertension, but further studies are required.

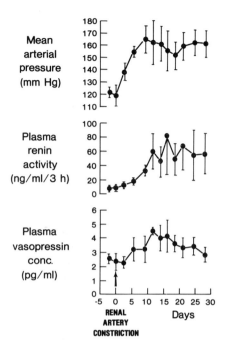

Fig. 2. Changes in arterial pressure, plasma renin activity and plasma vasopressin concentration during the development of two-kidney, one-clip Goldblatt hypertension in dogs. Values represent the mean ± S.E. of observations made in four dogs.

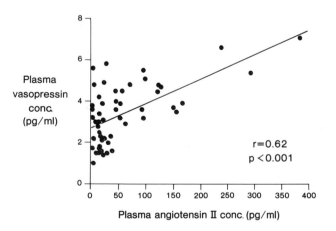

Fig. 3. Correlation between plasma vasopressin and angiotensin concentrations in two-kidney, one-clip Goldblatt hypertensive dogs.

INHIBITION OF RENIN SECRETION BY VASOPRESSIN

Many investigators have observed that vasopressin inhibits the release of renin by the kidneys (Keeton and Campbell, 1980). This inhibitory effect has been the subject of considerable research during the past decade and several interesting and important observations have been made. The aim of this section is to review the effects of vasopressin on renin secretion in man and experimental animals and to discuss the evidence concerning the mechanism of this inhibitory effect.

Dog

Bunag et al. (1967) were the first to demonstrate that vasopressin inhibits the secretion of renin. They observed inhibition of renin release during i.v. or intrarenal infusion of vasopressin in anaesthetized dogs in which renal perfusion pressure had been lowered by suprarenal aortic constriction. In some cases, the inhibition was accompanied by increased arterial pressure and decreased renal blood flow; in others, the inhibition occurred in the absence of measurable haemodynamic changes. Oxytocin was also found to inhibit renin release but only when infused in large doses.

The findings of Bunag et al. were confirmed and extended by Vander (1968), who showed that i.v. infusion of vasopressin in anaesthetized dogs suppressed basal renin release and the elevated renin levels produced by ureteral occlusion. He also observed that the inhibition of renin release was accompanied by a natriuresis and raised the possibility that the inhibition might be mediated by the macula densa mechanism.

Vasopressin has also been reported to inhibit renin secretion in conscious dogs, in normal sodium balance or during sodium depletion (Johnson et al., 1979; Malayan et al., 1980; Tagawa et al., 1971). The degree of inhibition is related to the dose of vasopressin and can be produced by elevations in plasma vasopressin concentration within the range occurring in situations such as water deprivation and non-hypotensive haemorrhage. With low doses of vasopressin, the inhibition of renin secretion occurs in the absence of changes in arterial pressure or heart rate.

Most studies of the effect of vasopressin on renin secretion have involved short-term experiments of up to several hours duration. However, inhibition of renin secretion has also been observed during long-term infusions (Smith et al., 1979). It appears that the inhibition is secondary to body fluid expansion since it does not occur when water intake is restricted (Young and McCaa, 1981).

Renin secretion may be inhibited by endogenous as well as by exogenous vasopressin. For example, bilateral cervical vagotomy in anaesthetized dogs undergoing a water diuresis causes a decrease in renin secretion (Schrier et al., 1975). This decrease is accompanied by an increase in vasopressin secretion and is abolished by hypophysectomy, suggesting that it is mediated via vasopressin. We have also observed that the increase in renin secretion produced by i.v. isoproterenol is greater in hypophysectomized dogs than in intact animals (Reid et al., 1972). This difference probably results from an increase in plasma vasopressin concentration as isoproterenol is a potent stimulus to vasopressin secretion. Finally, we have presented evidence that the inhibition of renin secretion by intracerebroventricular injection of angiotensin II is mediated via vasopressin (Malayan et al., 1979).

Rat

Several investigators have reported that vasopressin decreases plasma renin and angiotensin II levels in rats (Gutman and Benzakein, 1971; Henderson et al., 1978; Morton et al., 1982).

In this species, vasopressin decreases basal renin secretion and also suppresses the renin secretory responses to administration of isoproterenol (Meyer et al., 1975) and furosemide (Lauterwein et al., 1975). As in the dog, renin secretion can be suppressed by low doses of vasopressin. For example, Morton and associates (1982) observed a marked suppression in plasma angiotensin II concentration when plasma vasopressin concentration was increased to 10 fmol/ml in conscious rats.

To investigate the importance of vasopressin in the control of renin secretion, a number of investigators have studied rats with hereditary diabetes insipidus (DI rats). It has been shown consistently that plasma renin levels in these animals are higher than those in normal rats (Gutman and Benzakein, 1971, 1974). Renal renin content is also elevated (Gutman and Benzakein, 1974). These observations suggest that vasopressin normally exerts a tonic inhibitory effect on renin secretion in rats, but it is possible that the elevated renin levels in DI rats are due, at least in part, to hypovolaemia. Recently, Knepel and Meyer (1981) reported that the attenuation of the renin secretory response to isoproterenol by bilateral vagotomy in rats is mediated by vasopressin.

The effect of vasopressin on renin secretion in rats is partly dependent on sex. For example, Gutman and Benzakein (1974) observed that plasma renin levels are increased in male but not female DI rats. However, they did find that renal renin content is increased in female DI rats and that plasma renin levels decrease when vasopressin is infused in these animals. More recently, Henderson et al. (1978) reported that, whereas injections of vasopressin decreased plasma renin activity in male rats, they increased plasma renin activity in female rats. The suppression of plasma renin activity by vasopressin in male rats could be abolished by castration or cyproterone acetate administration, but the increase in female rats was not blocked by ovariectomy. Further studies are required to clarify the sex difference in the renin response to vasopressin.

Human

An inhibitory effect of vasopressin on renin secretion in humans was first reported by Newsome and Bartter (1968). They observed that administration of Pitressin, together with an increase in water intake, led to a decrease in plasma renin activity. Goodwin et al. (1970) also observed that long-term treatment with vasopressin decreased plasma renin activity during overhydration in normal men; in the absence of overhydration, vasopressin failed to suppress renin activity.

Subsequently, there have been reports that acute administration of vasopressin suppresses renin secretion in normal subjects and in patients on maintenance diuretic treatment. Khökhar et al. (1976) reported suppression of plasma renin activity with low doses of vasopressin which had little or no effect on arterial pressure or heart rate. The plasma vasopressin levels resulting from these infusions were within the range of values observed during fluid deprivation and orthostatic stress.

There is also evidence that endogenous vasopressin can inhibit renin secretion in man. For example, Davies et al. (1976) reported that plasma renin activity and plasma vasopressin concentration both increased during head-up tilt in normal volunteers but then became dissociated, with plasma vasopressin increasing further and plasma renin activity decreasing. They suggested that the fall in plasma renin activity resulted from the high plasma vasopressin levels. In patients with the syndrome of inappropriate antidiuretic hormone secretion, basal renin secretion and the renin response to upright posture are both markedly suppressed (Fichman et al., 1974).

Thus there is abundant evidence that vasopressin inhibits the secretion of renin in the rat, dog and man. This effect can be produced by physiological levels of vasopressin and it is likely that the peptide plays an important role in the control of renin secretion in physiological and pathological states.

Mechanism of action

The rate at which renin is secreted by the kidneys is responsive to changes in body fluid volume and composition, renal function, haemodynamics and sympathetic neural activity (Davis and Freeman, 1976; Keeton and Campbell, 1980). Each of these variables can be influenced by vasopressin, either directly or indirectly, and could mediate the suppression of renin secretion by vasopressin. More specifically, the suppression could be the result of volume expansion, vasoconstriction or altered renal handling of sodium. It is also possible that vasopressin acts directly on the juxtaglomerular apparatus to inhibit renin secretion. The evidence for each of these possibilities is discussed next.

Volume expansion

Studies in humans and dogs suggest that the inhibition of renin secretion which occurs during long-term administration of vasopressin is secondary to volume expansion. In dogs, the expansion of extracellular fluid volume produced by chronic treatment with vasopressin is accompanied by suppression of plasma renin activity to undetectable values (Smith et al., 1979). However, when the volume expansion is prevented by restriction of fluid intake, plasma renin activity remains unchanged (Young and McCaa, 1981). Similarly, Goodwin et al. (1970) observed that administration of markedly antidiuretic doses of vasopressin to normal men for five to ten days failed to suppress plasma renin activity when water intake was restricted.

Expansion of body fluid volume is less likely to be involved in the suppression of renin secretion observed during acute administration of vasopressin. However, Khökhar et al. (1976) reported that the decrease in plasma renin activity which occurred during a two-hour vasopressin infusion in normal men was accompanied by a decrease in plasma protein concentration and haematocrit without a change in plasma sodium concentration or osmolality. On the basis of this observation, they suggested that the suppression of plasma renin activity was due to an increase in plasma volume at the expense of extravascular volume. However, other investigators have presented evidence that acute administration of vasopressin can suppress plasma renin activity without changing plasma volume (Hesse and Nielsen, 1977). Taken together, these observations suggest that the suppression of renin secretion by vasopressin is secondary to volume changes in some situations, but that different mechanisms are involved in others.

Vasoconstriction

Vasopressin is a potent vasoconstrictor which plays an important role in blood pressure regulation (Cowley et al., 1980; Montani et al., 1980; Schwartz and Reid, 1981). Vasopressin causes vasoconstriction even in doses lower than those necessary for maximum urine concentration. At these low doses, blood pressure does not increase because of a reflex decrease in cardiac output. With higher doses, blood pressure increases despite decreased cardiac output. Thus, vasopressin could inhibit renin secretion by increasing arterial pressure and/or reflexly decreasing sympathetic neural activity.

Vasopressin can inhibit renin secretion in doses which do not increase arterial pressure (see above). Indeed, most investigators have reported suppression of renin secretion with subpres-

484

sor doses of the peptide. Thus, although high doses of vasopressin may suppress renin secretion by increasing blood pressure, other factors must be involved with lower doses.

In some situations, the suppression of renin secretion by vasopressin may be a reflex response to vasoconstriction. We recently observed that [1-(β-mercapto-β,β-cyclopentame-thylene proprionic acid),2-(O-methyl)tyrosine]arginine-vasopressin (d(CH$_2$)$_5$ Tyr(Me)AVP), a specific antagonist of the vasoconstrictor action of vasopressin, inhibits the suppression of renin secretion by vasopressin in conscious dogs (Fig. 4). We have also reported that vasopressin blockade in water-deprived dogs with elevated plasma vasopressin levels increases plasma renin activity (Schwartz and Reid, 1982). It could be argued that these effects resulted from blockade of a direct action of vasopressin on renin secretion. This seems unlikely, however, because the increase in renin secretion produced by the antagonist in water-deprived dogs could be blocked by the β-adrenergic blocking drug propranolol (Schwartz and Reid, 1982).

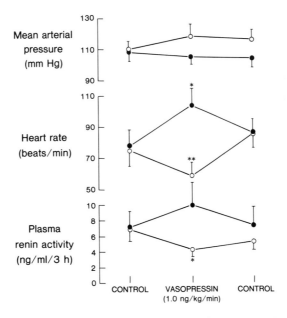

Fig. 4. Effect of the vasopressin antagonist d(CH$_2$)$_5$ Tyr(Me)AVP (10 μg/kg i.v.) on the changes in arterial pressure, heart rate and plasma renin activity produced by infusion of vasopressin (1.0 ng/kg/min i.v.) in conscious dogs. Values represent the mean ± S.E. of observations made in four dogs. o , Vasopressin alone; • , vasopressin plus antagonist. *$P < 0.05$; **$P < 0.01$.

Propranolol has also been reported to attenuate (but not abolish) the suppression of renin secretion by vasopressin in rats (Henderson et al., 1978) and we recently made the same observation in dogs. Taken together, these data indicate that, at least in some situations, the suppression of renin secretion by vasopressin is a reflex response to vasoconstriction.

Nevertheless, there is also convincing evidence that the inhibitory effect of vasopressin on renin secretion is not solely dependent on vasoconstrictor activity. For example, intrarenal infusion of vasopressin can inhibit renin secretion without decreasing renal blood flow (Bunag et al., 1967; Shade et al., 1973). More direct evidence has come from studies with analogues of vasopressin which lack vasoconstrictor activity but retain substantial antidiuretic activity. There have now been several reports that such analogues suppress renin secretion; indeed, in this respect they appear to be as potent as vasopressin.

One analogue that has been studied is 1-deamino[8-D-arginine]vasopressin (dDAVP). Joppich and Weber (1976) reported that administration of dDAVP in babies and children suppressed plasma renin activity to one-third of the control value. The suppression of renin activity was accompanied by a decrease in urinary aldosterone secretion and an increase in urinary sodium excretion. Konrads et al. (1978) studied the effect of dDAVP in an isolated perfused rat kidney preparation. The analogue did not decrease basal renin secretion; however, when the rate of renin release had been stimulated by addition of isoproterenol, the analogue decreased renin release by 30 %. Renal vascular resistance was unaltered and it was therefore suggested that the inhibition of renin release by vasopressin is not related to its vasoconstrictor activity.

The effects of analogues of vasopressin which lack vasoconstrictor activity have also been studied in dogs, but conflicting results have been obtained. We observed that 1-deamino[4-threonine,8-D-arginine]vasopressin (dTDAVP) suppressed renin release and increased sodium excretion in anaesthetized dogs undergoing water diuresis (Malayan and Reid, 1982; Fig. 5).

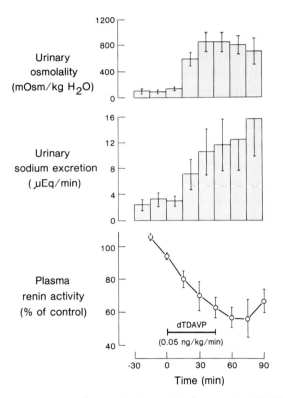

Fig. 5. Effect of i.v. infusion of 1-deamino[4-threonine,8-D-arginine]vasopressin (dTDAVP) on urinary osmolality, urinary sodium excretion and plasma renin activity in water-loaded anaesthetized dogs. (Data from Malayan and Reid, 1982.)

dTDAVP suppressed plasma renin activity as effectively as vasopressin (Fig. 6) but its effect on plasma renin activity was more prolonged than that of vasopressin, as were its effects on sodium and water excretion. On the other hand, Johnson et al. (1979) reported that administration of dDAVP in conscious dogs failed to inhibit renin secretion or increase urinary sodium excretion; infusion of vasopressin produced the expected results. The failure of

486

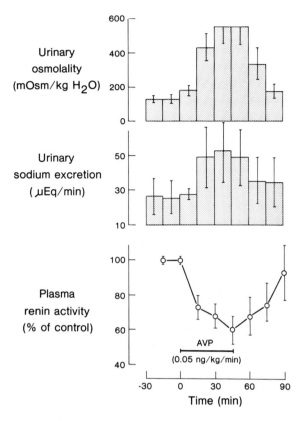

Fig. 6. Effect of i.v. infusion of arginine-vasopressin (AVP) on urinary osmolality, urinary sodium excretion and plasma renin activity in water-loaded anaesthetized dogs. (Data from Malayan and Reid, 1982.)

dDAVP to influence renin secretion or sodium excretion may have been due in part to the fact that the analogue was infused at 0.05 ng/kg/min whereas vasopressin was infused at 1.1 ng/kg/min. In support of this, we have recently observed that infusion of dDAVP in anaesthetized dogs at 1.0 ng/kg/min suppresses plasma renin activity to 47 % of the control value (Fig. 7).

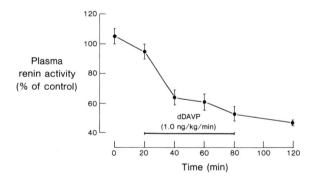

Fig. 7. Effect of i.v. infusion of 1-deamino[8-D-arginine]vasopressin (dDAVP) on plasma renin activity in water-loaded anaesthetized dogs.

In summary, analogues of vasopressin which lack vasoconstrictor activity can suppress renin secretion as effectively as vasopressin. This provides additional evidence that the suppression of renin secretion by vasopressin is not solely due to vasoconstriction.

Sodium excretion

Under some circumstances, vasopressin increases the excretion of sodium (Humphreys et al., 1970) and, as noted above, several investigators have observed that the suppression of renin secretion by vasopressin and vasopressin analogues is accompanied by natriuresis. Although the site at which vasopressin acts to increase sodium excretion has not been conclusively identified, most evidence suggests a site proximal to the distal tubule, possibly the proximal tubule or loop of Henle (Humphreys et al., 1970; Reid and Ganong, 1974). Thus vasopressin would increase the delivery of sodium to the macula densa and this would be expected to decrease the secretion of renin (Davis and Freeman, 1976).

However, there is little evidence that the macula densa plays an important role in the inhibition of renin secretion by vasopressin. Indeed, Shade et al. (1973) reported that vasopressin inhibits renin secretion when infused into non-filtering kidneys in which the macula densa mechanism controlling renin secretion is non-functional. Nevertheless, the relationship between the renin inhibitory and natriuretic actions of vasopressin is striking, and further investigation would seem worthwhile. Comparison of the effects on renin secretion of analogues of vasopressin with differing actions on sodium excretion should help resolve this issue.

Direct action

It has been suggested that vasopressin may inhibit renin secretion by direct action on the juxtaglomerular apparatus. Studies involving intrarenal infusion of vasopressin in vivo (Shade et al., 1973) or in isolated perfused kidneys (Konrads et al., 1978; Vandongen, 1975) have provided support for this possibility although it is difficult to eliminate the influence of changes in renal haemodynamics or function. The effect of vasopressin on renin release has also been studied using renal cortical slices in vitro where the influence of tubular or haemodynamic factors is minimized or absent. Conflicting results have been obtained. Two groups have reported that vasopressin inhibits renin release in vitro (Brooks et al., 1980; Park et al., 1981), while another two groups observed no effect (Knepel et al., 1982; Rosset and Veyrat, 1971). The reason for this discrepancy is not clear and further detailed studies are required.

In summary, current evidence indicates that vasopressin can suppress renin secretion by a variety of mechanisms. During long-term administration, the suppression appears to be secondary to retention of water and expansion of body fluids. With short-term administration, the suppression of renin secretion may be partly secondary to vasoconstriction; however, other mechanisms almost certainly play a role since analogues of vasopressin which lack vasoconstrictor activity also suppress renin secretion. Finally, there is some evidence that vasopressin can inhibit renin secretion by direct action on the juxtaglomerular apparatus. The relative importance of these different mechanisms is not clear.

SUMMARY AND CONCLUSIONS

(1) Vasopressin and the renin–angiotensin system interact in two major ways. Angiotensin II, the physiologically active component of the renin–angiotensin system, acts centrally to

490

Morton, J.J., Semple, P.F., Ledingham, I. McA., Stuart, B., Tehrani, M.A., Garcia, A.R. and McGarrity, G. (1977) Effect of angiotensin-converting enzyme inhibitor (SQ 20881) on the plasma concentration of angiotensin I, angiotensin II and arginine vasopressin in the dog during hemorrhagic shock. *Circulat. Res.*, 41: 301–308.

Morton, J.J., Garcia del Rio, C. and Hughes, M.J. (1982) Effect of acute vasopressin infusion on blood pressure and plasma angiotensin II in normotensive and DOCA-salt hypertensive rats. *Clin. Sci.*, 62: 143–149.

Newsome, H.H. and Bartter, F.C. (1968) Plasma renin activity in relation to serum sodium concentration and body fluid balance. *J. clin. Endocr.*, 28: 1704–1711.

Nicoll, R.A. and Barker, J.L. (1971) Excitation of supraoptic neurosecretory cells by angiotensin II. *Nature (Lond.)*, 233: 172–174.

Padfield, P.L. and Morton, J.J. (1977) Effects of angiotensin II on arginine-vasopressin in physiological and pathological situations in man. *J. Endocr.*, 74: 251–259.

Park, C.S., Han, D.S. and Fray, J.C.S. (1981) Calcium in the control of renin secretion: Ca^{2+} influx as an inhibitory signal. *Amer. J. Physiol.*, 240: F70–F74.

Ramsay, D.J. (1982) Effects of circulating angiotensin II on the brain. In W.F. Ganong and L. Martini (Eds.), *Frontiers in Neuroendocrinology*, Raven Press, New York, pp. 263–285.

Ramsay, D.J., Keil, L.C., Sharpe, M.C. and Shinsako, J. (1978) Angiotensin II infusion increases vasopressin, ACTH and 11-hydroxycorticosteroid secretion. *Amer. J. Physiol.*, 234: R66–R71.

Reid, I.A. (1979) The brain renin–angiotensin system: a critical analysis. *Fed. Proc.*, 38: 2255–2259.

Reid, I.A. and Ganong, W.F. (1974) The hormonal control of sodium excretion. In S.M. McCann (Ed.), *Endocrine Physiology*, Butterworths, University Park Press, pp. 205–237.

Reid, I.A., Schrier, R.W. and Earley, L.E. (1972) An effect of extrarenal beta-adrenergic stimulation on the release of renin. *J. clin. Invest.*, 51: 1861–1869.

Reid, I.A., Brooks, V.L., Rudolph, C.D. and Keil, L.C. (1982) Analysis of the actions of angiotensin on the central nervous system of conscious dogs. *Amer. J. Physiol.*, 243: R82–R91.

Rosset, E. and Veyrat, R. (1971) Effect of vasopressin (ADH), aldosterone, norepinephrine (NE), angiotensin I (AI) and II (AII) on renin release (RR) by human kidney (HK) slices in vitro. *Acta endocr.*, 155: 179.

Sakai, K.K., Marks, B.H., George, J. and Koestner, A. (1974) Specific angiotensin II receptors in organ-cultured canine supraoptic nucleus cells. *Life Sci.*, 14: 1337–1344.

Schrier, R.W., Reid, I.A., Berl, T. and Earley, L.E. (1975) Mechanism of suppression of renin secretion by cervical vagotomy. *Clin. Sci. Molec. Med.*, 48: 83–89.

Schwartz, J. and Reid, I.A. (1981) Effect of vasopressin blockade on blood pressure regulation during hemorrhage in conscious dogs. *Endocrinology*, 109: 1778–1780.

Schwartz, J. and Reid, I.A. (1982) Role of vasopressin in blood pressure regulation during water deprivation in conscious dogs. *Amer. J. Physiol.*, 244: R74–R77.

Severs, W.B. and Daniels-Severs, A.E. (1973) Effects of angiotensin on the central nervous system. *Pharmacol. Rev.*, 25: 415–449.

Shade, R.E., Davis, J.O., Johnson, J.A., Gotshall, R.W. and Spielman, W.S. (1973) Mechanism of action of angiotensin II and antidiuretic hormone on renin secretion. *Amer. J. Physiol.*, 224: 926–929.

Share, L. (1979) Interrelations between vasopressin and the renin–angiotensin system. *Fed. Proc.*, 38: 2267–2271.

Shimizu, K., Share, L. and Claybaugh, J.R. (1973) Potentiation by angiotensin II of the vasopressin response to an increasing plasma osmolality. *Endocrinology*, 93: 42–50.

Simmonet, G., Rodriguez, F., Fumoux, F., Czernichow, P. and Vincent, J.D. (1979) Vasopressin release and drinking induced by intracranial injection of angiotensin II in monkey. *Amer. J. Physiol.*, 237: R20–R25.

Simpson, J.B., Reed, M., Keil, L.C., Thrasher, T.N. and Ramsay, D.J. (1979) Forebrain analysis of vasopressin (AVP) secretion and water intake induced by angiotensin II (AII). *Fed. Proc.*, 38: 982.

Smith, Jr., M.J., Cowley, Jr., A.W., Guyton, A.C. and Manning, Jr., R.D. (1979) Acute and chronic effects of vasopressin on blood pressure, electrolytes and fluid volumes. *Amer. J. Physiol.*, 237: F 232–R240.

Sterling, G.H., Chee, O., Riggs, R.V. and Keil, L.C. (1980) Effect of chronic intracerebroventricular angiotensin II infusion on vasopressin release in rats. *Neuroendocrinology*, 31: 182–188.

Tagawa, H., Vander, A.J., Bonjour, J.P. and Malvin, R.L. (1971) Inhibition of renin secretion by vasopressin in unanesthetized sodium-deprived dogs. *Amer. J. Physiol.*, 220: 949–951.

Thibonnier, M., Soto, M.E., Menard, J., Aldiger, J.C., Corvol, P. and Milliez, P. (1981) Reduction of plasma and urinary vasopressin during treatment of severe hypertension by captopril. *Europ. J. clin. Invest.*, 11: 449–453.

Uhlich, E., Weber, P., Eigler, J. and Gröschel-Stewart, U. (1975) Angiotensin stimulated AVP-release in humans. *Klin. Wschr.*, 53: 177–180.

Vander, A.J. (1968) Inhibition of renin release in the dog by vasopressin and vasotocin. *Circulat. Res.*, 23: 605–609.

Vandongen, R. (1975) Inhibition of renin secretion in the isolated rat kidney by antidiuretic hormone. *Clin. Sci. Molec. Med.*, 49: 73–76.

Yamaguchi, K., Hama, H., Sakaguchi, T., Negoro, H. and Kamoi, K. (1980) Effects of intraventricular injection of Sar^1-Ala^8-angiotensin II on plasma vasopressin level increased by angiotensin II and by water deprivation in conscious rats. *Endocrinologia*, 93: 407–412.

Young, D.B. and McCaa, R.E. (1981) Lack of prolonged effect of antidiuretic hormone on the renin–aldosterone system in the dog. *Clin. exp. Pharmacol., Physiol.*, 8: 267–271.

vasopressin pathway to the zona externa arises from the paraventricular nucleus, and is separate from the one to the posterior pituitary. It is also of interest that a similar CRF pathway is now being described (Paull et al., 1982) which is apparently different from that containing vasopressin (Bloom et al., 1982; Bugnon et al., 1982).

In addition to some role in corticotropin and adrenal cortical stimulation, there is evidence that glucocorticoids in turn inhibit vasopressin secretion. It is a well known clinical observation that administration of cortisone-like drugs potentiates partial diabetes insipidus. Furthermore, the inability of patients with Addison's disease to secrete a water load, seems at least in part to be related to the effects of excessive vasopressin secretion. Adrenalectomy increases the activity of the vasopressin pathway to the zona externa (Russell et al., 1980; Silverman et al., 1980) as well as the activity of the pathway to the posterior pituitary (Seif et al., 1978).

NEUROPHYSIN AND VASOPRESSIN IN THE ZONA EXTERNA

The first immunohistochemical studies of hypothalamic neurosecretory pathways were carried out in the early 1970s using various antisera to the neurophysins (Alvarez-Buylla et al., 1973). As expected, these proteins were found in the perikarya of the supraoptic and paraventricular nuclei and in their pathway to the posterior pituitary (Alvarez-Buylla et al., 1973; Zimmerman et al., 1973b). In these experiments reactive fibres were also found in the zona externa of sheep (Parry and Livett, 1973), monkeys (Zimmerman et al., 1973a), and rats (Vandesande et al., 1974). The neurophysin was subsequently shown to be that which is predominantly associated with vasopressin (Vandesande et al., 1974; Antunes et al., 1977; Zimmerman et al., 1977). It was also recently demonstrated that the carboxy terminus of the precursor molecule of vasopressin and its neurophysin is present in zona externa fibres (Watson et al., 1982). In ox (Vandesande et al., 1975) and monkey (Antunes et al., 1977) there appear to be more oxytocin fibres than in rat, in which they are difficult to demonstrate even after adrenalectomy (Stillman et al., 1977; Zimmerman et al., 1977) when the numbers of demonstrable vasopressin fibres markedly increase. That vasopressin is primarily formed in this pathway, and not oxytocin or some other peptide, was suggested by the absence of both vasopressin and neurophysin in the zona externa in vasopressin-deficient homozygous Brattleboro rats with diabetes insipidus (DI rat) even after adrenalectomy (Sokol et al., 1976). These studies also provided evidence that the increases in neurophysin after adrenalectomy were not primarily associated with CRF as suggested by Watkins et al. (1974). The DI rat has CRF activity, although the type and character is still debated (Gillies and Lowry, 1982). Immunohistochemical studies at the ultrastructural level revealed that vasopressin and its neurophysin are contained in the smaller granules in nerve terminals characteristic of this region in guinea pig (Silverman and Zimmerman, 1975) and rat (LeClerc and Pelletier, 1974; Zimmerman et al., 1977). It is now known from histochemical studies that nerve terminals in this region contain a variety of peptides, including the known hypothalamic releasing factors and somatostatin (Hökfelt et al., 1978). It therefore became apparent that there is a vasopressin neurosecretory system to the hypophysial portal capillaries. The next questions to be answered concerned whether vasopressin was secreted into portal blood, and the organization and functions of such a system.

VASOPRESSIN IN PORTAL BLOOD

The presence of neurophysin in palisading fibres to portal capillaries in the zona externa of rhesus monkeys prompted us to collect and assay blood from individual portal veins in that animal (Zimmerman et al., 1973a). Vasopressin concentrations measured by radioimmunoassay averaged 13.5 ng/ml, about 1000-fold higher than peripheral blood values. Neurophysin concentrations were also increased, suggesting a neurosecretory process involving exocytosis of granule contents for this system similar to that previously shown for the posterior pituitary system (Sachs et al., 1969). Similar concentrations of vasopressin (1–2 ng/ml) were subsequently reported in individual portal vein blood of rats (Oliver et al., 1977; Recht et al., 1981). The source of the high concentrations of vasopressin in hypophysial portal blood is still not clear. The highly specialized pathway from the paraventricular nucleus ending directly on these capillaries would appear to be the obvious source. The work of Oliver et al. (1977) suggested, however, that most of the hormone arises from the posterior pituitary and reaches the long portal veins by retrograde flow. They found that vasopressin concentrations were 10-fold lower in portal blood after removal of the posterior lobe of the pituitary. We repeated their study in the rat and found no difference in vasopressin values between intact and operated rats (Recht et al., 1981). We have also measured oxytocin levels by radioimmunoassay in portal vein blood in a few rats and found them to be as high as vasopressin. This is surprising as very few oxytocin fibres can be found in the zona externa by immunohistochemistry. Either there may be a high rate of secretion from zona externa fibres, or it may come from the posterior pituitary. To resolve this issue portal vein vasopressin concentrations should be measured in animals with bilateral lesions of the paraventricular nucleus, which destroys the zona externa system. The main source of fibres to the posterior pituitary is the supraoptic nucleus, as will be described later. The differential stimulation studies of Dornhorst et al. (1981) in the cat, however, suggested that the paraventricular nucleus rather than the supraoptic nucleus may be the source of vasopressin-mediated corticotropin release. Corticotropin was released into the general circulation only by stimulation of the paraventricular nucleus, while vasopressin responded to activation of both nuclei. Evidence that the corticotropin response was due to vasopressin, at least in part, and not CRF, was provided by the studies of Carlson et al. (1982) in which the corticotropin responses from many of the stimulation points in the paraventricular nucleus were blocked by antiserum to vasopressin given into the cerebral ventricles.

It seems unlikely that the antisera generated to vasopressin reacted with CRF in paraventricular neurones which project to zona externa (Bloom et al., 1982; Bugnon et al., 1982; Makara et al., 1981). The CRF molecule does not share amino acid sequences with vasopressin (Vale et al., 1981).

ORGANIZATION OF THE VASOPRESSIN NEUROSECRETORY SYSTEM TO MEDIAN EMINENCE

When the neurophysin projections to zona externa were discovered, it was correctly predicted that they arose from the paraventricular nucleus (Parry and Livett, 1973). By immunohistochemistry, vasopressin is found in perikarya in the paraventricular (Fig. 1A), supraoptic (Fig. 1B) and suprachiasmatic (Fig. 1C) nuclei of the hypothalamus, all of which might be the sources of vasopressin terminals to the portal capillary plexus in the zona externa of the median eminence (Fig. 1D). The suprachiasmatic nucleus was eliminated as a candidate

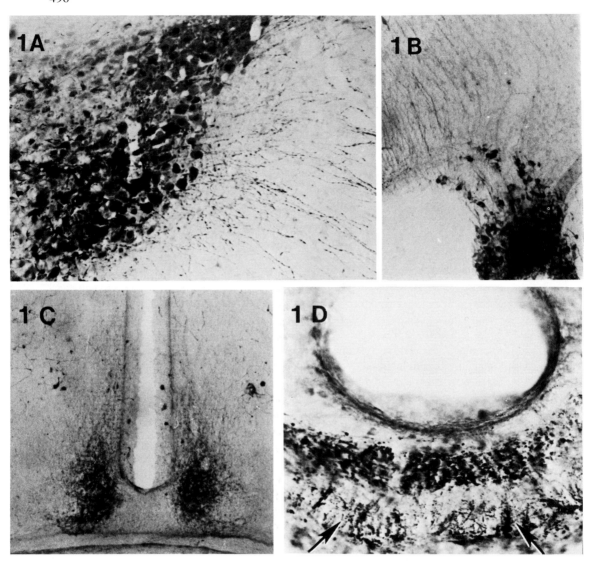

Fig. 1. Photomicrographs of coronal vibratome sections (100 μm) of normal rat hypothalamus immunoreacted for vasopressin using a monoclonal antibody to vasopressin and an immunoperoxidase technique. A: magnocellular vasopressin neurones concentrated in the lateral portion of the major wing of the paraventricular nucleus and beaded axonal processes exiting laterally. × 300. B: vasopressin neurones concentrated in the ventral part of the supraoptic nucleus. × 150. C: parvocellular vasopressin neurones concentrated in the medial and dorsal parts of the suprachiasmatic nucleus. × 70. D: median eminence vasopressin fibres in the internal zone forming a dense band. Reactive fibres can also be seen to extend into the external zone and the hypophysial portal capillary bed (arrows). × 600. (From Hou-Yu et al., 1982, with permission.)

by experiments in rats in which its bilateral destruction did not reduce the number of these fibres (Vandesande et al., 1977). Lesions of the paraventricular nucleus in rats (Vandesande et al., 1977) and monkeys (Antunes et al., 1977) caused the disappearance of this projection. By difference, therefore, the supraoptic nucleus probably does not project to the zona externa. Its fibres terminate in the posterior pituitary as shown by selective retrograde tracing studies (Armstrong and Hatton, 1980; Swanson et al., 1980; Wiegand and Price, 1980): most or all supraoptic neurones take up the tracer, as well as some of the paraventricular neurones (mainly cells in the magnocellular regions). Tracers placed in the median eminence label neurones concentrated in the anterior periventricular and medial aspects of the paraventricular nucleus where smaller (parvocellular) neurones predominate (Lechan et al., 1980, 1981; Swanson et al., 1980; Wiegand and Price, 1980). Therefore, smaller vasopressin neurones in this part of the nucleus may be the source of the zona externa fibre system which may be separate from the magnocellular vasopressin system to the posterior pituitary (Swanson and Sawchenko, 1980). This may explain why the vasopressin granules in terminals of the two systems differ in size. That these two systems function separately is also suggested by the observation that the parvocellular portion of the paraventricular nucleus, and the magnocellular neurones in both nuclei, receive different ascending noradrenergic inputs from the brainstem (Sawchenko and Swanson, 1981). In addition, adrenalectomy and dehydration have different effects on the two systems.

Recent immunohistochemical and tracing studies also shed light on the observations of Rasmussen (1940) that all of the neurones in the supraoptic nucleus, but only some of those in the paraventricular, are destroyed by hypophysectomy or pituitary stalk section, since fibres from paraventricular neurones also terminate at sites spared by such lesions including median eminence and extrahypothalamic regions (see Sofroniew, this volume). An anterograde study using [^{3}H]amino acids also demonstrated that the supraoptic nucleus projects only to the posterior pituitary, while paraventricular fibres were traced both to this terminal region and to the posterior pituitary (Alonso and Assenmacher, 1981). Retrograde tracing studies using different dyes simultaneously placed in the two terminal secretory regions suggested that different neurones in the paraventricular nucleus are the source of the two fibre systems (Swanson and Sawchenko, 1980). Electrophysiological analysis, however, demonstrated that at least some neurones in the paraventricular nucleus may innervate both the zona externa and the posterior pituitary (Pittman et al., 1978, 1981). ·

The precise source of zona externa vasopressin fibres and their anatomical relationship with other peptides in the medial parvocellular paraventricular and periventricular nuclear regions remain to be determined by studies using simultaneous localization techniques for tracers and peptides (Lechan et al., 1981; Swanson and Sawchenko, 1980). Neurotensin (Kahn et al., 1980), somatostatin (Hökfelt et al., 1978), TRH (Lechan and Jackson, 1982), and CRF (Bloom et al., 1982; Bugnon et al., 1982) are all concentrated in this region and send fibres to the zona externa. Whether vasopressin co-exists with these and other peptides in this system is not yet certain. There is a report that some CRF-containing fibres in the median eminence contain neurophysin in the guinea pig (Tramu and Pillez, 1982).

INTERACTION WITH THE ADRENAL GLAND

Thus considerable evidence suggests that a vasopressin pathway to the hypophysial portal system is probably a source of concentrations of the hormones in portal blood high enough to play some role in the release of corticotropin. The physiological contribution of vasopressin to adrenal cortical regulation is not fully understood, however. The adrenal cortex of the DI rat functions relatively normally (Sokol and Zimmerman, 1982), although its responses to certain stresses (Yates et al., 1971) and to angiotensin II given into the cerebral ventricles (Ganong et al., 1982) are deficient. It seems unlikely that vasopressin is the major CRF as suggested by

498

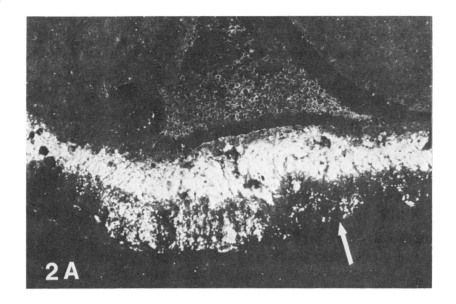

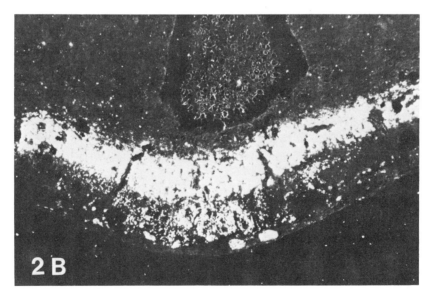

studies in which the CRF activity of hypothalamic extracts was blocked by antiserum to vasopressin (Gillies and Lowry, 1982). Furthermore, another molecule has been isolated by Vale et al. (1981) from sheep hypothalami which is 5–10 times more potent in releasing corticotropin than vasopressin. Whether this or a structurally related molecule accounts for the CRF activity in the DI rat remains to be established. It seems likely that there are several factors regulating corticotropin, acting in concert or complementarily with each other. Such overlaps are common in endocrine systems. The most potent CRF may function to maintain the minute-to-minute normal adrenal cortical function, and the vasopressin subsystem to the portal vessels may provide a back-up system for the further potentiation of corticotropin release in

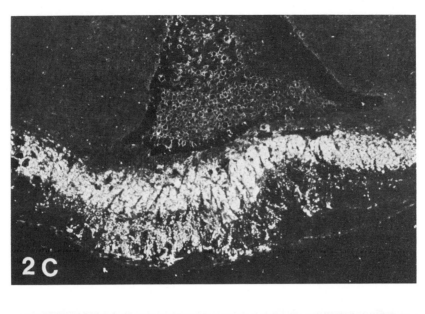

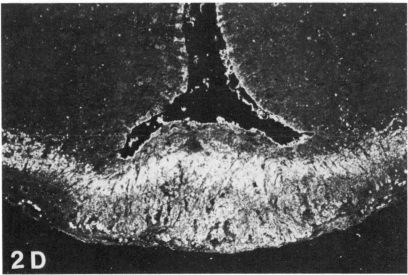

Fig. 2. Photomicrographs of the median eminence of experimental rats illustrating the time course of denervation and sprouting of neurophysin-reactive fibres in animals adrenalectomized for two weeks prior to placement of an electrolytic lesion confined to one side of the paraventricular nucleus (not shown). A: 6 days after the lesion there is a marked loss of fibres in the ipsilateral zona externa (arrow). B and C: by 21 days some fibres have begun to grow across from the intact side. D: at 26 days after the lesion reinnervation of the side ipsilateral to the lesion is almost complete. All × 136. (From Silverman and Zimmerman, 1982, with permission.)

times of extreme stress or adrenal insufficiency. The concentrations of vasopressin in hypophysial portal blood in a resting non-stressed animal are not known, as they had to be collected during the stress of radical surgery. They might be much lower under normal conditions. The vasopressin subsystem to the median eminence appears to behave differently from the one to the posterior pituitary. Granules are not stored very much in zona externa terminals compared with the large amounts stored in the posterior pituitary. Dehydration depletes posterior pituitary vasopressin but has no effect on the zona externa (Stillman et al., 1977; Seybold et al., 1981). Adrenalectomy, on the other hand selectively increases the RNA turnover in the vasopressin cells of the paraventricular nucleus (Silverman et al., 1980), and vasopressin biosynthesis (Russell et al., 1980). In addition to being smaller neurones with smaller granules, the vasopressin neurones which secrete into portal blood may function as a slower system, producing the hormones on demand in response to adrenal cortical needs. The posterior pituitary, mainly concerned with the antidiuretic actions of vasopressin, is prepared for the minute-to-minute demands for hormone with its large stores of granules immediately available. It remains to be shown by measurements of vasopressin in hypophysial portal blood of adrenalectomized rats whether more vasopressin is secreted when median eminence fibres contain large numbers of vasopressin granules. We failed to accomplish portal collections in adrenalectomized rats because they could not tolerate the procedure. This may now be possible with mineralocorticoid replacement. Deoxycorticosterone administration had no effect on the increases in vasopressin in zona externa after adrenalectomy in doses 5-fold higher than the amounts of replacement corticosterone which totally suppresses the phenomenon (Silverman et al., 1980).

How and where glucocorticoids inhibit the increases in zona externa vasopressin after adrenalectomy is not known. Although this could occur at the level of the paraventricular nucleus, few glucocorticoid receptors have been found at this site in autoradiographic studies (Warembourg, 1975). It seems more likely that limbic inputs to the paraventricular nucleus, which are known to contain glucocorticoid receptors (McEwen et al., 1975; Warembourg, 1975), mediate these effects. Recent studies of afferent inputs to the paraventricular nucleus have revealed projections from a number of receptor-rich areas: lateral septum, medial amygdala and ventral subiculum (Berk and Finkelstein, 1981; Silverman et al., 1981; Tribollet and Dreifuss, 1981). Noradrenaline may mediate some of these effects as its depletion by reserpine reduces vasopressin-containing zona externa fibres, but causes no apparent change in the posterior pituitary (Seybold et al., 1981).

The relatively long time course for the increase in the number and intensity of neurophysin and vasopressin in nerve terminals in the zona externa of the rat raise questions as to whether this represents filling of pathways already present, or sprouting of fibres. The increases are first visible at about 5 days and increase from 3–4 weeks. Sprouting occurs in the hypothalamo-hypophysial pathway after section of the pituitary stalk (Rothballer and Skaryna, 1960; Antunes et al., 1979). We have recently shown by an anterograde tracing method that the labelled ipsilateral pathway from the paraventricular nucleus to the zona externa on one side of the hypothalamus does not cross to the opposite zona externa in adrenalectomized rats, or in normal animals after electrolytic destruction of the paraventricular nucleus on the opposite side (Silverman and Zimmerman, 1982). Therefore adrenalectomy or a unilateral lesion does not result in sprouting. The combination of adrenalectomy and a unilateral lesion is associated with sprouting of intact zona externa axons to the denervated side (Fig. 2). Five days after the unilateral lesion in the paraventricular nucleus in adrenalectomized animals, fibres have disappeared from the zona externa on the side of the lesion (Fig. 2A). By 21 days neurophysin-reactive axons begin to cross over from the normal median eminence (Fig. 2B, C), and after 26 days reinnervation of the zona externa ipsilateral to the lesion is nearly complete. Inhibition of axonal growth and/or sprouting by glucocorticoids has been described previously in two glucocorticoid-sensitive neuronal systems: the hippocampus (Scheff et al., 1980) and adrenal medullary cells in culture (Unsicker et al., 1978).

SUMMARY

A role of vasopressin in the regulation of adrenal cortical function has been debated for more than 25 years. In the last decade, it has been established, by immunohistochemical techniques, that there is a vasopressin neurosecretory system that originates in the paraventricular nucleus and terminates on the hypophysial portal system. It appears that this is a separate pathway from the magnocellular projection to the posterior pituitary gland. The terminals contain smaller granules and probably arise from parvocellular neurones. In the monkey and rat, it has been shown that the projection is ipsilateral. Release of vasopressin into the portal blood in concentrations high enough to participate in ACTH release may arise from these secretory terminals. Glucocorticoid deficiency has been found to be associated with increases in RNA turnover in paraventricular nucleus vasopressin neurones, in vasopressin biosynthesis and in the content of vasopressin in the cell bodies. It remains to be established whether this metabolic activation reflects increased release of the neurohormone into the portal blood. Also unknown is the site of negative glucocorticoid feedback on this system: directly on the paraventricular nucleus or indirectly via synaptic connections with other steroid concentrating cells. It has been established, however, that the marked increase in the numbers of vasopressin terminals in the zona externa of the median eminence between days 5 and 21 following adrenalectomy is not due to the sprouting of pre-existing terminals. Sprouting does occur, however, in response to a unilateral lesion of the paraventricular nucleus in adrenalectomized animals. Within three weeks vasopressin fibres from the intact side reinnervate the denervated side of the zona externa. These results suggest a complex interaction between this vasopressin neurosecretory system and adrenal glucocorticoid levels.

ACKNOWLEDGEMENTS

The authors thank Joan U. Bergin for assistance with the manuscript. Supported by NIH Grant AM 20337 and the Whitehall Foundation.

REFERENCES

Alonso, G. and Assenmacher, I. (1981) Radioautographic studies on the neurophysial projections of the supraoptic and paraventricular nuclei in the rat. *Cell Tiss. Res.*, 219: 525–534.

Alvarez-Buylla, Livett, B.G., Uttenthal, L.O., Hope, D.B. and Milton, S.H. (1973) Immunological evidence for the transport in the hypothalamo-neurohypophysial system of the dog. *Z. Zellforsch.*, 137: 435–450.

Antunes, J.L., Carmel, P.W. and Zimmerman, E.A. (1977) Projections from the paraventricular nucleus to the zona externa of the median eminence of the rhesus monkey: an immunohistochemical study. *Brain Res.*, 137: 1–10.

Antunes, J.L., Carmel, P.W., Zimmerman, E.A. and Ferin, M. (1979) Regeneration of the magnocellular system of the rhesus monkey following hypothalamic lesions. *Ann. Neurol.*, 15: 462–569.

Armstrong, W.E. and Hatton, G.I. (1980) The localization of projection neurons in the rat hypothalamic paraventricular nucleus following vascular and neurophypophysial injections of HRP. *Brain Res. Bull.*, 5: 473–477.

Bargmann, W. and Scharrer, E. (1951) The site of origin of the hormones of the posterior pituitary. *Amer. Sci.*, 39: 255–259.

Berk, M.L. and Finkelstein, J.A. (1981) Afferent projections to the preoptic area and hypothalamic regions in the rat brain. *Neuroscience*, 6: 1601–1624.

Blackwell, R.E. and Guillemin, R. (1973) Hypothalamic control of adenohypophysial secretions. *Ann. Rev. Physiol.*, 35: 357–390.

Bloom, F.E., Battenberg, E.L.F., Rivier, J. and Vale, W. (1982) Corticotropin releasing factor (CRF): immunoreactive neurones and fibers in rat hypothalamus. *Regulat. Peptides*, 4: 43–48.

Bugnon, C., Fellmann, D., Gouget, A. and Cardot, J. (1982) Ontogeny of the corticoliberin neuroglandular system in rat brain. *Nature (Lond.)*, 298: 159–161.

Carlson, D.E., Dornhorst, A., Seif, S.M., Robinson, A.G. and Gann, D.S. (1982) Vasopressin-dependent and -independent control of the release of adrenocorticotropin. *Endocrinology*, 110: 680–682.

Dornhorst, A., Carlson, D.E., Seif, S.M., Robinson, A.G., Zimmerman, E.A. and Gann, D.S. (1981) Control of release of adrenocorticotropin and vasopressin by the supraoptic and paraventricular nuclei. *Endocrinology*, 108: 1420–1424.

Ganong, W.F., Shinsako, J., Reid, I.A., Keil, L.C., Hoffman, D.L. and Zimmerman, E.A. (1982) Role of vasopressin in the renin and ACTH responses to intraventricular angiotensin II. *Ann. N.Y. Acad. Sci.*, 394: 619–624.

Gillies, G. and Lowry, P.J. (1982) Corticotropin releasing hormone and its vasopressin component. In W.F. Ganong and L. Martini (Eds.), *Frontiers in Neuroendocrinology, Vol. 7*, Raven Press, New York, pp. 45–75.

Goldman, H. and Lindner, L. (1962) Antidiuretic hormone concentration in blood perfusing the adenohypophysis. *Experientia*, 18: 289.

Hökfelt, T., Elde, T., Fuxe, K., Johansson, O., Ljungdahl, A., Goldstein, M., Luft, R., Efendic, S., Nilsson, G., Terenius, L., Gaten, D., Jeffcoate, S.L., Rehfeld, J., Said, S. Perez de la Mora, M., Possani, L., Tapia, R., Teran, L. and Palacios, R. (1978) Aminergic and peptidergic pathways in the nervous system with special reference to the hypothalamus. In S. Reichlin, R.J. Baldessarini and J. B. Martin (Eds.), *The Hypothalamus*, Raven Press, New York, pp. 69–135.

Hou-Yu, A., Ehrlich, P.H., Valiquette, G., Engelhardt, D.L., Sawyer, W.H., Nilaver, G. and Zimmerman, E.A. (1982) A monoclonal antibody to vasopressin: preparation, characterization and application in immunocyto-chemistry. *J. Histochem. Cytochem.*, 30: 1249–1260.

Kahn, D., Abrams, G.M., Zimmerman, E.A., Carraway, R. and Leeman, S. (1980) Neurotensin neurons in the rat hypothalamus: an immunocytochemical study. *Endocrinology*, 107: 47–54.

Knigge, K.M. and Scott, D.E. (1970) Structure and function of the median eminence. *Amer. J. Anat.*, 129: 223–228.

Kobayashi, H., Matsui, T. and Ishii, S. (1970) Functional electron microscopy of the hypothalamic median eminence. *Int. Rev. Cytol.*, 29: 281–381.

Krieger, D.T. and Zimmerman, E.A. (1977) The nature of CRF and its relationship to vasopressin. In M. Besser and L. Martini (Eds.), *Clinical Neuroendocrinology*, Academic Press, New York, pp. 363–391.

Lechan, R.M. and Jackson, I.M.D. (1982) Immunohistochemical localization of thyrotropin-releasing hormone in rat hypothalamus and pituitary. *Endocrinology*, 111: 55–65.

Lechan, R.M., Nestler, J.L., Jacobson, S. and Reichlin, S. (1980) The hypothalamic tuberoinfundibular system of the rat as demonstrated by horseradish peroxidase (HRP) microiontophoresis. *Brain Res.*, 195: 13–27.

Lechan, R.M., Nestler, J.L. and Jacobson, S. (1981) Immunohistochemical localization of retrogradely and antero-gradely transported wheat germ agglutinin (WGA) within the central nervous system of the rat: application to immunostaining of a second antigen within the same neuron. *J. Histochem. Cytochem.*, 29: 1255–1262.

LeClerc, R. and Pelletier, G. (1974) Electron microscope localization of vasopressin in the hypothalamus and neurohypophysis of the normal and Brattleboro rat. *Amer. J. Anat.*, 140: 583–588.

Makara, G.B., Stark, E., Karteszi, M., Palkovitz, M. and Rappay, G.Y. (1981) Effects of paraventricular lesions on stimulated ACTH release and CRF in stalk-median eminence of the rat. *Amer. J. Physiol.*, 240: E441–E446.

Martini, L. (1966) Neurohypophysis and anterior pituitary activity. In G.W. Harris and B.T. Donovan (Eds.), *The Pituitary Gland, Vol. 3*, University of California Press, Berkeley, pp. 535–577.

McCann, S.M. (1957) The ACTH releasing activity of extracts of the posterior lobe of the pituitary in vivo. *Endocrinology*, 60: 664–676.

McCann, S.M. and Brobeck, J.R. (1954) Evidence for a role of the supraopticohypophysial system in the regulation of adrenocorticotropin secretion. *Proc. Soc. exp. Biol. Med.*, 87: 318–324.

McEwen, B.S., Gerlach, J.L. and Micco, D.J. (1975) Putative glucocorticoid receptors in hippocampus and other brain regions of the rat brain. In S. Isaacson and J. Pribram, *The Hippocampus, Vol. 1*, Plenum Press, New York, N.Y., pp. 285–322.

Oliver, C., Mical, R.S. and Porter, J.C. (1977). Hypothalamic–pituitary vasculature: evidence for retrograde blood flow in the pituitary stalk. *Endocrinology*, 101: 598–604.

Parry, H.B. and Livett, B.G. (1973) A new hypothalamic pathway to the median eminence containing neurophysin and its hypertrophy in sheep with natural scrapie. *Nature (Lond.)*, 242: 63–65.

Paull, W.K., Schöler, J., Arimura, A., Meyers, C.A., Chiang, J.K., Chiang, D. and Shimizu, M. (1982) Immunocy-tochemical localization of CRF in the ovine hypothalamus. *Peptides*, 3: 183–191.

Pittman, Q.J., Blume, H.W. and Renaud, L.P. (1978) Electrophysiological indications that individual hypothalamic neurons innervate both median eminence and neurohypophysis. *Brain Res.*, 157: 364–368.

Pittman, Q.J., Blume, H.W. and Renaud, L.P. (1981) Connections of the hypothalamic paraventricular nucleus with the neurohypophysis, median eminence, amygdala, lateral septum and midbrain periaqueductal grey. *Brain Res.*, 215: 15–28.

Rasmussen, A.T. (1940) Effects of hypophysectomy and hypophysial stalk section on the hypothalamic nuclei of animals and man. *Res. Publ. Assoc. nerv. ment. Dis.*, 20: 245–269.

Recht, L.D., Hoffman, D.L., Haldar, J., Silverman, A.-J. and Zimmerman, E.A. (1981) Vasopressin concentrations in hypophysial portal plasma: insignificant reduction following removal of the posterior pituitary gland. *Neuroendocrinology*, 33: 88–90.

Rothballer, A.B. and Skaryna, S.C. (1960) Morphological effects of pituitary stalk section in the dog with special reference to neurosecretory material. *Anat. Rec.*, 136: 5–11.

Russell, J.T., Brownstein, M.J. and Gainer, H. (1980) [^{35}S]Cysteine-labeled peptides transported to the neurohypophysis of adrenalectomized, lactating and Brattleboro rats. *Brain Res.*, 201: 227–234.

Sachs, H., Fawcett, P., Takabatake, Y. and Portanova, R. (1969) Biosynthesis and release of vasopressin and neurophysin. *Rec. Progr. Horm. Res.*, 25: 447–484.

Sawchenko, P.E. and Swanson, L.W. (1981) Central noradrenergic pathways for the integration of hypothalamic neuroendocrine and autonomic responses. *Science*, 214: 685–687.

Schally, A.V., Arimura, A. and Kastin, A.J. (1973) Hypothalamic regulatory hormones. *Science*, 179: 431–450.

Scheff, S.W., Benardo, L.S. and Cotman, C.W. (1980) Hydrocortisone administration retards axon sprouting in the rat dentate gyrus. *Exp. Neurol.*, 68: 195–201.

Seif, S.M., Robinson, A.G., Zimmerman, E.A. and Wilkins, J. (1978) Plasma neurophysin and vasopressin in the rat: response to adrenalectomy and steroid replacement. *Endocrinology*, 103: 109–113.

Seybold, V., Elde, R. and Hökfelt, T. (1981) Terminals of reserpine-sensitive vasopressin neurophysin neurons in the external layer of the rat median eminence. *Endocrinology*, 108: 1803–1809.

Silverman, A.-J. and Zimmerman, E.A. (1975) Ultrastructural localization of neurophysin and vasopressin in the median eminence and posterior of the guinea pig. *Cell Tiss. Res.*, 159: 291–301.

Silverman, A.-J. and Zimmerman, E.A. (1982) Adrenalectomy increases sprouting in a peptidergic neurosecretory system. *Neuroscience*, 7: 2705–2714.

Silverman, A.-J., Gadde, C.A. and Zimmerman, E.A. (1980) The effects of adrenalectomy on the incorporation of ^{3}H-cytidine into RNA in neurophysin and vasopressin containing neurons of the rat hypothalamus. *Neuroendocrinology*, 30: 285–290.

Silverman, A.-J., Hoffman, D.L. and Zimmerman, E.A. (1981) The descending afferent connections of the paraventricular nucleus of the hypothalamus. *Brain Res. Bull.*, 6: 47–61.

Sokol, H.W. and Zimmerman, E.A. (1982) The hormonal status of Brattleboro rat. *Ann. N.Y. Acad. Sci.*, 394: 535–548.

Sokol, H.W., Zimmerman, E.A., Sawyer, W.H. and Robinson, A.G. (1976) The hypothalamo-neurohypophysial system of the rat: localization and quantification of neurophysin by light microscopic immunocytochemistry in normal rat and in Brattleboro rats deficient in vasopressin and a neurophysin. *Endocrinology*, 98: 1176–1188.

Stillman, M.A., Recht, L.D., Rosario, S.L., Seif, S.M., Robinson, A.G. and Zimmerman, E.A. (1977) The effects of adrenalectomy and glucocorticoid replacement on vasopressin and vasopressin-neurophysin in the zona externa of the rat. *Endocrinology*, 101: 42–49.

Swanson, L.W. and Sawchenko, P.E. (1980) Paraventricular nucleus: a site for the integration of neuroendocrine and autonomic mechanisms. *Neuroendocrinology*, 31: 410–417.

Swanson, L.W., Sawchenko, P.E., Wiegand, S.J. and Price, J.L. (1980) Separate neurons in the paraventricular nucleus project to the median eminence and to the medulla or spinal cord. *Brain Res.*, 198: 190–195.

Tramu, G. and Pillez, A. (1982) Localization, immunohistochimique des terminaisons nerveuses a corticoliberine (CRF) dans l'eminence mediane du Cobaye et du rat. *C.R. Acad. Sci. (Paris)*, 294: 107–114.

Tribollet, E. and Dreifuss, J.J. (1981) Localization of neurones projecting to the hypothalamic paraventricular nucleus area of the rat: a horseradish peroxidase study. *Neuroscience*, 6: 1315–1328.

Unsicker, K., Krisch, B., Otten, U. and Theonen, H. (1978) Nerve growth factor-induced fiber outgrowth from isolated rat adrenal chromaffin cells: impairment by glucocorticoids. *Proc. nat. Acad. Sci. U.S.A.*, 75: 3498–3502.

Vale, W., Spiess, J., Rivier, C. and Rivier, J. (1981) Characteristics of a 41-residue ovine hypothalamic peptide that stimulates the secretion of corticotropin and β-endorphin. *Science*, 213: 1394–1397.

Vandesande, F., DeMey, J. and Dierickx, K. (1974) Identification of neurophysin producing cells. I. The origin of the neurophysin-like substance-containing nerve fibers of the external region of the median eminence of the rat. *Cell Tiss. Res.*, 151: 187–200.

Vandesande, F., Dierickx, K. and De Mey, J. (1975) Identification of the vasopressin-neurophysin II and the oxytocin-neurophysin I producing neurons in the bovine hypothalamus. *Cell Tiss. Res.*, 156: 189–200.

Vandesande, F., Dierickx, K. and DeMey, J. (1977) The origin of the vasopressin and oxytocinergic fibers of the external region of the median eminence of the rat hypophysis. *Cell Tiss. Res.*, 180: 443–452.

504

Warembourg, M. (1975) Radioautographic study of the rat brain after injection of [1,2-^{3}H]corticosterone. *Brain Res.*, 89: 61–70.

Watkins, W.B., Schwabedal, P. and Bock, R. (1974) Immunohistochemical demonstration of a CRF-associated neurophysin in the external zone of the rat median eminence. *Cell Tiss. Res.*, 152: 411–421.

Watson, S.J., Seidah, N.G. and Chrétien, M. (1981) The carboxy terminus of the precursor to vasopressin and neurophysin: immunocytochemistry in rat brain. *Science*, 217: 853–855.

Wiegand, S.J. and Price, J.L. (1980) Cells of origin of the afferent fibers to the median eminence in the rat. *J. comp. Neurol.*, 192: 1–19.

Wittowski, W. and Bock, R. (1972) Electron microscopical studies of the median eminence following interference with the feedback system anterior pituitary–adrenal cortex. In K.M. Knigge, D.E. Scott and A. Weindl (Eds.), *Brain–Endocrine Interaction: Median Eminence Structure and Function*, Karger, Basel, pp. 171–180.

Yates, F.E., Russell, S.M., Dallman, M.F., Hedge, G.A., McCann, S.M. and Dhariwal, A.P.S. (1971) Potentiation by vasopressin of corticotropin release induced by corticotropin-releasing factor. *Endocrinology*, 88: 3015.

Zimmerman, E.A., Carmel, P.W., Husain, M.K., Ferin, M., Tannenbaum, M., Frantz, A.G. and Robinson, A.G. (1973a) Vasopressin and neurophysin: high concentrations in monkey hypophyseal portal blood. *Science*, 182: 925–957.

Zimmerman, E.A., Hsu, K.C., Robinson, A.G., Carmel, P.W., Frantz, A.G. and Tannenbaum, M. (1973b) Studies on neurophysin secreting neurons with immunoperoxidase techniques employing antibody to bovine neurophysin. I. Light microscopic findings in monkey and bovine tissues. *Endocrinology*, 92: 931–940.

Zimmerman, E.A., Stillman, M.A., Recht, L.D., Antunes, J.L., Carmel, P.W. and Goldsmith, P.C. (1977) Vasopressin and corticotropin-releasing factor: an axonal pathway to portal capillaries in the zona externa of the median eminence containing vasopressin and its interaction with adrenal corticoids. *Ann. N.Y. Acad. Sci.*, 297: 405–419.

The Neurohypophysis: Structure, Function and Control, Progress in Brain Research, Vol. 60, edited by B.A. Cross and G. Leng

Vasopressin, Corticoliberins and the Central Control of ACTH Secretion

A.J. BAERTSCHI, J.-L. BÉNY, B.H. GÄHWILER [1] and E. KOLODZIEJCZYK

Department of Animal Biology, University of Geneva, 1211 Geneva 4 and [1]Preclinical Research, Sandoz Ltd., 4002 Basle (Switzerland)

INTRODUCTION

The role of vasopressin and other factors in the control of ACTH secretion has been a subject of intense research for the past 25 years (Saffran and Schally, 1977; Baertschi and Bény, 1982). This chapter gives a progress report on the hypothalamic localization of corticoliberins (corticotropin-releasing factor, CRF), and describes the sites where vasopressin and CRF may be released into portal vessels and their action on corticotrophic cells. Complementary information can be gathered in the recently published proceedings from a recent symposium on vasopressin, corticoliberins and opiomelanocortins (Baertschi and Dreifuss, 1982).

HYPOTHALAMIC ORIGINS OF CRF PATHWAYS

Although classic concepts hold that CRF-producing neurones are located diffusely throughout the basal hypothalamus, recent evidence points to the paraventricular nucleus (PVN) as a main source of CRF pathways. It has been known for some time that vasopressin-containing nerve fibres of the external median eminence originate within the PVN and that manipulation of adrenocortical function alters the intensity of immunocytochemical staining for vasopressin in that region (Zimmerman et al., 1977). It was realized subsequently that CRFs distinct from vasopressin may also originate from, or be transported through, the PVN, as PVN lesions result four days later in a diminished corticosterone response to ether stress, and in a diminished CRF content of the median eminence in normal rats (Makara et al., 1981). These results are confirmed in Brattleboro rats with diabetes insipidus (DI rats) (Baertschi et al., 1983). Tissue culture studies showed that CRFs distinct from vasopressin are released from the PVN (Baertschi et al., 1982a, b): PVN tissue punched from hypothalamic slices and cultured for four weeks induced a several-fold increase of ACTH secretion from co-cultured hemi-pituitary (Fig. 1), whereas supraoptic or basal hypothalamic explants had little or no effect. The levels of vasopressin and ACTH in the culture media were highly correlated ($r - 0.91$), yet vasopressin alone added to the hemi-pituitary weekly for four weeks had little effect on ACTH secretion.

To detect additional sites of CRF synthesis, the hypothalami of 7-day-old rats were sliced in the frontal plane from the preoptic area to the mammillary bodies into 400μm thick sections (Gähwiler, 1981). These slices were cultured for four weeks with one hemi-pituitary. Fig. 1 displays the mean levels of vasopressin and ACTH in the medium from six such culture series.

[505]

Slice number five presumably included the PVN, as suggested by the peak levels of vasopressin in the medium; peak levels for ACTH in the medium were also found in this slice. More surprisingly, a second peak level of ACTH was consistently found in the medium of slices of the posterior hypothalamus, suggesting that CRF neurones may also be located in that region.

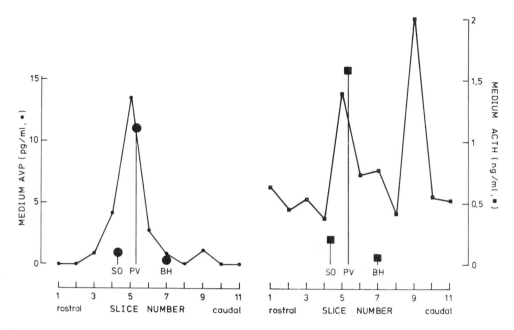

Fig. 1. Vasopressin (AVP) and ACTH levels in medium from co-cultures of hypothalamic explants and anterior pituitary gland. Either punched nuclei (large full squares and circles) or frontal hypothalamic slices (solid lines) were cultured (see Gähwiler, 1981) for 4 weeks with one hemi-pituitary. The medium was collected every week for assays (RIA for AVP, RIA and bioassay for ACTH) and renewed. All data points are mean values from 5–6 sliced hypothalami or punched hypothalamic regions. For details of methods and results, see Baertschi et al. (1982a, b).

Since a synthetic ovine CRF (sCRF) (Vale et al., 1981) became available, several immuno-cytochemical studies have been conducted to locate CRF neurones in the PVN of colchicine-treated rats and of normal sheep (cited in Kolodziejczyk et al., 1983). These cell bodies were not stained by anti-neurophysin (I + II) antisera. In our study on the sheep hypothalamus, we identified a second group of sCRF-immunoreactive neurones in the dorsolateral posterior hypothalamus. These were distinguished by their small size (10–15 μm) and smooth cytoplasm, and could only be stained by diluting the anti-sCRF less than 400 times. In contrast, sCRF-immunoreactive neurones in the PVN were larger, had a granular cytoplasm, and could be stained even when the antiserum was diluted more than 800 times. As only the immuno-reactivity in the posterior hypothalamus was abolished by preincubating the antiserum with sauvagine, we suggest that this region contains a CRF distinct from the ovine CRF described previously (Vale et al., 1981). In addition, numerous nerve fibres were stained by the sCRF antiserum in the external median eminence, around the anterior commissure, in the caudal neural lobe and in the vicinity of the intermediate lobe (Fig. 2), suggesting that sCRF-like peptides act not only on the anterior pituitary, but also on central neurones, the intermediate lobe and peripheral target organs.

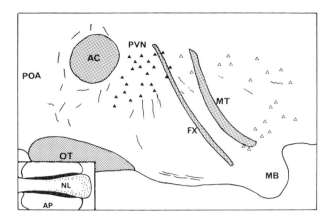

Fig. 2. Immunocytochemical localization of CRF neurones in sheep hypothalamus (for details, see Kolodziejczyk et al., 1983). Neurones were stained by the indirect immunocytochemical procedure with antiserum directed against synthetic ovine CRF and anti-rabbit goat gammaglobulin coupled to FITC. Filled triangles stand for cells 15–20 μm in diameter, with a granular cytoplasm, slightly off-centre nucleus, that were revealed even when antiserum was diluted more than 800 times; open triangles stand for smaller cells (10–15 μm diameter), with smooth cytoplasm and well centred nucleus, that were revealed only when dilutions of antiserum were less than or equal to 1:400. Immuno-reactive nerve fibres are marked by black lines. Section is in parasagittal plane. Insert shows horizontal section through sheep pituitary gland (NL, neural lobe; AP, anterior pituitary; in black, intermediate lobe). Immunoreactive nerve terminals marked by black dots. Other abbreviations: AC, anterior commissure; FX, fornix; MB, mammillary bodies; MT, mammillo-thalamic tract; PV, paraventricular nucleus. Shaded areas represent non-immunoreactive tracts.

PEPTIDE RELEASE AND TRANSPORT IN PORTAL BLOOD

Despite the immunocytochemical visualization and biological detection (Fig. 3) of CRF distinct from vasopressin in the median eminence and neural lobe, it has proved difficult to demonstrate the release of CRF.

The amounts of CRF released from the posterior pituitary by electrical stimulation in vitro could be totally ascribed to vasopressin in normal rats and to oxytocin in DI rats, whereas CRF released from the median eminence could also be totally accounted for by the concomitant release of vasopressin (work cited in Baertschi and Bény, 1982). However, extracts from these structures contained from 50 to 300 % more CRF than could be accounted for by vasopressin alone (Fig. 3). Thus CRF distinct from vasopressin is protected from oxidation by some other substance contained in the extracts. Released CRF distinct from vasopressin could only be detected when ascorbic acid was added to the medium (Fig. 3), and this may perhaps be explained by the lability of sCRF-like substances to oxidation (Vale et al., 1981).

Release of vasopressin into the hypophysial portal blood has been shown in both the monkey (Zimmerman et al., 1973) and rat (Oliver et al., 1977). Experiments to measure sCRF-like substances in portal blood are in progress. Peptide release is probably not confined to the median eminence, as electrical stimulation of the neural lobe promotes a vasopressin-mediated ACTH secretion in rats (Baertschi et al., 1980), and posterior lobectomy reduces the amounts of vasopressin detected in portal blood (Oliver et al., 1977). Moreover, neural lobe stimulation is followed after 2–5 sec by the appearance of large quantities of potassium in the rostral regions of the anterior pituitary gland, even when the long portal vessels have been lesioned (Baertschi, 1980). This suggests the scheme of Fig. 4, showing how hypothalamic factors are

508

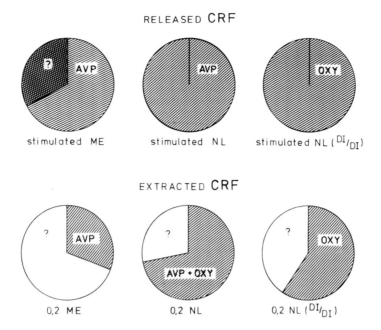

RELEASED CRF

stimulated ME   stimulated NL   stimulated NL ($^{DI}/_{DI}$)

EXTRACTED CRF

0,2 ME   0,2 NL   0,2 NL ($^{DI}/_{DI}$)

Fig. 3. Released (top panel) and extracted (lower panel) CRF from median eminence (ME) or neural lobe (NL) in Wistar rats and in DI rats. CRF was measured by bioassay. All circles stand for 100 % of all CRF activity. Hatched areas correspond to the percentage of CRF activity accounted for by vasopressin (AVP) alone or by vasopressin plus oxytocin (AVP + OXY). White areas (?) correspond to CRF activities distinct from those of vasopressin and oxytocin. Double-hatched area in upper left is CRF distinct from vasopressin detected when ascorbic acid is added to medium of electrically-stimulated ME. For details, see Bény and Baertschi (1981) and other work cited in Baertschi and Bény (1982).

thought to be conveyed from the median eminence and the stalk/neural lobe region towards the anterior pituitary gland. With the same methodology, it is possible to infer that anterior pituitary hormones may travel to the neural lobe through short interconnecting vessels, as has been suggested from scanning microscopy of hypophysial vascular casts (Page and Bergland, 1977).

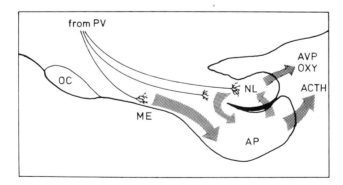

Fig. 4. Blood flow patterns in the pituitary gland, as deduced from microelectrode recordings of extracellular potassium activity during electrical stimulation of the stalk and neural lobe (for details, see Baertschi, 1980). Shaded areas indicate directions of blood flow. OC, optic chiasm; PV, paraventricular nucleus; NL, neural lobe; AP, anterior pituitary; in black, intermediate lobe.

PEPTIDE ACTIONS ON CORTICOTROPHS

On a molar basis, vasopressin was 3–5 times less effective than sCRF in releasing ACTH from acutely dispersed anterior pituitary cells, but could double the ACTH secretion by sCRF when both peptides were added in combination (Bény and Baertschi, 1982; Gillies et al., 1982). When vasopressin was injected in vivo in rats, it had almost the same effect as sCRF in raising the corticosterone levels in plasma (Rivier et al., 1982). The results above are compatible with a hypothesis that vasopressin potentiates the action of another releasing factor (Gillies and Lowry, 1979).

The cellular actions of vasopressin and other peptides on the corticotrophs have so far been little studied. Our preliminary results suggest that stimulation of ACTH secretion is mediated, in part, by cAMP, calmodulin and intracellular proteases (Bény and Baertschi, unpublished observations).

DISCUSSION

CRF-producing neurones have been localized by two independent experiments (Figs. 1 and 2) in both the PVN and the posterior hypothalamus. Direct evidence that these neurones project onto the external median eminence is not yet available. In view of the numerous peptidergic (non-vasopressin) fibres that run from the PVN to the external median eminence (Swanson and Sawchenko, 1980), and in consideration of physiological data (detailed in Baertschi and Dreifuss, 1982), it is most likely that CRF neurones in the PVN are mainly concerned with the direct control of anterior pituitary ACTH secretion. The lack of evidence for median eminence projections from many posterior hypothalamic areas (Renaud, 1980) where a second group of CRF neurones was detected, as well as the differential shapes and staining characteristics of PVN and posterior hypothalamic CRF neurones (Kolodziejczyk et al., 1982), all make it questionable whether these posterior hypothalamic CRF neurones are *directly* involved in the control of ACTH secretion.

The complex circulatory patterns (Fig. 4) within the hypothalamo-hypophysial system are far from being completely elucidated. Knowledge of the exact sites of peptide release and of the circulatory routes has to be gained before the mechanisms for pituitary secretions can be fully understood. Is there a short-loop feedback of opiomelanocortins on vasopressin- and CRF-secreting nerve terminals? Do anterior pituitary hormones modulate neural lobe secretions, and may they even act on hypothalamic neurones?

Finally, most studies conclude that ovine CRF (Vale et al., 1981) is a potent releasing factor in rats, and that vasopressin should be regarded as a potent modulator of CRF-induced ACTH secretion. However, the relative amounts of vasopressin and ovine CRF-like substances that act on the corticotrophs under various physiological situations are not yet known, and the cellular actions of these hypothalamic peptides remain to be established.

SUMMARY

Tissue culture and immunocytochemical studies suggest that two distinct hypothalamic areas contain CRF-producing neurones: (1) the PVN, which probably accounts for a large part of the CRF fibres to the external median eminence; and (2) the posterior, mainly dorsolateral, hypothalamus for which the projection sites have not yet been established. Immunocytochemical evidence suggests that corticoliberin and neurophysin are produced in distinct neurones. Investigations of blood flow patterns suggest that vasopressin, and to a lesser degree perhaps also corticoliberin, may reach the corticotrophs from both the median eminence and the pituitary stalk/rostral neural lobe regions, and that anterior pituitary hormones may reach the caudal neural lobe. Possible actions such as "presynaptic" modulation of neural lobe hormone secretions or short feedback on median eminence and neural lobe nerve terminals have not been examined. Vasopressin and peptides resembling ovine corticoliberin enhance each other's action on corticotrophs, but the hypophysial plasma levels of these hypothalamic peptides under various physiological conditions and their cellular mode of action remain to be established.

ACKNOWLEDGEMENTS

These studies were supported by the Swiss National Science Foundation (Grant 3.581-0.79 and 3.898.0.81). We thank Ms. M. Friedli, K. Constantin and C. Estoppey, Geneva, and Ms. L. Rietschin, Basle, for excellent technical assistance.

REFERENCES

Baertschi, A.J. (1980) A portal vascular route from neural lobe to adenohypophysis. *Amer. J. Physiol.*, 239: R463–R469.

Baertschi, A.J. and Bény, J.L. (1982) Central control of ACTH secretion: Role of vasopressinergic pathways and of the hypothalamohypophysial circulation. *Front. Horm. Res.* 10: 126–140.

Baertschi, A.J. and Dreifuss, J.J. (Eds.) (1982) *Neuroendocrinology of Vasopressin, Corticoliberin and Opiomelanocortins*, Academic Press, London.

Baertschi, A.J., Vallet, P., Baumann, J.B. and Girard, J. (1980) Neural lobe of pituitary modulates corticotropin release in the rat. *Endocrinology*, 106: 878–882.

Baertschi, A.J., Bény, J.L. and Gähwiler, B. (1982a) Hypothalamic paraventricular nucleus is a privileged site for brain–pituitary interaction in long-term tissue culture. *Nature (Lond.)*, 295: 145–147.

Baertschi, A.J., Bény, J.L. and Gähwiler, B. (1982b) The hypothalamo-hypophysial system in long-term tissue culture. In A.J. Baertschi and J.J. Dreifuss (Eds.), *Neuroendocrinology of Vasopressin, Corticoliberin and Opiomelanocortin.*, Academic Press, London, pp. 259–271.

Baertschi, A.J., Bény, J.L. and Makara, G.B. (1983) Hypothalamic paraventricular nucleus region controls pituitary–adrenal function in diabetes insipidus rats. *Amer. J. Physiol.*, in press.

Bény, J.L. and Baertschi, A.J. (1981) Corticotropin releasing factors (CRF) secreted by the rat median eminence in vitro in the presence or absence of ascorbic acid: quantitative role of vasopressin and catecholamines. *Endocrinology*, 109: 813–817.

Bény, J.L. and Baertschi, A.J. (1982) Synthetic corticoliberin needs arginine vasopressin for full corticotropin releasing activity. *Experientia*, 38: 1078-1079.

Gähwiler, B. (1981) Organotypic monolayer cultures of nervous tissue. *J. Neurosci. Meth.*, 4: 329–342.

Gillies, G. and Lowry, P.J. (1979) Corticotropin releasing factor may be modulated vasopressin. *Nature (Lond.)*, 278: 463–464.

Gillies, G., Linton, E. and Lowry, P.J. (1982) Vasopressin and the corticoliberin complex. In A.J. Baertschi and J.J. Dreifuss (Eds.), *Neuroendocrinology of Vasopressin, Corticoliberin and Opiomelanocortins*, Academic Press, London, pp. 239–248.

Kolodziejczyk, E., Baertschi, A.J. and Tramu, G. (1983) Corticoliberin-immunoreactive cell bodies localised in two distinct areas of the sheep hypothalamus. *Neuroscience*, in press.

Makara, G.B., Stark, E., Karteszi, M., Palkovits, M. and Rappay, Gy. (1981) The effect of paraventricular lesions on stimulated ACTH release and CRF in stalk-median eminence of the rat. *Amer. J. Physiol.*, 240: E441–E446.

Oliver, C., Mical, R.S. and Porter, J.C. (1977) Hypothalamic-pituitary vasculature: evidence for retrograde blood flow in the pituitary stalk. *Endocrinology*, 101: 598–604.

Page, R.B. and Bergland, R.M. (1977) The neurohypophysial capillary bed. *Amer. J. Anat.*, 148: 345–357.

Renaud, L.P. (1980) A neurophysiological approach to the identification, connections and pharmacology of the hypothalamic tuberoinfundibular system. *Neuroendocrinology*, 33: 186–191.

Rivier, C., Brownstein, M., Rivier, J. and Vale, W. (1982) In vivo corticotropin releasing factor-induced secretion of adrenocorticotropin, β-endorphin and corticosterone. *Endocrinology*, 110: 272–278.

Saffran, M. and Schally, A.V. (1977) The status of the corticotropin-releasing factor (CRF). *Neuroendocrinology*, 24: 359–375.

Swanson, L.W. and Sawchenko, P.E. (1980) Paraventricular nucleus: a site for the integration of neuroendocrine and autonomic mechanisms. *Neuroendocrinology*, 31: 410–417.

Vale, W., Spiess, J., Rivier, C. and Rivier, J. (1981) Characterisation of a 41 residue ovine hypothalamic peptide that stimulates secretion of corticotropin and β-endorphin. *Science*, 213: 1394–1397.

Zimmerman, E.A., Carmel, P.W., Husain, M.K., Ferin, M., Tannenbaum, M., Frantz, A.B. and Robinson, A.G. (1973) Vasopressin and neurophysin: high concentration in monkey hypophysial portal blood. *Science*, 182: 925–927.

Zimmerman, E.A., Stillman, M.A., Recht, L.D., Antunes, J.L., Carmel, P.W. and Goldsmith, P.C. (1977) Vasopressin and corticotropin-releasing factor. An axonal pathway to portal capillaries in the zona externa of the median eminence containing vasopressin and its interaction with corticoids. *Ann. N.Y. Acad. Sci.*, 297: 405–419.

The Neurohypophysis: Structure, Function and Control, Progress in Brain Research, Vol. 60, edited by B.A. Cross and G. Leng

Gonadal Sources of the Posterior Pituitary Hormones

D.C. WATHES, R.W. SWANN, M.G.R. HULL[1], J.O. DRIFE[1],
D.G. PORTER and B.T. PICKERING

Department of Anatomy, The Medical School, Bristol BS8 1TD and [1]University Department of Obstetrics and Gynaecology, Bristol Maternity Hospital, Bristol (U.K.)

INTRODUCTION

The importance of oxytocin in lactation and labour is well known, and in both cases its release from the neurohypophysis following the appropriate sensory stimulation has been demonstrated. In addition, oxytocin is thought to be involved in the regulation of the oestrous cycle as it induces regression of the corpus luteum on administration to the cow, sheep and goat (Armstrong and Hansel, 1959; Sheldrick et al., 1980; Cooke and Knifton, 1981). This effect is probably caused indirectly by stimulating the release of prostaglandin $F_{2\alpha}$ from the uterine endometrium (McCracken, 1980). However recent evidence shows that oxytocin can also directly inhibit steroidogenesis by luteal and testicular cells in vitro (Adashi and Hsueh, 1981; Tan et al., 1981) although in both cases inhibition was achieved only at peptide concentrations considerably in excess of circulating levels.

It has generally been assumed that the actions of oxytocin and related peptides on the reproductive system are achieved via release from the neurohypophysis into the peripheral circulation. However recent work suggests that the ovary itself may be a major source of oxytocin in some species and raises the possibility that oxytocin could act as a local hormone within the gonads.

NEUROHYPOPHYSIAL HORMONES IN THE OVARY

Sheep

Our initial observations were made using corpora lutea obtained from the ovaries of non-pregnant sheep (Wathes and Swann, 1982). These were extracted by the method of Walsh and Niall (1980) and purification was carried out using a column of Sephadex G-50 with 0.1 M ammonium acetate as the eluate. Material eluting in the position characteristic of oxytocin showed oxytocin-like activity in two bioassays. In a bioassay employing an electrically stimulated rat uterine strip it caused an increase in the resting tension and stimulated additional contractions (Fig. 1), and in a rat milk-ejection assay it caused pressure changes in a cannulated mammary gland (Fig. 2). When the extract was measured by radioimmunoassay (RIA) it showed parallelism with the oxytocin standard curve. Further purification was carried out by high performance liquid chromatography (HPLC). A single peak of immunoreactive material eluted in the same position as the oxytocin standard (Wathes and Swann, 1982).

[513]

514

These data suggest that the material extracted was authentic oxytocin. The concentration in the corpora lutea of non-pregnant sheep was estimated at 2.6 μg/g wet weight of tissue, equivalent to a total ovarian content of about 1–4 μg in a cyclic non-pregnant ewe. This can be compared with the figure of 18.2 μg which Lederis (1961) calculated to be the content of the ovine neurohypophysis and hypothalamus. We have also shown that corpora lutea of pregnant sheep contained only 34 ng/g, indicating that pregnancy leads to a marked decrease in the ovarian oxytocin content.

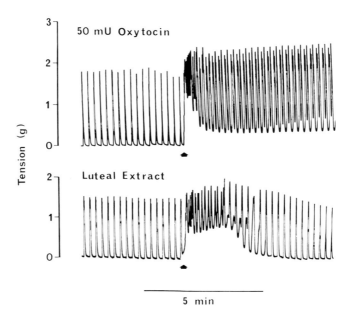

Fig. 1. Tension development in two uterine strips obtained from pro-oestrous rats. The strips were immersed in Krebs–Henseleit buffer at 37°C and stimulated electrically every 45 sec at 4 V amplitude and 50 Hz. (From Bradshaw et al., 1981). The traces show the effect of introducing: (a) 84 ng oxytocin (50 mU) and (b) luteal extract containing an estimated 95 ng oxytocin diluted from a Sephadex G-50 fraction on the basis of the RIA results.

The oxytocin in the corpora lutea could be the result of either uptake from the circulation or local synthesis. A number of points favour the latter hypothesis. The concentration in the ovary is about five orders of magnitude greater than that measured in peripheral plasma during the oestrous cycle which ranges from < 5 to about 70 pg/ml. During the cycle the oxytocin and progesterone levels in the circulation increase and decrease in synchrony (Sheldrick and Flint, 1981; Webb et al., 1981; Schams et al., 1982) and the oxytocin concentration becomes undetectable after ovariectomy (Schams et al., 1982). Finally Flint and Sheldrick (1982) have measured arterio-venous differences across the ovary in cyclic sheep and have shown that the oxytocin concentration is higher in the ovarian vein and that additional oxytocin is released into the ovarian vein following treatment with the prostaglandin $F_{2\alpha}$ analogue Estrumate (ICI, Macclesfield). There were no detectable differences between oxytocin concentrations in the carotid artery and jugular vein either before or after Estrumate treatment.

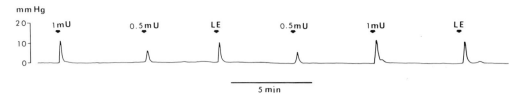

Fig. 2. Trace to show changes in intramammary pressure following the intravenous infusion of oxytocin or luteal extract to a lactating rat anaesthetized with urethane and pretreated with 0.1 mg propranolol (ICI, Macclesfield). (From Lincoln et al., 1973.) Oxytocin (Syntocinon, Sandoz) was infused at a concentration of 1.7 ng or 0.85 ng per 100 μl (1 or 0.5 mU). Luteal extract (LE) was one G-50 fraction diluted on the basis of the RIA results to give 1.7 ng oxytocin per 100 μl.

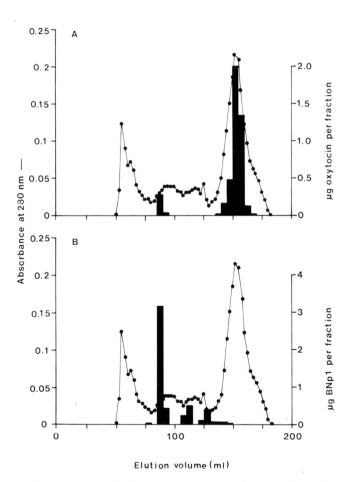

Fig. 3. Elution profile of a crude extract of 16.7 g bovine corpora lutea applied to a column of Sephadex G-75 (80 × 2 cm) measured as absorbance at 280 nm. The eluant was 0.1 M formic acid and the flow rate was 20 ml/h. Fractions (2.5 ml) were collected and lyophilized in pairs, before measurement of oxytocin (A) and bovine neurophysin I (B) by RIA.

Cow

To look for further evidence of local biosynthesis we repeated our initial experiments using bovine material. In the hypothalamus, oxytocin and oxytocin-related neurophysin are both released from the same precursor molecule (Pickering, 1978). Neurophysins have been more highly characterized in the cow than in the sheep, making this a suitable species for further study (Pickering and Jones, 1978). In three separate extractions the average yield of oxytocin from the corpora lutea of non-pregnant cows was 794 ng/g (see Table I). This material eluted at the appropriate position for oxytocin on Sephadex G-50, Sephadex G-75 and HPLC (Figs. 3 and 4) and showed characteristic activity in a uterine strip bioassay. The yield from pregnant cows was again considerably reduced (Table I).

TABLE I

OVARIAN OXYTOCIN CONCENTRATIONS IN DIFFERENT SPECIES

Each extration involved tissue of wet weight 11.0–21.5 g pooled from a number of individuals except for the figures marked with an asterisk, which represent the content of a single corpus luteum.

Species	No. of extractions	Tissue	Reproductive status	Oxytocin content (ng/g wet wt of tissue)
Sheep	2	Corpus luteum	Non-pregnant	2600, 227*
Sheep	1	Corpus luteum	Pregnant	34
Cow	3	Corpus luteum	Non-pregnant	1140, 980, 261
Cow	1	Corpus luteum	Pregnant	0.8
Human	2	Ovary	Non-pregnant	38*, 30.

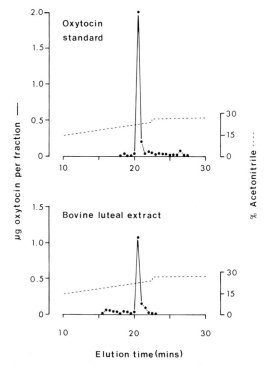

Fig. 4. Profiles obtained by adding bovine luteal extract or oxytocin standard to an HPLC system (Altex Model 322) and measuring aliquots of each 0.5 ml fraction by oxytocin RIA. For details of methodology see Wathes and Swann (1982).

Bovine neurophysin I was measured by RIA in the fractions from the Sephadex G-50 and G-75 columns. Using Sephadex G-50 with 0.1 M ammonium acetate as the eluant, a single peak of immunoreactive material eluted in the same position as the bovine neurophysin standard. Material from this peak also eluted at the same position as the standard on HPLC. Using Sephadex G-75 with 0.1 M formic acid as the eluant, three peaks of neurophysin were measured, the main one corresponding with a minor peak of oxytocin immunoreactivity (Fig. 3). The yield of bovine neurophysin I from non-pregnant cow corpora lutea was 307 ng/g. Its presence in the bovine ovary suggests that synthesis of oxytocin may occur at this site.

In the hypothalamo-neurohypophysial system, oxytocin and neurophysin are derived from a common precursor molecule, and the pituitary contains equimolar amounts of the two poly-peptides (see Pickering, 1978). Such a stoichiometry was not seen in the present study, so if the biosynthetic pathways in brain and ovary are similar, either there have been differential losses in the extraction procedure, or the ovarian and neurohypophysial neurophysins are not identical.

Human

In the cow and goat exogenous oxytocin is known to be luteolytic (Armstrong and Hansel, 1959; Cooke and Knifton, 1981) and in the human it has been shown that high concentrations of oxytocin (10^{-6} M) inhibit basal and human chorionic gonadotrophin (hCG)-stimulated progesterone production by human luteal cells in vitro. Luteolysis in the human is not well understood and so a possible role for oxytocin in this process is of particular interest.

Oxytocin was measured in ovarian tissue obtained from six women at laparotomy (Wathes et al., 1982). The oxytocin concentration in two separate extractions was 37.7 and 29.6 ng/g. This is less than the level measured in the sheep and cow but there are a number of reasons why these figures should not be compared directly. The human tissue contained ovarian stroma as well as corpus luteum, and was obtained from women aged 32–47 years whose reproductive potential was probably declining, and at various stages of the menstrual cycle. Nevertheless, the oxytocin concentration in the human ovary was four orders of magnitude greater than that in the peripheral circulation of non-pregnant women, which ranges from 0.3 to 7 pg/ml (Amico et al., 1981). These figures again suggest that the ovary either sequesters or produces oxytocin.

The arginine-vasopressin concentration in peripheral plasma also varies during the men-strual cycle (Forsling et al., 1981) and so the vasopressin content of the ovarian extracts was measured. In tissue obtained from a single ovary soon after ovulation, the concentration was 15.4 ng/g, whereas in tissue pooled from five ovaries at various stages of the cycle the concentration was only 281 pg/g (Wathes et al., 1982). These levels were again greater than the published concentrations of vasopressin in the circulation of between 0.5 and 2.5 pg/ml (Forsling et al., 1981).

NEUROHYPOPHYSIAL HORMONES IN THE TESTIS

Rat

Adashi and Hsueh (1981) reported that a variety of neurohypophysial hormones inhibited hCG-stimulated testosterone production by rat testicular cells in primary culture. Those peptides with the greatest antidiuretic and vasopressor activities (arginine-vasopressin, lysine-vasopressin and arginine-vasotocin) were about 100-fold more effective than oxytocin, valito-cin and mesotocin. The median effective doses for arginine-vasopressin and oxytocin were 2.5×10^{-10} M and 7.1×10^{-8} M, respectively. As already stated, circulating levels in various mammals are of the order of 10^{-12} M, so that if one is considering a neurohypophysial source these effective doses appear pharmacological.

Preliminary experiments in our laboratory have indicated that the concentrations of both oxytocin and vasopressin in rat testis are of the order of 10^{-9} M. Thus the tissue content is within the concentration range known to be physiologically active. Both oxytocin- and vasopressin-related neurophysins are also present indicating that synthesis of these neuropeptides may occur in the testis as well as the ovary.

CONCLUSIONS

In the three species so far examined, the ovarian oxytocin content is considerably in excess of circulating levels (Table I). Preliminary evidence suggests that vasopressin is also present in both the ovary and testis. The presence of neurophysin within the bovine corpus luteum and rat testis and the report by Flint and Sheldrick (1982) that the ovary of the ewe secretes oxytocin in response to prostaglandin $F_{2\alpha}$ stimulation both support the hypothesis that this oxytocin results from local synthesis.

The primary roles of gonadal oxytocin and vasopressin remain undetermined, although several possibilities warrant serious consideration. Both hormones can stimulate the contraction of the smooth muscle of the male and female reproductive tracts and they could therefore play a role in such processes as egg transport and spacing, or sperm transport. Oxytocin releases $PGF_{2\alpha}$ from the uterine endometrium of the ewe and is probably involved in the control of luteolysis in this species (McCracken, 1980). The most exciting possibility which has been suggested by recent in vitro data (Adashi and Hsueh, 1981; Tan et al., 1981) is that these peptides may provide a local feedback control system on steroid biosynthesis within the gonad.

ACKNOWLEDGEMENTS

The financial support of the M.R.C., the A.R.C. and the Wellcome Trust is gratefully acknowledged.

REFERENCES

Adashi, E.Y. and Hsueh, A.J.W. (1981) Direct inhibition of testicular androgen biosynthesis revealing antigonadal activity of neurohypophysial hormones. *Nature (Lond.)*, 293: 650–652.

Amico, J.A., Seif, S.M. and Robinson, A.G. (1981) Elevation of oxytocin and oxytocin-associated neurophysin in the plasma of normal women during midcycle. *J. clin. Endocr. Metab.*, 53: 1229–1232.

Armstrong, D.T. and Hansel, W.J. (1959) Alteration of the bovine estrous cycle with oxytocin. *J. Dairy Sci.*, 42: 533–542.

Bradshaw, J.M.C., Downing, S.J., Moffatt, A., Hinton, J.C. and Porter, D.G. (1981) Demonstration of some of the physiological properties of rat relaxin. *J. Reprod. Fert.*, 63: 145–153.

Cooke, R.G. and Knifton, A. (1981) Oxytocin-induced oestrus in the goat. *Theriogenology*, 16: 95–97.

Flint, A.P.F. and Sheldrick, E.L. (1982) Ovarian secretion of oxytocin is stimulated by prostaglandin. *Nature (Lond.)*, 297: 587–588.

Forsling, M.L., Åkerlund, M. and Strömberg, P. 1981) Variations in plasma concentrations of vasopressin during the menstrual cycle. *J. Endocr.*, 89: 263–266.

Lederis, K. (1961) Vasopressin and oxytocin in the mammalian hypothalamus. *Gen comp. Endocr.*, 1: 80–89.

Lincoln, D.W., Hill, A. and Wakerley, J.B. (1973) The milk ejection reflex of the rat an intermittent function not abolished by surgical levels of anaesthesia. *J. Endocr.*, 57: 459–476.

McCracken, J.A. (1980) Hormone receptor control of prostaglandin $F_{2\alpha}$ and secretion by the ovine uterus. *Advanc. Prostaglandin Thromb. Res.*, 8: 1329–1344.

Pickering, B.T. (1978) The neurohypophysial neurone: a model for the study of secretion. *Essays Biochem.*, 14: 45–81.

Pickering, B.T. and Jones, C.W. (1978) The neurophysins. In C.H. Li (Ed.), *Hormonal Proteins and Peptides, Vol. 5*, Academic Press, New York, pp. 103–158.

Schams, D., Lahlou-Kassi, A. and Glatzel, P. (1982) Oxytocin concentrations in peripheral blood during the oestrous cycle and after ovariectomy in two breeds of sheep with high and low fecundity. *J. Endocr.*, 92: 9–13.

Sheldrick, E.L. and Flint, A.P.F. (1981) Circulating concentrations of oxytocin during the estrous cycle and early pregnancy in sheep. *Prostaglandins*, 22: 631–636.

Sheldrick, E.L., Mitchell, M.D. and Flint, A.P.F. (1980) Delayed luteal regression in ewes immunized against oxytocin. *J. Reprod. Fert.*, 59: 37–42.

Tan, G.J.S., Tweedale, R. and Biggs, J.S.G. (1981) Oxytocin may have a role in the regulation of the human corpus luteum. *J. Steroid Biochem.* 14: xiii (abstract).

Walsh, J.R. and Niall, H.D. (1980) Use of an octadecylsilica purification method minimizes proteolysis during isolation of porcine and rat relaxins. *Endocrinology*, 107: 1258–1260.

Wathes, D.C. and Swann, R.W. (1982) Is oxytocin an ovarian hormone? *Nature (Lond.)*, 297: 225–227.

Wathes, D.C., Swann, R.W., Pickering, B.T., Porter, D.G., Hull, M.G.R. and Drife, J.O. (1982) Neurohypophysial hormones in the human ovary. *Lancet*, II: 410–412.

Webb, R., Mitchell, M.D., Falconer, J. and Robinson, J.S. (1981) Temporal relationships between peripheral plasma concentrations of oxytocin, progesterone and 13,14-dihydro-15-keto-prostaglandin $F_{2\alpha}$ during the oestrous cycle and early pregnancy in the ewe. *Prostaglandins*, 22: 443–453.

The Neurohypophysis: Structure, Function and Control, Progress in Brain Research, Vol. 60, edited by B.A. Cross and G. Leng

Secretion of Oxytocin by the Corpus Luteum in Sheep

A.P.F. FLINT and E.L. SHELDRICK

A.R.C. Institute of Animal Physiology, Babraham, Cambridge CB2 4AT (U.K.)

INTRODUCTION

The role of oxytocin in the processes controlling luteal regression has interested reproductive endocrinologists since early reports of the luteolytic effect of administered oxytocin in heifers (Armstrong and Hansel, 1959; Hansel and Wagner, 1960). Oxytocin has since been shown to shorten the oestrous cycle in goats (Cooke and Knifton, 1981) and to have a similar but relatively limited luteolytic effect in sheep (Milne, 1963). The fact that oxytocin stimulates uterine secretion of $PGF_{2\alpha}$, the luteolysin (Sharma and Fitzpatrick, 1974; Mitchell et al., 1975; McCracken et al., 1981) is consistent with this luteolytic action, and the possibility that endogenous oxytocin may be involved in luteal regression is confirmed by the delay in luteolysis observed in ewes that have been actively immunized against oxytocin (Sheldrick et al., 1980; Schams et al., 1982a). The uterus responds to oxytocin with increased secretion of $PGF_{2\alpha}$ only close to oestrus, when oxytocin would be expected to act if it were involved in luteal regression (Roberts et al., 1975), and this sensitivity has been accounted for in terms of increased levels of an endometrial oxytocin receptor at this time (Roberts et al., 1976). Furthermore, the episodic release of $PGF_{2\alpha}$ from the uterus is accompanied by transient increases in circulating levels of oxytocin-neurophysin (Fairclough et al., 1980); this is consistent with the observed stimulation of oxytocin secretion (presumed to be from the posterior pituitary) by $PGF_{2\alpha}$ in the pig (Ellendorf et al., 1978), cow (Schams and Karg, 1982) and man (Gillespie et al., 1972). There is therefore a considerable body of evidence implicating oxytocin in the control of uterine secretion of $PGF_{2\alpha}$ at luteal regression. The recently discovered secretion of oxytocin by the corpus luteum has, however, led to a re-interpretation of some of these ideas.

CIRCULATING CONCENTRATIONS OF OXYTOCIN DURING THE OESTROUS CYCLE

Measurement of oxytocin in jugular venous plasma samples obtained once daily from cycling sheep shows that levels rise with the formation of the corpus luteum and fall at luteal regression, being lowest at oestrus (Fig. 1). Similar results have been obtained with radioimmunoassays using different antisera and standards and in different breeds of sheep (Webb et al., 1981; Sheldrick and Flint, 1981; Schams et al., 1982b). These data suggest that the corpus

522

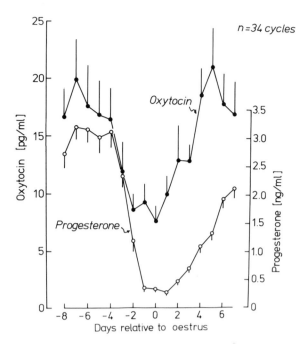

Fig. 1. Concentrations of oxytocin (●) and progesterone (○) in jugular venous plasma samples taken once per day (usually between 14.00 and 16.00 h). Values are means ± S.E.M. for two cycles from each of 17 ewes, plotted with reference to the day of behavioural oestrus (mating with a vasectomized ram). (From Flint and Sheldrick, 1983, with permission.)

luteum may be a source of oxytocin, and this conclusion is supported by changes in circulating oxytocin levels after luteal regression induced in mid-cycle with the luteolytic 16-aryl-oxyprostaglandin F analogue, cloprostenol (Estrumate; I.C.I. 80996; Fig. 2). Cloprostenol treatment causes a short-lived release of oxytocin, resulting in a surge of oxytocin in jugular venous plasma lasting about 30 min, followed some 24 h later by a fall in the concentration of oxytocin by about 50 % (Flint and Sheldrick, 1983). Note that oxytocin levels exhibit a diurnal rhythm on days 6–9 after oestrus that is not immediately interrupted by induced luteal regression; this rhythm is absent on days 11–15 of the cycle.

Further investigation of the transient release of oxytocin following cloprostenol showed that it was absent in sheep that had been either ovariectomized or hysterectomized (Fig. 3a). To investigate the source of this oxytocin, blood samples were taken from anaesthetized sheep in which the ovarian and utero-ovarian veins were cannulated; data from one such animal (Fig. 3b) show that, following administration of cloprostenol, levels of oxytocin increased in both vessels, but that the peak concentration reached in the ovarian vein exceeded that in the utero-ovarian vein by approximately 6-fold. This is consistent with the ratio of ovarian to utero-ovarian blood flow, which is in the range 5–8, and indicates that release is predominantly from the ovary. Any contribution by the pituitary to elevated oxytocin secretion following cloprostenol appeared to be ruled out by similar experiments in which arterio-venous concentration differences were measured across the head and the ovary simultaneously (Flint and Sheldrick, 1982a). These results confirm that the ovary is capable of secreting oxytocin.

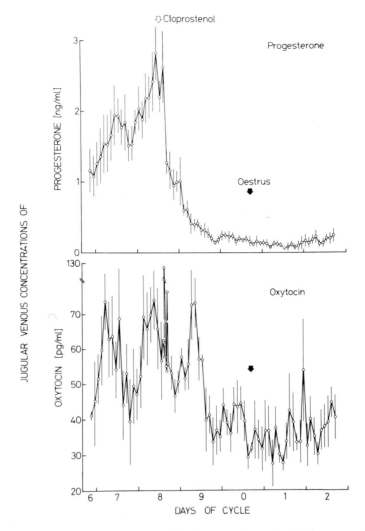

Fig. 2. Concentrations of oxytocin and progesterone in jugular venous plasma from four ewes treated with cloprostenol (Estrumate, 125 µg i.m.) on day 8 after oestrus. Samples were obtained at 2-h intervals, and at 20-min intervals between 50 min before and 110 min after treatment. Values are means ± S.E.M. All animals displayed behavioural oestrus within 48 h after treatment. (From Flint and Sheldrick, 1983, with permission.)

524

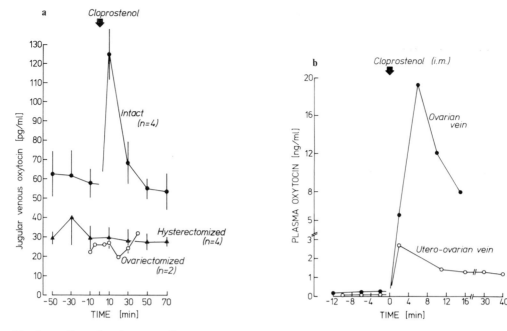

Fig. 3. a: effects of ovariectomy and hysterectomy on oxytocin release in response to cloprostenol. Values are means ± S.E.M. for jugular venous plasma concentrations of oxytocin before and after administration of cloprostenol (as Fig. 2). b: concentrations of oxytocin in plasma from the ovarian and utero-ovarian veins from a single anaesthetized animal (pentobarbitone, halothane) in which catheters were inserted into the vessels before cloprostenol treatment. The veins sampled were those draining an ovary bearing two corpora lutea. No oxytocin release was detected in control experiments in which saline was administered or when samples were collected from veins draining an ovary without a corpus luteum.

MEASUREMENT OF ARGININE-VASOPRESSIN IN OVARIAN VEIN BLOOD

To determine whether the ovary secretes arginine-vasopressin in addition to oxytocin after cloprostenol treatment, levels of vasopressin in ovarian venous blood before and after treatment with cloprostenol were compared with those of oxytocin. In one sheep, mean (± S.E.M.) levels of vasopressin measured by specific radioimmunoassay were 18.9 ± 1.75 (n = 3) and 17.1 ± 0.70 (n = 3) pg/ml in ovarian venous and carotid arterial plasma, respectively, before administering cloprostenol. After treatment these levels increased to reach 62 and 58 pg/ml, respectively, 40 min later; however at no time was there any preferential release into the ovarian vein. Levels in a second animal again showed no secretion by the ovary. In these animals peak ovarian venous levels of oxytocin reached after cloprostenol exceeded those of vasopressin by more than 20-fold. Therefore it was concluded that the ovary does not secrete vasopressin in response to prostaglandin, although there may be some release by the pituitary.

NATURE OF THE OXYTOCIN-LIKE COMPOUND IN THE CORPUS LUTEUM AND OVARIAN VENOUS BLOOD

In the absence of data describing the extraction, purification and sequence analysis of the immunologically active material present in ovarian venous blood after treatment with cloprostenol, it is not possible to be certain that ovarian oxytocin is identical to that in the pituitary. However the extensive analysis carried out on the oxytocic material from the corpus luteum by Wathes and Swann (1982), including HPLC, gel filtration, milk-ejection and uterine strip bioassays and radioimmunoassay, provides persuasive evidence that the corpus luteum contains oxytocin, and it seems most likely that the secreted material is identical to this.

From a consideration of the specificity of the antiserum used in the radioimmunoassay developed by us (Flint and Sheldrick, 1983) it seems unlikely that there are major differences between the luteal compound and oxytocin; the low cross-reactions of mesotocin (Ile^8-oxytocin, 4.1 %) and vasotocin (Arg^8-oxytocin, < 0.02 %) show that the antiserum recognizes the C-terminal end of the molecule, and the absence of cross-reactions with Pro–Leu–GlyNH$_2$ (oxytocin$_{7-9}$) and isotocin (Ser^4,Ile^8-oxytocin), < 0.01 and < 1 % respectively, indicate that the ring structure is also recognized. However the antiserum does cross-react with two derivatives of oxytocin, asulpho-oxytocin (49.6 %) and propionyl-oxytocin (48.9 %), and asulpho-oxytocin has some activity in the isolated rat uterine strip bioassay. Therefore limited differences between the secreted compound and authentic oxytocin are possible. Such differences are not ruled out by our demonstration (Fig. 4) that the compound in ovarian venous plasma is active in the rat milk-ejection assay.

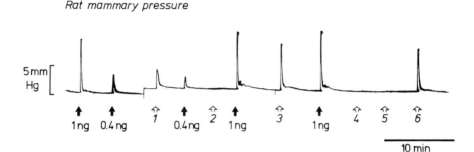

Fig. 4. Rat mammary pressure bioassay for oxytocin activity in ovarian venous plasma. Samples were administered via a jugular vein catheter to a rat under pentobarbitone anaesthesia 18 h after weaning on day 21 of lactation. Administration of oxytocin standards are shown by closed arrows. Open arrows indicate: 1, ovarian venous plasma from a sheep treated with cloprostenol (0.5 ml, equivalent to 0.5 ng oxytocin by radioimmunoassay); 2, carotid arterial plasma taken at the same time as sample 1 (content of sample by radioimmunoassay, 25 pg); 3, ovarian venous plasma after cloprostenol (0.48 ng); 4, jugular venous plasma taken at same time as sample 3 (14.8 pg); 5, ovarian venous plasma after administration of cloprostenol to a hysterectomized sheep (0.5 ml, 35 pg); 6, same sample as 5 after adding 1 ng oxytocin.

CONCENTRATION OF OXYTOCIN IN THE CORPUS LUTEUM — INFLUENCE OF THE UTERUS

Concentrations of oxytocin in luteal tissue from cycling sheep have been reported to be 1500 (Flint and Sheldrick, 1982b) to 2600 (Wathes and Swann, 1982) ng/g wet weight (see also Table I). The data of Flint and Sheldrick (1982b) were corrected for extraction losses by addition of tracer quantities of [^{3}H]propionyl-oxytocin during homogenization. Using the same technique other ovarian and uterine tissues contain relatively little immunologically active oxytocin (follicles and other non-luteal ovarian tissues, < 0.01 ng/g; myometrium, 3.5

ng/g and endometrium, 0.55 ng/g). Oxytocin has also been measured in luteal tissue after treatment with cloprostenol, which causes loss from the corpus luteum of more than 98 % of the oxytocin it contains within 40 min (Table I).

As indicated above, luteal release of oxytocin in response to cloprostenol is much reduced after hysterectomy, although in intact sheep secretion by the uterus is probably low. Measurement of oxytocin in corpora lutea from hysterectomized ewes has accounted for this inconsistency by revealing that almost all the oxytocin disappears from the corpora lutea after hysterectomy (Table I and Fig. 4; Sheldrick and Flint, 1983). The reason for this is unknown, although it does suggest some influence of the uterus in the control of luteal oxytocin synthesis, rather than a lack of responsiveness to cloprostenol after hysterectomy. It is not certain, however, whether the uterus controls expression of the gene for (a presumed) pro-oxytocin/neurophysin, or the subsequent processing of such a precursor.

LUTEAL OXYTOCIN DURING PREGNANCY

Maternal circulating concentrations of oxytocin during late gestation are low in sheep (Webb et al., 1981) and measurement of luteal oxytocin in pregnant animals is consistent with this; tissue levels are low relative to those in non-pregnant ewes by day 14 after mating and decline to less than 1 % of levels during the cycle by day 50 (Fig. 5). Circulating concentrations decline on day 15 after fertile mating (Sheldrick and Flint, 1981), and this is consistent with the drop in luteal levels; however levels in plasma subsequently rise, on days 16 and 17, suggesting increased secretion by another organ.

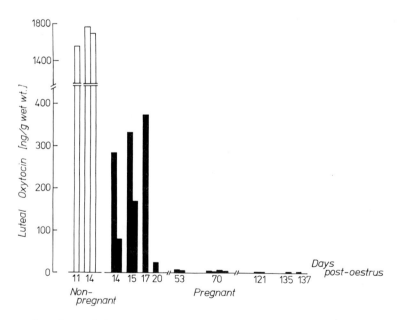

Fig. 5. Concentrations of oxytocin in corpora lutea from non-pregnant cycling (open bars) and pregnant (closed bars) ewes. Each bar indicates concentration determined by radioimmunoassay in an acid extract of one corpus luteum. Extraction recoveries were monitored by addition of [³H]propionyl-oxytocin at homogenization.

PROPORTION OF CIRCULATING OXYTOCIN ACCOUNTED FOR BY OVARIAN SECRETION

Rates of secretion of oxytocin calculated from metabolic clearance rates (total production rate) exceed ovarian secretion rates determined from arterio-venous differences across the organ in anaesthetized animals by approximately 10-fold. Values reported by Flint and Sheldrick (1983) are: for total production rate (data for day 11 of the oestrous cycle) 29.6 pg/ml $\times$ 300 ml/min $= 8880$ pg/min $= 0.53\,\mu$g/h; for ovarian secretion in the same ewe, $220.2 - 29.6$ pg/ml (arterio-venous difference) $\times$ 4 ml/min (typical ovarian venous plasma flow; Short et al., 1963; Mattner and Thorburn, 1969) $= 0.044\,\mu$g/h. From the decline in circulating concentrations of oxytocin at oestrus, when levels drop from approx. 20 to approx. 10 pg/ml (Fig. 1), it would appear that 50 % of circulating oxytocin is secreted by the corpus luteum. However the data calculated above would indicate a considerably lower proportion is luteal in origin.

These discrepancies may be accounted for in a number of ways. Anaesthesia reduces hepatic blood flow (Paterson and Harrison, 1972), and therefore probably also metabolic clearance rate; in addition a significant proportion of the oxytocin leaving the ovary may do so in the lymphatic drainage (see Setchell et al., 1983, for data on testicular lymphatic secretion of charged molecules). These factors would lead to underestimation of the proportion of oxytocin derived from the ovary. That such an underestimation may occur is further suggested by the failure to account for more than 20 % of the oxytocin content of the corpus luteum in ovarian venous blood after treatment with cloprostenol (Flint and Sheldrick, 1982a), when almost all the luteal content is released (Table I).

TABLE I

EFFECTS OF CLOPROSTENOL TREATMENT AND HYSTERECTOMY ON CONCENTRATIONS OF OXYTOCIN MEASURED BY RADIOIMMUNOASSAY IN CORPORA LUTEA FROM NON-PREGNANT SHEEP

Values are means $\pm$ S.E.M. for the number of animals in parentheses. For 'after cloprostenol' values, samples were taken 45 min following administration of 125 μg of cloprostenol i.m.

Animals	Oxytocin concentration (ng/g wet wt)	
	Untreated	After cloprostenol
Intact (days 11–14 after oestrus)	1714 ± 27 (3)	39 ± 16 (5)
Hysterectomized (days 53–76 after oestrus)	5, 7 (2)	4.3 ± 0.7 (6)

Despite this probable underestimation of ovarian contribution to circulating oxytocin levels, additional extra-pituitary sources cannot be dismissed. Lack of any arterio-venous concentration difference across the head (Flint and Sheldrick, 1982a) would appear to rule out the posterior pituitary as a major source of oxytocin during the cycle; on the other hand the diurnal rhythm in plasma oxytocin levels (Fig. 2) may indicate some contribution by the pineal gland (or sub-commissural organ?). Similar rhythms for neurohypophysial hormones have been reported in the CSF in a variety of species and the secretion of melatonin in a diurnal fashion by the pineal (Rollag et al., 1978) also implies that this organ may be a source of oxytocin. It is uncertain however whether pineal oxytocin would enter the circulation by a route other than via the external jugular vein.

FUNCTIONS OF LUTEAL OXYTOCIN

The data implicating oxytocin in the control of uterine secretion of $PGF_{2\alpha}$ at luteal regression, summarized in the Introduction, are further supported by the demonstration of coincident episodic surges of oxytocin and $PGF_{2\alpha}$ release on days 13–15 of the cycle (Flint and Sheldrick, 1983). These spontaneous surges are quantitatively comparable to the peaks of release observed after giving cloprostenol at this stage of the cycle (i.e. reaching 100–150 pg/ml in peripheral plasma), and since 98 % of the oxytocin in the corpus luteum is lost in response to cloprostenol (Table I), it seems likely that each spontaneous episode of release may represent total secretion of the luteal content of oxytocin. In view of this it has been suggested (Flint and Sheldrick, 1983) that luteal oxytocin is involved both in stimulating uterine production of $PGF_{2\alpha}$ (so ensuring maximal release and, in consequence, rapid and complete luteal regression) and bringing about the cessation of each individual episode of $PGF_{2\alpha}$ secretion.

In addition to such a systemic action, oxytocin may also be involved in regulating steroid synthesis in a local manner. In rat Leydig cells in culture, vasopressin and vasotocin at concentrations of $2-5 \times 10^{-9}$ M (oxytocin at 7×10^{-8} M) reduce human chorionic gonadotrophin-stimulated testosterone synthesis by approximately one-half (Adashi and Hsueh, 1981). A similar effect on progesterone synthesis has been reported for oxytocin in isolated bovine and human luteal cells (Tan et al., 1982). The effect of neurohypophysial hormones on testosterone synthesis is exerted through inhibition of 17α-hydroxylase and C-17,20 lyase (Adashi and Hsueh, 1982).

The concentration of oxytocin in the corpus luteum (1500 ng/g wet weight, or 5×10^{-6} M, assuming an intracellular water space of $300 \mu l/g$), exceeds that found to reduce steroid synthesis in isolated testicular cells. Therefore oxytocin may either exert a chronic antisteroidogenic action in the corpus luteum, or mediate the luteolytic effects of prostaglandins. The latter effect would appear to be consistent with the "mobilizing" action of cloprostenol on luteal oxytocin described above. However the corpora lutea of hysterectomized ewes, which contain low levels of oxytocin (Table I), are as susceptible to the luteolytic action of cloprostenol as those of intact animals, and this possible mode of action must therefore be considered unlikely (Flint and Sheldrick, 1982c; Sheldrick and Flint, 1983).

CONCLUSIONS

The demonstration that the corpus luteum contains and secretes large quantities of oxytocin is remarkable not only because it provides evidence for the ectopic production in normal animals of a hormone previously considered to be limited to the neurohypophysis, but also because of the role oxytocin may play in the regression and lysis of the tissue that secretes it. The evidence for such a role for oxytocin in ruminants is persuasive; however the possible involvement of oxytocin or related compounds in the regression of the human corpus luteum is of greater potential importance because of the lack of information at present available on the factors leading to luteolysis in man.

ACKNOWLEDGEMENTS

We would like to thank Dr. R.J. Bicknell for performing vasopressin assays and Dr. G. Leng for assistance with the rat mammary pressure bioassay.

REFERENCES

Adashi, E.Y. and Hsueh, A.J.W. (1981) Direct inhibition of testicular androgen biosynthesis revealing antigonadal activity of neurohypophysial hormones. *Nature (Lond.)*, 293: 650–652.

Adashi, E.Y. and Hsueh, A.J.W. (1982) Direct inhibition of rat testicular androgen biosynthesis by arginine vasotocin. *J. Biol. Chem.*, 257: 1301–1308.

Armstrong, D.T. and Hansel, W. (1959) Alteration of the bovine estrous cycle with oxytocin. *J. Dairy Sci.*, 42: 533–542.

Cooke, R.G. and Knifton, A. (1981) Oxytocin-induced oestrus in the goat. *Theriogenology*, 16: 95–97.

Ellendorf, F., Forsling, M.L., Parvizi, N., Smidt, D., Taverne, M. and Williams, H. (1978) Prostaglandin $F_{2\alpha}$ administration and oxytocin release in the pig and miniature pig. *Brit. J. Pharmacol.*, 62: 412P.

Fairclough, R.J., Moore, L.G., McGowan, L.T., Petersen, A.J., Smith, J.F., Tervit, H.R. and Watkins, W.B. (1980) Temporal relationships between plasma concentrations of 13,14-dihydro-15-keto-prostaglandin F and neurophysin I/II around luteolysis in sheep. *Prostaglandins*, 20: 199–208.

Flint, A.P.F. and Sheldrick, E.L. (1982a) Ovarian secretion of oxytocin is stimulated by prostaglandin. *Nature (Lond.)*, 297: 587–588.

Flint, A.P.F. and Sheldrick, E.L. (1982b) Ovarian secretion of oxytocin in the sheep. *J. Physiol. (Lond.)*, 330: 61P–62P.

Flint, A.P.F. and Sheldrick, E.L. (1982c) Is ovarian oxytocin involved in luteal regression? *J. Endocr.*, 94: 50P.

Flint, A.P.F. and Sheldrick, E.L. (1983) Evidence for a systemic role for ovarian oxytocin in luteal regression in sheep. *J. Reprod. Fert.*, 67: 215–225.

Gillespie, A., Brummer, H.C. and Chard, T. (1972) Oxytocin release by infused prostaglandin. *Brit. med. J.*, 1: 543–544.

Hansel, W. and Wagner, W.C. (1960) Luteal inhibition in the bovine as a result of oxytocin injections, uterine dilatation, and intrauterine infusions of seminal and preputial fluids. *J. Dairy Sci.*, 43: 796–805.

Mattner, P.E. and Thorburn, G.D. (1969) Ovarian blood flow in sheep during the oestrous cycle. *J. Reprod. Fert.*, 19: 547–549.

McCracken, J.A., Schramm, W., Barcikowski, B. and Wilson, L. (1981) The identification of prostaglandin $F_{2\alpha}$ as a uterine luteolytic hormone in the sheep and the endocrine control of its synthesis. *Acta vet. scand.*, Suppl. 77: 71–88.

Milne, J.A. (1963) Effects of oxytocin on the oestrous cycle of the ewe. *Aust. vet. J.*, 39: 51–52.

Mitchell, M.D., Flint, A.P.F. and Turnbull, A.C. (1975) Stimulation by oxytocin of prostaglandin F levels in uterine venous effluent in pregnant and puerperal sheep. *Prostaglandins*, 9: 47–56.

Paterson, J.Y.F. and Harrison, F.A. (1972) The splanchnic and hepatic uptake of cortisol in conscious and anaesthetized sheep. *J. Endocr.*, 55: 335–350.

Roberts, J.S., Barcikowski, B., Wilson, L., Skarnes, R.C. and McCracken, J.A. (1975) Hormonal and related factors affecting the release of prostaglandin $F_{2\alpha}$ from the uterus. *J. Steroid Biochem.*, 6: 1091–1097.

Roberts, J.S., McCracken, J.A., Gavagan, J.E. and Soloff, M.S. (1976) Oxytocin stimulated release of prostaglandin $F_{2\alpha}$ from ovine endometrium in vitro: correlation with estrous cycle and oxytocin-receptor binding. *Endocrinology*, 99: 1107–1114.

Rollag, M.D., O'Callaghan, P.L. and Niswender, G.D. (1978) Serum melatonin concentrations during different stages of the annual reproductive cycle in ewes. *Biol. Reprod.*, 18: 279–285.

Schams, D. and Karg, H. (1982) Hormonal responses following treatment with different prostaglandin analogues for estrous cycle regulation in cattle. *Theriogenology*, 17: 499–513.

Schams, D., Prokopp, A. and Schmidt-Adamopoulou, B. (1982a) The effect of active immunization against oxytocin on ovarian cyclicity in ewes. *Acta endocr.*, 246, Suppl. 7 (abstract).

Schams, D., Lahlou-Kassi, A. and Glatzel, P. (1982b) Oxytocin concentrations in peripheral blood during the oestrous cycle and after ovariectomy in two breeds of sheep with low and high fecundity. *J. Endocr.*, 92: 9–13.

Setchell, B.P., Laurie, M.S., Flint, A.P.F. and Heap, R.B. (1983) The transport of free and conjugated steroids from the boar testis in lymph, venous blood and rete testis fluid. *J. Endocr.*, 96: 127–136.

Sharma, S.C. and Fitzpatrick, R.J. (1974) Effect of oestradiol-17β and oxytocin treatment on $PGF_{2\alpha}$ release in the anoestrous ewe. *Prostaglandins*, 6: 97–105.

Sheldrick, E.L. and Flint, A.P.F. (1981) Circulating concentrations of oxytocin during the estrous cycle and early pregnancy in sheep. *Prostaglandins*, 22: 631–636.

Sheldrick, E.L. and Flint, A.P.F. (1983) Regression of the corpora lutea in sheep in response to cloprostenol is not affected by loss of luteal oxytocin after hysterectomy. *J. Reprod. Fert.*, 68: 155–160.

Sheldrick, E.L., Mitchell, M.D. and Flint, A.P.F. (1980) Delayed luteal regression in ewes immunized against oxytocin. *J. Reprod. Fert.*, 59: 37–42.

Short, R.V., McDonald, M.F. and Rowson, L.E.A. (1963) Steroids in ovarian venous blood of ewes before and after gonadotrophic stimulation. *J. Endocr.*, 26: 155–167.

Tan, G.J.S., Tweedale, R. and Biggs, J.S.G. (1982) Effects of oxytocin on the bovine corpus luteum of early pregnancy. *J. Reprod. Fert.*, 66: 75–78.

Wathes, D.C. and Swann, R.W. (1982) Is oxytocin an ovarian hormone? *Nature (Lond.)*, 297: 225–227.

Webb, R., Mitchell, M.D., Falconer, J. and Robinson, J.S. (1981) Temporal relationships between peripheral plasma concentrations of oxytocin, progesterone and 13,14-dihydro-15-keto prostaglandin $F_{2\alpha}$ during the oestrous cycle and early pregnancy in the ewe. *Prostaglandins*, 22: 443–453.

The Neurohypophysis: Structure, Function and Control, Progress in Brain Research, Vol. 60, edited by B.A. Cross and G. Leng
© *1983 Elsevier Science Publishers B.V.*

The General Discussion: A Reflection

R.G. DYER

A.R.C. Institute of Animal Physiology, Babraham, Cambridge CB2 4AT (U.K.)

Hal Gainer chaired the discussion. His forethought and skillful planning ensured that this last session of the meeting was a lively and successful occasion.

First he brought two important technical points to our attention. Boer was asked to review his poster with Kruisbrink, which described a novel method for infusing small peptides at a constant rate for periods of up to 60 days. This involves subcutaneous implantation of microporous Accurel polypropylene tubing, of such small size (0.7 mm o.d.) that it can be used in situations where the Alzet minipump is impracticable, for example in foetal and neonatal rats. The second experimental matter to be discussed concerned the usefulness of mice with nephrogenic diabetes insipidus. Valtin described how these mice urinate about eight times their body mass daily, despite normal concentrations of vasopressin in both their plasma and neurohypophysis. Valtin referred to an earlier publication of his for a description of these mice (Kettyle and Valtin, *Kidney Int.,* 1 (1972) 135) and offered to send a nucleus for a breeding programme to anyone who could find a use for them. Comments from Morris and J. Sladek indicated that several laboratories had already realized that this animal was a valuable adjunct to the Brattleboro rat.

The discussion then turned to electrophysiology and Andrew and Dudek were both asked to describe parts of their excellent poster which had attracted much informed attention and admiration the previous day. They had studied, with intracellular micropipettes, the basic mechanisms underlying phasic firing in the presumptive vasopressin secreting cells. In seven out of 26 magnocellular neurones recorded in a hypothalamic slice preparation, graded depolarization was found to induce phasic generation of action potentials. These periods of spike generation were associated with a plateau potential and were followed by a period of hyperpolarization. Dudek and Andrew suggested that this hyperpolarization occurred because the rapid intraburst firing caused a calcium activated potassium conductance to open and that this mechanism was responsible for switching off each burst of activity. However, Nordmann and others found it difficult to accept that this alone was responsible since there would then be the problem of how the phases lengthen and continuous firing commences. A key question in this area concerns the ubiquity of phasic firing — i.e. is phasic firing observed only in the presumptive vasopressin cells because they have particular membrane properties, or only because they have a unique synaptic input? It was to seek an answer to this problem that Poulain questioned the proportion of cells in which graded depolarizations failed to induce phasic firing. However, neither Dudek or Andrew would be drawn into stating that they thought phasic firing was restricted to one clan of magnocellular neurones. Before curtailing further discussion on this topic, Gainer pointed out that a definitive answer to this question about phasic firing could be best obtained by immunocytochemical identification of the cells from which intracellular recordings are made. The following day, at an informal meeting in our laboratory at Babraham, Yamashita caused great interest by showing unpublished data obtained from magnocellular neurones which showed that he had immunohistochemically identified seven out of ten phasically firing cells to contain vasopressin. Were the other three different or did they just fail to react with the vasopressin antisera?

The discussion then focussed on two posters presented by Leake and her colleagues concerning the presence of arginine-vasotocin (AVT) in the blood of children at two and 24 hours post-partum, and the inhibitory action of this hormone in the ovine foetus on transfer of water to the ewe when she is given an osmotic stimulus. These experiments on sheep seemed rather interesting, but most comments were directed at the methodology and whether or not AVT is in fact found in mammals at all!

The last major point for discussion concerned the possible roles (if any) of the peptides that are found in the cerebrospinal fluid. Since Robinson's talk on the first morning of the meeting this had been a recurring topic but, like many other problems in the history of biology, lack of knowledge about function seemed to become equated with lack of function. Thus a number of speakers described the CSF as no more than a "sewer" for transport of "waste" or "excess" peptide. How many, I wonder, appreciated the irony that some 1800 years earlier Galen had attributed a similar "waste disposal" role to the pituitary itself — a misconception that was to survive for one and a half millenia until Schneider (1655) observed that nasal secretions were not filtered waste derived from the hypophysis. Fortunately current misconceptions about CSF peptides are likely to be corrected much more quickly because we know already some of the circumstances that cause their concentration to change. For example, brain stimulation and time of day. For the present, however, the last word on this topic should be left to Pickering who, at the end of much speculative discussion, remarked that "one can tell a great deal about a town by inspecting the contents of the sewer!".

Subject Index

[533]

534